8/03

Structural Fetal
Abnormalities

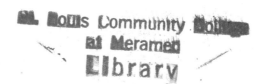

Structural Fetal Abnormalities

The Total Picture

Second Edition

EDITOR

Roger C. Sanders, MD

Research Professor of Radiology
Thomas Jefferson University School of Medicine
Philadelphia, Pennsylvania
Consultant at Los Alamos Women's Health Center
Los Alamos, New Mexico
Clinical Professor of Radiology
University of New Mexico
Albuquerque, New Mexico

ASSISTANT EDITORS

Lillian R. Blackmon, MD

Associate Professor of Pediatrics
University of Maryland School of Medicine
Department of Perinatology/Neonatology
University of Maryland Medical Center
Baltimore, Maryland

W. Allen Hogge, MD

Associate Professor, Obstetrics, Gynecology and Reproductive Sciences
University of Pittsburgh School of Medicine
Medical Director, Department of Genetics
Magee-Women's Hospital
Pittsburgh, Pennsylvania

Philip Spevak, MD

Associate Professor
The Johns Hopkins University School of Medicine
Division of Cardiology
Department of Pediatrics
The Johns Hopkins Hospital
Baltimore, Maryland

Eric A. Wulfsberg, MD

Professor of Pediatrics
University of Maryland School of Medicine
Department of Human Genetics and Pediatrics
University of Maryland Medical Center
Baltimore, Maryland

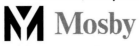

Mosby

An Affiliate of Elsevier Science

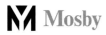
Mosby

An Affiliate of Elsevier Science

11830 Westline Industrial Drive
St. Louis, Missouri 63146

NOTICE

Medicine is an ever-changing field. Standard safety precautions must be followed, but as new research and clinical experience broaden our knowledge, changes in treatment and drug therapy may become necessary or appropriate. Readers are advised to check the most current product information provided by the manufacturer of each drug to be administered to verify the recommended dose, the method and duration of administration, and contraindications. It is the responsibility of the treating physician, relying on experience and knowledge of the patient, to determine dosages and the best treatment for each individual patient. Neither the publisher nor the editor assumes any liability for any injury and/or damage to persons or property arising from this publication.

The Publisher

Library of Congress Cataloging-in-Publication Data

Structural fetal abnormalities: the total picture. Roger C. Sanders ...[et al.].—2nd ed.
    p. cm.
  ISBN 0-323-01476-3
   1. Fetus—Abnormalities. 2. Fetus—Ultrasonic imaging. I. Sanders, Roger C.
RG626 .S78 2002
618.3'2—dc21   2002016674

Acquisitions Editor: Judith Fletcher
Project Manager: Tina Rebane
Design Coordinator: Gene Harris

MX

Printed in the United States of America.

Last digit is the print number: 9 8 7 6 5 4 3 2

Contributors

Lillian R. Blackmon, MD
Associate Professor of Pediatrics
University of Maryland School of Medicine
Department of Perinatology/Neonatology
University of Maryland Medical Center
Baltimore, Maryland

Timothy M. Cromblehome, MD
Associate Professor of Surgery
Center for Fetal Diagnosis and Treatment
Children's Hospital of Philadelphia
Philadelphia, Pennsylvania

Craig R. Dufresne, MD, FACS
Co-Director, Center for Facial Rehabilitation
Fairfax Hospital, Inova Medical Institution
Fairfax, Virginia
Clinical Assistant Professor, Departments of
  Neurosurgery and Plastic Surgery
The Johns Hopkins University School of Medicine
Baltimore, Maryland
Clinical Assistant Professor of Plastic Surgery
Georgetown University School of Medicine
Washington, D.C.

John Gearhart, MD, FRCSC
Professor of Pediatric Urology
The Johns Hopkins University School of Medicine
Baltimore, Maryland

John Herzenberg, MD, FRCSC
Associate Professor of Orthopaedic Surgery and
  Pediatrics
University of Maryland School of Medicine and
  Rubin Institue for Advanced Orthopedics, Sinai
  Hospital
Baltimore, Maryland

W. Allen Hogge, MD
Associate Professor, Obstetrics, Gynecology and
  Reproductive Sciences
University of Pittsburgh School of Medicine
Medical Director, Department of Genetics
Magee-Women's Hospital
Pittsburgh, Pennsylvania

Charles N. Paidas, MD
Associate Professor of Surgery, Pediatrics, Oncology,
  Anesthesia, and Critical Care Medicine
Director, Pediatric Trauma
The Johns Hopkins University School of Medicine
Baltimore, Maryland

E. Dror Paley, MD, FRCSC
Associate Professor of Orthopaedic Surgery and
  Pediatrics
University of Maryland School of Medicine and Rubin
  Institute for Advanced Orthopedics, Sinai Hospital
Baltimore, Maryland

John Ragheb, MD
Assistant Professor
Chief of Neurosurgery
University of Miami
Miami, Florida

Roger C. Sanders, MD
Research Professor of Radiology
Thomas Jefferson University School of Medicine
Philadelphia, Pennsylvania
Consultant, Los Alamos Women's Health Center
Los Alamos, New Mexico

Philip Spevak, MD
Associate Professor
The Johns Hopkins University School of Medicine
Division of Cardiology
Department of Pediatrics
The Johns Hopkins Hospital
Baltimore, Maryland

Eric A. Wulfsberg, MD
Professor of Pediatrics
University of Maryland School of Medicine
Department of Human Genetics and Pediatrics
University of Maryland Medical Center
Baltimore, Maryland

Preface

Most fetal anomalies discovered in utero are found in the course of a diagnostic ultrasound examination. On occasion, sonograms are performed in a specific effort to find an anomaly because of family history or a positive screening test such as an abnormal alpha-fetoprotein. More often, ultrasound examinations that uncover anomalies are performed for unrelated reasons. For instance, many sonograms are requested when there is a date versus examination discrepancy or vaginal bleeding is present. This book is designed to provide a comprehensive picture of the genetics, epidemiology, ultrasonic features, and obstetrical, neonatal, and surgical management, as well as the prognosis, of the more common anomalies discovered by ultrasound examination. Many conditions discovered with invasive prenatal testing, but which do not have ultrasonic features, such as Tay-Sachs disease and Fragile X syndrome, are not considered in this text.

When ultrasound reveals a fetus with an unusual appearance, many questions arise. Parents may experience varying levels of grief, guilt, and worry. Often there is no correlation between the level of concern and the ultrasonic findings. However, these concerns stimulate spoken and unspoken questions about the pregnancy and neonatal consequences. The obstetrician who encounters fetal malformations infrequently is faced with unfamiliar dilemmas concerning the pregnancy management, such as delivery timing, route, and site. Whoever discovers the abnormality, whether it be a sonographer, radiologist, or obstetrician, encounters some unplanned worrisome responsibilities. Is the finding real or merely an artifact? Is the diagnosis specific, or is there a wide differential? Is it lethal? Is it correctable? Is it hereditary? This book attempts to answer many of these questions.

Prenatal care of both mother and fetus is a team effort. Today, most prenatal centers have established fetal anomaly management groups. These groups meet at regular intervals to coordinate care. Depending on the nature and severity of the finding, responsibility for care is shared by the obstetrician, perinatologist, neonatologist, and surgeon. In practice, clinical staff such as sonographers, nurses, and genetic counselors play a very significant role in both diagnosis and care. In addition, consultations with specialty experts, such as those in pediatric cardiology, dysmorphology, or maxillofacial surgery, may be required. The patient in this way is assured a more caring, comprehensive care plan. Each care provider must have some knowledge of the other specialties involved and of the long-term prognosis. This volume includes sections written by experts in each area. Sonologist Roger C. Sanders provides the ultrasonic findings of each anomaly followed by the perspective of each involved expert. Eric A. Wulfsberg, pediatric geneticist and dysmorphologist; W. Allen Hogge, perinatologist; Lillian Blackmon, neonatologist; Philip Spevak, pediatric and fetal cardiologist; and several surgeons (Timothy Cromblehome, Craig DuFresne, John Gearhart, John Herzenberg, Chuck Paidas, E. Dror Paley, and John Ragheb) have joined forces to complete this comprehensive picture of diagnosis and management of the more common structural fetal anomalies detected by obstetrical ultrasound.

There are thousands of conditions and syndromes that cause fetal deformities. Conditions presented here were chosen either because they are frequently recognized with ultrasound or because a distinct ultrasonic feature exists that allows definitive diagnosis and prognosis (e.g., the "hitchhiker" thumb of diastrophic dwarfism distinguishes this syndrome from other dwarfisms). Some of the more common sonographic dilemmas that sometimes indicate underlying fetal problems, such as amniotic bands or cord masses, are also included. Many rare malformations or syndromes are mentioned in the discussion of differential diagnosis.

Each anomaly is considered in a similar manner. The template for each entity has been designed to facilitate location of a specific feature of any condition, whether it be the recurrence rate, ultrasonic differential diagnosis, or surgical complications. Included in the first appendix is a brief description of the ultrasonic appearance of many of the more rare syndromes or abnormalities. In the second appendix there is a list of the differential diagnoses of fetal ultrasonic findings. I hope that this book will be used during prenatal care in the same fashion in which Smith's *Recognizable Patterns of Human Malformation* is used post-delivery, as an easy reference when an anomaly is found. There is a sizable bibliography following each anomaly to afford the reader greater detail for each condition.

New in this edition is a discussion of many additional entities, including syndromes such as Beckwith-Wiedemann syndrome. A more comprehensive and detailed cardiac section include several entities not discussed in the first edition.

Several sonography colleagues have donated images of entities that I have either not seen or for which I have only a poor example. I am grateful to Drs. Sandy Isbister, Sheila Sheth, and Gary Thieme for these images.

Roger C. Sanders, MD

Contents

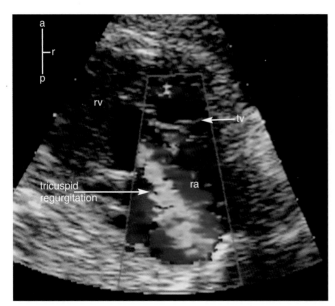

Severe tricuspid regurgitation in Ebstein's anomaly. A broad jet of tricuspid regurgitation is seen in the markedly dilated right atrium (ra). Machine settings are optimized to increase temporal and spatial resolution. rv, right ventricle; tv, tricuspid valve.

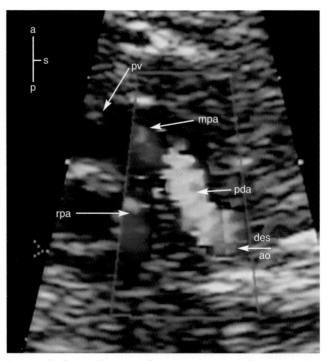

Retrograde flow in the patent ductus arteriosus in pulmonary atresia. With severe pulmonary stenosis or with pulmonary atresia, ductal flow is reversed. Here, one sees retrograde flow in the patent ductus arteriosus (pda) representing flow from the descending aorta (des ao) to the main pulmonary artery (mpa). Normal antegrade flow is seen in the right pulmonary artery (rpa). pv, pulmonary vein.

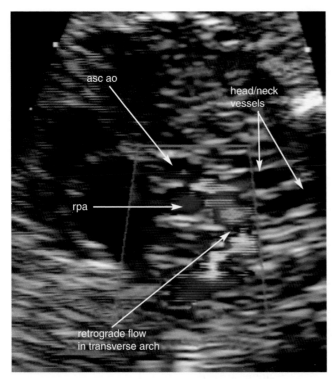

Hypoplastic left heart syndrome with retrograde flow in the transverse aortic arch. Same image but with color Doppler interrogation showing retrograde flow in the transverse arch. This is an ominous finding and strongly suggests a ductus dependent lesion postnatally. asc ao, ascending aorta; rpa, right pulmonary artery.

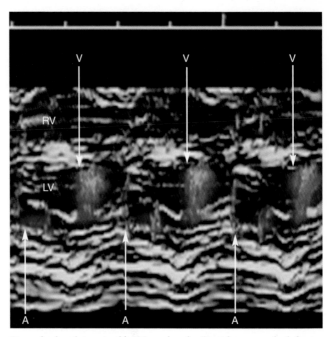

Sinus rhythm determined by M-mode color Doppler across the left ventricular outflow tract. One can easily see the one-to-one relationship between each atrial (A) and ventricular (V) contraction and that ventricular rate is 142 beats per minute. One can also time ventricular contraction by noting the motion of the right ventricular free wall on the M-mode recording. In this fetus, the atrioventricular interval is increased.

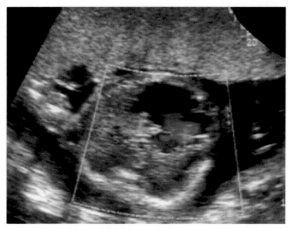

Color flow Doppler image of hemangioendothelioma in the liver. The mass is basically cystic with a large vascular component.

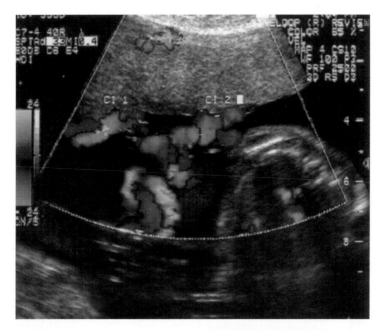

Monoamniotic monochorionic twins. Single placenta with adjacent cord insertions (C1 and C2). Only minimal cord entanglement has occurred so far.

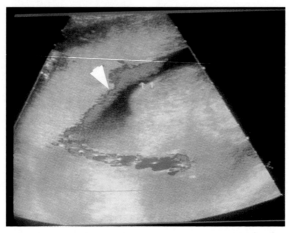

Color flow view showing large communicating vessel between the placental circulations of identical twins, running along the surface of the placenta (*arrowhead*).

Chromosomes 1

1.1 Triploidy

Epidemiology/Genetics

Definition   Rare, lethal chromosomal abnormality. An entire extra haploid set of chromosomes results in 69 chromosomes instead of the usual 46. Severe growth retardation affects the skeleton more than the head.

Epidemiology   One to 2% of human conceptions are triploid, but most end in spontaneous miscarriage. Very rare at birth (M1.5:F1).

Embryology   A complete extra set of chromosomes results in 69 XXX (digynic) or XXY (diandric). Sixty percent result from fertilization with two sperm, 40% result from fertilization of a diploid egg. Central nervous system malformations include hydrocephalus, holoprosencephaly, and neural tube defects. Hypertelorism, cleft lip/cleft palate, syndactyly of fingers three and four, and congenital heart defects are typical features.

Inheritance Patterns   Sporadic.

Teratogens   None.

Screening   Serum levels of human chorionic gonadotrophin may be extremely high in triploidy with dispermy as the cause. Very low levels of alpha-fetoprotein, estriol, and human chorionic gonadotropin are seen in pregnancies in which fertilization of diploid egg occurs.

Prognosis   Lethal antenatally or in the newborn period. Rare mosaic cases survive with moderate to severe mental retardation.

Sonography

FINDINGS

1. **Fetus:** The sonographic findings include:
   a. Severe early onset of intrauterine growth retardation (IUGR). Asymmetric IUGR with a large fetal head is associated with digynic triploidy, whereas symmetric IUGR is typical of digynic triploidy.
   b. Central nervous system abnormalities such as holoprosencephaly, isolated ventriculomegaly, Arnold-Chiari malformation with spina bifida, or Dandy-Walker syndrome.
   c. Nuchal thickening in the first trimester and hydrops are common.
   d. Micrognathia may be seen.
   e. Congenital heart disease.
   f. Renal anomalies such as hydronephrosis.
   g. Omphalocele.
   h. Limb abnormalities such as clubfeet and syndactyly.
2. **Amniotic Fluid:** Oligohydramnios is often seen.
3. **Placenta:** The placenta is often abnormal. There is either an enlarged placenta with normal texture or an enlarged placenta with cystic spaces, similar to a molar pregnancy (partial mole) in cases of paternal origin (XXY). In cases in which the extra set of chromosomes is of maternal origin (XXX), a very small placenta (similar to trisomy 18) may be seen. Multiple theca lutein cysts in the adnexa may be present.
4. **Measurement Data:** Severe early onset of IUGR is usually seen. IUGR may develop as early as 12 to 14 weeks. This is particularly common in triploidy of maternal origin.
5. **When Detectable:** Placental changes and some of the more severe structural changes may be seen as early as 12 to 14 weeks.

Pitfalls   Structural changes are highly variable, and the placenta may be tiny and senescent.

Differential Diagnosis   Trisomy 13 and 18.

Where Else to Look   The lead finding (placentomegaly or IUGR) mandates a careful look at the rest of the fetus.

Pregnancy Management

Investigations and Consultations Required   Traditional karyotyping with or without aneuploid fluorescent in situ hybridization (FISH) analysis via amniocentesis,

1

chorionic villi sampling (CVS), or umbilical blood sampling establishes the diagnosis. Once a cytogenetic diagnosis has been established, no further investigations or consultations are necessary.

Monitoring If pregnancy termination is not an option, monitor for preeclampsia or hyperthyroidism.

Pregnancy Course Molar changes in the placenta predispose to hyperemesis gravidarum, early preeclampsia, theca lutein cysts, and, on occasion, hyperthyroidism.

Pregnancy Termination Issues Suction dilatation and evacuation is appropriate once a cytogenetic diagnosis has been established.

Delivery Fetal monitoring and caesarian section are both contraindicated for the pregnancy complicated by a triploid gestation.

Neonatology

Resuscitation Contraindicated if the diagnosis is definite because of the established lethal prognosis.

Transport Indicated only if diagnostic confirmation, counseling, and long-term care planning are not available locally.

Testing and Confirmation Lymphocyte karyotype can confirm the chromosome abnormality.

Nursery Management Provision of basic supportive care—warmth, hygiene, nourishment, and comfort only—until prognosis for protracted survival is defined and long-term care decisions can be addressed by family.

REFERENCES

Crane JP, Beaver HA, Cheung SW: Antenatal ultrasound findings in fetal triploidy syndrome. J Ultrasound Med 1985;4:519–524.

Edwards MT, Smith WL, Hanson J, Abu Yousef M: Prenatal sonographic diagnosis of triploidy. J Ultrasound Med 1986;5:279–281.

Eiben B, Trawicki W, Hammans W, et al: Rapid prenatal diagnosis of aneuploidies in uncultured amniocytes by fluorescence in situ hybridization. Evaluation of >3,000 cases. Fetal Diagn Ther 1999;14:193–197.

Gorlin RJ, Cohen MM, Hannekan RCM (eds): Syndromes of the Head and Neck, 4th ed. New York, Oxford University Press, 2001, pp 68–71.

Jauniaux E, Brown R, Rodeck C, Nicolaides KH: Prenatal diagnosis of triploidy during the second trimester of pregnancy. Obstet Gynecol 1996;88:983–989.

Jauniaux E, Brown R, Snijders RJM, et al: Early prenatal diagnosis of triploidy. Am J Obstet Gynecol 1997;176:550–554.

Jones KL (ed): Smith's Recognizable Patterns of Human Malformations. Philadelphia, WB Saunders, 1988, pp 10–15.

Lewin P, Kleinfinger P, Bazin A, et al: Defining the efficiency of fluorescence in situ hybridization on uncultured amniocytes on a retrospective cohort of 27,407 prenatal diagnoses. Prenat Diagn 2000;20:1–6.

Lockwood C, Scioscia A, Stiller R, Hobbins J: Sonographic features of the triploid fetus. Am J Obstet Gynecol 1987;157:285–287.

Matias A, Montenegro N, Areias JC, Brandao O: Anomalous fetal venous return associated with major chromosomopathies in the late first trimester of pregnancy. Ultrasound Obstet Gynecol 1998;11:209–213.

McFadden DE, Pantzar JT, Placental pathology of triploidy. Hum Pathol 1996;27:1018–1020.

Mittal TK, Vujanic GM, Morrissey BM, Jones A: Triploidy: Antenatal sonographic features with post-mortem correlation. Prenat Diagn 1998;18:1253–1262.

Pircon RA, Porto M, Towers CV, et al: Ultrasound findings in pregnancies complicated by fetal triploidy. J Ultrasound Med 1989;8:507–511.

Shepard TH, Fantel AG: Embryonic and early fetal loss. Clin Perinatol 1979;6:219–243.

Wertecki W, Graham JM Jr, Sergovich GP: The clinical syndrome of triploidy. Obstet Gynecol 1976;47:69.

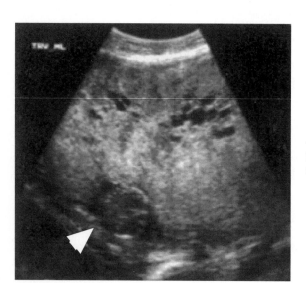

Triploidy. The placenta is enlarged and contains numerous cystic areas. A small but otherwise normal-appearing fetus can be seen (*arrow*). There is oligohydramnios. In other examples of triploidy, the placenta may be large but without cysts.

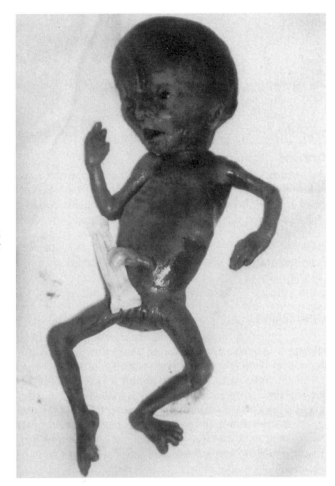

A 24-week fetus with triploidy (69,XXX) and severe intrauterine growth retardation showing relative macrocephaly and three- to four-finger syndactyly.

1.2 Trisomy 13

Epidemiology/Genetics

Definition   Trisomy 13 is the third most common multiple-malformation autosomal trisomy syndrome recognized at birth. Infants have a characteristic phenotype that includes major cardiac, brain, gastrointestinal, and limb malformations.

Epidemiology   One in 5000 to 10,000 births.

Embryology   The phenotype is due to full trisomy 13. Increased maternal age has been documented in this disorder. Rare mosaic partial trisomy 13 syndromes (with varying phenotypes) and translocation patients have been reported. Microcephaly, holoprosencephaly, microphthalmia, polydactyly, facial clefts, and abnormal helices are found in more than 50% of patients. Eighty percent of patients have congenital heart defects with atrial septal defects (ASDs) and ventricular septal defects (VSDs) being the most common, but many patients have complex heart lesions. Other distinctive abnormalities include polycystic kidneys (30% of patients) and omphalocele (<50% of patients).

Inheritance Patterns   Most cases are sporadic, with a 1 in 100 risk of recurrence in future pregnancies. Rare familial translocations have a higher recurrence risk, depending on the specific translocation.

Teratogens   None.

Screening   Maternal serum biochemical marker screening ("triple screen") is not helpful in detecting trisomy 13 fetuses.

Prognosis   This condition is lethal or has a very poor prognosis in all cases. Seventy percent of affected infants are stillborn or die by the age of 6 months, and 85% die in the first year. All survivors with full trisomy 13 have profound mental retardation. In infancy, severe failure to thrive, feeding difficulties, seizures, apneic attacks, and visual and hearing deficits occur in the majority of infants, secondary to the orofacial and central nervous system defects.

Sonography

FINDINGS

1. An ultrasonographically visible abnormality is seen in about 90% of cases. Sonographic findings may include the following:
   a. Holoprosencephaly (40%) (see Chapter 2.11).
   b. Central cleft lip and palate (45%) (see Chapter 7.1).
   c. Enlarged cisterna magna (15%).
   d. Eyes—Close-set eyes with many variations, e.g., hypotelorism, single orbit with two globes, cyclops, or microphthalmia.
   e. Nose—The nose may have a single nostril or be absent and replaced by a proboscis.
   f. Hand and feet problems—Polydactyly, club and rocker-bottom feet, club hands, and overlapping fingers may occur.
   g. Increased nuchal translucency is common at 11 to 14 weeks (72%). Cystic hygroma are also seen (21%).
   h. Congenital heart disease—Numerous different abnormalities are seen such as large ventricular defects and coarctation of the aorta.
   i. Cystic kidneys—The kidneys may be more echogenic and enlarged and contain a few small cysts.
   j. Omphalocele (see Chapter 6.8).
   k. Neural tube defects (see Chapter 2.18). Basal ganglia calcification may occur.
2. **Amniotic Fluid:** Polyhydramnios is seen in 15%, oligohydramnios in 13%.
3. **Placenta:** Normal.
4. **Measurement Data:** IUGR is often present (50%). Microcephaly may occur (12%).
5. **When Detectable:** With vaginal probe at about 11 weeks by increased nuchal translucency. Holoprosencephaly is already present at 12 weeks and is easily recognizable.

Differential Diagnosis

1. Meckel-Gruber syndrome: polydactyly, echogenic enlarged kidneys, and cranial abnormalities are common in both entities.
2. Holoprosencephaly with facial abnormalities without trisomy 13.

Where Else to Look   A detailed look at all organs is required when this karyotype abnormality is suspected.

Pregnancy Management

Investigations and Consultations Required   Traditional karyotyping with or without aneuploidy, FISH analysis via amniocentesis, CVS, or umbilical blood sampling establishes the diagnosis. For patients in whom the diagnosis is made beyond the point of legal pregnancy termination or in those who decide to continue the pregnancy, a neonatologist should consult with the family about appropriate perinatal and neonatal management.

Monitoring   Only routine prenatal care should be performed. The family should be offered supportive psychological care throughout the pregnancy.

Pregnancy Course   Intrauterine growth retardation is common, and aggressive management such as monitoring or early delivery is inappropriate.

Pregnancy Termination Issues   Suction dilatation and evacuation is appropriate once a cytogenetic diagnosis has been established.

Delivery   Electronic fetal monitoring and caesarean section should be avoided unless requested by the family after a thorough discussion of the prognosis for infants with trisomy 13.

Neonatology

Resuscitation   A decision about whether to give life support should be made prior to delivery when the diagnosis is established. If the diagnosis is unknown prior to birth, providing life support is appropriate until diagnosis can be established.

Transport   Indicated only if diagnostic confirmation, counseling, and long-term care planning are not available locally.

Testing and Confirmation   Birth weight is frequently normal. Lymphocyte karyotype can confirm the chromosome abnormality.

Nursery Management   Full life support is appropriate until the diagnosis is confirmed and the family has time for weighing options for duration and intensity of support. Care requirements will be contingent on associated organ involvement and the long-term goals of the family. Central nervous system, cardiac, and orofacial defects are usually the major problems. Feeding mode and respiratory drive are most commonly the key issues for interim care.

REFERENCES

Benacerraf BR, Frigoletto FD Jr, Greene MF: Abnormal facial features and extremities in human trisomy syndromes: Prenatal US appearance. Radiology 1986;159:243–246.

Benacerraf BR, Miller WA, Frigoletto FD Jr: Sonographic detection of fetuses with trisomy 13 and 18: Accuracy and limitations. Am J Obstet Gynecol 1988;158:404–409.

Carey JC: Health Supervision and anticipatory guidance for infants with congenital defects. In Ballard RA (ed): Pediatric Care of the ICN Graduate. Philadelphia, WB Saunders, 1988.

Eiben B, Trawicki W, Hammans W, et al: Rapid prenatal diagnosis of aneuploidies in uncultured amniocytes by fluorescence in situ hybridization. Evaluation of >3,000 cases. Fetal Diagn Ther 1999;14:193–197.

Gorlin RJ, Cohen MM, Hennekan RCM (eds): Syndromes of the Head and Neck, 4th ed. New York, Oxford University Press, 2001, pp 42–45.

Greene MF, Benacerraf BR, Frigoletto FD Jr: Reliable criteria for the prenatal sonographic diagnosis of alobar holoprosencephaly. Am J Obstet Gynecol 1987;156:687–689.

Hodes ME, Cole J, Palmer CG, Reed T: Clinical experience with trisomies 18 and 13. J Med Genet 1978;15:48–60.

Jones KL (ed): Smith's Recognizable Patterns of Human Malformations. Philadelphia, WB Saunders, 1988, pp 20–21.

Lehman CD, Nyberg DA, Winter TC 3rd, et al: Trisomy 13 syndrome: Prenatal US findings in a review of 33 cases. Radiology 1995;194:217–222.

Lewin P, Kleinfinger P, Bazin A, et al: Defining the efficiency of fluorescence in situ hybridization on uncultured amniocytes on a retrospective cohort of 27,407 prenatal diagnoses. Prenat Diagn 2000;20:1–6.

Martich Kriss V, Kriss TC: Doppler sonographic confirmation of thalamic and basal ganglia vasculopathy in three infants with trisomy 13. J Ultrasound Med 1996;15:523–526.

Matias A, Montenegro N, Areias JC, Brandao O: Anomalous fetal venous return associated with major chromosomopathies in the late first trimester of pregnancy. Ultrasound Obstet Gynecol 1998;11:209–213.

Snijders RJ, Sebire NJ, Nayar R, et al: Increased nuchal translucency in trisomy 13 fetuses at 10–14 weeks of gestation Am J Med Genet 1999;86:205–207.

Taylor AI: Autosomal trisomy syndromes: A detailed study of 27 cases of Edwards' syndrome and 27 cases of Patau's syndrome. J Med Genet 1968;5:227–252.

Warkany J, Passarge E, Smith LB: Congenital malformations in autosomal trisomy syndromes. Am J Dis Child 1966;112:502–517.

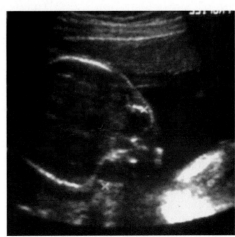

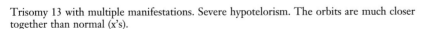

Trisomy 13 with multiple manifestations. Severe hypotelorism. The orbits are much closer together than normal (x's).

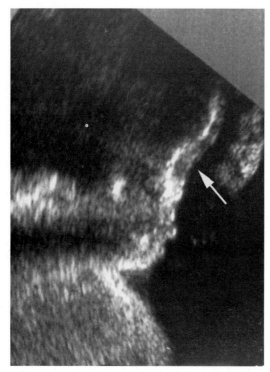

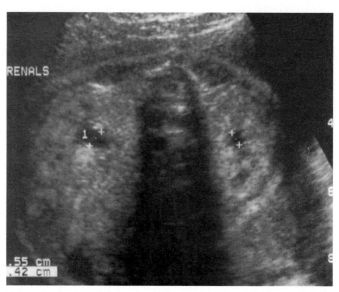

Profile view of fetus with trisomy 13 showing recessed nasal area and a common orbit above the nasal area (*arrow*).

Enlarged echogenic kidneys due to trisomy 13. There is mild renal pelvic dilation (between the x's).

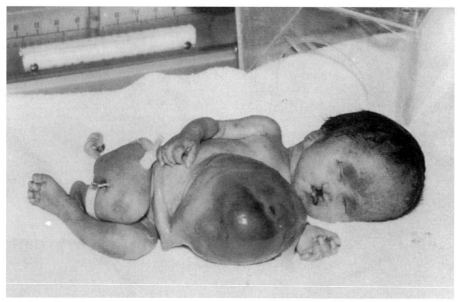

A 19-week fetus with trisomy 13 (47,XX,T13) exhibiting the classic features, including midline facial cleft, omphalocele, and polydactyly.

1.3 Trisomy 18

Epidemiology/Genetics

Definition Trisomy 18 is the second most common multiple-malformation autosomal trisomy syndrome. It presents with IUGR, microcephaly, and congenital heart defects (80%).

Epidemiology One in 3000 to 5000 (M1:F3).

Embryology Most infants have full trisomy 18. Rare patients with mosaic karyotypes, partial trisomy 18 syndromes (with varying phenotypes), and translocation cases have been reported. Infants with trisomy 18 present with severe IUGR, microdolichocephaly with a prominent occiput, malformed ears, micrognathia, clenched hands, and congenital heart defects (80%) that are characterized by complex polyvalvular abnormalities with VSDs. Malformations that occur in less than 50% of cases include cleft lip and palate, limb defects, omphalocele, and diaphragmatic hernias.

Inheritance Patterns Most cases are sporadic, with a 1 in 100 risk of recurrence in future pregnancies. Rare familial translocations have a higher recurrence risk depending on the specific translocation.

Teratogens None.

Screening Maternal serum biochemical marker screening (the "triple screen") may detect as many as 60% of trisomy 18 fetuses.

Prognosis Trisomy 18 is lethal or has a very poor prognosis in all cases. Fifty percent of affected infants will die in the first 2 months of life and 90% will die in the first year. All survivors with full trisomy 18 have profound mental retardation. Associated cardiac and gastrointestinal anomalies are usually life-threatening and definitely life-limiting, if not corrected or palliated by surgery. Failure to thrive and feeding difficulties occur in all who survive the immediate neonatal period.

Sonography

FINDINGS

1. **Fetus:** Sonographic findings that point to trisomy 18 include the following:
    a. Limbs—Persistently clenched hands with overlapping of the fourth digit is a common but not invariable finding. Club and rocker-bottom feet are typical. Unusually positioned or absent thumbs or radial agenesis occurs. Persistently extended legs may be seen.
    b. Face—Micrognathia is common (a good-quality profile view is desirable). Unilateral or bilateral cleft lip and/or palate may occur.
    c. Congenital heart disease—Ventricular septal defect, coarctation of the aorta, and polyvalvular redundancy are most common.
    d. Omphalocele usually containing only bowel is seen in about 25%.
    e. Diaphragmatic hernia (about 10%).
    f. Neural tube defects (20%).
    g. Choroid plexus cysts (25%). Between 2% and 9% of choroid plexus cysts are associated with trisomy 18. A choroid plexus cyst as the sole feature of trisomy 18 is very rare. The number of cysts does not influence the likelihood of trisomy 18. Larger cysts are thought by some to be more likely due to trisomy 18.
    h. Single umbilical artery. Umbilical cord cysts may be seen. Other vascular abnormalities such as a persistent right umbilical vein may be present.
    i. Cystic hygroma (15%). Increased nuchal translucency is usually present between 11 and 14 weeks.
    j. Enlarged (greater than 10 mm) cisterna magna.
    k. Lemon-like head shape with or without spinal dysraphism. A strawberry-shaped head may also be seen.
2. **Amniotic Fluid:** Twenty-five percent have polyhydramnios with IUGR. Oligohydramnios may occur.
3. **Placenta:** Normal.
4. **Measurement Data:** Early onset of IUGR is seen in more than 50% (prior to 18 weeks).
5. **When Detectable:** At 11 to 14 weeks, if increased nuchal translucency is present. At 12 to 14 weeks, other anomalies such as clubfeet or omphalocele can be seen.

Pitfalls A medial indentation on the border of the choroid plexus may be mistaken for a choroid plexus cyst.

Differential Diagnosis

1. Pena-Shokeir syndrome (see Chapter 11.5).
2. Arthrogryposis (see Chapter 8.4).

Where Else to Look May affect any organ.

Pregnancy Management

Investigations and Consultations Required Traditional karyotyping with or without aneuploid FISH analysis via amniocentesis, CVS, or umbilical blood sampling establishes the diagnosis. Once a cytogenetic diagnosis has been established, consultation should be obtained from a neonatologist to discuss a plan for management of the newborn with the family. An isolated choroid plexus cyst with a normal triple screen is considered by many as so unlikely to be due to trisomy 18 that karyotyping is not essential.

Monitoring   Maternal status should be monitored in standard fashion. Fetal evaluation is not appropriate, since emergency intervention is not warranted. The family should be offered supportive psychological care.

Pregnancy Course   Fetuses with trisomy 18 are likely to develop severe IUGR and, if monitored, evidence of fetal distress in labor.

Pregnancy Termination Issues   Suction dilatation and evacuation techniques are appropriate once a cytogenetic diagnosis has been established.

Delivery   Electronic fetal monitoring and cesarean section should be avoided unless requested by the family after a thorough discussion of the prognosis for infants with trisomy 18.

Neonatology

Resuscitation   A decision about whether to give life support should be considered prior to delivery when the diagnosis is definite. If the diagnosis is unknown prior to birth, providing life support is appropriate until the diagnosis can be established.

Transport   Indicated only if diagnostic confirmation, counseling, and long-term care planning are not available locally.

Testing and Confirmation   Lymphocyte karyotype can confirm the abnormality.

Nursery Management   Decisions regarding surgical intervention for cardiac and gastrointestinal defects are the primary concerns in the postnatal period. If no surgical intervention is desired by the family, care requirements are determined primarily by feeding difficulties.

REFERENCES

Benacerraf BR, Miller WA, Frigoletto FD Jr: Sonographic detection of fetuses with trisomies 13 and 18: Accuracy and limitations. Am J Obstet Gynecol 1988;158:404–409.

Bundy AL, Saltzman DH, Pober B, et al: Antenatal sonographic findings in trisomy 18. J Ultrasound Med 1986;5:361–364.

Carey JC: Health supervision and anticipatory guidance for infants with congenital defects. In Ballard RA (ed): Pediatric Care of the ICN Graduate. Philadelphia, WB Saunders, 1988.

Chitty LS, Chudleigh P, Wright E, et al: The significance of choroid plexus cysts in an unselected population: Results of a multicenter study. Ultrasound Obstet Gynecol 1998;12:391–397.

Eiben B, Trawicki W, Hammans W, et al: Rapid prenatal diagnosis of aneuploidies in uncultured amniocytes by fluorescence in situ hybridization. Evaluation of >3,000 cases. Fetal Diagn Ther 1999; 14:193–197.

Gorlin RJ, Cohen MM, Hennekan RCM (eds): Syndromes of the Head and Neck, 4th ed. New York, Oxford University Press, 2001, pp 45–78.

Hepper PG, Shahidullah S: Trisomy 18: Behavioral and structural abnormalities. An ultrasonographic case study. Ultrasound Obstet Gynecol 1992;2:48–50.

Hodes ME, Cole J, Palmer CG, Reed T: Clinical experience with trisomies 18 and 13. J Med Genet 1978;15:48–60.

Jones KL (ed): Smith's Recognizable Patterns of Human Malformations. Philadelphia, WB Saunders, 1988, pp 16–17.

Lam YH, Tang MHY: Sonographic features of fetal trisomy 18 at 13 and 14 weeks: Four case reports. Ultrasound Obstet Gynecol 1999;13: 366–369.

Lewin P, Kleinfinger P, Bazin A, et al: Defining the efficiency of fluorescence in situ hybridization on uncultured amniocytes on a retrospective cohort of 27,407 prenatal diagnoses. Prenat Diagn 2000;20: 1–6.

Matias A, Montenegro N, Areias JC, Brandao O: Anomalous fetal venous return associated with major chromosomopathies in the late first trimester of pregnancy. Ultrasound Obstet Gynecol 1998;11:209–213.

Nadel AS, Bromely BS, Frigoletto FD Jr, et al: Isolated choroid plexus cysts in the second trimester fetus: Is amniocentesis really indicated? Radiology 1992;185:545–548.

Nyberg DA, Kramer D, Resta RG, et al: Prenatal sonographic findings of trisomy 18: Review of 47 cases. J Ultrasound Med 1993;2:103–113.

Palomaki GE, Knight GJ, Haddow JE, et al: Prospective intervention trial of a screening protocol to identify fetal trisomy 18 using maternal serum alpha-fetoprotein, unconjugated oestriol, and human chorionic gonadotropin. Prenat Diagn 1992;12:925–930.

Petrikovsky B, Smith-Levitin M, Gross B: A honeycomb appearance of the fetal choroid plexus. J Diagn Med Sonogr 1999;15:189–191.

Sepulveda W, Treadwell MC, Fisk NM: Prenatal detection of preaxial upper limb reduction in trisomy 18. Obstet Gynecol 1195;85:847–850.

Steiger RM, Porto M, Lagrew DC, Randall R: Biometry of the fetal cisterna magna: Estimates of the ability to detect trisomy 18. Ultrasound Obstet Gynecol 1995;5:384–390.

Sullivan A, Giudice T, Vavelidis F, Thiagarajah S: Choroid plexus cysts: Is biochemical testing a valuable adjunct to targeted ultrasonography? Am J Obstet Gynecol 1999;181:260–265.

Swan TJ, Rouse GA, DeLange M: Sonographic findings in Trisomy 18: A pictorial essay. JDMS 1991;7:255–263.

Taylor AI: Autosomal trisomy syndromes: A detailed study of 27 cases of Edwards' syndrome and 27 cases of Patau's syndrome. J Med Genet 1968;5:227–252.

Gratton RJ, Hogge WA, Aston CE: Choroid plexus cysts and trisomy 18: Risk modification based on maternal age and multiple marker screening. Am J Obstet Gynecol 1996;175:1493–1497.

Thurmond AS, Nelson DW, Lowensohn RI, et al: Enlarged cisterna magna in trisomy 18: Prenatal ultrasonographic diagnosis. Am J Obstet Gynecol 1989;161:83–85.

Tul N, Spencer K, Noble P, et al: Screening for trisomy 18 by fetal nuchal translucency and maternal serum free B-hCG and PAPP-A at 10–14 weeks of gestation. Prenat Diagn 1999;19:1035–1042.

Warkany J, Passarge D, Smith LB: Congenital malformations in autosomal trisomy syndromes. Am J Dis Child 1966;112:502–517.

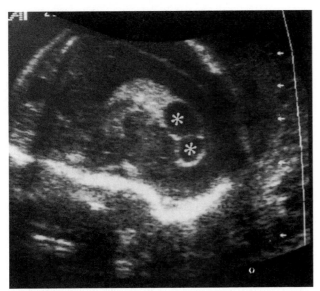

Choroid plexus cysts. Two large cysts (*asterisks*) are present in the choroid plexus. This finding, if isolated, has a slight but statistically significant association with trisomy 18.

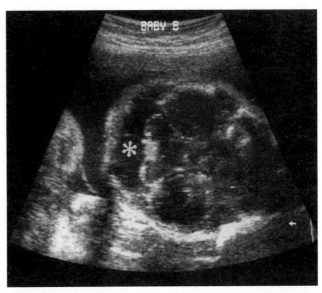

Large cisterna magna over 10 mm wide (*asterisk*). Although associated with trisomy 18, this finding has not so far been the only abnormality seen in a trisomy 18 case.

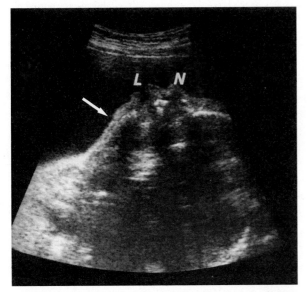

Micrognathia. The chin (*arrow*) is unduly small and recessed posterior to the forehead. This is a frequent finding in trisomy 18. L, lips; N, nose.

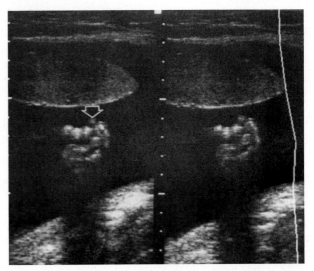

Abnormal hand in trisomy 18. The hand is clenched and the fingers are crowded with the third finger overriding (*arrow*).

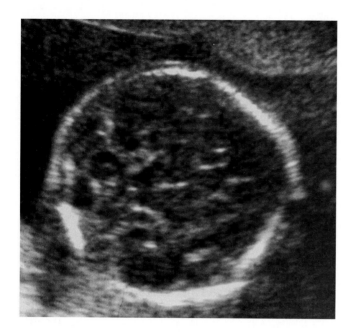

Strawberry-shaped head in a case of trisomy 18.

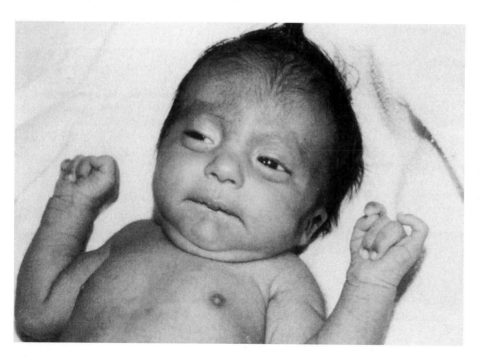

Newborn with trisomy 18 (47,XY,+18) exhibiting classic features, including round face with short nose and clenched fists.

1.4 Trisomy 21 DOWN SYNDROME

Epidemiology/Genetics

Definition Trisomy 21 (Down syndrome) is the most common multiple-malformation chromosome abnormality in newborns, and it results in a characteristic phenotype with major malformations, including congenital heart disease and duodenal atresia.

Epidemiology Occurs in 1 in 800 live births (M1:F1). No racial differences have been noted, but there is a significant increase in incidence with increasing maternal age.

Embryology The phenotype is due to trisomy for all or part (21q22) of chromosome 21. Ninety-five percent of cases are due to full trisomy 21, 3% are translocation, and 2% are mosaic. Infants with trisomy 21 have a characteristic craniofacial appearance that includes microbrachycephaly, midface hypoplasia, excess nuchal skin, and small overfolded ears. There is generalized shortening of the limbs, with small hands, clinodactyly of the fifth fingers (60%), single palmar creases (45%), and wide spacing between the first and second toes. Approximately 50% of patients have congenital heart disease, with endocardial cushion defects and VSDs being the most common lesions. Two thirds of cases of endocardial cushion defects have trisomy 21. Alimentary tract defects—duodenal atresia, tracheoesophageal fistula, imperforate anus, Hirschprung's disease—occur in approximately 10% of infants with trisomy 21.

Inheritance Patterns Most cases are sporadic, with a 1 in 100 risk of recurrence in future pregnancies. Rare familial translocations have a higher recurrence risk depending on the specific translocation.

Teratogens None.

Screening Assuming all women would elect to have CVS or amniocentesis, the use of advanced maternal age as a risk factor would detect approximately 25% of trisomy 21 fetuses. Combining maternal age with maternal serum biochemical markers raises the detection rate to 60%. An additional 20% can be identified using sonographic markers.

Prognosis Cardiac abnormalities are the major cause of increased mortality in infancy. Mortality between infancy and the age of 40 years is not much increased over mortality in the general population, but it then increases because of premature aging. IQs range from 25 to 50 in childhood but fall in adulthood. Alimentary tract obstructions are generally corrected in the neonatal period.

Sonography

FINDINGS

1. **Fetus:**
   a. Thickened nuchal fold or nuchal translucency—About 60% of Down syndrome fetuses have increased "nuchal translucency" (nuchal edema) of greater than 3 mm at 11 to 14 weeks. There is an echopenic area extending from the back of the skull to the sacrum. This finding is also seen in other chromosomal abnormalities. By 18 weeks, the nuchal fold has regressed into "nuchal thickening." A standard cerebellar view will show nuchal thickening of greater than 6 mm. About one in seven fetuses with nuchal thickening of this type will have Down syndrome.
   b. Although Down syndrome is typically associated with nuchal edema, cystic hygroma may also be seen (10%).
   c. Congenital heart disease—Fetuses with Down syndrome often have congenital heart disease (about 50%). Endocardial cushion defect with extensive ASD and VSD and abnormal mitral and tricuspid valve is typical of Down syndrome. VSD alone is also common. Tetralogy of Fallot can occur.
   d. Duodenal atresia—The stomach and duodenal bulb are dilated. Appropriate transducer angulation shows the pyloric connection. The small and large bowel are empty. Other gut atresias such as tracheoesophageal fistula with or without atresia may occur (2%).
   e. Omphalocele—Although more typical of trisomy 13 and 18, omphalocele may be seen (2%).
   f. Short humerus and femur—Both femur and humerus are mildly shortened to 0.91 of the biparietal diameter value. This sign has about a 1 in 10 likelihood of being associated with Down syndrome and is seen in 26% of Down syndrome cases.
   g. Mild renal pelvic dilation—Renal pelvic dilation to greater than 3 mm prior to 20 weeks has a weak but convincing association with Down syndrome and is seen in 5% of Down syndrome cases.
   h. Short middle phalanx of fifth finger—This structure is difficult to measure, but there is an association with Down syndrome.
   i. Flattened facial profile—The nose is small and recessed.
   j. Posterior urethral valve syndrome—Particularly when the onset of posterior urethral valve syndrome occurs very early, e.g., 12 weeks, Down syndrome may be responsible.

k. Isolated pleural effusion and isolated fetal ascites with retained lymph fluid have an approximately 5% association with Down syndrome.

l. Nonimmune hydrops—One of the numerous causes is trisomy 21 (2%). Transient ascites may occur.

m. Echogenic bowel—A group of adjacent small bowel loops with an echogenicity as great as bone increases the risk of Down syndrome.

n. The big toe may be separated from the remaining toes (a "sandal" foot).

o. Choroid plexus cysts have been reported with Down syndrome, but it is doubtful that they raise the risk of trisomy 21.

p. Mild lateral ventriculomegaly increases the risk of Down syndrome. The frontothalamic distance is reduced and the transcerebellar distance is smaller in fetuses with Down syndrome.

q. Echogenic focus in the papillary muscles. There is a slight increase in the risk of aneuploidy, particularly trisomy 21. Bilateral foci increase the risk.

r. Some fetuses with Down syndrome have an iliac crest angle of greater than 90% (one third).

s. Macroglossia, a rare sonographic finding, is associated with Down syndrome.

t. A shortened ear length has been reported in Down syndrome.

u. Enlargement of the liver and spleen due to a leukemia or a transient leukemoid reaction can be seen. The echogenicity of the liver is markedly decreased.

2. **Amniotic Fluid:** Normal. Delayed fusion of the amnion and chorion is associated with trisomy 21.

3. **Placenta:** Normal.

4. **Measurement Data:** Growth is usually normal. IUGR occurs only occasionally. Brachycephaly may be seen with decreased frontothalamic distance.

5. **When Detectable:** Some manifestations, e.g., nuchal edema and posterior urethral valves, are detectable at 11 weeks; cushion defects have been detected at 13 weeks with endovaginal echocardiography. Duodenal atresia is usually detected after 24 weeks.

Pitfalls

1. Nuchal folds at 18 weeks are difficult to measure accurately and can easily be overmeasured. Make sure that the cerebellar and cortical brain structures are satisfactorily visualized at the same time. Extension of the fetal neck can increase nuchal fold thickness measurements.

2. Increased nuchal translucency has been associated with many other abnormalities apart from chromosomal abnormalities, including cardiac malformations, diaphragmatic hernia, omphalocele, multicystic kidney, and fetal akinesia.

3. Duodenal atresia usually presents late (after 24 weeks).

4. An unfused amniotic membrane may be confused with nuchal edema if the fetus is lying on its back.

5. Use of a high-frequency transducer may give an impression of echogenic bowel.

6. Echogenic foci in the papillary muscles of the heart are a common variant in Asian mothers.

7. Echogenic bowel is also seen in cystic fibrosis, in intra-amniotic bleeding, as a normal variant, in IUGR, and in cytomegalovirus.

Differential Diagnosis

1. Other chromosomal anomalies can have some of the same findings, e.g., cystic hygroma and nuchal folds.

2. Macroglossia is also seen in Beckwith-Wiedemann syndrome and hypothyroidism.

Where Else to Look   Any component of the fetus can be affected by Down syndrome.

Pregnancy Management

Investigations and Consultations Required   Traditional karyotyping with or without aneuploid FISH analysis via amniocentesis, CVS, or umbilical blood sampling establishes the diagnosis. The high incidence of cardiac defects requires fetal echocardiography, which also may be helpful in assessing prognosis.

Monitoring   No alterations in prenatal care are necessary.

Pregnancy Course   Duodenal atresia results in severe polyhydramnios and resultant preterm labor.

Pregnancy Termination Issues   Suction dilatation and evacuation techniques are appropriate once a cytogenetic diagnosis has been established.

Delivery   The fetus with Down syndrome should be managed like a fetus with normal chromosomes. Cesarean section should be performed if there are obstetric indications. If structural malformations are present, delivery should be in a tertiary center.

Neonatology

Resuscitation   Rarely contraindicated unless multiple complex associated anomalies have been confirmed antenatally and a prior decision has been made by family not to begin life support measures. If the diagnosis is not known prior to birth, providing life support is appropriate initially.

Transport   Indicated if cardiac or alimentary tract anomalies are suspected or if diagnostic confirmation, counseling, and long-term care planning are not available locally.

Testing and Confirmation   Children with trisomy 21 present in the newborn period with hypotonia and a characteristic craniofacial appearance. Lymphocyte karyotype can confirm the chromosome abnormality.

Nursery Management   The major objectives of care are comprehensive evaluation to identify all associated problems and the development of a post-nursery plan of care to facilitate parental adaptation. The initial priorities are to determine the presence and type of cardiac and alimentary defects and plan surgical interventions. Short-term issues include polycythemia in 25%, feeding difficulties, particularly if preterm or with concurrent cardiac or alimentary anomalies, and neutrophil abnormalities, which are uncommon and usually transient.

REFERENCES

Appleman Z, Zalel Y, Fried S, Caspi B: Delayed fusion of amnion and chorion: Possible association with trisomy 21. Ultrasound Obstet Gynecol 1998;11:303–305.

Baird PA, Sadovnick AD: Life expectancy in Down syndrome. J Pediatr 1987;110:849–854.

Benacerraf BR, Barss VA, Laboda LA: A sonographic sign for the detection in the second trimester of the fetus with Down's syndrome. Am J Obstet Gynecol 1985;151:1078–1079.

Benacerraf BR, Cnaan A, Gelman R, et al: Can sonographers reliably identify anatomic features associated with Down syndrome? Radiology 1989;173:377–380.

Benacerraf BR, Neuberg D, Bromley B, Frigoletto FD Jr: Sonographic scoring index for prenatal detection of chromosomal abnormalities. J Ultrasound Med 1992;11:449–458.

Bromley B, Lieberman E, Laboda L, Benacerraf BR: Echogenic intracardiac focus: A sonographic sign for fetal down syndrome. Obstet Gynecol 1995;86:998–1001.

Bronshtein M, Bar-Hava I, Blumenfeld I, et al: The difference between septated and nonseptated nuchal cystic hygroma in the early second trimester. Obstet Gynecol 1993;81:683–687.

Brumfield CG, Hauth JC, Cloud GA, et al: Sonographic measurements and ratios in fetuses with Down syndrome. Obstet Gynecol 1989;73:644–646.

Carey JC: Health supervision and anticipatory guidance for infants with congenital defects. In Ballard RA (ed): Pediatric Care of the ICN Graduate. Philadelphia, WB Saunders, 1988.

Eiben B, Trawicki W, Hammans W, et al: Rapid prenatal diagnosis of aneuploidies in uncultured amniocytes by fluorescence in situ hybridization. Evaluation of >3,000 cases. Fetal Diagn Ther 1999;14:193–197.

Gorlin RJ, Cohen MM, Hennekan RCM (eds): Syndromes of the Head and Neck, 4th ed. New York, Oxford University Press, 2001, pp 35–42.

Hamada H, Yamada N, Watanabe H, et al: Hypoechoic hepatomegaly associated with transient abnormal myelopoiesis provides clues to trisomy 21 in the third trimester fetus. Ultrasound Obstet Gynecol 2001;17:442–444.

Jones KL: Smith's recognizable patterns of human malformations, 4th ed. Philadelphia, WB Saunders, 1988.

Kliewer MA, Hertzberg BS, Freed KS, et al: Dysmorphologic features of the pelvis in Down syndrome: Prenatal sonographic depiction and diagnostic implications of the iliac angle. Radiology 1996;201:681–684.

Lewin P, Kleinfinger P, Bazin A, et al: Defining the efficiency of fluorescence in situ hybridization on uncultured amniocytes on a retrospective cohort of 27407 prenatal diagnoses. Prenat Diagn 2000;20:1–6.

Lynch L, Berkowitz GS, Chitkara U, et al: Ultrasound detection of Down syndrome: Is it really possible? Obstet Gynecol 1989;73:267–270.

Matias A, Montenegro N, Areias JC, Brandao O: Anomalous fetal venous return associated with major chromosomopathies in the late first trimester of pregnancy. Ultrasound Obstet Gynecol 1998;11:209–213.

Miller M, Cosgriff JM: Hematological abnormalities in newborn infants with Down syndrome. Am J Med Genet 1983;16:173–177.

Nicolaides KH, Azar G, Snijders RJ, Gosden CM: Fetal nuchal oedema: Associated malformations and chromosomal defects. Fetal Diagn Ther 1992;7:123–131.

Nyberg DA, Resta RG, Luthy DA, et al: Prenatal sonographic findings of Down syndrome: Review of 94 cases. Obstet Gynecol 1990;76:370–377.

Paladini D, Tartaglione A, Agangi A, et al: The association between congenital heart disease and Down syndrome in prenatal life. Ultrasound Obstet Gynecol 2000;15:104–108.

Penna L, Bower S: Hyperechogenic bowel in the second trimester fetus: A review. Prenat Diagn 2000;20:909–913.

Roberts D, Walkinshaw SA, McCormack MJ, Ellis J: Prenatal detection of trisomy 21: Combined experience of two British hospitals. Prenat Diagn 2000;20:17–22.

Sepulveda W, Romero D: Significance of echogenic foci in the fetal heart. Ultrasound Obstet Gynecol 1998;12:445–449.

Shipp TD, Bromley B, Lieberman E, Benacerraf BR: The second-trimester fetal iliac angle as a sign of Down syndrome. Ultrasound Obstet Gynecol 1998;12:15–18.

Simpson J: The cardiac echogenic focus. Prenat Diagn 1999;19:972–975.

Snijders RJ, Noble P, Sebire N, et al: UK multicentre project on assessment of risk of trisomy 21 by maternal age and fetal nuchal translucency thickness at 10–14 weeks of gestation. Lancet 1998;352:343–346.

Souka AP, Snijders RJM, Novakov A, et al: Defects and syndromes in chromosomally normal fetuses with increased nuchal translucency thickness at 10–14 weeks of gestation. Ultrasound Obstet Gynecol 1998;11:391–400.

Warkany J, Passarge E, Smith LB: Congenital malformations in autosomal trisomy syndromes. Am J Dis Child 1966;112:502–517.

Weissman A, Mashiach S, Achiron R: Macroglossia: Prenatal ultrasonographic diagnosis and proposed management. Prenat Diagn 1995;15:66–69.

Wilkins I: Separation of the great toe in fetuses with Down syndrome. J Ultrasound Med 1999;13:229–231.

Winter TC, Ostrovsky AA, Komarniski CA, Uhrich SB: Cerebellar and frontal lobe hypoplasia in fetuses with trisomy 21: Usefulness of combined US markers. Radiology 2000;214:533–538.

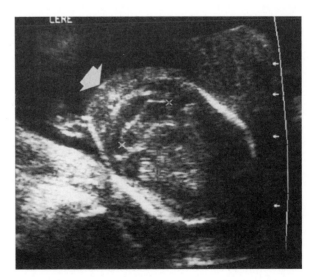

Nuchal thickening. At the level of an intracranial view, which shows the cerebellum (between the x's), thickened skin is seen at the back of the neck (*arrow*).

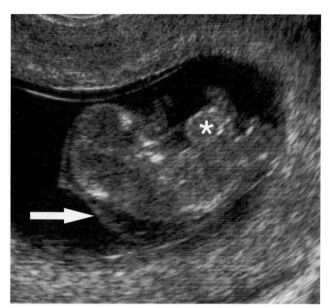

An 11-week fetus later shown to have Down syndrome. There is increased nuchal translucency (*arrow*). Note physiologic gut herniation (*).

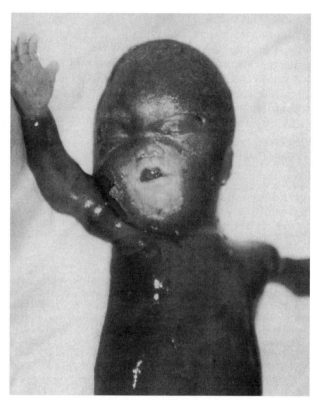

A 23-week fetus with Down syndrome. Note midface hypoplasia with short nose and small hand.

1.5 Turner Syndrome (45XO Syndrome)

Epidemiology/Genetics

Definition Turner syndrome is a rare sex chromosome abnormality characterized by a complete or partial monosomy for one X chromosome.

Epidemiology Occurs in 1 in 5000 births (M0:F1).

Embryology Turner syndrome is due in most cases to a 45XO karyotype that results from chromosomal nondisjunction. No maternal age effect has been noted. Forty percent of newborns with Turner syndrome are mosaic or have variant chromosome patterns, as opposed to only 7% of those spontaneously aborted. Over 95% of 45XO conceptions are spontaneously aborted. Characteristic cardiac abnormalities (20%) include a bicuspid aortic valve and coarctation of the aorta. Horseshoe kidney and other renal structural abnormalities occur in 60% of patients. A nuchal cystic hygroma with or without hydrops is the most common antenatal presentation.

Inheritance Patterns Sporadic.

Teratogens None.

Screening Maternal serum biochemical screening (triple screen) will detect cases with cystic hygroma and hydrops. The markers will suggest an increased risk for Down syndrome (low alpha-fetoprotein, high human chorionic gonadotropin, and low estriol).

Prognosis If hydrops is present, fetal death will almost always occur during pregnancy. Isolated cystic hygromas, without hydrops, regress during pregnancy. Early death in infancy results from associated cardiac defects and is infrequent with current surgical and postoperative intensive care. The potential life span is normal, and those who survive early infancy usually reach adulthood. Skeletal growth retardation occurs in all and perceptive hearing impairment in 50%. Absence of secondary sexual characteristics and infertility are uniformly present. Hormone replacement therapy will be necessary for maturational changes in adolescence. Most Turner syndrome women have normal or near normal intelligence.

Sonography

FINDINGS

1. **Fetus:**
   a. Cystic hygromas, or collections of lymph (see Chapter 7.2), develop in the late first to early second trimester. Bilateral cysts develop in the pos-

terolateral aspect of the neck. Later, skin thickening with cystic spaces separated by septa is seen in the skin. Hydrops often develops.
   b. Lymph collections may occur in other sites, such as isolated fetal ascites, pleural effusion, or lymphangiomata. Pleural effusions may be transient.
   c. Congenital heart disease most likely involving the left side of the heart, such as coarctation of the aorta or valvular aortic stenosis can occur. Secondary right heart enlargement may occur.
   d. Renal anomalies, such as renal agenesis, horseshoe kidney, and pelvic kidney, are seen.
2. **Amniotic Fluid:** There may be oligohydramnios.
3. **Placenta:** Normal.
4. **Measurement Data:** Usually not affected.
5. **When Detectable:** Cystic hygromas are detectable from 10 weeks on.

Pitfalls Cystic hygromas may be seen in fetuses that are eventually normal (20% to 30%).

Differential Diagnosis

1. Noonan syndrome—Cystic hygromas with hydrops are often seen. Fetuses may be male or female, often with cardiac anomalies such as hypoplastic pulmonary valves. Short femur and polyhydramnios are other features. Chromosomes are normal.
2. Multiple pterygium syndrome (see Chapter 8.12).
3. Down syndrome (see Chapter 1.4).
4. Achondrogenesis (see Chapter 8.1).

Where Else to Look

1. Look for flexed arms and extended legs—Features of multiple pterygium syndrome.
2. Look at the gender—Turner syndrome fetuses have female genitalia, but Noonan fetuses can be either male or female.

Pregnancy Management

Investigations and Consultations Required Traditional karyotyping with or without aneuploid FISH analysis via amniocentesis, CVS, or umbilical blood sampling establishes the diagnosis. Once a cytogenetic diagnosis has been established, fetal echocardiography should be performed because of the high incidence of congenital heart disease. Consultations with surgical specialists will be dependent on the types of structural malformations seen.

Monitoring No change in standard obstetric care is needed.

Pregnancy Course   Whereas cystic hygroma with hydrops is virtually always fatal, cystic hygroma without hydrops slowly regresses and leaves a webbed neck.

Pregnancy Termination Issues   Should a family choose pregnancy termination, suction dilatation and evacuation techniques are appropriate once a cytogenetic diagnosis has been established.

Delivery   If congenital heart disease is present, delivery should occur in a tertiary center. In other cases, the site of delivery can be the family's and physician's choice.

Neonatology

Resuscitation   There is no contraindication to full resuscitation. As coarctation of the aorta is the most frequently occurring cardiac defect, peripheral perfusion may be dependent on flow through the ductus arteriosus. Prolonged exposure to high oxygen concentrations is not advisable until the cardiac anatomy is known.

Transport   Indicated if a cardiac malformation is suspected and counseling and long-term care planning are not available locally. If asymptomatic and no cardiac involvement is suspected, outpatient evaluation in early infancy is appropriate.

Testing and Confirmation   Newborns present with a short webbed neck (50%) with a low hairline (80%), lymphedema of hands and feet, prominent ears (80%), and cardiac abnormalities. Patients not detected in infancy are detected in childhood with short stature and delayed puberty due to ovarian dysgenesis. Lymphocyte karyotype with special attention to possible mosaicism confirms the diagnosis.

Nursery Management   Diagnostic evaluation should include an echocardiogram and renal sonogram irrespective of symptomatology. No intervention is usually required for lymphedema. Peripheral invasive procedures should be minimized to decrease the potential for systemic infection.

REFERENCES

Brown BSJ, Thompson DL: Ultrasonographic features of the fetal Turner syndrome. J Can Assoc Radiol 1984;35:40–46.

Carey JC: Health supervision and anticipatory guidance for infants with congenital defects. In Ballard RA (ed): Pediatric Care of the ICN Graduate. Philadelphia, WB Saunders, 1988.

Chervenak FA, Isaacson G, Blakemore KJ, et al: Fetal cystic hygroma: Cause and natural history. N Engl J Med 1983;309:822–825.

Eiben B, Trawicki W, Hammans W, et al: Rapid prenatal diagnosis of aneuploidies in uncultured amniocytes by fluorescence in situ hybridization. Evaluation of >3,000 cases. Fetal Diagn Ther 1999;14:193–197.

Gorlin RJ, Cohen MM, Hennekan RCM (eds): Syndromes of the Head and Neck, 4th ed. New York, Oxford University Press, 2001, pp 57–62.

Haddad HM, Wilkins L: Congenital anomalies associated with gonadal aplasia: Review of 55 cases. Pediatrics 1959;23:885.

Hall G, Weston MJ, Campbell DJ: Transitory pleural effusion associated with mosaic Turner syndrome. Prenat Diagn 2001;21:421–422.

Jones KL (ed): Smith's Recognizable Patterns of Human Malformations. Philadelphia, WB Saunders, 1988, pp 10–15.

Lewin P, Kleinfinger P, Bazin A, et al: Defining the efficiency of fluorescence in situ hybridization on uncultured amniocytes on a retrospective cohort of 27,407 prenatal diagnoses. Prenat Diagn 2000;20:1–6.

Litvak AS, Rousseau TG, Wrede LD, et al: The association of significant renal anomalies with Turner's syndrome. J Urol 1978;120:671–672.

Matias A, Montenegro N, Areias JC, Brandao O: Anomalous fetal venous return associated with major chromosomopathies in the late first trimester of pregnancy. Ultrasound Obstet Gynecol 1998;11:209–213.

Nisbet DL, Grimm DR, Chitty L: Prenatal features of Noonan syndrome. Prenat Diagn 1999;19:642–647.

Robinow M, Spisso K, Buschi AJ, Brenbridge AN: Turner syndrome: Sonography showing fetal hydrops simulating hydramnios. Am J Roentgenol 1980;135:846–848.

Sculerati N, Ledesma-Medina J, Finegold DN, Stool SE: Otitis media and hearing loss in Turner syndrome. Arch Otolaryngol Head Neck Surg 1990;116:704–707.

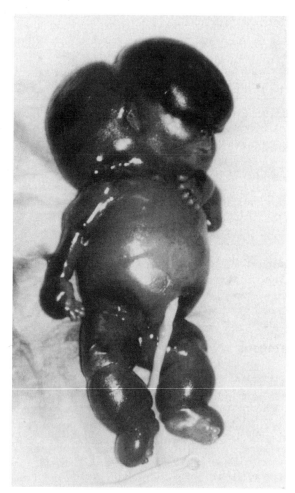

An 18-week fetus with massive cystic hygroma and lymphedema as a result of Turner syndrome (45XO).

Central Nervous System 2

2.1 Agenesis of the Corpus Callosum (ACC)

Epidemiology/Genetics

Definition   Complete or partial failure of the callosal commisural fibers to cross in the midline and form the corpus callosum between the two cerebral hemispheres.

Epidemiology   Incidence may be as high as 1% with many asymptomatic individuals.

Embryology   The corpus callosum develops between the 12th and the 22nd week of gestation. Vascular disruption or failure of formation may cause complete or partial agenesis. Associated abnormalities include hydrocephalus, microcephaly, pachygyria, and lissencephaly. More than 80 sporadic, genetic, and chromosomal syndromes have been described with agenesis of the corpus callosum (ACC), including trisomies 13 and 18. Agenesis of the corpus callosum, combined with intracranial cysts and/or eye anomalies, should suggest Aicardi syndrome, an X-linked dominant disorder with male lethality.

Inheritance Patterns   Most isolated defects are sporadic. Autosomal dominant, recessive, and X-linked syndromes have been described.

Teratogens   None known.

Prognosis   Isolated ACC may be asymptomatic unless associated with other brain abnormalities. The prognosis of some syndromes such as the Dandy-Walker syndrome is worsened when there is concomitant ACC. Associated brain or extracranial abnormalities suggest a guarded prognosis.

Sonography

FINDINGS

1. **Fetus:**
   a. Since the corpus callosum is absent, the third ventricle lies high between widely separated lateral ventricles. The lateral ventricles are more parallel to the midline than usual, so the medial wall is well seen at a more superior level.
   b. There may be a cyst arising from the superior aspect of the third ventricle, which communicates with the lateral ventricles. It usually has a more or less round shape with multiple projections. A mass—the bundles of Probst—causes an impression on the lateral aspects of the cystic area.
   c. The gyri are normally horizontally aligned. They assume a vertical orientation with agenesis. A sagittal view through the midline (difficult to obtain) will show absence of the normal corpus callosum and the radiating gyri.
   d. The occipital horns of the lateral ventricle are usually locally dilated (colpocephaly), forming an appearance on axial views similar to bulls' horns.
   e. The pericallosal artery is absent or does not follow its usual course.
   f. Partial forms in which only a portion of the corpus callosum is absent may occur.
2. **Amniotic Fluid:** Normal, unless there is an associated anomaly.
3. **Placenta:** Normal, unless there is an associated anomaly.
4. **Measurement Data:** Normal.
5. **When Detectable:** At about 18 weeks—the corpus callosum usually forms by this time.

Pitfalls

1. The sonographic findings are technically difficult to detect. A coronal view is the best for seeing the relationship to the lateral ventricles. A sagittal view, if obtainable, will show gyri radiating from the lateral ventricle and the absence of the corpus callosum. This view may best be obtained using an endovaginal approach if the fetus is vertex.
2. The cavum pellucidum and cavum verga can be mistaken for ACC, but there will be a third ventricle in normal position. Magnetic resonance imaging (MRI) helps in confusing cases.

3. Development of the corpus callosum may not be complete until 18 weeks, so the diagnosis may be missed on earlier examinations.

Differential Diagnosis

1. Lobar holoprosencephaly—The lateral ventricles and apparent third ventricle are joined. There is no midline falx, and the lateral ventricles are squared off. The corpus callosum is absent.
2. Arachnoid cyst—Irregular shape and unlikely to be exactly midline. There is usually no ventricular dilation.
3. Mild lateral ventriculomegaly—The entire ventricle is dilated and the third ventricle will be mildly dilated and in a normal position.
4. Enlarged cavum septum pellucidum and vergae. The corpus callosum is present and the cyst is symmetrical.

Where Else to Look

1. Dandy-Walker syndrome is the most common association. The vermis of the cerebellum will be small and will be surrounded by a fourth ventricular cyst.
2. Additional brain abnormalities such as asymmetry of the cerebral hemispheres, gyri abnormalities, and heterotopia are common. Lipoma of the corpus callosum seen as a brightly echogenic mass is strongly associated with ACC (50%).
3. Encephalocele or myelomeningocele—There will be no visible cisterna magna and the cerebellum will be banana-shaped.
4. Aicardi syndrome: females or 47XXY karyotype—Arachnoid cysts and vertebral anomalies are often seen in addition to the agenesis.
5. Chromosomal anomalies (trisomies 8, 13, and 18)—Look for the stigmata.
6. Diaphragmatic hernia (see Chapter 5.2).
7. Cardiac malformations.
8. Lung agenesis or dysplasia.
9. Absent or dysplastic kidneys are more frequent with ACC.

Pregnancy Management

Investigations and Consultations Required
Chromosome studies of the fetus are essential. Evaluation of the parents for signs of autosomal dominant conditions, such as basal cell nevus syndrome and tuberous sclerosis, should be performed by a dysmorphologist. Fetal echocardiography should be performed to detect congenital heart disease. Maternal serum TORCH titers should be drawn. Additional consultations will depend on the associated abnormalities found.

Monitoring
No change in standard obstetric practice is indicated for isolated ACC. The aggressiveness of fetal intervention must be based on the underlying cause, if that can be determined. Isolated ACC should not progress, but if associated with a cyst, a third-trimester examination is desirable to make sure the cyst has not enlarged and that other processes have not been missed.

Pregnancy Course
Obstetric complications are not expected on the basis of ACC alone.

Pregnancy Termination Issues
Because many conditions have ACC as a component, an intact fetus should be delivered in an institution with expertise in dysmorphology and fetal pathology.

Delivery
Because of the high association with other non–central nervous system (CNS) abnormalities, delivery should occur in a tertiary center with full capabilities for diagnosis and management of infants with multiple malformations.

Neonatology

Resuscitation
No specific issues except in those infants with additional CNS defects, in which case the associated defect will be the dominant factor in decisions regarding intervention.

Transport
Referral to a tertiary center after birth is not indicated with an isolated lesion and asymptomatic course. With any neurologic symptoms present or associated CNS lesions, the infant should be referred promptly to a tertiary perinatal center with pediatric neurology capabilities for definitive evaluation.

Testing and Confirmation
Postnatal confirmation of the defect and evaluation for other associated lesions is best achieved with MRI. Screening for inherited metabolic disorders is indicated with isolated lesions of the corpus callosum.

Nursery Management
Subsequent course and management are dictated by the associated lesion(s).

REFERENCES

Achiron R, Achiron A: Development of the human fetal corpus callosum: A high-resolution, cross-sectional sonographic study. Ultrasound Obstet Gynecol 2001;18:343–347.

Bamforth F, Bamforth S, Poskitt K, et al: Abnormalities of corpus callosum in patients with inherited metabolic diseases. Lancet 1988; 2:451.

Bertino RE, Nyberg DA, Cyr DR, Mack LA: Prenatal diagnosis of agenesis of the corpus callosum. J Ultrasound Med 1988;7:251–260.

Bromley B, Krishnamoorthy KS, Benacerraf BR: Aicardi syndrome: Prenatal sonographic findings. A report of two cases. Prenat Diagn 2000;20:344–346.

Cohen MM Jr, Kreiborg S: Agenesis of the corpus callosum: Its associated anomalies and syndromes with special reference to the Apert syndrome. Neurosurg Clin North Am 1991;2:565–568.

Comstock CH, Culp D, Gonzalez J, Boal DB: Agenesis of the corpus callosum in the fetus: Its evolution and significance. J Ultrasound Med 1985;4:613–616.

D'Ercole C, Girard N, Cravello L, et al: Prenatal diagnosis of fetal corpus callosum agenesis by ultrasonography and magnetic resonance imaging. Prenat Diagn 1998;18:247–253.

Dobryns WB: Agenesis of the corpus callosum and gyral malformations are frequent manifestations of nonketotic hyperglycinemia. Neurology 1989;39:817.

Franco I, Kogan S, Fisher J, et al: Genitourinary malformations associated with agenesis of the corpus callosum. J Urol 1993;149:1119–1121.

Gupta JK, Lilford RJ: Assessment and management of fetal agenesis of the corpus callosum. Prenat Diagn 1995;15:301–312.

Malinger G, Zakut H: The corpus callosum: Normal fetal development as shown by transvaginal sonography. Am J Roentgenol 1993;161:1041–1043.

Marszal E, Jamroz E, Pilch J, et al: Agenesis of corpus callosum: Clinical description and etiology. J Child Neurol 2000;15:401–405.

Monteagudo A: Fetal neurosonography: Should it be routine? Should it be detailed? Ultrasound Obstet Gynecol 1998;12:1–5.

Pilu G, Sandri F, Perolo A, et al: Sonography of fetal agenesis of the corpus callosum: A survey of 35 cases. Ultrasound Obstet Gynecol 1993;3:318–329.

Vergani P, Ghidini A, Mariani S, et al: Antenatal sonographic findings of agenesis of corpus callosum. Am J Perinatol 1988;5:105–108.

Vergani P, Ghidini A, Strobelt N, et al: Prognostic indicators in the prenatal diagnosis of agenesis of corpus callosum. Am J Obstet Gynecol 1994;170:753–758.

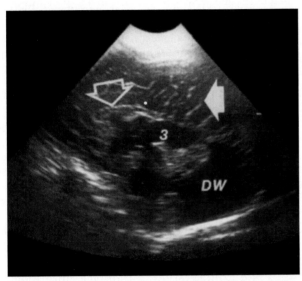

Partial agenesis of the corpus callosum, midline sagittal view. The anterior portion of the corpus callosum is present (*arrow*). Posteriorly, where the corpus callosum is absent, the gyri are aligned vertically (*solid arrow*). The patient also had Dandy-Walker syndrome with an enlarged third ventricle (3) and a posterior fossa cyst (DW).

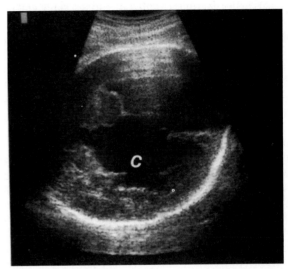

Axial view. A centrally placed cyst (c) communicates with both lateral ventricles. Such a centrally placed cyst is not uncommon with agenesis of the corpus callosum.

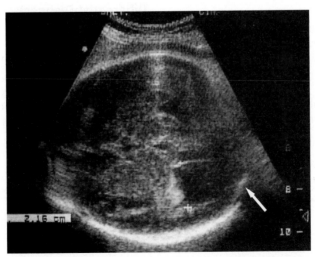

Axial view showing marked colpocephaly. Note the large size of the occipital horn (between the x's), whereas the anterior horn (*arrow*) is very narrow.

2.2 Anencephaly

Epidemiology/Genetics

Definition   Anencephaly is a defect in closure of the anterior neural tube characterized by complete or partial absence of the forebrain, overlying meninges, skull, and skin.

Epidemiology   The incidence is geographically and population dependent and ranges from about 1 in 1000 births in the United States to 1 in 100 in parts of the British Isles (M1:F3.7). Preconceptual supplementation with folic acid has been shown to decrease the incidence of open neural tube defects.

Embryology   Neural tube closure occurs between 20 and 28 days of pregnancy, with abnormalities of cephalic closure, which occurs late, resulting in anencephaly. Anencephaly is characterized by the absence of the cranial vault with exposed neural tissue and is associated with spina bifida, facial and nasal clefts, and omphalocele. Amniotic band disruptions are also an unusual cause of anencephaly.

Inheritance Patterns   Multifactorial inheritance with both genetic and environmental factors is implicated. Recurrence risk after one affected pregnancy is 2 to 3% for any open neural tube defect. Rare families have been reported with X-linked inheritance. It is estimated that periconceptional folic acid supplementation of 0.4 mg/day would decrease the incidence of spina bifida and anencephaly by 50%.

Teratogens   Valproic acid, folic acid antagonists, such as methotrexate and aminopterin, maternal diabetes, hyperthermia, and folic acid deficiency are associated with an increased risk for neural tube defects.

Screening   Maternal serum alpha-fetoprotein screening or fetal ultrasonographic screening will detect most cases of anencephaly.

Prognosis   Anencephaly is invariably lethal, with about 50% of cases being stillborn, and the remainder dying in the newborn period.

Sonography

FINDINGS

1. **Fetus:**
   a. Skull development, usually completed by 10 weeks, never occurs. The exposed brain is gradually eliminated after exposure to the amniotic fluid. When diagnosed between 10 and 14 weeks, the brain is still present to a variable extent. The remaining brain has an irregular outline and is often bilobulated, forming the "Mickey Mouse" sign. By about 17 weeks, the brain has been eliminated, but intracranial vessels remain as a superior bulge. The earlier stages of anencephaly when some brain remains are sometimes known as acrania (when all the brain appears present) or exencephaly (when part of the brain appears present).
   b. Facial and brain stem structures persist, so there is a typical frog-like appearance to the fetal face.
   c. Myelomeningoceles in the lumbosacral or cervical region are quite frequent.
2. **Amniotic Fluid:** Polyhydramnios is common but not invariable (about 75%). Because of the polyhydramnios, there can be increased fetal movement.
3. **Placenta:** Normal.
4. **Measurement Data:** Appropriate for dates.
5. **When Detectable:** First detectable at 11 weeks when all of the brain will be present. The brain will have an irregular "floppy" outline, since the skull is absent.

Pitfalls

1. An irregular fetal head outline at 10 to 12 weeks can easily be overlooked.
2. If the head is deep in the pelvis and no endovaginal probe study is done, the defect may be overlooked and the absence of the skull thought to be a technical problem.

Differential Diagnosis

1. Large encephalocele—The skull will be visible on close inspection.
2. Microcephaly—A small skull will be present.
3. Iniencephaly is often seen with anencephaly. Because of the delivery complications that may be associated with iniencephaly, this condition must be ruled out before deciding on an appropriate management plan.

Where Else to Look

1. Look at the cervical spine for shortening and rachischisis. Iniencephaly is commonly associated with anencephaly.
2. Myelomeningocele may also be present in the lumbosacral region.
3. Diaphragmatic hernia, hydronephrosis, cleft lip, and cardiac malformations have been reported with anencephaly. Since the condition is lethal, an extensive search for additional malformations seems futile.
4. Occasional cases of anencephaly are due to the amniotic band syndrome. The amniotic bands may be visible on careful ultrasonographic inspection.

Pregnancy Management

Investigations and Consultations Required No specific antenatal evaluations or consultations are necessary.

Monitoring In pregnancies that are continued, clinical assessment for the presence of polyhydramnios is indicated. The most important component of the prenatal care is emotional support for the family.

Pregnancy Course Always lethal at or shortly after birth.

Pregnancy Termination Issues Suction dilatation and evacuation techniques are appropriate. Karyotyping abortus material is worthwhile to detect the rare case caused by chromosome anomaly, such as trisomy 18.

Delivery There are no special conditions regarding delivery. The majority of anencephalic infants will deliver in the breech presentation.

Neonatology

Resuscitation Given the lethal prognosis, neonatal resuscitation is never indicated. Prenatal diagnosis and counseling should focus on preparing the family for nonintervention.

Transport Not an issue.

Testing and Confirmation The abnormality is obvious at birth. Evidence of amniotic band disruptions should be sought.

Nursery Management Provision of warmth, hygiene, and facilitation of parental grief are the principal elements of care. Some infants may survive for several days with intermittent periods of stable cardiorespiratory function, which parents and staff may find disturbing.

REFERENCES

Bronshtein M, Ornoy A: Acrania: Anencephaly resulting from secondary degeneration of a closed neural tube: Two cases in the same family. J Clin Ultrasound 1991;19:230–234.

Centers for Disease Control and Prevention: Recommendations for use of folic acid to reduce number of spina bifida cases and other neural tube defects. JAMA 1993;369:1236–1238.

Chatzipapas IK, Whitlow BJ, Economides DL: The "Mickey Mouse" sign and the diagnosis of anencephaly in early pregnancy. Ultrasound Obstet Gynecol 1999;13:196–199.

Goldstein RB, Filly RA: Prenatal diagnosis of anencephaly: Spectrum of sonographic appearances and distinction from the amniotic band syndrome. Am J Roentgenol 1988;151:547–550.

Hendricks SK, Cyr DR, Nyberg DA, et al: Exencephaly: Clinical and ultrasonic correlation to anencephaly. Obstet Gynecol 1988;72:898–900.

Melnick M, Myrianthopoulos NC: Studies in neural tube defects. II. Pathologic findings in a prospectively collected series of anencephalics. Am J Med Genet 1987;26:797–810.

Salamanca A, Gonzalez-Gomez F, Padilla MC, et al: Prenatal ultrasound semiography of anencephaly: Sonographic-pathological correlations. Ultrasound Obstet Gynecol 1992;2:95–100.

Van Allen MI, Kalousek DK, Chernoff GF, et al: Evidence for multisite closure of the neural tube in humans. Am J Med Genet 1993;47:723–743.

Vergani P, Ghidini A, Sirtori M, Roncaglia N: Antenatal diagnosis of fetal acrania. J Ultrasound Med 1987;6:715–717.

Wilkins-Haug L, Freedman W: Progression of exencephaly to anencephaly in the human fetus: An ultrasound perspective. Prenat Diagn 1991;11:227–233.

Worthen NJ, Lawrence D, Bustillo M: Amniotic band syndrome: Antepartum ultrasonic diagnosis of discordant anencephaly. J Clin Ultrasound 1980;8:453–455.

Yang YC, Wu CH, Chang FM, et al: Early prenatal diagnosis of acrania by transvaginal ultrasonography. J Clin Ultrasound 1992;20:343–345.

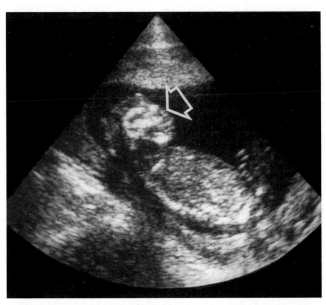

Anencephaly at 16 weeks. Little brain and no skull is present superior to the orbits (*arrow*).

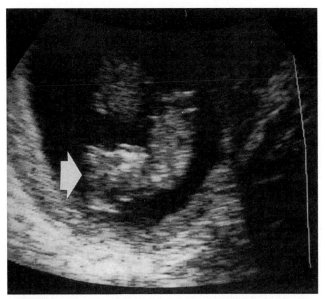

Acrania at 11 weeks. Although the brain is present (*arrow*), the skull is absent. If this fetus is followed, by approximately 16 weeks the brain tissue will no longer be visible.

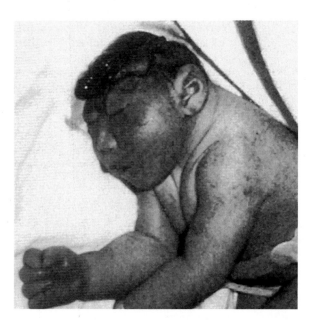

Newborn with isolated anencephaly.

2.3 Aqueductal Stenosis

Epidemiology/Genetics

Definition Aqueductal stenosis is an obstruction or maldevelopment of the aqueduct of Sylvius resulting in congenital hydrocephalus.

Epidemiology One in 2000 (M1.8:F1). Ninety percent of cases of congenital hydrocephalus are the result of Arnold-Chiari malformations, whereas 3 to 5% have aqueductal stenosis.

Embryology The aqueduct of Sylvius is the connection between the third and fourth ventricles in the brain and develops at about 6 weeks' gestation. Histologic evidence of gliosis is found in approximately 50% of cases of aqueductal stenosis, suggesting inflammatory or infectious causes. The etiology is heterogeneous and includes congenital tumors, hemorrhage, infections, and genetic syndromes. Flexion and adduction deformities of the thumbs are seen in 20% of boys with X-linked aqueductal stenosis.

Inheritance Patterns Most cases are sporadic. Estimates suggest that 2 to 5% of cases of hydrocephalus, not associated with neural tube defects, have X-linked recessive inheritance. The gene for X-linked aqueductal stenosis has been mapped to Xq28. Because of the rapid progress in mapping of genes and subsequent development of genetic testing, consultation with a medical geneticist or genetic counselor to determine the availability of clinical genetic testing for this disorder is advised.

Teratogens Congenital infections including cytomegalovirus (CMV), rubella, toxoplasmosis.

Prognosis There is a 10 to 30% neonatal mortality rate, partly dependent on associated abnormalities. Approximately 50% of survivors will have an IQ greater than 70. The X-linked recessive form is associated with profound mental retardation and a poor prognosis. Cases diagnosed in utero have a worse prognosis; in one series, there was normal development in only 14%.

Sonography

FINDINGS

1. **Fetus:**
   a. With aqueductal stenosis, there is enlargement of the lateral and third ventricles, but not of the fourth ventricle. A dilated proximal aqueduct of Sylvius may occasionally be visible. Unless the ventriculomegaly is very severe, the cisterna magna and cerebellum are normal. With very severe lateral ventricular enlargement, the cisterna magna may not be seen and the cerebellum may be technically difficult to find.
   b. Mild asymmetry of the lateral ventricular dilation is possible. Facial structures remain of a size appropriate for gestational age.
   c. Mild lateral ventricular dilation (10–15 mm) may not progress and may indicate a chromosomal anomaly (trisomy 21) rather than early aqueductal stenosis. The "hanging choroid" sign is a helpful indication that a mild increase in lateral ventricle size indicates hydrocephalus with increased intracranial pressure.
   d. Measurement of the remaining cortical mantle has some relationship to prognosis. The cortical mantle is customarily measured at the occipital, parietal, and frontal areas. The occipital mantle thickness is usually the smallest.
   e. Flexion and adduction of the thumb is seen in some boys with the X-linked form.
2. **Amniotic Fluid:** Usually normal.
3. **Placenta:** Normal.
4. **Measurement Data:** The head size is larger than predicted for gestational age. If the head size is not increased, other causes such as cerebral atrophy need to be considered. Intrauterine growth retardation may be seen.
5. **When Detectable:** Usually detectable by 17 weeks, but may develop later.

Pitfalls

1. Ventriculomegaly is present in many different entities. When ventriculomegaly is very severe, aqueductal stenosis can be confused with Arnold-Chiari malformation or holoprosencephaly.
2. If there is ventriculomegaly, but a head circumference measurement that is decreased or appropriate for gestational age, consider cerebral atrophy or Arnold-Chiari malformation with myelomeningocele.
3. Do not mistake the echogenic blush superior to the lateral ventricle, previously termed the lateral border of the lateral ventricle, for the true lateral ventricles. The choroid plexus should be visible within the lateral ventricle.
4. Mantle thickness measurement looks much more severe in utero. Once a shunt is in place, the cortical mantle regains thickness. Mantle thickness is especially thin posteriorly.
5. Anterior horn enlargement is a normal variant at the 13- to 15-week stage.

Differential Diagnosis

1. Arnold-Chiari malformation—Look for absence of cisterna magna and cerebellar deformity.

2. Holoprosencephaly—Look for a fused thalamus and absent third ventricle.
3. Unilateral ventriculomegaly. Isolated unilateral ventriculomegaly is often a normal variant but is associated with obstruction, chromosomal aberrations, cerebral hemorrhage, and lissencephaly.
4. Mild ventriculomegaly (10–15 mm) usually has a benign prognosis but is associated with aneuploidy and long-term retardation.

Where Else to Look

1. Up to 16% of aqueductal stenosis cases have other anomalies elsewhere. There is a moderate but definite association with karyotypic abnormalities.
2. Look for the gender of the fetus, since there is an X-linked form of aqueductal stenosis.
3. Look for stigmata of CMV, a known cause of mild hydrocephalus. Calcification in the lateral aspect of the lateral ventricular border is characteristic.

Pregnancy Management

Investigations and Consultations Required   Chromosome evaluation and viral studies (both maternal serum and amniotic fluid) should be performed. Pediatric neurosurgical consultation should be obtained to plan management.

Fetal Intervention   Theoretically, aqueductal stenosis should be the perfect situation for in utero shunt placement. However, the experience to date has been quite disappointing. There are many reasons for the relatively poor outcomes that have been seen. Misdiagnosis has been a common finding in all series, as has been failure to detect associated abnormalities. Morbidity has been high, reflecting the difficulties of exact shunt placement in the fetus. For these reasons, and the lack of data to support a clear benefit of fetal surgical intervention, in utero ventriculo-amniotic shunts are not indicated in the management of fetal ventriculomegaly.

Monitoring

1. Ventriculomegaly, caused by aqueductal stenosis, may abruptly increase in severity over a few weeks, so ultrasonographic monitoring every 2 or 3 weeks is desirable.
2. Spontaneous resolution of mild to moderate hydrocephalus has been reported.
3. Aqueductal stenosis is a condition that should have few complications given a carefully managed pregnancy with early intervention, if necessary.

Pregnancy Termination Issues   The method should be a nondestructive one and undertaken at a site with special expertise in neuropathology.

Delivery   In theory, early delivery followed by shunt placement could improve outcome. However, the centers utilizing this approach have limited data to support the benefits of this approach over the risks of prematurity from delivery at 32 to 37 weeks' gestation. Further study is needed before clear recommendations can be made. Mode of delivery can be vaginal, if the head is of relatively normal size and the fetus is in a vertex presentation. Occasionally, excessive head growth and fetal position may require cesarean section. Delivery should occur where appropriate neonatal and neurologic support services are available.

Neonatology

Resuscitation   The decision regarding support of the onset of respiration should be discussed with the family prior to delivery. Except in circumstances of extreme enlargement of the head or presence of other severe CNS abnormalities, initial resuscitation is indicated. Delay in spontaneous onset of respiration secondary to fetal distress from dystocia because of macrocephaly occurs frequently. Prematurity, if early delivery is chosen because of rapidly advancing hydrocephalus, may also cause respiratory distress.

Transport   Immediate referral to a tertiary perinatal center with pediatric neurology and neurosurgery capabilities is always indicated. Precautions during transport are dictated by the maturity of the infant, presence of respiratory distress, and other associated abnormalities.

Testing and Confirmation   Both cranial computed tomography (CT) and MRI are useful to establish a definite anatomic diagnosis.

Further imaging studies to be considered are echocardiography and abdominal sonography if physical examination findings suggest other abnormalities and studies were not obtained prenatally.

Nursery Management   The first priority is to determine the severity of the increased intracranial pressure, as immediate reduction may be needed to achieve clinical stability.

Surgery

Preoperative Assessment   Issues of importance with respect to the surgical management of aqueductal stenosis are as follows:

1. The presence of other anomalies (i.e., cardiac, renal, spinal, or limb deformities), which may be associated with a poor overall prognosis.
2. The presence of a posterior fossa mass or compressive lesion such as congenital tumor or tectal mass.
3. Rate of ventricular enlargement and head growth.

Operative Indications   Evidence of progressive ventricular enlargement or accelerated head growth is indication for surgical intervention.

Types of Procedures   Standard surgical therapy for aqueductal stenosis is ventricular shunting with either a ventriculoperitoneal or a ventriculoatrial shunt using a pressure-regulated valve system. Ventricular shunts are

Section 2.3—Aqueductal Stenosis

associated with high failure rate (60% of newly placed shunts will require revision within 2 years). An alternative therapy available since the reinvigoration of endoscopic techniques is fenestration of the floor of the third ventricle. This procedure, called an endoscopic third ventriculostomy, opens an alternative pathway for cerebrospinal fluid to exit the third ventricle by a fenestration in the tuber cinereum of the floor of the third ventricle. Although success is limited when performed within the first year of life (<20%), third ventriculostomy is extremely successful in treating obstructive hydrocephalus without a shunt in children older than 2 years of age. The success rate is nearly 80% in properly selected patients.

Surgical Results/Prognosis In the absence of associated CNS or non-CNS abnormalities, children with aqueductal stenosis have a good overall prognosis. It is the cause of the hydrocephalus, not the degree of ventricular enlargement, and the complications associated with shunting, that have the greatest impact on long-term prognosis.

REFERENCES

Benacerraf BR, Birnholz JC: The diagnosis of fetal hydrocephalus prior to 22 weeks. J Clin Ultrasound 1987;15:531–536.

Bowerman RA, DiPietro MA: Erroneous sonographic identification of fetal lateral ventricles: Relationship to the echogenic periventricular "blush." AJNR 1987;8:661–664.

Callen PW, Hashimoto BE, Newton TH: Sonographic evaluation of cerebral cortical mantle thickness in the fetus and neonate with hydrocephalus. J Ultrasound Med 1986;5:251–255.

Cardoza JD, Filly RA, Podrasky AE: The dangling choroid plexus: A sonographic observation of value in excluding ventriculomegaly. Am J Roentgenol 1988;151:767–770.

Cochrane DD, Myles ST, Nimrod C, et al: Intrauterine hydrocephalus and ventriculomegaly: Associated anomalies and fetal outcome. Can J Neurol Sci 1985;12:51–59.

Holmes LB, Nash A, ZuRhein GM, et al: X-linked aqueductal stenosis: Clinical and neuropathological findings in two families. Pediatrics 1973;51:697–704.

Levitsky DB, Mack LA, Nyberg DA, et al: Fetal aqueduct stenosis diagnosed sonographically: How grave is the prognosis? AJR 1995;164:725–730.

Lipitz S, Yagel S, Malinger G, et al: Outcome of fetuses with isolated borderline unilateral ventriculomegaly diagnosed at mid-gestation. Ultrasound Obstet Gynecol 1998;12:23–26.

McClone DSG, Naidich TP, Cunningham T: Posterior fossa cysts: Management and outcome. Conc Ped Neurosurg 1987;7:134.

McCullough DC, Balzer-Martin LA: Current prognosis in overt neonatal hydrocephalus. J Neurosurg 1982;57:378–383.

Pilu G, Falco P, Gabrielli S, et al: The clinical significance of fetal isolated cerebral borderline ventriculomegaly: Report of 31 cases and review of the literature. Ultrasound Obstet Gynecol 1999;14:320–326.

Pretorius DH, Davis K, Manco-Johnson ML, et al: Clinical course of fetal hydrocephalus: 40 cases. Am J Roentgenol 1985;144:827–831.

Rosenthal A, Jouet M, Kenwrick S: Aberrant splicing of neural cell adhesion molecule L1 mRNA in a family with X-linked hydrocephalus. Nat Genet 1992;2:107–112.

Senat MV, Bernard JP, Schwarzler P, et al: Prenatal diagnosis and follow-up of 14 cases of unilateral ventriculomegaly. Ultrasound Obstet Gynecol 1999;14:327–332.

Tomlinson MW, Treadwell MC, Bottoms SF: Isolated mild ventriculomegaly: Associated karyotypic abnormalities and in utero observations. J Matern Fetal Med 1997;6:241–244.

Vergani P, Locatelli A, Strobelt N, et al: Clinical outcome of mild fetal ventriculomegaly. Am J Obstet Gynecol 1998;178:218–222.

Vintzileos AM, Campbell WA, Weinbaum PJ, Nochimson DJ: Perinatal management and outcome of fetal ventriculomegaly. Obstet Gynecol 1987;68:5–11.

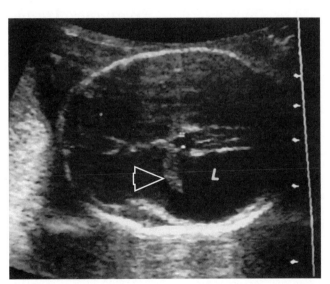

Aqueductal stenosis. There is a dilated lateral ventricle (L) showing the hanging choroids sign of ventriculomegaly (*arrow*). The third ventricle is dilated (*small x's*).

2.4 Arachnoid Cyst

Epidemiology/Genetics

Definition Arachnoid cysts are membrane-lined fluid-filled cavities that may occur anywhere within the brain or spinal cord in association with the arachnoid or ventricular lining.

Epidemiology Very rare (M1:F1).

Embryology Arachnoid cysts can occur anywhere in the lining of the brain or spinal cord. They may arise postnatally and are associated with trauma or infection. The cause of congenital cysts is unclear. They may represent maldevelopment of the leptomeninges or acquired destructive events.

Inheritance Patterns Rare autosomal recessive families with isolated arachnoid cysts have been described.

Teratogens Congenital infections.

Prognosis Since these cysts generally compress normal brain structures, the outcome is usually favorable unless it is associated with other congenital anomalies or there are significant complications related to treatment. The association of intracranial cysts with agenesis of the corpus callosum should suggest the Aicardi syndrome, an X-linked dominant disorder with male lethality.

Sonography

FINDINGS

1. **Fetus:** Intrabrain cystic collections with a random shape and size, which abut the meninges. Cysts located in the midbrain (50–65%), suprasellar, and quadrigeminal regions may expand and cause secondary ventriculomegaly. A subtentorial form known as an extra-axial cyst can compress the cerebellum (5%). A cyst has been reported to rupture and disappear spontaneously in utero.
2. **Amniotic Fluid:** Normal.
3. **Placenta:** Normal.
4. **Measurement Data:** Head size may be enlarged or normal.
5. **When Detectable:** Arachnoid cysts have been seen as early as 23 weeks.

Pitfalls If the cyst is in the dependent part of the skull and the nondependent portion of the brain can never be seen because of acoustic shadowing, arachnoid cysts can be confused with bilateral processes such as holoprosencephaly. They may be missed altogether if they lie in the portion of the brain closest to the transducer. MRI is helpful if the cyst is partially obscured by reverberation artifact.

Differential Diagnosis

1. Porencephalic cyst—The cystic area will border on the ventricle.
2. Vein of Galen aneurysm—There will be blood flow in a centrally placed cyst.
3. Intracranial bleed—There will be internal echoes in the apparent cyst if the gain is increased.
4. Schizencephaly—Disorganized cystic area extending across the midline involving both hemispheres.

Depending on the location of the cyst, obstructive hydrocephalus may develop. An attempt should be made to exclude conditions not associated with a risk of significant in utero ventriculomegaly.

Where Else to Look Assess for presence of the corpus callosum, as Aicardi syndrome has been reported in two cases of fetal arachnoid cysts. Usually arachnoid cyst is an isolated finding.

Pregnancy Management

Investigations and Consultations Required Despite the low reported incidence of chromosome abnormalities, cytogenetic studies should be performed. No other diagnostic evaluations are indicated. Consultation with a pediatric neurosurgeon should be arranged.

Fetal Intervention Invasive fetal intervention is not indicated because of the relatively benign course of this malformation.

Monitoring Serial ultrasonographic examinations should be performed every 3 to 4 weeks to detect or follow ventriculomegaly.

Pregnancy Course Obstetric complications are not to be expected.

Pregnancy Termination Issues The method should be a nondestructive procedure undertaken at a site with expertise in neuropathology.

Delivery The site of delivery should be at a location with expertise in the management of neonates with CNS malformations.

Neonatology

Resuscitation   The most likely intrapartum risk is for distress secondary to head compression and/or hemorrhage into the cyst. Prematurity, from early delivery because of rapidly advancing hydrocephalus, may also have an impact on early adaptation.

Transport   Referral to a tertiary center with pediatric neurology and neurosurgery capabilities is always indicated.

Testing and Confirmation   Presentations at birth include macrocephaly or a bulging fontanelle with widened sutures. The cysts cause their symptoms through pressure and mass effect. Small to moderate cysts are frequently asymptomatic. Postnatal CT or MRI will accurately define these abnormalities.

Determination of the degree of increased intracranial pressure governs the urgency of surgical intervention.

Nursery Management   Hemorrhage into the cyst may complicate the course at any point and should be suspected if an abrupt clinical deterioration occurs. Preoperative and postoperative course is determined by the location of the cyst and the neurologic dysfunction that results.

Surgery

Preoperative Assessment   Location of the arachnoid cyst with respect to the ventricular system, the basal cisterns, and the structures of the posterior fossa is important for surgical planning. Computed tomographic scan or MRI scanning is useful to define the surgical anatomy.

Operative Indications   Small arachnoid cysts without mass effect on surrounding neural structures warrant observation only with periodic CT or MRI. If stable over time, then no surgical intervention is indicated. Larger cysts that present with hydrocephalus, the presence of a neurologic deficit, increase in cyst size, or poorly controlled seizures require surgical intervention.

Types of Procedures

1. Shunting of the cyst to the peritoneal cavity or the right atrium.
2. Marsupialization of the cyst into the basal cisterns or surrounding subarachnoid space. This technique is useful only for arachnoid cysts that present at the skull base adjacent to the basal cisterns.
3. Fenestration of the cyst into an adjacent ventricle, which may be accomplished endoscopically.

Surgical Results/Prognosis   Arachnoid cysts in general have an excellent outcome and are not typically associated with neurologic or cognitive impairment. Children who present with poorly controlled epilepsy respond well to cyst decompression. Controversy exists as to the best surgical approach, although most surgeons will choose to avoid shunt placement if at all possible. In some situations, fenestration or marsupialization may fail, ultimately requiring placement of a shunt.

REFERENCES

Bannister CM, Russell SA, Rimmer S, Mowle DH: Fetal arachnoid cysts: Their site, progress, prognosis and differential diagnosis. Eur J Pediatr Surg 1999;1:27–28.

Blaicher W, Prager D, Kuhle S, et al: Combined prenatal ultrasound and magnetic resonance imaging in two fetuses with suspected arachnoid cysts. Ultrasound Obstet Gynecol 2001;18:166–168.

Bromley B, Krishnamoorthy K, Benacerraf BR: Aicardi syndrome: Prenatal sonographic findings. A report of two cases. Prenat Diagn 2000;20:344–346.

Chen CY, Chen FH, Lee CC, et al: Sonographic characteristics of the cavum velum interpositum. Am J Neuroradiol 1998;19:1631–1635.

Diakoumakis EE, Weinberg B, Mollin J: Prenatal sonographic diagnosis of a suprasellar arachnoid cyst. J Ultrasound Med 1986;5:529–530.

Elbers SEL, Furness ME: Resolution of presumed arachnoid cyst in utero. Ultrasound Obstet Gynecol 1999;14:353–355.

Meizner I, Barki Y, Tadmor R, Katz M: In utero ultrasonic detection of fetal arachnoid cyst. J Clin Ultrasound 1988;16:506–509.

Pilu G, Falco P, Perolo A, et al: Differential diagnosis and outcome of fetal intracranial hypoechoic lesions: Report of 21 cases. Ultrasound Obstet Gynecol 1997;9:229–236.

Rafferty PG, Britton J, Penna L, Ville Y: Prenatal diagnosis of a large fetal arachnoid cyst. Ultrasound Obstet Gynecol 1998;12:358–361.

Wilson WG, Deponte KA, McIlhenny J, Dreifuss FE: Arachnoid cysts in a brother and sister. J Med Genet 1988;25:714–715.

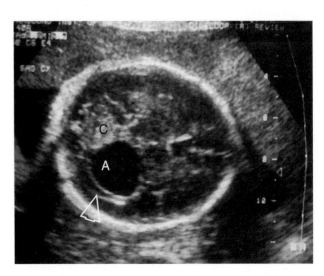

Arachnoid cyst. A cyst (A) lies alongside the tentorium, displacing the lateral ventricle (*arrow*) laterally. The cyst arises in a cistern and displaces but does not destroy brain tissue.

2.5 Caudal Aplasia/Dysplasia (Regression) Sequence

Epidemiology/Genetics

Definition Caudal aplasia-dysplasia sequence is the total or partial agenesis of the distal neural tube resulting in sacral agenesis/dysgenesis with associated abnormalities of the lower extremities and gastrointestinal and/or genitourinary tracts.

Epidemiology Occurs in about 1 to 5 in 100,000 births (M1:F1).

Embryology Differentiation of the lower spine is usually complete before the seventh week of pregnancy. The term caudal "regression" is probably inaccurate, as the caudal defects in this condition are primary malformations rather than the result of regression of structures. Sirenomelia may represent one end of the spectrum of this condition or may be etiologically separate. Heart defects are common associated malformations. This condition may overlap with the VACTERL assocation, making evaluation for other VACTERL association findings important.

Inheritance Patterns Most often sporadic. Rare families showing autosomal and X-linked dominant inheritance have been reported. Often seen in association with maternal diabetes.

Teratogens Approximately 16% of cases are seen in infants of diabetic mothers.

Prognosis Dependent on the severity of the defect and presence of associated abnormalities. Bowel and urinary complications are common and may not be compatible with life. If not part of a genetic or chromosomal syndrome, cognitive function is usually normal.

Sonography

FINDINGS

1. **Fetus:**
   a. Shortened spine with missing sacral and lower lumbar vertebrae. Normally the superior aspect of the iliac crest lies at the level of L5; in this condition, no vertebrae are seen at this level.
   b. The femurs are fixed in a V pattern, giving a typical "Buddha's pose." There is decreased or absent movement of the lower extremities. Clubfeet may be seen.
   c. A dilated bladder, ureter, or collecting system may be seen.
2. **Amniotic Fluid:** Normal.
3. **Placenta:** Normal.
4. **Measurement Data:** Normal.
5. **When Detectable:** The syndrome has been detected as early as 9 to 11 weeks.

Pitfalls

1. Since the sacrum does not calcify until 22 weeks, the syndrome may be difficult to identify before that time.
2. The legs are often flexed over the abdomen, so if the fetus is in a supine position, the femur may obscure the lower spine.

Differential Diagnosis

1. Myelomeningocele with cord tethering.
2. Sirenomelia is a related condition in which both legs are fused. In sirenomelia, there is oligohydramnios or absent fluid and the kidneys may appear to be absent, obstructed, or dysplastic. There may be a single lower extremity, or both legs may be fused and lie alongside each other. (See Chapter 4.14.)

Where Else to Look

1. Look at the cranium for hydrocephalus.
2. Look at the kidneys for hydronephrosis and multicystic kidney.
3. Look at the legs for movement and clubfeet. (In sirenomelia, both legs are close together and straight.) Both legs may be crossed and positioned over the abdomen.
4. Look at the spine for hemivertebrae and cord tethering.

Pregnancy Management

Investigations and Consultations Required Evaluation of the mother for diabetes should be performed. Fetal echocardiography should be performed to evaluate for associated cardiac defects. Pediatric surgical consultations should be obtained to plan with the family for neonatal management.

Monitoring No specific alterations in obstetric care are necessary. The diagnosis is difficult, so a repeat ultrasonogram in the third trimester is worthwhile.

Pregnancy Termination Issues In the patient with known diabetes, no special autopsy requirements are necessary. In the absence of maternal diabetes, full autopsy of an intact fetus should be performed to establish the diagnosis.

Delivery The high likelihood of neonatal complications requires delivery at a tertiary site. Breech presentation may warrant cesarean section because of the marked body/head discrepancy that may be present.

Neonatology

Resuscitation Beyond the issues of prematurity and of infants of diabetic mothers, there are no special concerns in planning for resuscitation. In a small number of cases, there may be other serious anomalies (CNS or cardiac) that could govern approach.

If other life-threatening and potentially uncorrectable defects are known to be present, prenatal discussion with the parents regarding nonintervention is appropriate.

Transport Referral to a tertiary center with multiple pediatric subspecialty capabilities is indicated.

Testing and Confirmation The physical findings are apparent at birth. Echocardiography, to exclude concomitant cardiac anomalies, and cranial CT scan or MRI, for CNS defects, should be obtained prior to invasive interventions.

Nursery Management Approach and management are governed by both the suspected cause (i.e., maternal diabetes, associated anomalies) and the location of the defect. In general, with the exception of hydrocephalus, the long-term issues of ambulation and bowel and bladder function are very similar to those of a patient with a high to mid-lumbar myelomeningocele.

REFERENCES

Adra A, Cordero D, Mejides A, et al: Caudal regression syndrome: Etiopathogenesis, prenatal diagnosis, and perinatal management. Obstet Gynecol Surv 1994;49:508–516.

Andrish J, Kalamchi A, MacEwen GD: Sacral agenesis: A clinical evaluation of its management, heredity and associated anomalies. Clin Orthop 1979;139:52–57.

Loewy JA, Richards DG, Toi A: In-utero diagnosis of the caudal regression syndrome: Report of three cases. J Clin Ultrasound 1987;15:469–474.

Mills JL: Malformations in infants of diabetic mothers. Teratology 1982;25:381–394.

Price DL, Dooling EC, Richardson EP Jr: Caudal dysplasia (caudal regression syndrome). Arch Neurol 1970;23:212–220.

Rusnak SL, Driscoll SG: Congenital spinal anomalies in infants of diabetic mothers. Pediatrics 1965;35:989.

Subtil D, Cosson M, Houfflin V, et al: Early detection of caudal regression syndrome: Specific interest and findings in three cases. Eur J Obstet Gynecol Reprod Biol 1998;80(1):109–112.

Twickler D, Budorick N, Pretorius D, et al: Caudal regression versus sirenomelia: Sonographic clues. J Ultrasound Med 1993;12:323–330.

Valenzano M, Paoletti R, Rossi A, et al: Sirenomelia: Pathological features, antenatal ultrasonographic clues, and a review of current embryogenic theories. Hum Reprod Update 1999;5:82–86.

Welch JP, Aterman K: The syndrome of caudal dysplasia: A review, including etiologic considerations and evidence of heterogeneity. Pediatr Pathol 1984;2:313–327.

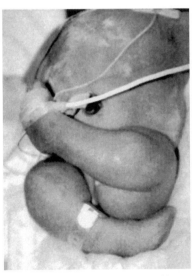

Newborn with caudal regression and lower limb deformities from maternal diabetic embryopathy.

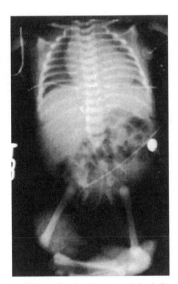

Radiograph showing caudal deficiency with absent sacrum.

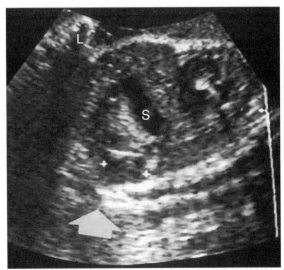

Caudal regression. The lumbar spine ends at about L2 (*arrow*). Note how close the stomach (S) is to the lower end of the spine. The legs (L) are crossed over the anterior aspect of the abdomen.

2.6 Cranial Tumors Other Than Intracranial Teratoma

Epidemiology/Genetics

Definition The majority of antenatally detected cranial tumors are teratomas derived from totipotent cells, including embryonic ectodermal, endodermal, and mesodermal tissue derivatives. It is difficult, however, to reliably separate these tumors from other intracranial neoplasms and benign cystic lesions.

Epidemiology Intracranial tumors are very rare, with 50% of antenatally detected tumors being teratomas that show a 5:1 male to female preponderance.

Embryology Teratomas occur most often in a midline location and have mixed solid and cystic areas. Only 3% of all teratomas occur intracranially.

Inheritance Patterns Sporadic.

Teratogens None.

Differential Diagnosis Benign intracranial cystic lesions such as arachnoid cysts and other benign lesions such as lipomas. Teratomas and other intracranial neoplasms generally show progression and distortion of normal structures.

Prognosis Dependent on the size and location of the tumor. Most antenatally detected tumors have been lethal.

Sonography

FINDINGS

1. **Fetus:**
   a. Craniopharyngioma
      1. A central, highly echogenic mass is seen near the base of the skull. A cystic area within the mass may develop and represent areas of necrosis.
      2. Secondary ventriculomegaly is common.
   b. Glioblastoma multiforme (astrocytoma)
      1. A highly echogenic unilateral mass that may be central or peripheral. Within a few weeks, the mass replaces the cerebral hemisphere on one side of the brain. Intramass hemorrhage causes echogenic areas, whereas central necrosis may lead to echo-free areas. Calcification may occasionally be seen within the mass.
      2. Severe midline shift to the opposite side occurs.
      3. Dilation of contralateral lateral ventricle is almost always seen.
      4. Color flow will show vascularity within the mass.
   c. Choroid plexus papilloma
      1. An echogenic mass is seen that involves the choroid plexus on one side. The mass can grow to a large size and fill the lateral ventricle. A third ventricular choroid plexus papilloma has been reported.
      2. Secondary ventriculomegaly of the involved side occurs with mild midline shift.
      3. Color flow studies will show flow with the mass, distinguishing it from an intraventricular bleed.
   d. Lipoma
      1. A brightly echogenic mass is present in the region of the anterior genu of the corpus callosum. Bilateral extension of the mass into the region of the lateral ventricle choroid plexus in the caudothalamic groove may occur (25%). Calcifications along the margin of the intrahemispheric lipoma are common but difficult to appreciate because the mass itself is so echogenic.
      2. Agenesis of the corpus callosum is a frequent association.
      3. Secondary lateral ventriculomegaly occurs.
2. **Amniotic Fluid:** Polyhydramnios usually occurs.
3. **Placenta:** Normal.
4. **Measurement Data:** Increased head size occurs in the third trimester. Remaining measurements are normal.
5. **When Detectable:** Tumors have been first detected in the third trimester.

Pitfalls

1. Intracranial hemorrhage can resemble a tumor when first seen. Color flow Doppler will show no flow in a hemorrhage and there will be a rapid change in appearance within a few days with a hemorrhage.
2. Masses adjacent to the near side of the skull may be difficult to see because of the skull reverberations. An endovaginal probe view in a vertex presentation can be very helpful.
3. MRI may be helpful in delineating lesions that are difficult to see because of the skull artifact on the near side of the brain.

Where Else to Look Consider the possibility that the mass represents neuroblastoma metastases and look in the adrenal region.

Pregnancy Management

Investigations and Consultations Required Consultation with the neurosurgeon and neonatologist is essential to provide the family full information regarding the grave prognosis for the neonate, and to develop a plan of management.

Fetal Intervention   None is indicated.

Monitoring   Fetal hydrops and polyhydramnios have been common complications of intracranial tumors. Serial ultrasonographic evaluations are useful to monitor for the development of these complications, as well as to assess fetal head size.

Pregnancy Course   The pregnancy may be complicated by polyhydramnios and resulting preterm labor.

Pregnancy Termination Issues   The excessive growth of the head may complicate both forms of pregnancy termination. An intact fetus is not necessary for confirmation of the diagnosis.

Delivery   The significant head size reported in these infants may require elective cesarean section, despite the grave prognosis. Attempts at cranial decompression are not likely to be successful. The decision to use a vertical or horizontal incision on the uterus will depend on the fetal lie and the status of the lower uterine segment.

Neonatology

Resuscitation   Because progressive cranial enlargement is the primary fetal manifestation of an intracranial tumor, operative delivery prior to full gestation may be indicated. Assistance with the onset of respiration will be determined by both the gestational age at delivery and the difficulties encountered intrapartum. The most common intracranial mass presenting in fetal life is a teratoma, which has an almost uniform perinatal mortality. Therefore, if prenatal diagnosis suggests that the mass is a teratoma, it is appropriate for the option of nonintervention to establish respiration following delivery to be presented to the parents.

Transport   Transfer to a tertiary center with pediatric and pediatric neurosurgical subspecialty capabilities is essential. If there is evidence of cardiorespiratory compromise, the transport should be conducted by experienced neonatal personnel.

Testing and Confirmation   Computed tomography and MRI are used to determine the location, degree of anatomical distortion, and presence of ventricular enlargement. On occasion, Doppler flow studies are useful to define the impact on cerebral vasculature. The definitive diagnosis requires tissue histopathologic examination from either tumor resection or biopsy.

Nursery Management   The management of a neonate with an intracranial tumor in general involves three issues beyond those that are relative to preterm delivery, if such has been required. These are as follows:

- hydrocephalus—if and when to place a shunt
- tumor removal—timing, approach, and feasibility of complete resection
- adjuvant therapy—chemotherapy or radiotherapy or both

The most common clinical presentation is increased cranial size with or without hydrocephalus. In addition, certain tumors, are frequently complicated by intraventricular hemorrhage, which can be severe. The approach chosen for a given infant depends directly on the specific tumor cell type, the size and location of the mass, and the general condition of the infant.

Surgery

Preoperative Assessment   Congenital tumors usually occur in the midline and may reach astonishing size. Tumors diagnosed antenatally are usually very aggressive and have a poor prognosis; therefore, a careful assessment to determine the extent of disease as well as a search for metastatic deposits in the spine or outside the CNS is necessary preoperatively. MRI and CT of the brain as well as a general oncology evaluation may be indicated depending on the particular tumor.

Operative Indications and Procedures   The decision to proceed with surgery depends on the preoperative assessment and the predicted histology. Neonates with large tumors that involve vital structures or that have replaced the majority of the developing brain are usually not surgical candidates because of their poor prognosis. Some tumors, such as lipomas or hamartomas of the brain, may not require surgical intervention unless symptomatic. Choroid plexus tumors in infants are extremely vascular, and surgery may be associated with significant morbidity and mortality from blood loss. Tumors that are highly vascular or of malignant histology may be treated with chemotherapy prior to attempted definitive resection.

Surgical Results/Prognosis   The prognosis of infants with antenatally diagnosed brain tumors is poor. There are case reports of long-term (i.e., 5-year) survival but no large series exist in the literature. The size and histologic type of the tumor and the neurologic status of the child at birth will ultimately determine prognosis.

REFERENCES

Anderson DR, Falcone S, Bruce JH, et al: Radiologic-pathologic correlation: Congenital choroid plexus papillomas. Am J Neuroradiol 1995;16:2072.

Broeke ED, Verdonk GW, Roumen FJ: Prenatal ultrasound diagnosis of an intracranial teratoma influencing management: Case report and review of the literature. Eur J Obstet Gynecol Reprod Biol 1992;45:210–214.

D'Addario V, Pinto V, Meo F, Resta M: The specificity of ultrasound in the detection of fetal intracranial tumors. J Perinat Med 1998;26:480–485.

Fort DW, Rushing EJ: Congenital central nervous system tumors. J Child Neurol 1997;12:157.

Haddad SF, Menezes AH, Bell WE, et al: Brain tumors occurring before 1 year of age: A retrospective review of 22 cases in an 11-year period. Neurosurgery 1991;29:8.

Mapstone TB, Warf BC: Intracranial tumor in infants: Characteristics, management, and outcome of a contemporary series. Neurosurgery 1991;28:343.

Pezzotta S, Locatelli D, Arico M: Brain tumors in infants: Preferred treatment options. Drugs 1992;44:368.

Sherer DM, Onyeije CL: Prenatal ultrasonographic diagnosis of fetal intracranial tumors: A review. Am J Perinatol 1998;15:319–328.

Sherer DM, Abramowicz JS, Eggers PC, et al: Prenatal ultrasonographic diagnosis of intracranial teratoma and massive craniomegaly with associated high output cardiac failures. Am J Obstet Gynecol 1993;168:97–99.

Tomita T, McLone DG, Flannery AM: Choroid plexus papillomas of neonates, infants and children. Pediatr Neurosci 1988;14:23.

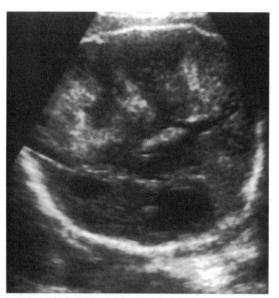

Axial view of large anterior mass with mixed echo texture. This was a glioblastoma multiforme.

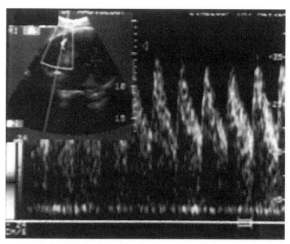

Doppler study showing flow within the mass, distinguishing it from a large bleed.

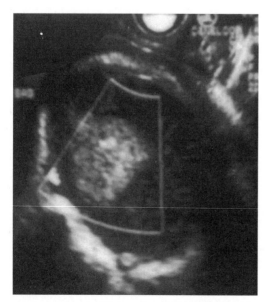

Echogenic mass within the left lateral ventricle. Color flow shows flow within the mass, which was a choroid plexus papilloma at surgery.

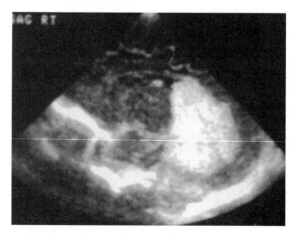

Neonatal head scan showing the choroid plexus papilloma lying in the left ventricle.

2.7 Craniosynostosis

Epidemiology/Genetics

Definition Abnormal development or premature closure of one or more of the cranial sutures resulting in an abnormal head shape. More than 150 syndromes with craniosynostosis have been described.

Epidemiology Isolated craniosynostosis is relatively common (3.4 in 1000 live births, M2:F1), but most craniosynostosis syndromes are rare (<1 in 50,000–100,000).

Embryology Abnormal head shape detectable antenatally and ranging from plagiocephaly caused by a single fused suture to a trilobar skull deformity referred to as a cloverleaf skull (kleeblattschädel) caused by multiple suture synostosis. There is often associated syndactyly of the hands and feet and/or other abnormalities. Currently, six syndromes are associated with abnormalities of fibroblast growth factor receptors (FGFRs) for which molecular testing is available. These include Crouzon, Jackson-Weiss, Apert, and Pfeiffer syndromes (FGFR2); Adelaide type, Crouzon with acanthosis nigricans (FGFR3); and Pfeiffer II (FGFR1). Thanatophoric dysplasia, type II (FGFR3) can have a cloverleaf skull but is distinguished by the severe short-limbed dwarfism.

Inheritance Patterns Most isolated cases of craniosynostosis have multifactorial or sporadic inheritance, although some families show autosomal dominant or autosomal recessive inheritance. Craniosynostosis as part of a syndrome is often autosomal dominant. The inheritance pattern depends on the specific syndrome diagnosis.

Teratogens Aminopterin, methotrexate, hydantoin, retinoic acid, valproic acid, and intra-uterine mechanical restraint can cause craniosynostosis.

Additional Investigations Ultrasonographic monitoring, looking for other birth defects, including shortened limbs, fused fingers or toes, and cleft lip or palate. DNA testing via amniocentesis or chorionic villus sampling is available for certain genetic conditions that feature craniosynostosis, and genetic consultation should be sought. Karyotype and aneuploid fluorescent in situ hybridization (FISH) should be considered to rule out any chromosome abnormalities.

Prognosis Prognosis for isolated craniosynostosis is usually very good with reconstructive surgery. Prognosis for individuals with a genetic syndrome featuring craniosynostosis varies from very good (Crouzon, Jackson-Weiss syndromes) to developmental delay and mental retardation (Apert and Pfeiffer syndromes) or lethality (thanatophoric dysplasia, type II).

Sonography

FINDINGS

1. **Fetus:**
   a. Crouzon syndrome
      1. Premature fusion of the coronal sutures leads to brachycephaly and elongated skull height. Severe cases have cloverleaf skull.
      2. Midface hypoplasia with hypertelorism and proptosis is typical.
      3. There may be micrognathia and maxillary hypoplasia.
   b. Apert syndrome
      1. Brachycephaly with short occipitofrontal diameter with cloverleaf deformity of the skull.
      2. The orbits are shallow and there is hypertelorism with a prominent forehead and recessed nose, giving a flat face.
      3. Ventriculomegaly may develop, and there is an association with agenesis of the corpus callosum.
      4. Fusion of cervical vertebrae may be present.
      5. A nuchal fold is present in the first trimester.
      6. "Mitten hands" related to osseous and/or cutaneous syndactyly of second, third, and fourth fingers are present.
   c. Pfeiffer syndrome
      1. Brachycephaly and acrocephaly related to fusion of the coronal and sometimes the sagittal sutures are present.
      2. There is a depressed nasal bridge and hypertelorism.
      3. The thumbs are broad, and there is syndactyly of hands and feet.
   d. Carpenter's syndrome
      1. Brachycephaly and acrocephaly due to fusion of coronal sagittal and/or lambdoid sutures.
      2. Depressed nasal bridge and micrognathia are facial features.
      3. Syndactyly, polydactyly, and clinodactyly are findings in hands and feet.
      4. Heart abnormalities such as septal defects, tetralogy, and transposition affect 50% of individuals.
2. **Amniotic Fluid:** Polyhydramnios is often present.
3. **Placenta:** Normal.

4. **Measurement Data:** The head size is small for gestational age.
5. **When Detectable:** Apert syndrome has been detected at 18 weeks, Crouzon syndrome at 21 weeks, and Pfeiffer syndrome at 35 weeks. Carpenter's syndrome has been diagnosed at 17 weeks.

Pitfalls   In milder cases, the changes are subtle even in the third trimester. 3-D ultrasound helps determine if sutures are fused.

Differential Diagnosis

1. Thanatophoric dwarfism—In type II, which is associated with cloverleaf skull, limbs are straight but significantly shortened, and the chest is narrow.
2. Ectrodactyly-ectodermal dysplasia clefting syndrome—Deformed split hands are present but the cranium is normal.

Where Else to Look

1. Cleft lip and palate may be seen with Crouzon syndrome.
2. All types may be associated with ventriculomegaly and vertebral abnormalities.
3. Heart defects such as tetralogy of Fallot and genitourinary abnormalities such as hydronephrosis and cryptorchidism may be seen with Apert syndrome.
4. Heart defects, omphalocele, and genital abnormalities occur in Carpenter's syndrome.

Pregnancy Management

Investigations and Consultations Required   Depending on the shape of the head, chromosome studies to exclude trisomy 18 may be indicated. Many of the craniosynostosis syndromes have been found to be based on mutations in FGFR2. For some, such as Apert syndrome, the limited number of responsible mutations may allow a precise molecular diagnosis. Collaboration between the sonologist and a pediatric dysmorphologist may be helpful in determining what molecular studies may be useful for a more definitive diagnosis.

Fetal Intervention   None is indicated.

Monitoring   Because of the association of ventriculomegaly with many of the disorders, serial ultrasonograms should be performed to monitor ventricular size.

Pregnancy Course   Polyhydramnios has been reported in a number of syndromes with craniosynostosis and may result in preterm labor.

Pregnancy Termination Issues   Unless a precise diagnosis has been established prenatally, an intact fetus should be delivered for complete pathologic evaluation.

Delivery   Abnormal head shape and/or significant enlargement of the head due to ventriculomegaly may prevent vaginal delivery.

Neonatology

Resuscitation   In general, respiratory depression at birth is not expected with isolated craniosynostosis, and therefore there is no contraindication to full resuscitation following delivery. If the premature suture closure is one manifestation of a rare syndrome or systemic disorder, the need for resuscitation is predicated on the specific disorder and its implications for long-term prognosis.

Transport   In the absence of systemic disease, immaturity, or other need for neonatal intensive care, transfer to a tertiary center is not indicated in the immediate neonatal period. Early referral to a center with pediatric neurosurgery and preferably with a multidisciplinary craniofacial reconstructive program is recommended.

Testing and Confirmation   Identification of a closed suture or sutures can be suspected from the physical findings of a non-mobile suture, a closed or firm feeling fontanelle, and/or an abnormal cranial shape. CT scanning with bone windows is the recommended imaging technique for confirming suture closure. A careful physical examination will reveal concomitant abnormalities, suggesting a syndromal or metabolic cause, the incidence of which is related to the specific sutural involvement. Additional diagnostic testing and imaging will be dictated by the concomitant abnormalities.

Nursery Management   Beyond careful assessment to exclude multiple congenital anomaly syndromes, no special care requirements are indicated in the immediate newborn period. The decision for surgical correction and the appropriate timing are influenced by the anatomic involvement (single or multiple suture), the apparent pathophysiology and associated anomalies (isolated or syndrome associated), and the presence of increased intracranial pressure.

Surgery

Preoperative Assessment   Some mild forms of single suture craniosynostosis may not be readily appreciated at birth but become more apparent as the cranium grows and a more unusual cranial configuration becomes evident. Ridging along the involved suture often will accompany this process. Early obliteration of the anterior and posterior fontanelles can also occur with this process and signal possible increased intracranial pressure.

In cases of multiple suture craniosynostosis and syndromic forms of craniosynostosis, the physical and neurologic problems are often evident. Many of these will involve the coronal sutures and the cranial base. Frontal bone bossing may also be seen in conjunction with an abnormal cranial configuration.

Operative Indications   The association of craniosynostosis with other functional problems dictates the indications for surgical intervention. Evidence of "thumbprinting" on plain films of the calvarium is one indirect way of assessing the possibility of disparity between intracranial volume and brain volume, resulting in an increase in intracranial pressure. Studies have shown that increased intracranial pressure is found in 42% of cases of multiple craniosynostosis and in 13% of single suture craniosynostosis.

Hydrocephalus is found in many cases, but the true incidence is unknown. The communicating and noncommunicating forms are observed, with the communicating being more common. The incidence is lowest in scaphocephaly and unilateral and bilateral coronal synostosis. It is highest in multiple suture synostosis, especially the kleeblattschädel deformity, in which there is evidence of obstruction of cerebrospinal fluid flow at the level of the fourth ventricle.

The incidence of mental retardation in craniosynostosis syndromes is difficult to quantify. The risk is higher than in the general population and is attributed to increased intracranial pressure (unrelieved) with cerebral atrophy, hydrocephalus, associated intracranial anomalies, meningitis, prematurity, or a family history of mental retardation. The incidence is lowest in patients with involvement of a single suture, except in metopic synostosis, in which it is observed more frequently. The incidence is highest in Apert syndrome and in the kleeblattschädel deformity.

Types of Procedures Surgical intervention is employed either early (within the first year of life) or late (after 1 year of life), with the trend in recent years toward earlier intervention. This will often correct the potential neurologic problems and mental retardation as well as spare the psychological and social trauma associated with craniofacial disfigurement.

The goals of the surgery for the newborn with craniosynostosis are to (1) decompress the intracranial space (to reduce the intracranial pressure, to prevent visual problems and promote normal mental development), and (2) achieve satisfactory craniofacial form, growth, and aesthetics. The simplest procedures at the earliest times of intervention involve strip craniectomies. These work best on isolated sagittal synostosis with either a sagittal or a parasagittal strip craniectomy. Unilateral or bilateral coronal craniosynostosis is best corrected by a strip craniectomy combined with frontal bone advancement and/or recontouring.

Surgical Results/Prognosis Surgical results are good and usually restore normal craniofacial aesthetics and reduce any possibility of neurologic sequelae. With single suture craniosynostosis, only one operation is usually required, whereas multiple synostosis syndromes will require multiple procedures. Complications from surgery are generally low, in the range of 4 to 5%, and the mortality rate is less than 1%.

REFERENCES

Anderson FM: Treatment of coronal and metopic synostosis: 107 cases. Neurosurgery 1981;8:143.

Boop FA, Chadduck WM, Shewmake K, Teo C: Outcome analysis of 85 patients undergoing the pi procedure for correction of sagittal synostosis. J Neurosurg 1996;85:50.

Carson B, Dufresne C: Craniosynostosis and neurocranial asymmetry. In Dufresne C, Carson B, Zinreich J (eds): Complex Craniofacial Problems. New York, Churchill Livingstone, 1992, p 167.

Chenoweth-Mitchell C, Cohen G: Prenatal sonographic finding of Apert syndrome. J Clin Ultrasound 1994;22:510.

Chumas PD, Cinalli G, Arnaud E, et al: Classification of previously unclassified cases of craniosynostosis. J Neurosurg 1997;86:177.

Cohen M: Craniosynostosis: Diagnosis, Evaluation and Management. New York, Raven Press, 1986.

Cohen MM: Craniosynostoses: Phenotypic/molecular correlations. Am J Med Genet 1995;56:334.

Cohen SR, Persing JA: Intracranial pressure in single-suture craniosynostosis. Cleft Palate Craniofac J 1998;35:194.

Dufresne C, Jelks G: Classification of craniofacial anomalies. In Smith B (ed): Ophthalmic Plastic and Reconstructive Surgery. Philadelphia, Mosby-Year Book, 1987, p 1185.

Ferreira JC, Carter SM, Bernstein PS, et al: Second trimester molecular prenatal diagnosis of sporadic Apert syndrome following suspicious ultrasound findings. Ultrasound Obstet Gynecol 1999;14:426.

Hollway GE, Suthers GK, Haan EA, et al: Mutation detection in FGFR2 craniosynostosis syndromes. Hum Genet 1997;99:251.

Huang MHS, Mouradian WE, Cohen SR, Gruss JS: The differential diagnosis of abnormal head shapes: Separating craniosynostosis from positional deformities and normal variants. Cleft Palate Craniofac J 1998;35:204.

Jabs EW: Toward understanding the pathogenesis of craniosynostosis through clinical and molecular correlates. Clin Genet 1998;53:79.

Kapp-Simon KA: Mental development and learning disorders in children with single suture craniosynostosis. Cleft Palate Craniofac J 1998;35:197.

Krakow D, Santulli T, Platt LD: Use of three-dimensional ultrasonography in differentiating craniosynostosis from severe fetal molding. J Ultrasound Med 2001;20:427–431.

Lajeunie E, LeMerrer M, Bonaiti-Pellie M, Marchac D: Genetic study of nonsyndromic coronal craniosynostosis. Am J Med Genet 1995;55:500.

Lajeunie E, LeMerrer M, Marchac D, Renier D: Syndromal and nonsyndromal primary trigonocephaly: Analysis of a series of 237 patients. Am J Med Genet 1998;75:211.

Liptak GS, Serletti JM: Pediatric approach to craniosynostosis. Pediatr Rev 1998;19:352.

Menashe Y, Baruch GB, Rabinovitch O, et al: Exophthalmus-prenatal ultrasonic features of Crouzon syndrome. Prenat Diagn 1989;9:805.

Munro IR: Reshaping the cranial vault. In Converse JM (ed): Reconstructive Plastic Surgery, vol 4. Philadelphia, WB Saunders, 1977.

Panchal J, Marsh JL, Park TS, et al: Sagittal craniosynostosis outcome: Assessment for two methods and timings of intervention. Plast Reconstruct Surg 1999;103:1574.

Virtanen R, Korhonen T, Fagerholm J, Viljanto J: Neurocognitive sequelae of scaphocephaly. Pediatrics 1999;103:791.

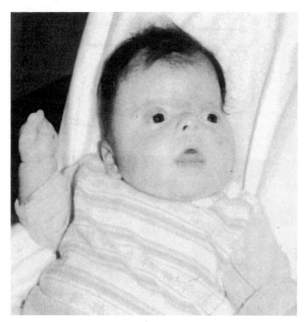

Facial appearance of an infant with Apert syndrome.

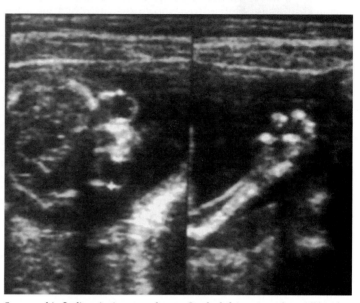

Sonographic findings in Apert syndrome. On the left is a view of a small brachycephalic cranium and exophthalmic orbits and on the right syndactyly in the fingers forming a "mitten hand" in an 18-week fetus.

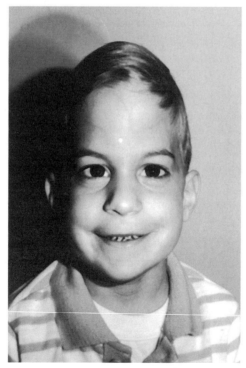

Two-year-old child with sagittal craniosynostosis. Note narrow elongated head at presentation.

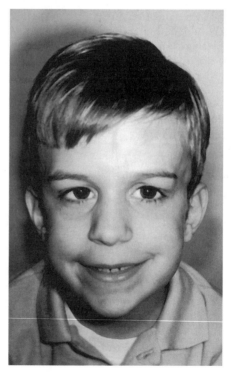

Same child 2 years after surgery.

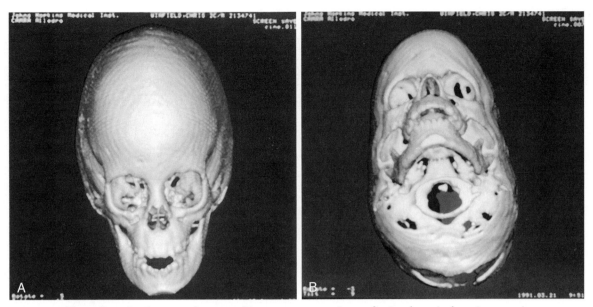

Three-dimensional computed tomographic scans at presentation confirming the sagittal craniosynostosis.

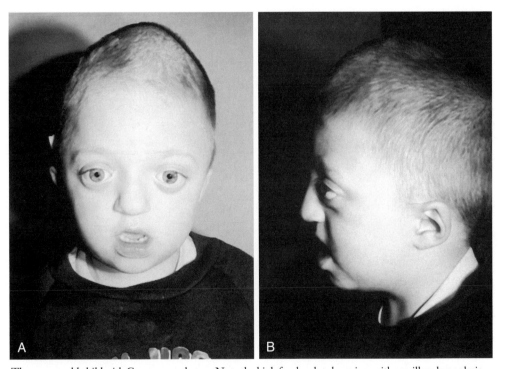

Three-year-old child with Crouzon syndrome. Note the high forehead and cranium with maxillary hypoplasia, class II maxillary malocclusion, and exorbitism.

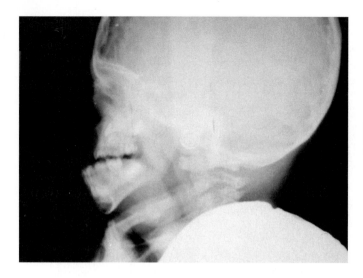

Lateral cephalometric radiograph of the same case. Note the "copper beaten" appearance of the anterior cranium secondary to increased intracranial pressure.

2.8 Dandy-Walker Malformations

Epidemiology/Genetics

Definition Dandy-Walker malformations are characterized by (1) a posterior fossa cyst, (2) a defect in the cerebellar vermis that provides a communication between the cyst and the fourth ventricle, and (3) variable hydrocephalus.

Epidemiology One in 25,000 to 35,000. Occurs in approximately 4% of cases of hydrocephalus.

Embryology The Dandy-Walker malformation is an abnormality in the development of the central nervous system that probably occurs before the sixth to seventh week of gestation. Associated intracranial abnormalities occur in about 50% of cases and associated extracranial abnormalities in 35% of cases. Common associated defects are agenesis of the corpus callosum, ventricular septal defect, and facial clefts. Chromosomal abnormalities are seen in approximately 15 to 30% of cases including trisomies 13, 18, and 21.

Inheritance Patterns Rare familial recurrence of isolated Dandy-Walker malformation has been seen with possible autosomal or X-linked recessive inheritance. The Dandy-Walker malformation can be a feature of mendelian genetic syndromes, including the Meckel-Gruber syndrome (autosomal recessive), Walker-Warburg syndrome (autosomal recessive), and the Aicardi syndrome (X-linked dominant with male lethality). Because of the rapid progress in mapping of genes and the subsequent development of genetic testing, consultation with a medical geneticist or genetic counselor to determine the availability of clinical genetic testing for this disorder or disorders is advised.

Teratogens Congenital infections.

Prognosis Postnatal mortality is approximately 35% and is dependent on the associated abnormalities. Twenty to 30% of survivors, with isolated abnormalities, have IQs above 80. Shunting is usually required for associated hydrocephalus.

Sonography

FINDINGS

1. **Fetus:**
   a. A Dandy-Walker cyst is seen as a fluid collection separating the lobes of the cerebellum. It represents an intracerebellar cyst connected to the fourth ventricle. Visualization is enhanced by using an exaggerated cerebellar view.
   b. The vermis of the cerebellum is variably hypoplastic and may be difficult to see with large Dandy-Walker cysts. The remainder of the cerebellum may also be partially or completely absent.
   c. With larger cysts, there is secondary dilation of the third and lateral ventricles and the tentorium is elevated.
2. **Amniotic Fluid:** Normal, unless the Dandy-Walker cyst is secondary to a chromosomal abnormality when oligohydramnios or polyhydramnios may occur.
3. **Placenta:** Normal.
4. **Measurement Data:** Biparietal diameter and head circumference are usually increased in size. There can be intrauterine growth retardation (IUGR) if associated syndromes are present.
5. **When Detectable:** The syndrome has been detected as early as 13 weeks by endovaginal probe use, but extreme caution must be used in making this diagnosis early because development of the vermis is not completed until 17 to 18 weeks of gestation.

Pitfalls

1. An enlarged cisterna magna of greater than 1 cm diameter, but with a normally formed cerebellum, is called a Dandy-Walker variant by some practitioners, although it does not carry the same generally gloomy prognosis.
2. A small cyst inferior to the cerebellum is frequently seen. This is an unimportant normal variant if small.
3. Isolated enlargement of the fourth ventricle at 14 to 16 weeks in the absence of vermian changes may be a normal variant.

Differential Diagnosis

1. When an infracerebellar arachnoid cyst becomes very large, it is known as an extra-axial cyst. Such cysts can be distinguished from Dandy-Walker cysts by the size and appearance of the cerebellum. Although compressed, a normal cerebellum is still present.
2. Enlarged cisterna magna. The cerebellum has a normal appearance.
3. If the posterior fossa is difficult to examine, the secondary findings of bilateral lateral and third ventricular dilation may be confused with aqueduct stenosis.

Where Else to Look

1. Up to 50% of cases have associated central nervous system abnormalities. Agenesis of the corpus callosum is commonly associated and markedly worsens the prognosis. The corpus callosum is best seen on midline sagittal views, but such views are difficult to obtain in utero. Transverse coronal views or endovaginal views may be helpful (see Chapter 2.1).

2. Look for stigmata of trisomy 18 and 13, which are associated with Dandy-Walker cysts in about 15 to 30% of cases.
3. Encephaloceles (including Meckel-Gruber and Walker-Warburg) often have Dandy-Walker cysts in addition.
4. Neural tube defects are associated with Dandy-Walker cysts.
5. Holoprosencephaly is associated with Dandy-Walker syndrome.
6. Joubert syndrome has the following sonographic characteristics: a Dandy-Walker–like appearance to the cerebellum and fourth ventricle with, in addition, micrognathia, multicystic kidneys, and polydactyly. It has a universally poor prognosis; either retardation or fetal death occurs.

Pregnancy Management

Investigations and Consultations Required   Chromosome studies should be performed at any gestational age at which the initial diagnosis is made. The high association with trisomy 18 and the dismal prognosis of this chromosome abnormality would preclude any aggressive obstetric management. Fetal echocardiography should be performed to detect the commonly associated cardiac lesions. A pediatric neurosurgeon should be consulted to discuss prenatal and neonatal management.

Fetal Intervention   Despite the reports of "successful" in utero placement of shunts for the Dandy-Walker malformation, fetal intervention is contraindicated because of the poor prognosis and high incidence of associated abnormalities in this disorder.

Monitoring   Serial ultrasonographic examinations should be performed every 3 to 4 weeks to assess for the presence and degree of ventriculomegaly.

Pregnancy Course   Many of the syndromes of which the Dandy-Walker malformation is a component may be associated with intrauterine growth retardation, and decisions regarding management of this complication will be highly dependent on the prognosis of the underlying condition.

Pregnancy Termination Issues   As with other CNS malformations, special expertise in neuropathology is essential for a precise diagnosis and the resultant counseling that will be necessary following this diagnosis.

Delivery   Early delivery after 32 weeks may be considered when there is progressive and severe ventriculomegaly. However, this approach is controversial because of the inherent poor prognosis for normal neurologic development in the infant with Dandy-Walker malformation.

Neonatology

Resuscitation   The major issues relate to (1) fetal distress secondary to dystocia from macrocephaly, and (2) prematurity, if early delivery is chosen because of rapidly advancing hydrocephalus. Given the very poor prognosis, if there are associated CNS and/or other organ system anomalies, a prenatal discussion with the family regarding intervention to initiate respiration is appropriate. No special techniques are required.

Transport   Referral to a tertiary center with pediatric neurosurgery capabilities is indicated.

Testing and Confirmation   The priority issue is the identification of associated CNS abnormalities by cranial CT and MRI. In the majority of infants, hydrocephalus develops by 2 months of age if not present prenatally.

If karyotyping was not performed on the fetus, it should be obtained after birth before invasive interventions are undertaken, especially if there are other dysmorphic features.

Nursery Management   Hemorrhage into the cyst can occur at any point and should be suspected with an abrupt clinical deterioration.

Surgery

Preoperative Assessment   Magnetic resonance imaging will differentiate a Dandy-Walker malformation from a mega cisterna magna or an arachnoid cyst of the foramen magnum and also rule out the presence of other associated intracranial anomalies.

Operative Indications   The Dandy-Walker malformation without hydrocephalus does not necessarily require treatment in asymptomatic infants. In infants who have hydrocephalus or who are symptomatic (i.e., poor feeding, recurrent aspiration, hoarse or weak cry, or a poor suck), the treatment is initially directed at the Dandy-Walker malformation. Subsequent treatment of the hydrocephalus is occasionally necessary.

Types of Procedures   Treatment of Dandy-Walker malformation in the absence of hydrocephalus usually involves shunting the cyst to the peritoneal cavity. In the presence of hydrocephalus, controversy exists about the management. Some practitioners advocate simultaneously shunting the ventricular system and the Dandy-Walker cyst, whereas others advocate shunting the Dandy-Walker cyst only, with the hope that the hydrocephalus will resolve once the posterior fossa cyst is decompressed. Should the child remain symptomatic or the ventricular size remain enlarged, ventriculoperitoneal shunting is performed.

Surgical Results/Prognosis   Outcome in children with Dandy-Walker malformation in isolation is reasonably good. These children can have normal cognitive development, although the risk of shunt malfunction and the need for revision is significantly greater with the presence of dual shunt systems (i.e., cyst and ventricular). The Dandy-Walker malformation with the presence of associated anomalies generally has a poor prognosis, with less than 25% of children demonstrating a normal IQ.

REFERENCES

Aletebi FA, Fung KF: Neurodevelopmental outcome after antenatal diagnosis of posterior fossa abnormalities. J Ultrasound Med 1999;18:683–689.

Bernard JP, Moscoso G, Renjar D, et al: Cystic malformations of the posterior fossa. Prenat Diagn 2001;21:1064–1069.

Bronshtein M, Zimmer EZ, Blazer S: Isolated large fourth ventricle in early pregnancy: A possible benign transient phenomenon. Prenat Diagn 1998;18:997–1000.

Cornford E, Twining P: The Dandy Walker syndrome: The value of antenatal diagnosis. Clin Radiol 1992;45:172–174.

Cowles T, Gurman P, Wilkins I: Prenatal diagnosis of Dandy-Walker malformation in a family displaying X-linked inheritance. Prenat Diagn 1993;13:87–91.

Ecker JL, Shipp TD, Bromley B, Benacerraf B: The sonographic diagnosis of Dandy-Walker and Dandy-Walker variant: Associated findings and outcome. Prenat Diagn 2000;20:328–332.

Estroff JA, Scott MR, Benacerraf BR: Dandy Walker variant: Prenatal sonographic features and clinical outcome. Radiology 1992;185:755–758.

Hart MN, Malamud N, Ellis WG: The Dandy Walker syndrome: A clinicopathological study based on 28 cases. Neurology 1972;22:771–780.

Hill LM, Martin JG, Fries J, Hixson J: The role of the transcerebellar view in the detection of fetal central nervous system anomaly. Am J Obstet Gynecol 1991;164:1220–1224.

Hirsch JF, Pierre-Kahn A, Renier D, et al: The Dandy Walker malformation: A review of 40 cases. J Neurosurg 1984;61:515–522.

Hudgins R, Edwards MSB: Management of hydrocephalus detected in utero. In Scott M (ed): Concepts of Neurosurgery: Hydrocephalus. Baltimore, Williams & Wilkins, 1990, pp 99–108.

Kolble N, Wisser J, Kurmanavicius J, et al: Dandy-Walker malformation: Prenatal diagnosis and outcome. Prenat Diagn 2000;20:318–327.

Kollias SS, Ball WS Jr, Prenger EC: Cystic malformations of the posterior fossa: Differential diagnosis clarified through embryologic analysis. Radiographics 1993;13:1211–1231.

McCullough DC, Balzer-Martin LA: Current prognosis in overt neonatal hydrocephalus. J Neurosurg 1982;57:378–383.

Murray JC, Johnson JA, Bird TD: Dandy Walker malformation: Etiologic heterogeneity and empiric recurrence risks. Clin Genet 1985;28:272–283.

NiScanaill S, Crowley P, Hogan M, Stuart B: Abnormal prenatal sonographic findings in the posterior cranial fossa: A case of Joubert's syndrome. Ultrasound Obstet Gynecol 1999;13:71–74.

Nyberg DA: The Dandy Walker malformation: Prenatal sonographic diagnosis and its clinical significance. J Ultrasound Med 1988;7:65–72.

Nyberg DA, Cyr DR, Mack LA, et al: The Dandy Walker malformation: Prenatal sonographic diagnosis and its clinical significance. J Ultrasound Med 1988;7:65–71.

Nyberg DA, Mahony BA, Hegge FN, et al: Enlarged cisterna magna and the Dandy Walker malformation: Factors associated with chromosome abnormalities. Obstet Gynecol 1991;77:436–442.

Nyberg DA, Pretorius DH: Cerebral malformations. In Nyberg DA, Mahony BS, Pretorius DH (eds): Diagnostic Ultrasound of Fetal Anomalies. Chicago, Yearbook, 1990, pp 83–145.

Obwegeser R, Deutinger J, Bernaschek G: Recurrent Dandy-Walker malformation. Arch Gynecol Obstet 1994;255:161–163.

Pilu G, Goldstein I, Reece EA, et al: Sonography of fetal Dandy Walker malformation: A reappraisal. Ultrasound Obstet Gynecol 1992;2:151–157.

Pilu G, Visantin A, Valeri B: The Dandy Walker complex and fetal sonography. Ultrasound Obstet Gynecol 2000;16:115–117.

Raman S, Rachagan SP, Lim CT: Prenatal diagnosis of a posterior fossa cyst. J Clin Ultrasound 1991;19:434–437.

Rekate H: Treatment of hydrocephalus. In Cheek W (ed): Pediatric Neurosurgery, 3rd ed. Philadelphia, WB Saunders, 1994, pp 202–220.

Russ PD, Pretorius DH, Johnson MJ: Dandy Walker syndrome: A review of fifteen cases evaluated by prenatal sonography. Am J Obstet Gynecol 1989;161:401–406.

Tal Y, Freigang B, Dunn HG, et al: Dandy Walker syndrome: Analysis of 21 cases. Dev Med Child Neurol 1980;22:189–201.

Ulm B, Ulm MR, Deutinger J, Bernaschek G: Isolated Dandy-Walker malformation: Prenatal diagnosis in two consecutive pregnancies. Am J Perinatol 1999;16:61–63.

Ulm B, Ulm MR, Deutinger J, Bernaschek G: Dandy-Walker malformation diagnosed before 21 weeks of gestation: Associated malformations and chromosomal abnormalities. Ultrasound Obstet Gynecol 1997;10:167–170.

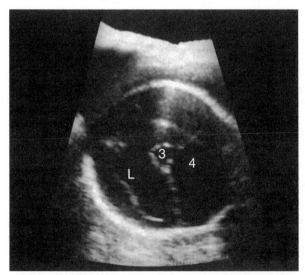

Dandy-Walker cyst. The axial view shows a large cystic structure below the tentorium (4). No cerebellar tissue remains. The lateral ventricle (L) and the third ventricles (3) are secondarily dilated.

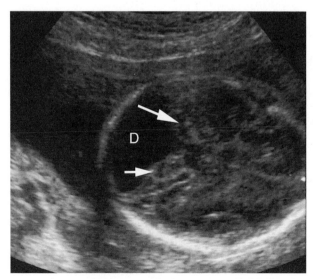

A more mild example shows a small dysplastic cerebellar configuration (*arrows*) adjacent to the Dandy-Walker cyst (D).

2.9 Diastematomyelia

Epidemiology/Genetics

Definition An abnormality of the spinal canal in which the dura is separated by a bony spike or fibrous band, leading to a splitting of a portion of the spinal cord, which rejoins below the abnormality.

Epidemiology Rare (M1:F2.4).

Embryology Although diastematomyelia is a defect in neural tube closure, the exact pathogenesis is unknown. Most cases have associated vertebral column abnormalities such as spina bifida (>50%), kyphoscoliosis, butterfly vertebrae, and hemivertebrae.

Inheritance Patterns Essentially all cases are sporadic. Two families with affected siblings suggest possible autosomal recessive inheritance in rare cases.

Teratogens None described.

Differential Diagnosis Other spinal dysraphia.

Prognosis Isolated diastematomyelia generally has an excellent prognosis with surgical repair, although untreated cases can have progressive signs of spinal cord tethering. Cases with associated spina bifida or other neural tube abnormalities have a prognosis more dependent on the severity of the associated abnormality.

Sonography

FINDINGS

1. **Fetus:**
   a. A bony or cartilaginous spur causing an echogenic focus splits the spinal cord, filum terminale, or conus medullaris. The spur is usually located at the level of the lumbar vertebra but can be at a higher or lower level. The spinal cord is tethered by the bony or cartilaginous spur.
   b. There is localized widening of posterior ossification centers at the level of the spur.
   c. Butterfly, fused, or hemivertebrae are usually present below the level of the spur, sometimes causing kyphoscoliosis.
   d. In a minority of cases, there is an associated myelomeningocele with secondary cranial changes of banana-shaped cerebellum and lemon-shaped skull.
2. **Amniotic Fluid:** Normal.
3. **Placenta:** Normal.
4. **Measurement Data:** Normal unless there is an associated myelomeningocele, in which case the cranium will be small unless hydrocephalus has developed.
5. **When Detectable:** Reported cases have been detected in the second trimester from 17 weeks on, but the echogenic focus should be detectable with the endovaginal probe at 13 weeks.

Pitfalls Marked distortion of the vertebrae in the region of the bony spur may make recognition of the process difficult.

Where Else to Look

1. Look at the skull for secondary Arnold-Chiari type 2 findings.
2. If there is an associated myelomeningocele, clubfeet may be present.

Pregnancy

Investigations and Consultations Required No further evaluations are necessary.

Fetal Intervention None is indicated.

Monitoring No change in normal obstetric management should be necessary.

Pregnancy Course No obstetric complications should be associated with this condition.

Pregnancy Termination Issues An intact fetus is necessary to confirm this diagnosis; therefore, induction of labor is indicated.

Delivery Given the uncertain prognosis for these infants, delivery in a tertiary center is prudent.

Neonatology

Resuscitation In the absence of an accompanying neural tube defect, there are no special concerns for assisting cardiorespiratory adaptation. With a neural tube defect, the management both pre- and post-natally is determined by the specific features of the defect.

Transport In the absence of an accompanying neural tube defect, transfer to a tertiary center in the immediate neonatal period is not indicated. Referral to a pediatric neurologist or a multidisciplinary team for outpatient evaluation and follow-up early in infancy is recommended.

Testing and Confirmation Diagnostic imaging—CT and MRI—is the best means of identifying and characterizing the disrupted anatomy.

Nursery Management Beyond the diagnostic assessment initially, no special management in the immediate neonatal period is required in the absence of an accompanying neural tube defect.

Surgical Management

Preoperative Assessment Diastematomyelia represents a spectrum of anomalies in which the spinal cord is split into two "hemicords." This anomaly has been termed the split cord malformation (SCM) and subdivided into two types. The type I SCM consists of two hemicords, each contained within separate dural tubes and divided by an osseous or cartilaginous septum. The type II SCM consists of the two hemicords, within a single dural sac, and the cords are separated by a membranous nonrigid septum. Magnetic resonance imaging, plain radiographs, and CT are all usually necessary preoperatively to define the type of lesion, level of the anomaly, position of the conus medullaris, and whether the two hemicords rejoin or remain separate.

Operative Indications Surgical management is necessary to prevent progressive loss of neurologic function and is usually performed electively within the first year of life. Management of the type II SCM is controversial, with some practitioners recommending observation only for patients with the conus at a normal level and normal findings on the neurologic examination.

Types of Procedures The nature of the surgical procedure depends on the anatomy of the specific anomaly.

In general, the septum (bone, cartilage, or fibrous) separating the hemicords must be resected as well as any dural investiture. The filum terminale must also be sectioned whenever the conus is low.

Surgical Results/Prognosis Surgical intervention is effective in preventing progressive neurologic deterioration and occasionally progressive scoliosis. Ultimate functional outcome is therefore dependent on early diagnosis and intervention before the appearance of significant neurologic dysfunction. The relative rarity of this anomaly necessitates referral of these children to an experienced surgeon for management.

REFERENCES

Allen LM, Silverman RK: Prenatal ultrasound evaluation of fetal diastematomyelia: Two cases of type 1 split cord malformation. Ultrasound Obstet Gynecol 2000;15:78–82.

Anderson NG, Jordan S, MacFarlane MR, Lovell-Smith M: Diastematomyelia: Diagnosis by prenatal ultrasound. Am J Roentgenol 1994; 163:911–914.

Caspi B, Gorbacz S, Appelman Z, Elchalal U: Antenatal diagnosis of diastematomyelia. J Clin Ultrasound 1990;18:721.

Harwood-Nash DC, McHugh K: Diastematomyelia in 172 children: The impact of modern neuroradiology. Pediatr Neurosurg 1991;16:247.

Miller A, Guille JT, Bowen JR: Evaluation and treatment of diastematomyelia. J Bone Joint Surg Am 1993;75:1308–1317.

Pachi A, Maggi E, Giancotti A, et al: Prenatal sonographic diagnosis of diastematomyelia in a diabetic woman. Prenatal Diagn 1992;12:535–539.

Pang D, Dias MS, Ahab-Barmada M: Split cord malformation: Part I. A unified theory of embryogenesis for double spinal cord malformations. Neurosurgery 1992;31:451.

Pang D: Split cord malformation: Part II. Clinical syndrome. Neurosurgery 1992;31:481–500.

Sepulveda W, Kyle PM, Hassan J, Weiner E: Prenatal diagnosis of diastematomyelia: Case reports and review of the literature. Prenat Diagn 1997;17:161–165.

Winter RK, McKnight R, Byrne RA, Wright CH: Diastematomyelia: Prenatal ultrasonic appearances. Clin Radiol 1989;40:291–294.

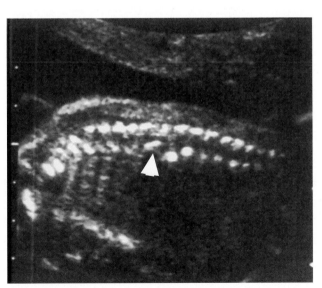

Coronal view of lumbosacral spine showing bony spur (*arrow*) due to diastematomyelia.

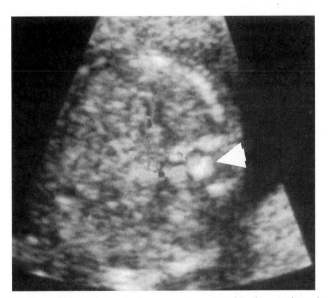

Transverse view showing the bony spur (*arrow*) within the spinal canal anterior to the vertebral ossification center.

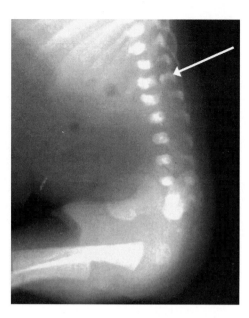

Radiographic view of the lower back showing bony spur (*arrow*) related to diastematomyelia.

2.10 Encephalocele

Epidemiology/Genetics

Definition   Encephaloceles are skin-covered neural tube defects affecting the cranium that result in a midline mass overlying a skull defect.

Epidemiology   One in 2000 live births (M1:F1). Varies with ethnic group and geographic region.

Embryology   Encephaloceles are the result of failure of neural tube closure in the cranial region during the first month of fetal development. They are frequently associated with other brain malformations, hydrocephalus, iniencephaly, facial clefts, cardiac abnormalities, and genital malformations. More than 30 genetic, sporadic, and chromosomal syndromes have been described with encephaloceles, including trisomy 13, amniotic band disruption syndrome, Meckel-Gruber syndrome (autosomal recessive disorder with encephalocele, polycystic kidneys, and polydactyly), and the Roberts pseudothalidomide syndrome (autosomal recessive). Because of the rapid progress in mapping of genes and subsequent development of genetic testing, consultation with a medical geneticist or genetic counselor to determine the availability of clinical genetic testing for this disorder or disorders is advised.

Inheritance Patterns   Often sporadic with multifactorial recurrence risks (2–5%). Otherwise related to specific syndrome diagnosis.

Teratogens   Cocaine, rubella, and maternal hyperthermia.

Prognosis   Dependent on the associated brain malformations and syndrome diagnosis. Large size is not important prognostically, as large encephaloceles may not contain neural elements. Microcephaly with the presence of neural elements in the encephalocele is associated with a poor prognosis.

Sonography

FINDINGS

1. **Fetus:**
   a. A paracranial mass is present. In 75% the mass is occipital, in 12% the mass is frontal, and in 13% it is parietal. The mass may be (1) fluid filled, (2) entirely brain filled, or (3) filled with both fluid and brain. If much or most of the brain is in the encephalocele, microcephaly occurs. A "cyst within a cyst" appearance indicates that the apparent cranial meningocele contains brain enclosing a prolapsed fourth ventricle.
   b. There is often hydrocephalus, which becomes more likely if much brain is in the encephalocele.
   c. It is important to decide how much and what area of brain tissue lies in the encephalocele, since both affect the prognosis. Often the brain substance within the mass is the cerebellum, since most encephaloceles are occipital.
   d. In a relatively rare subgroup, mainly those with encephalocele in a parietal location, the encephalocele is caused by the amniotic band syndrome. Amniotic bands may be visible attached to the encephalocele.
   e. The skull may assume the lemon shape normally thought to be characteristic of myelomeningocele.
2. **Amniotic Fluid:** Polyhydramnios may be present.
3. **Placenta:** Normal.
4. **Measurement Data:** The head size is usually small despite ventriculomegaly.
5. **When Detectable:** Usually detectable at 12 to 13 weeks using the vaginal probe.

Pitfalls

1. Occipital masses are especially likely to be overlooked, and the condition is thought to be hydrocephalus only.
2. Small amounts of brain in an apparently fluid-filled encephalocele may be overlooked.
3. The fetal ear has been mistaken for an encephalocele.

Differential Diagnosis

1. Nuchal edema—The skull will be intact.
2. Cystic hygroma—Bilateral posterolateral cysts with intact skull.
3. Dandy-Walker cyst—The skull will be intact.
4. Cephalohematoma—The skull will be intact and the brain normal. Cephalohematomas only occur in labor.
5. Frontal encephaloceles may be mistaken for facial teratoma (epignathus).
6. Cranial hemangioma—The skull is intact and the mass solid. Color flow power Doppler may show flow within the mass.
7. Fetal scalp cyst—The skull will be intact.

Where Else to Look

1. Look for Meckel-Gruber syndrome: (a) Large echogenic kidneys with visible cysts, (b) polydactyly, and (c) encephalocele attached by a thin neck. Less common findings are (a) congenital heart disease, (b) cleft lip and palate, (c) microcephaly, and (d) liver cysts. (See Chapter 11.4.)
2. Look for Walker-Warburg syndrome: (a) encephalocele, (b) ocular malformations, (c) Dandy-Walker malformations, and (d) ventriculomegaly.

3. Look for other findings of amniotic band syndrome, e.g., gastroschisis and absent limbs.
4. Agenesis of the corpus callosum is common with encephalocele and worsens the prognosis. (See Chapter 7.1.)
5. Dandy-Walker syndrome may occur with encephalocele, especially in Joubert syndrome. Other features of Joubert syndrome are polycystic kidneys and polydactyly. (See Chapter 2.8.)
6. Cervical rachischisis and cerebellar hypoplasia can be associated with encephalocele.

Pregnancy Management

Investigations and Consultations Required   In addition to the sonographic search for associated abnormalities, chromosome studies should be performed. Trisomy 13 is a cause for a few encephaloceles (1–5%). Fetal echocardiography should be done to exclude cardiac malformations, which are a common feature of many of the syndromes with encephalocele. The family should also be referred to a pediatric neurosurgeon for discussion regarding prognosis and neonatal management.

Fetal Intervention   No in utero therapy is indicated. Decompression of the encephalocele under ultrasonographic control prior to delivery may be required.

Monitoring   To assess the development and/or progression of ventriculomegaly and/or hydrocephalus, serial ultrasonographic examinations should be done monthly. Management of IUGR should be based on the overall prognosis of the primary condition. In the absence of an apparent syndrome to explain growth retardation, standard obstetric protocols are appropriate.

Pregnancy Course   Many of the syndromes, of which encephalocele is a feature, may also have prenatal growth deficiency as a component. Management should be based on the prognosis for the underlying condition, not the presence of IUGR.

Pregnancy Termination Issues   Because of the large number of syndromes that may have encephalocele as a component, and the wide range of inheritance patterns seen in these conditions, termination should be done by a nondestructive technique in an institution with special expertise in fetal pathology.

Delivery   Delivery management depends on the size of the defect, the amount of herniated brain, and associated abnormalities. Nonaggressive management is recommended when severe microcephaly is present. In cases with normal head size, caesarean section might improve prognosis by avoiding trauma to the herniated brain tissue.

Neonatology

Resuscitation   Most cases do not require assistance with the onset of respiration, unless the mass is very large and contains mostly brain tissue. Intubation may be difficult, with large posterior masses impeding proper positioning for visualization of the cords. Bag and mask-assisted ventilation with the infant in a side-lying position is often sufficient.

When prenatal diagnostic evaluations confirm associated intracranial malformations, microcephaly with the bulk of the brain tissue in the mass, or other severe organ abnormalities, a pre-delivery discussion should be undertaken with the family about nonintervention in the event that spontaneous onset of respiration does not occur.

Special care to avoid trauma to the mass is important when the attachment is pedunculated or there is only a membranous tissue covering the surface.

Transport   Referral to a tertiary center with pediatric neurology and neurosurgery capabilities is always indicated.

Testing and Confirmation   Diagnostic imaging, either cranial CT or MRI, to define the defect and to delineate any associated CNS abnormalities, is important. Chromosomal analysis, echocardiography, and abdominal sonography are indicated contingent on physical findings and clinical course if not obtained prenatally.

Nursery Management   Postoperatively, seizures and hydrocephalus are the more common neurologic complications requiring intervention.

Surgery

Preoperative Assessment   The size and location of the encephalocele, its contents, and relationship to major vascular structures are important for surgical planning. The volume of the remaining intracranial contents, hydrocephalus, and the head circumference are also important information.

Magnetic resonance imaging is useful to define the encephalocele contents and its relationship to vital structures. The relationship of the encephalocele to the structures of the posterior fossa and venous sinuses is important from the surgical standpoint and can be determined by MRI and magnetic resonance angiography.

Operative Indications   Small, entirely skin-covered lesions can be repaired electively. Large lesions or those that are leaking cerebrospinal fluid need to be repaired urgently.

Types of Procedures   Surgical treatment involves resection of the encephalocele contents and closure of the dura, scalp, and skull. Large encephaloceles such as those in which the majority of the brain is in the encephalocele sac, or in which vital structures such as the brain stem are extracranial, cannot be treated surgically and are associated with a very poor outcome. If hydrocephalus is present, then a ventricular shunt is placed at the same procedure.

Surgical Results/Prognosis   Outcome is dependent on the size, location, and contents of the encephalocele as well as the presence of other brain anomalies. Large lesions in which the majority of the brain is extracranial, or in which essential structures are included in the encephalocele sac have a very poor functional outcome and are treated expectantly. Despite this, a good overall prognosis is possible, regardless of the size of the encephalocele, when the encephalocele sac is devoid of vital neural or vascular structures.

REFERENCES

Bronshtein M, Bar-Hava I, Blumenfeld Z: Early second-trimester sonographic appearance of occipital haemangioma simulating encephalocele. Prenat Diagn 1992;12:695–698.

Brown MS, Sheridan-Pereira M: Outlook for the child with a cephalocele. Pediatrics 1992;90:914–919.

Budorick NE, Pretorius DH, McGahan JP, et al: Cephalocele detection in utero: Sonographic and clinical features. Ultrasound Obstet Gynecol 1995;5:77–85.

Curnes JT, Oakes WJ: Parietal cephaloceles: Radiographic and magnetic resonance imaging evaluation. Pediatr Neurosci 1988;14:71.

Fink IJ, Chinn DH, Callen PW: A potential pitfall in the ultrasonographic diagnosis of fetal encephalocele. J Ultrasound Med 1983;2:313–314.

Goldstein RB, LaPidus AS, Filly RA: Fetal cephaloceles: Diagnosis with US. Radiology 1991;180:803–808.

Graham D, Johnson TRB Jr, Winn K, Sanders RC: The role of sonography in the prenatal diagnosis and management of encephalocele. J Ultrasound Med 1982;1:111–115.

Jeanty P, Shah D, Zaleski W, et al: Prenatal diagnosis of fetal cephalocele: A sonographic spectrum. Am J Perinatol 1991;8:144–149.

Lay KL, Lang TN, Leung TY: Fetal scalp cysts: Challenge in diagnostic counseling. J Ultrasound Med 2001;20:175–177.

Monteaguido A, Alayon A, Mayberry P: Walker-Warburg syndrome: Case report and review of the literature. J Ultrasound Med 2001;20:419–426.

Ogle RF, Jauniaux E: Fetal scalp cysts: Dilemmas in diagnosis. Prenat Diagn 1999;19:1157–1159.

Nyberg DA, Hallesy D, Mahony BS, et al: Meckel-Gruber syndrome: Importance of prenatal diagnosis. J Ultrasound Med 1990;9:691–696.

Saw PD, Rouse GA, DeLange M: Meckel syndrome: Sonographic findings. JDMS 1991;7:8–11.

Wang P, Chang FM, Chang CH, et al: Prenatal diagnosis of Joubert syndrome complicated with encephalocele using two-dimensional and three-dimensional ultrasound. Ultrasound Obstet Gynecol 1999;14:360–364.

Wininger SJ, Donnenfeld AE: Syndromes identified in fetuses with prenatally diagnosed cephaloceles. Prenat Diagn 1994;14:839–843.

Wiswell TE, Tuttle DJ, Northan RS, Simonds GR: Major congenital neurologic malformations: A 17 year survey. Am J Dis 1990;144:61.

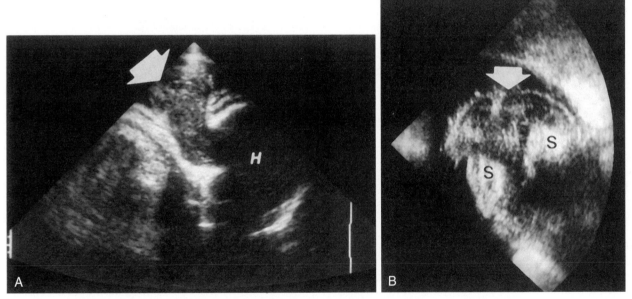

Longitudinal and transverse views of large midline occipital encephalocele (*arrow*). H, head; S, skull.

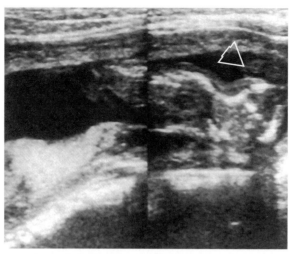

Parietal encephalocele due to amniotic bands. Note that the encephalocele (*arrow*) arises from the top of the head.

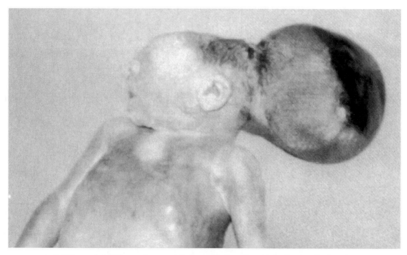

A 28-week stillborn fetus with large isolated occipital encephalocele.

2.11 Holoprosencephaly

Epidemiology/Genetics

Definition Holoprosencephaly is the term used for the spectrum of severe early abnormalities in forebrain cleavage. These cleavage abnormalities can occur both sagittally, resulting in fusion of the cerebral hemispheres, and horizontally, resulting in abnormalities of the optic and olfactory bulbs.

Epidemiology One to two per 10,000 liveborns. One in 250 embryos. (M1:F3 for alobar holoprosencephaly, M1:F1 for lobar form.)

Embryology Holoprosencephaly is an early arrest in prosencephalon cleavage. Most cases are sporadic, but chromosomal, genetic, and teratogenic causes have been described. One third of cases with multiple malformations are caused by chromosomal abnormality, with trisomy 13, trisomy 18, 13q-, and 18p- being the most common. An empirical recurrence risk for sporadic cases is approximately 6%. More than 12 genetic loci have been mapped for holoprosencephaly, but less than 5% of cases have detectable mutations. The current status of genetic testing should be discussed with a clinical geneticist or genetic counselor.

Inheritance Patterns Rare families showing autosomal dominant and autosomal recessive inheritance have been described. Mutations in the sonic hedgehog (SHH) gene, located at 7q36, have been found in familial and sporadic cases of holoprosencephaly, with familial cases more likely to have an SHH mutation than sporadic cases. Consultation with a medical geneticist or a laboratory offering this testing is advised. Multiple malformation syndromes, including Smith-Lemli-Opitz syndrome (autosomal recessive), the Meckel syndrome (autosomal recessive), the Aicardi syndrome (X-linked dominant), the Fryn syndrome (autosomal recessive), and the hydrolethalus syndrome (autosomal recessive), have been described with holoprosencephaly. Because of the rapid progress in mapping of genes and subsequent development of genetic testing, consultation with a medical geneticist or genetic counselor to determine the availability of clinical genetic testing for this disorder or disorders is advised.

Teratogens Alcohol, phenytoin, retinoic acid, maternal diabetes, and congenital infections have been reported with holoprosencephaly.

Prognosis Most severely affected patients die at birth or in the first 6 months of life. Survival, with variable mental retardation, occurs in mild cases.

Sonography

FINDINGS

1. **Fetus:**
   a. Brain changes. Three subtypes: (1) alobar—virtually no cortical mantle; (2) semilobar—single horseshoe-shaped ventricle with some mantle and partially separated cerebral hemispheres posteriorly; (3) lobar—the single ventricle is fused anteriorly only with incomplete falx and intrahemispheric fissure. The frontal horns are squared off. A third ventricle may be seen with a small echogenic area separating the third ventricle from the central ventricle.
   b. In the alobar and semilobar forms, the findings are (1) fused or partially fused thalamus with absence of the third ventricle; (2) single ventricle with a horseshoe configuration; (3) dorsal cyst—expansion of the posterior aspect of the common ventricle; (4) hippocampal ridge—a bulge on the lateral aspect of the common ventricle at the midpoint; and (5) absent cavum septum pellucidum, corpus callosum, and intrahemispheric fissure.
   c. Facial deformities are usually seen: (1) close-set eyes with either hypotelorism or a single orbit with one or two globes (cyclops deformity); (2) median cleft lip and palate (see Chapter 7.1); (3) flattened nose with a single nostril; and (4) possibly a proboscis superior to the level of the eyes with an absent nose and hypotelorism, yielding a markedly abnormal profile (ethmocephaly).
2. **Amniotic Fluid:** Polyhydramnios may occur.
3. **Placenta:** Normal.
4. **Measurement Data:**
   a. The fetal head size is often enlarged but may be normal or small despite ventricular enlargement.
   b. IUGR is often present.
   c. The intraorbital distance is usually reduced.
5. **When Detectable:** With the endovaginal probe from 9 weeks.

Pitfalls See differential diagnosis.

Differential Diagnosis

1. Hydranencephaly can be confused with the alobar form. The thalamus will not be fused and a third ventricle should be visible in hydranencephaly.
2. The alobar form can be confused with aqueductal stenosis if the posterior fusion of the ventricles and the absent third ventricle are overlooked.
3. Schizencephaly—The cystic defect in schizencephaly may involve both hemispheres, but it will be asym-

metrically shaped and the remaining ventricles will appear normal.

4. Dandy-Walker cyst—A massive Dandy-Walker cyst can give the impression of a dilated common ventricle, but the normal supratentorial system will be visible.

5. Agenesis of the corpus callosum can mimic the lobar form. The third ventricle will be separate from the lateral ventricles and will be at a high level. MRI is helpful in sorting out this confusion.

Where Else to Look   Look for the stigma of trisomy 13: abnormal hands, feet, and omphalocele. (See Chapter 1.2.) Other associated problems are congenital heart disease, particularly double outlet problems, omphalocele, and Dandy-Walker malformation. Trisomy 18 is also associated with holoprosencephaly.

Pregnancy Management

Investigations and Consultations Required   The high incidence of cytogenetic abnormalities makes chromosome evaluation of the fetus mandatory, even late in pregnancy. Maternal evaluation for diabetes should be done. Fetal echocardiography is useful only to document additional malformations but is not essential. Consultations with the neonatology staff should be arranged to discuss nonaggressive management at birth.

Fetal Intervention   In utero therapeutic procedures are contraindicated except to facilitate delivery (see below).

Monitoring   No pregnancy interventions such as early delivery or cesarean section are appropriate. All forms of holoprosencephaly have a very poor prognosis, so monitoring, except at the parents' request, is unwarranted. The head size needs to be assessed before delivery to make sure vaginal delivery is possible.

Pregnancy Course   Polyhydramnios may be associated with holoprosencephaly, resulting in preterm labor.

Pregnancy Termination Issues   The heterogeneous causes for holoprosencephaly require that a complete external and internal examination of the fetus be performed by individuals with training in fetal pathology and dysmorphology.

Delivery   Vaginal delivery should be accomplished in all cases. Cephalocentesis is appropriate in circumstances in which a large head results in dystocia.

Neonatology

Resuscitation   With an established diagnosis of holoprosencephaly, the decision to initiate resuscitative measures should be discussed with the family prior to delivery. If the diagnosis is uncertain or associated anomalies are not delineated, it is appropriate to support respiration to allow time for the diagnostic evaluation and parental adaptation to occur.

Transport   If the diagnostic evaluation has not been completed prior to delivery, transfer to a tertiary center with pediatric neurology capability is appropriate to confirm diagnosis and provide counseling and support to the family.

Testing and Confirmation   The clinical presentation of holoprosencephaly includes a spectrum of facial abnormalities including cyclopia, hypotelorism, and facial clefts. Newborns may have hydrocephalus and signs of neurologic dysfunction. Postnatal CT or MRI clearly defines these abnormalities.

Nursery Management   The priority is to obtain a definitive diagnosis as promptly as possible. If chromosomal analysis was not performed prenatally, blood should be collected prior to any major invasive procedure or blood transfusion.

Respiratory support is indicated pending confirmation of diagnosis and to give the family time to make a decision about life support and long-term care.

REFERENCES

Berry SM, Gosden C, Snijders RJ, Nicolaides KH: Fetal holoprosencephaly: Associated malformations and chromosomal defects. Fetal Diagn Ther 1990;5:92–99.

Blaas HK, Eik-Nes SH, Vainio T, et al: Alobar holoprosencephaly at 9 weeks gestational age visualized by two and three dimensional ultrasound. Ultrasound Obstet Gynecol 2000;15:62–65.

Cohen MM: Perspectives on holoprosencephaly. Part I. Epidemiology, genetics and syndromology. Teratology 1989;40:211–235.

Cohen MM Jr: An update on the holoprosencephalic disorders. J Pediatr 1982;101:865–869.

Croen LA, Shaw GM, Lammer EJ: Holoprosencephaly: Epidemiologic and clinical characteristics of a California population. Am J Med Genet 1996;64:465–472.

Filly RA, Chinn DH, Callen PW: Alobar holoprosencephaly: Ultrasonographic prenatal diagnosis. Radiology 1984;151:455–459.

Golden JA: Towards a greater understanding of the pathogenesis of holoprosencephaly. Brain Dev 1999;21:513–521.

Greene M, Benacerraf B, Frigoletto FD Jr: Reliable criteria for the sonographic diagnosis of alobar holoprosencephaly. Am J Obstet Gynecol 1987;156:687–689.

Kobori JA, Herrick MK, Urich H: Arhinencephaly: The spectrum of associated malformations. Brain 1987;110:237–260.

Munke M: Clinical, cytogenetic and molecular approaches to the genetic heterogeneity of holoprosencephaly. Am J Med Genet 1989;34:237–245.

Nanni L, Croen LA, Lammer EJ, Muenke M: Holoprosencephaly: Molecular study of a California population. Am J Med Genet 2000;90:315–319.

Nanni L, Ming JE, Bocian M, et al: The mutational spectrum of the sonic hedgehog gene in holoprosencephaly: SHH mutations cause a significant proportion of autosomal dominant holoprosencephaly. Hum Mol Genet 1999;8:2479–2488.

Nyberg DA, Mack LA, Bronstein A, et al: Holoprosencephaly: Prenatal sonographic diagnosis. Am J Roentgenol 1987;149:1051–1058.

Peebles DM: Holoprosencephaly. Prenat Diagn 1998;18:477–480.

Pilu G, Ambrosetto P, Sandri F, et al: Intraventricular fused fornices: A specific sign of fetal lobar holoprosencephaly. Ultrasound Obstet Gynecol 1994;4:65–67.

Pilu G, Sandri F, Perolo A, et al: Prenatal diagnosis of lobar holoprosencephaly. Ultrasound Obstet Gynecol 1992;2:88–94.

Turner CD, Silva S, Jeanty P: Prenatal diagnosis of alobar holoprosencephaly at 10 weeks of gestation. Ultrasound Obstet Gynecol 1999;13:360–362.

Wallis D, Muenke M: Mutations in holoprosencephaly. Hum Mutat 2000;16:99–108.

Wong HS, Lam YH, Tang MHY, et al: First-trimester ultrasound diagnosis of holoprosencephaly: Three case reports. Ultrasound Obstet Gynecol 1999;13:356–359.

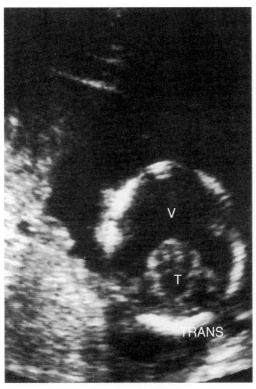

Alobar holoprosencephaly. The most severe form of holoprosencephaly with no cortical mantle and very large single ventricle (V). The thalamus (T) is fused on this coronal view.

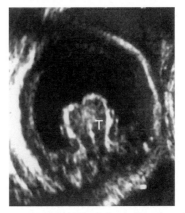

Semilobar holoprosencephaly. A single horseshoe-shaped ventricle with considerable cortical mantle is present. Again, there is a fused thalamus (T) with no septum pellucidum present.

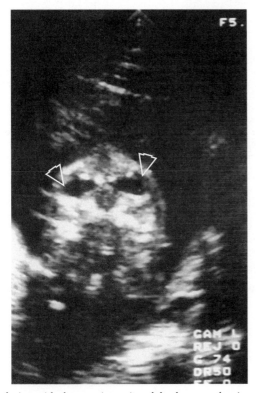

Hypotelorism with the eyes (*arrows*) unduly close together in a case of holoprosencephaly.

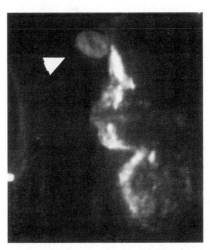

Profile view showing absence of nose with a proboscis (*arrow*).

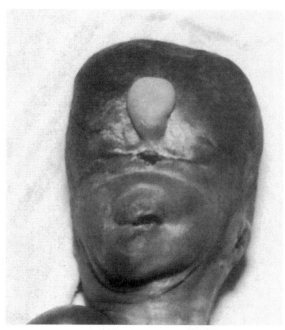

A 19-week fetus with isolated holoprosencephaly. Face shows proboscis, fused eyes, and absent nose.

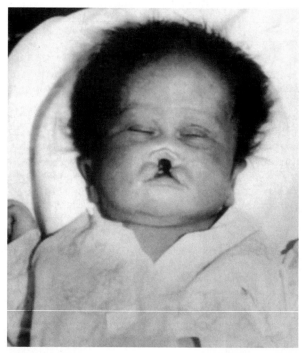

Newborn with median facial cleft, absent nose, and hypotelorism resulting from holoprosencephaly.

2.12 Hydranencephaly

Epidemiology/Genetics

Definition Hydranencephaly is a severe brain abnormality in which most or all of the cerebral hemispheres are absent and the cranium is filled with fluid.

Epidemiology Rare occurrence (M1:F1).

Embryology The etiology is heterogeneous, but most cases are thought to be due to generalized brain ischemia or overwhelming antenatal infection with resultant destruction of brain parenchyma. Ischemia may be due to hypotension, vascular agenesis/dysgenesis, arterial occlusion from twin-to-twin emboli, and occlusion of the vein of Galen. Maternal clotting disorders, seizures, and severe abdominal trauma are predisposing conditions. Most people differentiate hydranencephaly from extreme porencephaly by the former's symmetry and lack of cystic cavities, although they may represent a continuum. Extreme hydrocephalus differs from hydranencephaly in having a lining of cortex at the outside of its sac. Chromosomal abnormalities, especially trisomy 13, have been reported with hydranencephaly.

Inheritance Patterns Rare familial recurrence has been reported. About 20 multiple malformation syndromes have been reported with hydranencephaly or porencephaly.

Teratogens Congenital infections, including herpes, cytomegalovirus, and toxoplasmosis, and use of cocaine and warfarin.

Prognosis Hydranencephaly is usually lethal, with neonatal survivors having profound mental retardation.

Sonography

FINDINGS

1. **Fetus:**
   a. Almost all brain structures, above the brain stem and midbrain, are absent. The midbrain is variably present. In some instances, there is a central linear structure composed of the remnants of the brain, but usually even the falx and septum pellucidum are partially or completely absent. The choroid plexuses are absent. There is absence or hypoplasia of the supraclinoid portion of the internal carotid arteries.
   b. The brain stem, on coronal views, has a characteristic appearance as it protrudes into the completely fluid-filled calvarium. The roof of the third ventricle is absent, but paired thalami are seen.
   c. The absence of cortex is due to a global cortical infarct. Infarction takes place sometime between 12 and 30 weeks' gestation. During the phase when infarction occurs, the brain becomes echogenic, with loss of landmarks. The cortical brain, once infarcted, is fairly rapidly removed, and eventually fluid replaces the brain. During the dissolution process, a debris-fluid level may be seen.
2. **Amniotic Fluid:** Normal or increased.
3. **Placenta:** Normal.
4. **Measurement Data:** The head size is normal or slightly enlarged.
5. **When Detectable:** Some time between 20 and 30 weeks as a rule, although an example at 12 weeks has been described.

Pitfalls Since the dura and arachnoid are preserved, there may be confusion with very severe hydrocephalus. In the latter situation, the brain stem and midbrain are complete and the choroid plexuses are present. Usually, with severe hydrocephalus, the ventricular enlargement is asymmetrical and the third ventricle is dilated.

Differential Diagnosis

1. Lobar holoprosencephaly—The third ventricle will be absent, but the thalami are present.
2. Severe hydrocephalus—See Pitfalls.
3. Porencephaly—Only confusing if the normal brain (close to the transducer) is shadowed out by skull reverberations.
4. Hydrolethalis syndrome. In severe examples, no cortical structure is seen. Unlike hydranencephaly, the cerebellum and brain stem are absent and additional findings such as micrognathia and polydactyly are seen.

Where Else to Look Usually not associated with problems elsewhere.

Pregnancy Management

Investigations and Consultations Required Although rare, disseminated fetal viral infections, especially herpes, can cause extensive cerebral destruction. Therefore, viral titers should be done. Chromosome studies should also be performed because of the potential for a misclassification of severe hydrocephalus as hydranencephaly.

Monitoring Serial ultrasonographic examinations to monitor head size are quite appropriate. Because hydranencephaly should not be an "increased pressure" form of ventriculomegaly, an enlarging head relative to other fetal parameters should prompt a reassessment of the diagnosis.

Pregnancy Course   Hydranencephaly should not be associated with specific obstetric complications.

Pregnancy Termination Issues   Termination of pregnancy is an appropriate option, and it should be done by a nondestructive procedure at an institution with expertise in fetal neuropathology.

Delivery   Vaginal delivery is appropriate in all cases. In the presence of a relatively large head, cephalocentesis may be indicated to accomplish vaginal delivery of the infant.

Neonatology

Resuscitation   The decision to initiate resuscitative efforts should be discussed with the family prior to delivery. With a definitive diagnosis of hydranencephaly of known cause, nonintervention is appropriate if spontaneous onset of respiration does not occur. If the diagnosis is uncertain, support is indicated to allow time for confirmation.

Transport   Transfer to a tertiary center with pediatric neurology and neurosurgery capabilities is indicated for confirmation of diagnosis.

Testing and Confirmation   Affected infants may initially appear normal at birth or have signs of central nervous system dysfunction such as seizures, poor feeding, and

developmental delay. Postnatally, the diagnosis is confirmed by MRI or CT scan. Serologic and microbiologic testing for congenital infections is indicated if not obtained prenatally.

Nursery Management   The major priorities are the confirmation of the diagnosis and cause, and facilitation of parental adaptation to the severe prognosis.

Decisions regarding long-term custodial care may be required, as some infants may survive the neonatal period.

REFERENCES

Belfar HB, Kuller JA, Hill LM, Kislak S: Evolving fetal hydranencephaly mimicking intracranial neoplasm. J Ultrasound Med 1991;10:231–233.

Greene MF, Benacerraf B, Crawford JM: Hydranencephaly: US appearance during in utero evolution. Radiology 1985;156:779–780.

Halsey JH Jr, Allen N, Chamberlin HR: The morphogenesis of hydranencephaly. J Neurol Sci 1971;12:187–217.

Halsey JH Jr, Allen N, Chamberlin HR: Hydranencephaly. In Vinken PJ, Bruyn GW (eds): Congenital Malformations of the Brain and Skull. Handbook Clin Neurol 1977;30:661.

Lam YH, Tang MHY: Serial sonographic features of a fetus with hydranencephaly from 11 weeks to term. Ultrasound Obstet Gynecol 2000;16:77–79.

Lin YS, Chang FM, Liu CH: Antenatal detection of hydranencephaly at 12 weeks, menstrual age. J Clin Ultrasound 1992;20:62–64.

McGahan JP, Ellis W, Lindfors KK, et al: Congenital cerebrospinal fluid containing intracranial abnormalities: A sonographic classification. J Clin Ultrasound 1988;16:531–544.

Pilu G, Rizzo N, Orsini LF, Bovicelli L: Antenatal recognition of cerebral anomalies. Ultrasound Med Biol 1986;12:319–326.

Sherer DM, Anyaegbunam A, Onyeije C: Antepartum fetal intracranial hemorrhage, predisposing factors and prenatal sonography: A review. Am J Perinatol 1998;15:431–441.

Siffring PA, Forrest TS, Frick MP: Sonographic detection of hydrolethalus syndrome. J Clin Ultrasound 1991;19:43–47.

Spirt BA, Oliphant M, Gordon LP: Fetal central nervous system abnormalities. Radiol Clin North Am 1990;28:59–73.

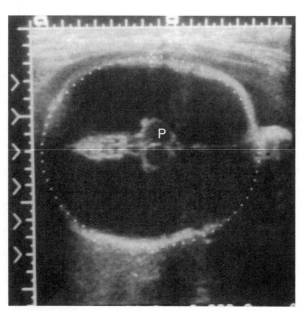

Hydranencephaly. No cortical mantle is present. No midline structures above the level of the cerebral peduncles (P) are present.

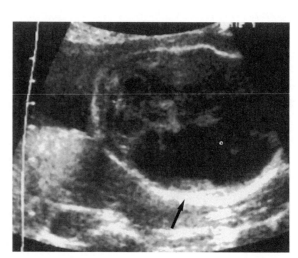

Developing hydranencephaly. The brain has recently infarcted, and the remains of the brain are seen as a debris fluid level in the dependent portion of the skull (*arrow*).

2.13 Iniencephaly

Epidemiology/Genetics

Definition   Iniencephaly is an abnormality in cervical vertebrae associated with an excessive lordosis of the cervicothoracic spine and neural tube closure defects.

Epidemiology   Rare (M1:F10). Preconceptual supplementation with folic acid may be of use in decreasing the incidence or recurrence of iniencephaly.

Embryology   The pathogenesis is unknown. It is possible that iniencephaly is a primary defect in fetal cervical development and the resulting lordosis causes a failure of neural tube closure. Alternatively, it may be a primary defect in neural tube closure. Anencephaly, encephalocele, microcephaly, and other anomalies have been associated with iniencephaly.

Inheritance Patterns   Sporadic, no known syndrome associations.

Teratogens   Folic acid antagonists (methotrexate and aminopterin), vitamin A, thalidomide, maternal diabetes, hyperthermia, and folate deficiency are associated with an increased risk for neural tube abnormalities.

Screening   Alpha-fetoprotein elevation may be present.

Prognosis   Iniencephaly, when diagnosed in utero, is almost always lethal.

Sonography

FINDINGS

1. **Fetus:**
   a. There is a very short cervical spine with missing vertebrae. The cervical spine may be acutely angled with a gibbus deformity.
   b. The cervical spine is almost always open (cervical rachischisis), often with a large cervical meningocele.
   c. There is fixed retroflexion of the head so the face looks upward in a "stargazing" position.
   d. Anencephaly or severe microcephaly is usually present.
   e. An additional lumbosacral meningomyelocele or caudal regression may be present.
2. **Amniotic Fluid:** Polyhydramnios is common.
3. **Placenta:** Normal.
4. **Measurement Data:** Normal apart from microcephaly.
5. **When Detectable:** At 10 weeks using the vaginal probe.

Pitfalls   Extended neck in a fetus for other reasons may be confused with iniencephaly, since the cervical spine vertebrae are often difficult to see when the head is extended. Since the number of vertebrae is reduced in iniencephaly, locating and counting vertebral bodies is essential.

Differential Diagnosis

1. Masses arising from the front of the neck, such as goiter or teratoma, also cause neck extension.
2. It can be hard to distinguish a low posterior encephalocele from iniencephaly. The vertebrae may be difficult to examine due to position.
3. Other causes of an extended head such as Klippel-Feil deformity, Jarcho-Levin syndrome, and arthrogryposis should be considered. The Klippel-Feil syndrome consists of a short neck with vertebral anomalies such as hemivertebrae and may be a mild form of iniencephaly. In the Jarcho-Levin syndrome, there are multiple vertebral anomalies and rib malformations.

Where Else to Look

1. Look at the lower spine for myelomeningocele.
2. Look at the intracranial structures; anencephaly, encephalocele, microcephaly, hydrocephalus, and holoprosencephaly have been reported with iniencephaly.
3. Extra CNS malformations seen with iniencephaly include diaphragmatic hernia, omphalocele, cardiac defects, genitourinary malformations, cleft lip and palate, imperforate anus, clubfoot, and single umbilical artery.

Pregnancy Management

Investigations and Consultations Required   The distinctive ultrasonographic features should preclude the need for any additional evaluation.

Monitoring   There are no special considerations for prenatal care, except supportive emotional care for the family. This is almost always a lethal anomaly, so ultrasonographic monitoring is inappropriate except to ensure that massive hydrocephalus preventing vaginal delivery does not occur.

Pregnancy Course   The incidence of complicated labor and delivery is high with iniencephaly because of the high likelihood of fetal malpresentation.

Pregnancy Termination Issues   There are no indications for special pathologic examination. Nondestructive methods of termination may be complicated by obstructed labor secondary to malpresentations of these fetuses.

Delivery   Cephalocentesis should be performed in the presence of severe hydrocephalus. In cases in which obstructed labor occurs, embryotomy may be necessary to avoid cesarean section.

Neonatology

Resuscitation   Not indicated, as the lesion is uncorrectable.

Transport   Not indicated, as the lesion is uncorrectable.

Testing and Confirmation   The abnormality is obvious at birth.

Nursery Management   Provision of comfort care and support of family are the only appropriate care measures.

REFERENCES

Aleksic S, Budzilovich G, Greco MA: Iniencephaly: A neuropathologic study. Clin Neuropathol 1983;2:55–61.

Foderaro AE, Abu-Yousef MM, Benda JA, et al: Antenatal ultrasound diagnosis of iniencephaly. J Clin Ultrasound 1987;15:550–554.

Katz VL, Aylsworth AS, Albright SG: Iniencephaly is not uniformly fatal. Prenat Diagn 1989;9:595–599.

Meizner I, Bar-Ziv J: Prenatal ultrasonic diagnosis of a rare case of iniencephaly apertus. J Clin Ultrasound 1987;15:200–203.

Meizner I, Press F, Jaffe A, Carmi R: Prenatal ultrasound diagnosis of complete absence of the lumbar spine and sacrum. J Clin Ultrasound 1992;20:77–80.

Sahid S, Sepulveda W, Dezeraga V, et al: Iniencephaly: Prenatal diagnosis and management. Prenat Diagn 2000;20:202–205.

Sherer DM, Hearn-Stebbins B, Harvey W, et al: Endovaginal sonographic diagnosis of iniencephaly apertus and craniorachischisis at 13 weeks, menstrual age. J Clin Ultrasound 1993;21:124–127.

Shipp TD, Bromley B, Benecerraf B: The prognostic significance of hyperextension of the fetal head detected antenatally with ultrasound. Ultrasound Obstet Gynecol 2000;15:391–396.

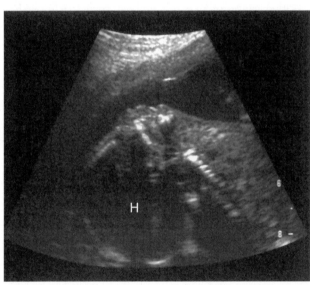

Iniencephaly. Retroverted head (H) with "stargazing" attitude because there were many missing cervical vertebrae. Cervical rachischisis was present.

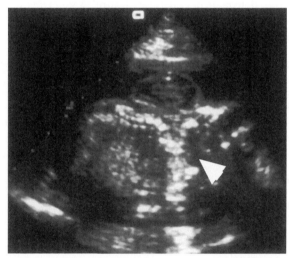

Severe gibbus deformity in iniencephaly with missing vertebrae and acute angle (*arrow*). A myelomeningocele was present at the level of the deformity. There was also anencephaly.

2.14 Intracranial Hemorrhage

Epidemiology/Genetics

Definition   Intracranial hemorrhage is the extravasation of blood from a blood vessel into the parenchyma or ventricles of the brain or spaces surrounding the brain.

Epidemiology   Unknown, but very rare.

Embryology   Maternal-fetal pregnancy complications, including hypotension and preeclampsia, are believed to be the most common etiologic factors. Twin-to-twin complications, antenatal infection, vascular malformations, alloimmune antibodies, and trauma are other possible causes of intracranial hemorrhage.

Inheritance Patterns   Sporadic.

Teratogens   Congenital infections, including cytomegalovirus, herpesvirus, and toxoplasmosis, and use of cocaine. Also, alloimmune and idiopathic thrombocytopenia and von Willebrand's disease.

Prognosis   Dependent on the severity of damage to the central nervous system. Extensive hemorrhages are fatal. Permanent neurologic damage, moderate to severe mental retardation, hydrocephalus, and porencephalic cysts may be seen in survivors.

Sonography

FINDINGS

1. **Fetus:**
   a. Intrabrain bleeds—Initially, an echogenic area within the brain is seen that later becomes cystic. If it borders on a lateral ventricle, a bulge from the lateral ventricle known as a porencephalic cyst develops.
   b. Intraventricular bleeds—Blood within the ventricles has low-level echoes for a brief period of time. Echogenic clots soon develop. An echogenic rim to the ventricular wall develops.
   c. Subdural bleeds—Echopenic and echogenic blood between the skull and the brain has been reported and is typically echofree when extradural.
   d. Reactive hydrocephalus—If the blood clot does not obstruct the aqueduct of Sylvius, only lateral ventricular dilation may be seen. With aqueduct blockage, the third and lateral ventricles are all dilated.
   e. Color Doppler is of help in showing absence of flow in bleeds and in showing diminished or absent flow in adjacent vessels. MRI is of value in confirming hemorrhage.
2. **Amniotic Fluid:** Normal.

3. **Placenta:** Normal.
4. **Measurement Data:** Normal.
5. **When Detectable:** Bleeding generally occurs in the third trimester. It is easily detectable as soon as clot develops.

Pitfalls

1. If blood clot is not seen, the ventricular dilation may be thought to be due to aqueduct stenosis.
2. A space between the brain and the skull is often seen as a normal variant in utero. Asymmetry and a local cranial bulge favor a subdural bleed. Doppler ultrasonography will show increased resistance in neighboring intracranial vessels.
3. Echogenic bleeds in the choroid plexus or the vermis of the cerebellum may be difficult to see because of the echogenicity of those structures.

Differential Diagnosis

1. Aqueductal stenosis—See Pitfalls. (See Chapter 2.3.)
2. An echogenic brain mass, due to clot, may be mistaken for tumor. No blood flow is seen with color flow Doppler.
3. A brain infarct may resemble clot.

Where Else to Look

1. Other sites of bleeding—Liver and lungs, look for evidence of a bleeding diathesis.
2. Hydrops—Secondary to fetal anemia.
3. Active hemorrhages may be associated with fetal distress manifested by fetal heart rate changes.

Pregnancy Management

Investigations and Consultations Required

1. Analysis of fetal platelet count and hematocrit by percutaneous umbilical blood sampling should be done.
2. TORCH titers and appropriate confirmation studies of abnormal results complete the work-up.
3. The family should be referred to a neonatologist for a thorough discussion of the neonatal management options and subsequent therapy.

Monitoring   In severe bleeds, the use of fetal assessment methods, such as non-stress testing, should not be used, as no benefit can be expected from early intervention. Frequent ultrasonographic studies are appropriate to observe evolution of bleeds, to make sure no other bleeds occur, and to monitor the head for size increases related to hydrocephalus.

Pregnancy Course   Intracranial bleeds with resultant hydrocephalus may result in macrocephaly.

Pregnancy Termination Issues   Termination should occur by nondestructive procedures in a center with expertise in neuropathology.

Delivery   The pregnancy complicated by a fetal intracranial bleed requires delivery in a center with capabilities for neonatal resuscitation. In the case of alloimmune thrombocytopenia, consideration should be given to caesarian section to prevent further hemorrhage. Consideration of cephalocentesis versus caesarian section may arise if the degree of cerebral destruction is severe and severe hydrocephalus develops.

Neonatology

Resuscitation   The decision to initiate resuscitation in the presence of documented antenatal intracranial hemorrhage is contingent on the extent of the hemorrhage, the degree of resultant brain destruction (porencephaly), the duration of the gestation at delivery, and the cumulative effect of the listed factors on long-term prognosis. Prenatally, it is appropriate to discuss nonintervention with the family, should there be no spontaneous onset of respirations and the prognosis for severe disability is certain.

If active resuscitation is to be instituted, there are no specific technical issues other than preparation for acute packed red blood cell transfusion if the hemorrhage is known to have been recent and severe.

Transport   Transfer to a tertiary perinatal center is appropriate to confirm diagnosis and prognosis.

Testing and Confirmation   Serologic testing for intrauterine coagulopathy secondary to congenital infections, coagulation defects, or alloimmune thrombocytopenia should be considered if the physical examination and clinical course are suggestive of any of the above disorders. The extent of the hemorrhage and resultant brain injury can be demonstrated by cranial CT or MRI. The latter may be preferable, as vascular lesions are more easily identified.

Nursery Management   The initial priority is to establish cardiorespiratory adaptation. Support of perfusion and oxygen delivery by transfusion as noted above may be required. Posthemorrhagic hydrocephalus may complicate the course both prenatally and in the neonatal period.

REFERENCES

Ben-Chetrit A, Anteby E, Lavy B, et al: Increased middle cerebral artery blood flow impedance in fetal subdural hematoma. Ultrasound Obstet Gynecol 1991;1:357–358.

Bowerman RA, Donn SM, Silver TM, Jaffe MH: Natural history of neonatal periventricular/intraventricular hemorrhage and its complications: Sonographic observations. Am J Roentgenol 1984;143:1041–1052.

Chinn DH, Filly RA: Extensive intracranial hemorrhage in utero. J Ultrasound Med 1983;2:285–287.

Cochrane DD, Myles ST, Nimrod C, et al: Intrauterine hydrocephalus and ventriculomegaly: Associated anomalies and fetal outcome. Can J Neurol Sci 1985;12:51–59.

Filly RA: The fetus with a central nervous system malformation: Ultrasound evaluation. In Harrison MR, et al (eds): The Unborn Patient: Prenatal Diagnosis and Treatment. Philadelphia, WB Saunders, 1991, pp 424–425.

Fogarty K: Sonography of fetal intracranial hemorrhage: Unusual causes and a review of the literature. J Clin Ultrasound 1989;17:366–370.

Guerriero S, Ajossa S, Mais V, et al: Color Doppler energy imaging in the diagnosis of fetal intracranial hemorrhage in the second trimester. Ultrasound Obstet Gynecol 1997;3:205–208.

Minkoff H, Schaffer RM, Delke I, Grunebaum AN: Diagnosis of intracranial hemorrhage in utero after a maternal seizure. Obstet Gynecol 1985;65:22S—24S.

Mintz MC, Arger PH, Coleman BG: In utero sonographic diagnosis of intracerebral hemorrhage. J Ultrasound Med 1985;4:375–376.

Naidu S, Messmore H, Caserta V, Fine M: CNS lesions in neonatal isoimmune thrombocytopenia. Arch Neurol 1983;40:552–554.

Sherer DM, Anyaegbunam A, Onyeije C: Antepartum fetal intracranial hemorrhage, predisposing factors and prenatal sonography: A review. Am J Perinatol 1998;15:431–441.

Stagnicni FML, Cuni G, Canapicchi R, et al: Fetal intracranial hemorrhage: Is minor maternal trauma a possible pathogenetic factor. Ultrasound Obstet Gynecol 2001;18:335–342.

Zalneraitis EL, Young RS, Krishnamoorthy KS: Intracranial hemorrhage in utero as a complication of isoimmune thrombocytopenia. J Pediatr 1979;95:611–614.

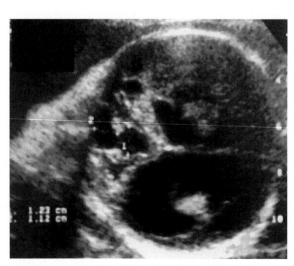

A 24-week pregnancy. Intracranial hemorrhage in the temporal region with blood clot collection within the dilated lateral ventricles. Both lateral ventricles and the third and fourth ventricles were dilated because of the hemorrhage. *Arrow* shows area of hemorrhage.

Same patient, coronal view. Dilated lateral ventricle can be seen. The fourth ventricle is massively dilated and contains clot.

2.15 Intracranial Teratoma

Epidemiology/Genetics

Definition Teratomas are germ cell tumors that are derived from totipotent stem cells. These tumors contain cells representing all three embryonic germ cell layers: ectoderm, endoderm, and mesoderm.

Epidemiology Very rare. M10:F1.

Embryology Although the pathogenesis is unknown, teratomas may represent abnormalities in twinning. Commonly, gastrointestinal, respiratory, and nervous system tissue elements are present. They occur most often in a para-axial location from the brain to the sacral area. Primary sites in infants and children include sacrococcyx (60%), gonads (20%), chest and abdomen (15%), and intracranial (3%). Fifty percent of brain tumors detected in utero are teratomas.

Inheritance Patterns Sporadic.

Teratogens None.

Prognosis Dependent on the size and location of the tumor. So far, all prenatally diagnosed intracranial teratomas have been lethal.

Sonography

FINDINGS

1. **Fetus:** Structures within the fetal head are disorganized, with areas of calcification and cystic areas. Few recognizable structures are visible. Almost all intracranial teratomas diagnosed in utero have been very advanced, filling much of the skull.
2. **Amniotic Fluid:** Amniotic fluid is often increased, since the tumor may involve swallowing control.
3. **Placenta:** The placenta is normal.
4. **Measurement Data:** The fetal head size may be greatly increased.
5. **When Detectable:** Most often in the late second and third trimester. Has been detected at 17 weeks.

Pitfalls Intracranial bleeds can cause echogenic areas that may be mistaken for areas of intracranial calcification.

Differential Diagnosis

1. Other forms of intracranial tumor, e.g., choroid plexus papilloma (characteristic intrachoroidal location), glioblastoma, craniopharyngioma, and neuroblastoma have

been reported (see Chapter 2.6). Calcifications and cystic areas are strongly suggestive of intracranial teratoma.
2. Focal infarction or bleed—The appearances of the apparent mass will change relatively quickly.
3. Choroid plexus and corpus callosum lipoma are benign lesions with a typical echogenic appearance and location.
4. Fetus in fetu. A viable embryo located in the posterior fossa of a 17-week pregnancy has been reported.

Where Else to Look Teratomas may involve the mouth (epignathus), so look closely at the face.

Pregnancy Management

Investigations and Consultations Required Because of the inability to make a precise diagnosis, other causes must be considered for the sonographic features. Disseminated viral infections and massive intracranial hemorrhage could present a similar picture. Maternal viral titers and percutaneous umbilical blood sampling for determination of fetal hematologic status may be helpful in excluding these conditions. A targeted CT scan with ultrasonic guidance can be helpful in establishing calcification and the presence of fat. Because of the grave prognosis, consultation with the neonatologist is essential for the planning of neonatal management. Likewise, a neurosurgical consult may provide the family additional information regarding the expected course in these infants.

Fetal Intervention If the tumor is associated with hydrocephalus and an enlarged head, consideration should be given to cephalocentesis prior to delivery.

Monitoring Since the head may grow to an unmanageable size, serial ultrasonographic studies to determine the time of delivery are desirable. Signs of fetal hydrops or polyhydramnios may be detected with ultrasonography.

Pregnancy Course Obstetric complications, including polyhydramnios, fetal hydrops, and cephalopelvic disproportion, are likely.

Pregnancy Termination Issues As with other CNS malformations, the method of choice should allow a precise pathologic diagnosis of the sonographic findings.

Delivery There are no benefits to cesarean section. Delivery should be vaginal, even with an enlarged head (see above). Consideration should be given to management of labor, without electronic heart rate monitoring, because evidence of "fetal distress" would not be unusual given the significant CNS malformations. Decisions regarding mode of delivery should not be made on the basis of fetal heart rate changes.

Neonatology

Resuscitation A prenatal discussion with the family regarding nonintervention is appropriate should there be fetal distress or delay in spontaneous onset of respiration. If the decision is made to intervene, no specific resuscitation techniques are required. The prenatal development of either hydrocephalus or hydrops can also complicate resuscitation.

Transport Referral to a tertiary center with pediatric neurosurgery capabilities is indicated.

Testing and Confirmation Intracranial teratomas can be associated with obstructive hydrocephalus, signs of increased intracranial pressure, and focal neurologic abnormalities. Half are found in the pineal region. Postnatal CT or MRI scan can confirm the diagnosis.

Nursery Management Because the mortality rate from this lesion is almost 100%, the major issue is the accessibility of the tumor to operative resection.

Surgery

Preoperative Assessment These tumors are found primarily in the midline, as are most congenital CNS tumors. The most common sites are the pineal region, the suprasellar region, and the fourth ventricle. There is a striking male predominance that has been reported to range between 5:1 and 10:1. MRI scanning of the head and spine is performed, plus a careful search for tumor outside the CNS.

Operative Indications All intracranial mass lesions suspicious for neoplasm require surgical treatment for the purpose of diagnosis and therapy.

Types of Procedures Some intracranial tumors, depending on the location and size, may warrant biopsy

alone. Open surgical biopsy and radical resection is indicated if a reasonable prognosis is anticipated.

Surgical Results/Prognosis Teratomas can be divided pathologically into mature and immature forms. Mature teratomas have well differentiated components and a good prognosis if complete resection is possible. Immature teratomas show evidence of germinomatous or poorly differentiated components. These tumors have a relatively poor prognosis with a significant recurrence rate and a tendency for tumor to spread along cerebrospinal fluid pathways. Teratomas that present in the pineal or suprasellar region are more likely to be of the mature type, whereas those in the fourth ventricle tend to be immature with a relatively poor prognosis. These tumors can attain tremendous size, and the size does not necessarily reflect the pathology.

REFERENCES

Billmore DF, Grosfeld JL: Teratomas in childhood: Analysis of 142 cases. Pediatr Surg 1986;21:548–551.

Body G, Darnis E, Pourcelot D, et al: Choroid plexus tumors: Antenatal diagnosis and follow-up. J Clin Ultrasound 1990;18:575–578.

Chervenak FA, Isaacson G, Touloukian R, et al: Diagnosis and management of fetal teratomas. Obstet Gynecol 1985;66:666–671.

Dolkart LA, Balcom RJ, Eisinger G: Intracranial teratoma: Prolonged neonatal survival after prenatal diagnosis. Am J Obstet Gynecol 1990; 162:768–769.

Ianniruberto A, Rossi P, Ianniruberto M, et al: Sonographic prenatal diagnosis of intracranial fetus in fetu. Ultrasound Obstet Gynecol 2001;18:67–68.

Lipman SP, Pretorius DH, Rumack CM, Manco-Johnson ML: Fetal intracranial teratoma: US diagnosis of three cases and a review of the literature. Radiology 1985;157:491–494.

McConachie NS, Twining P, Lamb MP: Case report: Antenatal diagnosis of congenital glioblastoma. Clin Radiol 1991;44:121–122.

Mulligan G, Meier P: Lipoma and agenesis of the corpus callosum with associated choroid plexus lipomas. J Ultrasound Med 1989;8:583–588.

Russel D, Rubinstein L: Pathology of Tumors of the Nervous System, 5th ed. Baltimore, Williams & Wilkins, 1989, p 681.

Schlembach D, Bornemann A, Rupprecht T, Beinder E: Fetal intracranial tumors detected by ultrasound: A report of two cases and review of the literature. Ultrasound Obstet Gynecol 1999;14:407–418.

Suresh S, Indrani S, Vijayalakshmi S, et al: Prenatal diagnosis of cerebral neuroblastoma by fetal brain biopsy. J Ultrasound Med 1993;12: 303–306.

Ulreich S, Hanieh A, Furness ME: Positive outcome of fetal intracranial teratoma. J Ultrasound Med 1993;3:163–165.

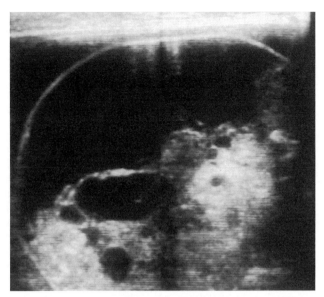

Intracranial teratoma. The entire brain was replaced by a tumor that was partially cystic and partially solid. The biparietal diameter was 18 cm.

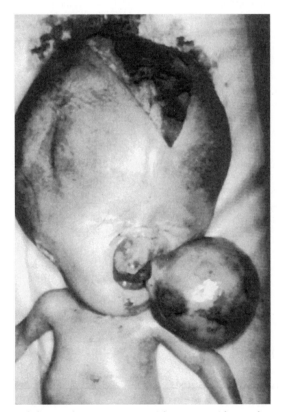

A 28-week fetus with massive intracranial teratoma with nasopharyngeal extension.

2.16 Microcephaly

Epidemiology/Genetics

Definition Microcephaly is defined as a head circumference three standard deviations below the mean (i.e., less than 5%). Most cases are secondary to a small brain.

Epidemiology One in 10,000 births (M1:F1) for isolated microcephaly. Much more common as an associated abnormality.

Embryology Microcephaly most often occurs secondary to a small brain. It can have antenatal or postnatal onset and is associated with various brain malformations, disruptions, and more than 300 sporadic, genetic, and chromosomal syndromes.

Inheritance Patterns Both autosomal recessive and autosomal dominant families have been reported with isolated microcephaly. A number of different loci have been identified. Because of the rapid progress in mapping of genes and subsequent development of genetic testing, consultation with a medical geneticist or genetic counselor to determine the availability of clinical genetic testing for this disorder or disorders is advised.

Teratogens Most human teratogens, including intrauterine infection (cytomegalovirus, rubella, and toxoplasmosis), radiation, drugs, hypoxia, and alcohol, can cause microcephaly.

Prognosis Dependent on the cause of the microcephaly and any associated brain malformations. Most microcephaly syndromes and isolated genetic microcephalies result in moderate to severe mental retardation.

Sonography

FINDINGS

1. **Fetus:** The head is small, yet the facial structures remain normal-sized. Diagnosis is easier if there is ventriculomegaly. Without ventriculomegaly, the diagnosis is difficult to make in utero unless the head size is at least three standard deviations below normal. A slanting forehead supports the diagnosis. Doppler ultrasonography may show reduced or absent flow in the intracranial arteries compared with the vertebral arteries, suggesting a vascular cause. Excessive fluid in the subarachnoid space and failure of development of the occipital horns are supporting features. Endovaginal views may help in making these observations if the fetus is vertex.
2. **Amniotic Fluid:** Usually normal.
3. **Placenta:** If the microcephaly is caused by cytomegalovirus, there may be placentomegaly and/or oligohydramnios.
4. **Measurement Data:** The biparietal diameter and the head circumference are below three standard deviations for a given gestational age. Measurement of the frontal lobe size is said to be helpful in the detection of microcephaly. A measurement is made from the medial wall of the lateral ventricle to the front of the skull on a standard biparietal diameter view.
5. **When Detectable:** Usually not detectable until after 24 weeks. The diagnosis becomes progressively easier as the pregnancy proceeds.

Pitfalls After 30 weeks, it is common to see the head circumference and the biparietal diameter below the tenth percentile as a normal variant. Usually, there is a family history of small heads.

Differential Diagnosis

1. Normal variant small head. Ask for a family history of a small hat size.
2. Anencephaly, since the base of the brain persists. (See Chapter 2.2.)

Where Else to Look

1. Cytomegalovirus—Look at the lateral ventricular walls; if they are unduly echogenic, calcification related to cytomegalovirus may be present. (See Chapter 9.1.)
2. Holoprosencephaly is associated with microcephaly. Look at the facial structures and ventricular structure. (See Chapter 2.11.)
3. Look to see that the intracranial structures and head shape are symmetrical. If they are not, consider brain infarction. The lateral ventricle on the involved side may be enlarged.
4. Microcephaly is associated with Arnold-Chiari malformation and myelomeningocele. Look at the cerebellum and skull shape and the lower lumbar spine.
5. Microcephaly is associated with many syndromes, e.g., Pena-Shokeir type 1, so look carefully at the rest of the fetus, especially the heart.
6. Neu-Laxova syndrome is characterized by IUGR, sloping forehead, externalized eyes, short neck, and microcephaly.
7. Maternal phenylketonuria—Microcephaly, cardiac anomalies, micrognathia.

Pregnancy Management

Investigations and Consultations Required

1. A careful history of drug or environmental exposures should be taken.

2. Biochemical evaluation of mother should be done to exclude maternal phenylketonuria.
3. Testing for maternal infections (e.g., cytomegalovirus, toxoplasmosis). Viral titers should be performed with appropriate confirmational studies, if positive titers are found.
4. Congenital heart defects are commonly associated with conditions having microcephaly as a feature; therefore, fetal echocardiography should be a part of the initial evaluation.
5. Fetal karyotype is recommended, especially if there is microcephaly or multiple malformations.

Monitoring There are no specific needs beyond usual obstetric care. Since the diagnosis is difficult to make, repeat ultrasonographic studies are helpful to confirm diminished cranial growth and may reveal additional anomalies.

Pregnancy Course No specific obstetric complications would be expected secondary to this fetal malformation.

Pregnancy Termination Issues If a diagnosis has not been established, a nondestructive procedure should be performed and a careful external examination of the fetus by a dysmorphologist should be a part of the autopsy protocol.

Delivery Delivery at a tertiary center is appropriate if a precise diagnosis has not been made prenatally. Special care and evaluation may be necessary following birth.

Neonatology

Resuscitation No specific measures are required with isolated microcephaly.

Transport Neonatal referral to a perinatal tertiary center for isolated microcephaly is not indicated. Subsequent referral to a pediatric neurologist for consultation is appropriate.

Testing and Confirmation In the genetic isolated microcephalies, brain growth may be normal throughout pregnancy or fall off shortly before term. Therefore, normal fetal sonograms are NOT necessarily reassuring. Measurement of head circumference and CT or MRI for brain morphology are indicated. Screening evaluations for isolated microcephaly include TORCH titers, blood and urinary testing for metabolic disorders, and cranial CT.

Nursery Management As noted above, microcephaly is often associated with other malformations or diseases that will dictate the neonatal management.

REFERENCES

Broderick K, Oyer R, Chatwani A: Neu-Laxova syndrome: A case report. Am J Obstet Gynecol 1988;158:574–575.

Bromley B, Benacerraf BR: Difficulties in the prenatal diagnosis of microcephaly. J Ultrasound Med 1995;14:303–306.

Chervenak FA, Rosenberg J, Brightman RC, et al: A prospective study of the accuracy of ultrasound in predicting fetal microcephaly. Obstet Gynecol 1987;69:908–910.

Den Hollander NS, Wessels MW, Los FJ, et al: Congenital microcephaly detected by prenatal ultrasound: Genetic aspects and clinical significance. Ultrasound Obstet Gynecol 2000;15:282–287.

Goldstein I, Reece A, Pilu G, et al: Sonographic assessment of the fetal frontal lobe: A potential tool for prenatal diagnosis of microcephaly. Am J Obstet Gynecol 1988;158:1057–1062.

Kurtz AB, Wapner RJ, Rubin CS, et al: Ultrasound criteria for in utero diagnosis of microcephaly. J Clin Ultrasound 1980;8:11–16.

Martin HP: Microcephaly and mental retardation. Am J Dis Child 1970;119:128–131.

Persutte WH: Microcephaly: No small deal. Ultrasound Obstet Gynecol 1998;11:317–318.

Pilu G, Falco P, Milano V, Bovicelli L: Prenatal diagnosis of microcephaly assisted by vaginal sonography and power Doppler. Ultrasound Obstet Gynecol 1998;11:357–360.

Rossi LN, Candini G, Scarlatti G, et al: Autosomal dominant microcephaly without mental retardation. Am J Dis Child 1987;141:655–659.

Rouse B, Matalon R, Koch R, et al: Maternal phenylketonuria syndrome: Congenital heart defects, microcephaly, and developmental outcomes. J Pediatr 2000;136:57–61.

Tolmie JL, McNay M, Stephenson JB, et al: Microcephaly: Genetic counseling and antenatal diagnosis after the birth of an affected child. Am J Med Genet 1987;27:583–594.

Volpe JJ: Neuronal proliferation, migration, organization, myelination. In Neurology of the Newborn. Philadelphia, WB Saunders, 1987, p35.

Warkany J, Lemire RJ, Cohen MM: Mental retardation and congenital malformations of the central nervous system. In Microcephaly. Chicago, Year Book Medical Publishers, 1981.

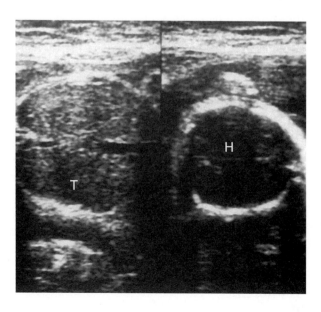

Microcephaly. The abdominal circumference (T) measurement, normally about the same size as the head circumference at term, is much larger. The head (H) circumference needs to be at least below the fifth percentile before microcephaly is considered, unless there is also ventriculomegaly (see example under cytomegalovirus).

2.17 Porencephaly and Schizencephaly

Epidemiology/Genetics

Definition   Porencephaly is generally thought to be destructive cystic lesions involving brain parenchyma resulting from antenatal hypotension, vascular accidents, or other disruptive processes.

Epidemiology   Uncommon (M1:F1).

Embryology   The brain may show cleft-like lesions (schizencephaly) or discrete cysts that may communicate with the ventricles. Most people differentiate extensive porencephaly from hydranencephaly by the latter's symmetry and lack of cavities, although they most likely represent varying severities of the same pathologic processes. The etiology of porencephaly and schizencephaly is heterogeneous, but most cases are thought to be due to generalized or localized brain ischemia caused by hypotension, vascular agenesis, twin-to-twin emboli, and overwhelming antenatal infection. Only rarely have chromosomal abnormalities, usually trisomy 13, been seen with porencephaly.

Inheritance Patterns   Generally sporadic with presumed low recurrence.

Teratogens   Congenital infections, including cytomegalovirus and toxoplasmosis, and use of cocaine.

Differential Diagnosis   Consideration of lissencephaly/pachygyria syndromes such as the Walker-Warburg syndrome, Miller-Dieber (microdeletion 17p) syndrome, arachnoid cysts, and other intracranial cystic abnormalities.

Prognosis   The prognosis for this group of conditions is dependent on the severity of CNS damage. Survivors generally have moderate to severe mental retardation with seizures and other focal signs of neurologic damage.

Sonography

FINDINGS

1. **Fetus:**
   a. Porencephalic cysts—Cystic bulges of the ventricle related to earlier intracranial bleeds. They generally occur in the watershed area adjacent to the ventricle in the temporoparietal area. Remnants of an intracranial bleed may be seen within the abnormal area as internal debris or an echogenic lining to the ventricular wall.
   b. Schizencephaly—A midline cleft is currently thought to be related to an old infarct, most likely of the middle cerebral artery. The lesion often connects to the lateral ventricles (when it is known as open-lipped), has a round eccentric shape, and is symmetrically bilateral. A second type may be unilateral and fail to communicate with the ventricle (close-lipped). This type has acutely angled borders. There is an association with ventriculomegaly, agenesis of the corpus callosum, and absence of the septum pellucidum.
2. **Amniotic Fluid:** Normal.
3. **Placenta:** Normal.
4. **Measurement Data:** Normal.
5. **When Detectable:** After approximately 18 weeks.

Pitfalls   When the lesion is unilateral, it may be difficult to see when it is on the side of the brain closest to the transducer owing to shadowing from the skull. MRI is helpful when the borders of the cystic area are ill defined.

Differential Diagnosis

1. Holoprosencephaly—The thalami in schizencephaly are normal, as is the third ventricle. (See Chapter 2.11.)
2. Bilateral arachnoid cysts—The cysts do not communicate with the ventricle, usually are asymmetric, and relate to the meninges. (See Chapter 2.4.)
3. Dilated cava septi pellucidi and vergae—These are midline structures within the septum pellucidum, which can grow to a size larger than the normal 5 mm. Bleeding into these normal cysts may be responsible for enlargement. Enlargement of the cavum septi pellucidi or vergae has been associated with mild hydrocephalus but has no other consequences.

Where Else to Look   Look for other signs of fetal hemorrhage, e.g., echogenic material in the ventricles, echogenic rims to the ventricles, and echogenic areas in the brain.

Pregnancy Management

Investigations and Consultations Required   Because of the limited number of cases of schizencephaly that have been diagnosed prenatally, and the potential for misdiagnosis, a complete evaluation should be done to exclude other causes of enlarged ventricles. Amniocentesis should be performed for chromosome analysis and for viral studies. For porencephaly, consideration should be given to alloimmune thrombocytopenia and appropriate maternal antibody studies.

Fetal Intervention   None is indicated.

Monitoring   Normal obstetric management is appropriate. Serial ultrasonograms are useful to document progression, which has been reported.

Pregnancy Course   Should be uncomplicated.

Pregnancy Termination Issues   Because of the rarity of making this diagnosis in the second trimester, an intact fetus should be delivered to confirm the diagnosis.

Delivery   Because of the significant likelihood of neurologic deficits, delivery in a tertiary center may be prudent.

Neonatology

Resuscitation   Generalization regarding appropriateness of intervention following birth for a non-breathing infant in whom an antenatal diagnosis of a cortical destructive lesion has been made is difficult at best. The timing in gestation of the vascular insult, the location and extent of the injury, and the intervening pregnancy history all have an effect on the potential for serious adverse neurologic outcomes. Discussion with the parents prior to delivery of treatment options in the event of initial respiratory depression is important. Such a discussion should be based on the specific clinical situation, taking into account all of the previously cited factors. There are no special technical aspects for initiating respiration in infants with these diagnoses.

Transport   Transfer of an infant to a tertiary center with pediatric neurology and neuroradiology diagnostic capabilities is appropriate to confirm the diagnosis and delineate the extent of cortical injury.

Testing and Confirmation   Computed tomography and MRI, in some circumstances with vascular contrast, are the imaging techniques of choice to describe the pathologic anatomy.

Nursery Management   Beyond a thorough diagnostic evaluation and routine supportive care for a newborn, the other elements of care are dictated by the specific neurologic deficits manifested by a given infant. These may, but do not always, include respiratory control, feeding difficulties, neonatal seizures, and focal motor deficits.

REFERENCES

Bronshtein M, Weiner Z: Prenatal diagnosis of dilated cava septi pellucidi et vergae: Associated anomalies, differential diagnosis, and pregnancy outcome. Obstet Gynecol 1992;80:838–842.

Chamberlain MC, Press GA, Bejar RF: Neonatal schizencephaly: Comparison of brain imaging. Pediatr Neurol 1990;6:382.

Deasy NP, Jarosz JM, Cox TC, Hughes E: Congenital varicella syndrome: Cranial MRI in a long-term survivor. Neuroradiology 1999;41:205–207.

Edmonson SR, Hallak M, Carpenter JR, Cotton DB: Evolution of hydranencephaly following intracerebral hemorrhage. Obstet Gynecol 1992;79:870–871.

Klingensmith WC III, Cioffi-Ragan DT: Schizencephaly: Diagnosis and progression in utero. Radiology 1986;159:617.

Komarniski CA, Cyr DR, Mack LA, Weinberger E: Prenatal diagnosis of schizencephaly. J Ultrasound Med 1990;9:305–307.

Larroche J-C: Fetal encephalopathies of circulatory origin. Biol Neonate 1986;50:61.

McGahan JP, Ellis W, Lindfors KK, et al: Congenital cerebrospinal fluid-containing intracranial abnormalities: A sonographic classification. J Clin Ultrasound 1988;16:531–544.

Sherer DM, Anyaegbunam A, Onyeije C: Antepartum fetal intracranial hemorrhage, predisposing factors and prenatal sonography: A review. Am J Perinatol 1998;15:431–441.

Suchet IB: Schizencephaly: Antenatal and postnatal assessment with colour-flow Doppler imaging. Can Assoc Radiol J 1994;45:193–200.

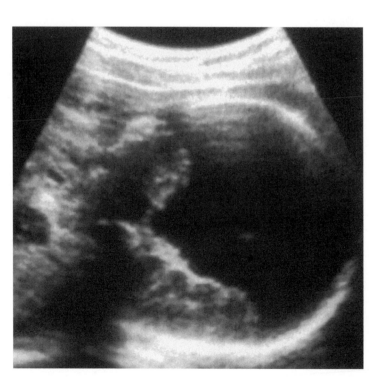

Severe open-lipped schizencephaly with destruction of most of the brain.

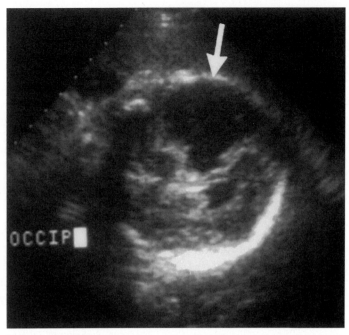

Large porencephalic cystic area (*arrow*) in the left parietotemporal area connecting to the left lateral ventricle presumed to be the long-term result of an infarct and hemorrhage.

2.18 Spinal Dysraphism (Myelomeningocele, Myeloschisis, Meningocele)

Epidemiology/Genetics

Definition Myelomeningocele, the most common type of neural tube defect, is defined by (1) protrusion of neural elements and meninges through open vertebral arches, and (2) associated neurologic deficits.

Epidemiology The incidence is very geography- and population-dependent and ranges from about 1 in 500 to 1 in 2000 births in the United States (M1:F>1).

Embryology Meningomyeloceles result from the failure of the vertebral arches to close prior to the sixth week of pregnancy secondary to a failure of normal neural ectodermal development. They most often occur in the lumbosacral area and are associated with hydrocephalus due to an Arnold-Chiari malformation in 90% of patients. Genitourinary tract and cardiac abnormalities are the most frequent associated malformations. Although most myelomeningoceles are isolated abnormalities, more than 25 genetic, sporadic, and chromosomal multiple malformation syndromes have been described, including trisomy 18.

Inheritance Patterns Isolated defects are due to multifactorial inheritance with a combination of genetic and environmental influences. The risk of recurrence, after one affected pregnancy, is about 2 to 3%. If part of an underlying genetic syndrome, the recurrence risk is that of the underlying syndrome.

Teratogens Two percent of fetuses exposed to valproic acid will have neural tube defects. Folic acid antagonists (methotrexate and aminopterin), vitamin A, thalidomide, maternal diabetes, hyperthermia, and folate deficiency are also associated with an increased risk for neural tube defects.

Screening Maternal serum alpha-fetoprotein screening will detect approximately 80% of meningomyeloceles.

Prognosis Dependent on the size and location of the defect, and the presence of associated abnormalities. In simple isolated defects, there is a 10% risk for mental retardation. Modern surgical and medical treatment has resulted in better long-term function, but urinary tract and orthopedic disability are common long-term problems.

Sonography

FINDINGS

1. **Fetus:**
   a. The cord is tethered and often split into two components. At the site of the cord abnormality, the bony canal is widened and forms a U shape. In the most common form of myelomeningocele, there is a cystic pouch posterior to the spine that contains some linear structures representing nerve fibers. In another form, the cystic pouch contains no nerves (meningocele) and may not be associated with cord tethering. In a third form (myeloschisis), there is no pouch, but the nerves are tethered and exposed to the amniotic fluid if they are not covered with skin. In closed spina bifida, the cord is tethered and split with bony splaying, but there is a thick membrane or skin covering the defect so the alpha-fetoprotein level is normal.
   b. Most spinal dysraphism occurs in the lower lumbar and upper sacral areas, but a few spinal defects are at a higher level. It is important to assess the level accurately, since it affects prognosis. All thoracic lesions are associated with paraparesis. Lesions below L4 are associated with normal ambulation. The prognosis with lesions between L1 and L4 is mixed. The iliac superior crest aspect is at L5 level. The superior vertebral level at which the abnormality first occurs can be established by counting up from this level.
   c. Findings that worsen the prognosis are a marked angulation of the spine at the level of the deformity (a gibbus deformity), a very large or long defect, or a defect at a higher vertebral level than L2.
   d. Technical aspects—Three bony structures make up the surroundings of the spinal canal: The posterior ossification center of the vertebral body and bilateral ossification centers related to the junction of the lamina and pedicle, known as the posterior elements. A transverse spinal view will show these latter structures as echogenic areas that are splayed. A sagittal, posterior view will show a cystic pouch posterior to the spine. If no pouch is present, a depression at the abnormal level will be seen. A coronal view of the spine will show the posterior elements more widely separated at the level of the defect. In a recent review, sonography was 97% sensitive and 100% specific in the diagnosis of open neural tube defect.
   e. Cranial changes
      1. Typically, the head is bilaterally flattened in the frontal region to give a "lemon" or "bullet" shape.
      2. The cerebellum is rounded to form a "banana" shape. Its width is decreased.
      3. The cisterna magna is effaced—This is the strongest sign.
      4. Bilateral lateral and third ventricular dilation may occur.
   f. Leg changes—With severe myelomeningocele, there is absent leg movement and clubfoot, prog-

nostic of poor long-term result. Good leg movement in utero may be followed by lower limb paralysis at birth and has no prognostic significance.

 g. Myelocystocele—This uncommon form of spinal dysraphism may occur at any level of the spine. An inner cyst is connected via a thin stalk to the central canal of the spinal cord through a defect in the posterior spinal cord. No vertebral anomaly is present. A cystic structure is seen alongside the spine, which has a second cyst within it.

2. **Amniotic Fluid:** Usually normal.
3. **Placenta:** Usually normal.
4. **Measurement Data:** Even though the lateral ventricles may be dilated, the head size is small. IUGR may occur.
5. **When Detectable:** Can be detected at 9 weeks by vaginal sonography, but usually detected at 16 to 18 weeks. Approximately 98% are detected by the recognition of the sonographic signs in the head and spine.

Pitfalls

1. Defects involving a single vertebral body or those located in the sacral vertebrae can be difficult to detect.
2. Sacral defects may not be detectable until later because the sacral bones are not ossified until 20 weeks.
3. Occasional spina bifida do not show a "lemon" deformity and even more rarely do not show a "banana" cerebellar change. The cerebellum may lie within the upper cervical canal. Conversely, a "lemon" sign may be seen in a normal fetus.
4. Oblique views through the lumbar spine region can make the gluteus muscles look like a myelomeningocele. 3-D ultrasound may help with confusing cases.
5. Oligohydramnios or maternal obesity may prevent the meningocele sac from being seen.
6. A slanting transducer angulation can create an impression of a widened interpedicular distance.

Differential Diagnosis Sacrococcygeal teratoma—A cystic mass posteroinferior or anterior to the coccyx may be the only finding in this entity, although usually there are solid components. The primary region of abnormality in myelomeningocele is superior to the coccyx, partially or completely fluid-filled, and more or less symmetrical.

Where Else to Look

1. The lower limbs (see above).
2. The head (see above).
3. The kidneys for hydronephrosis; however, the genitourinary system is almost always normal.
4. Other findings of trisomy 18 triploidy, and the VACTERL association, which are associated with myelomeningocele.

Pregnancy Management

Investigations and Consultations Required Amniocentesis should be performed for chromosome studies (approximately a 10% risk of aneuploidy), and confirmation of the diagnosis by amniotic fluid alpha-fetoprotein and acetylcholinesterase. A history of medication exposure should be taken, with special emphasis on anticonvulsants. Congenital heart malformations are associated with neural tube defects; therefore, fetal echocardiography should be done. Consultation with a neurosurgeon and a developmental pediatrician will prepare the family for the multidisciplinary approach necessary for the most favorable outcome in their child.

Fetal Intervention Recent reports have indicated that in utero repairs of myelomeningocele decrease the incidence of hindbrain herniation and may decrease the incidence of shunt-dependent hydrocephalus. Preterm delivery is a significant complication, however, with an average gestational age at delivery of 33 weeks. To date there is no evidence of improved neurologic function in infants undergoing in utero repairs. Parents should have extensive counseling regarding risk and benefits of experimental surgery before referral to a center with expertise in fetal surgery.

Monitoring Serial ultrasonographic examinations every 3 to 4 weeks to assess the degree and/or progression of ventriculomegaly are necessary.

Pregnancy Course For lesions above the lumbar area, the likelihood of progressive ventriculomegaly and macrocephaly is high.

Pregnancy Termination Issues If chromosome studies can be completed on abortus material and no associated anomalies are seen by ultrasonography, suction dilation and evacuation procedures are appropriate.

Delivery The presence of progressive and severe ventriculomegaly may be justification for early delivery after 32 weeks' gestation. The potential benefit of early shunting, however, must be weighed against the risk of prematurity. In the absence of progressive ventriculomegaly, delivery should be at term. The mode of delivery for the fetus with myelomeningocele is controversial. Recent information seems to favor cesarean section because of evidence suggesting a better prognosis for motor function in these infants. Unfortunately, no well-controlled prospective studies have been done.

Neonatology

Resuscitation In the third trimester and prior to the onset of labor, a discussion with the parents of the options for intervention is mandatory. By this point, the presence of other CNS and unrelated organ system anomalies affecting prognosis should be delineated, allowing for a more accurate assessment of potential outcome. Fetal distress in labor and respiratory depression at birth occur frequently, and an antepartum decision regarding resuscitation is helpful.

 Protection of the lesion from trauma and surface contamination is imperative. Use of sterile sheets on the resuscitation table and having one member of the team prepared to cover and pad the lesion using strict aseptic technique are important measures.

Transport   Referral to a tertiary center with a multidisciplinary team for management is always indicated. Protection of the lesion as described above during transport is essential.

Testing and Confirmation   The first priority is the complete assessment of the infant to identify all abnormalities and determine severity of dysfunction. This should include thorough neurologic examination, cranial CT to delineate associated CNS malformations, and evaluation for other organ system anomalies if there are other dysmorphic physical findings.

Nursery Management   The decision regarding direct intervention beginning with surgical closure should again be reviewed with the family as the projected outcome after full evaluation of the infant may not coincide with that from prenatal assessment.

Closure of the defect within 48 hours and/or broad-spectrum antibiotic treatment have been shown to preserve existing peripheral neurologic function.

Following closure of the defect, the three primary management issues, depending on the location and extent of the spinal defect, are concomitant hydrocephalus in 65 to 95% of infants, urinary tract structural and functional abnormalities, and orthopedic deformities and dysfunction. All require management by the appropriate subspecialties.

Surgery

Preoperative Assessment   The location and size of the myelomeningocele defect as well as the presence of a kyphotic deformity are important from the neurosurgical standpoint. The presence of associated cranial and extracranial anomalies, particularly hydrocephalus, is also important prenatal information.

General physical assessment with special attention to the cardiac, pulmonary, and renal systems is important in the decision to proceed with closure of the myelomeningocele and in determining the timing of surgery. A head sonogram is necessary to establish the ventricular size. In addition, careful inspection of the myelomeningocele lesion is essential. If the defect is open and leaking spinal fluid, then despite small ventricular size by sonogram, hydrocephalus may still be present and a ventricular shunt necessary.

Operative Indications   All open (i.e., not completely skin covered) defects require early closure to minimize the risk of infection.

Types of Procedures   Repair involves release of the exposed spinal cord placode from the surrounding skin with closure of the dural tube, muscle, and subcutaneous tissue over the cord. Ventricular shunting, if indicated, is performed at the same procedure.

The in utero repair of myelomeningocele is being performed at a few centers between the 24 and 30 weeks of gestation. Preliminary results suggest a lower incidence of symptomatic hydrocephalus as well as less anatomic distortion of the hindbrain from the Chiari II malformation. No objective improvement in neurologic function from in utero closure has been seen.

Surgical Results/Prognosis   The functional outcome of a child born with myelomeningocele is, in general terms, related to the size and level of the defect. The larger and higher (thoracic or thoracolumbar) lesions are associated with paraparesis or paraplegia, sphincter dysfunction, and a greater risk of spinal deformity. Careful monitoring for signs of lower cranial nerve or brain stem dysfunction can identify those children who develop symptomatic Chiari II malformation that may require surgical decompression. Children with myelomeningocele will require careful long-term follow-up from the neurosurgical, orthopedic, urologic, and pediatric standpoint.

REFERENCES

American Academy of Pediatrics, Committee on Genetics: Folic acid for the prevention of neural tube defects. Pediatrics 1999;104:325–327.

Ball RH, Filly RA, Goldstein RB, Callen PW: The lemon sign: Not a specific indicator of meningomyelocele. J Ultrasound Med 1993;3:131–134.

Benacerraf BR, Stryker J, Frigoletto FD Jr: Abnormal US appearance of the cerebellum (banana sign): Indirect sign of spina bifida. Radiology 1989;171:151–153.

Biggio JR, Owen J, Weinstrom KD: Can prenatal findings predict ambulatory status in fetuses with open spina bifida? Am J Obstet Gynecol 2001;185:1016–1020.

Blaas HK, Eik-Nes SH, Isaksen CV: The detection of spina bifida before 10 gestational weeks using two- and three-dimensional ultrasound. Ultrasound Obstet Gynecol 2000;16:25–29.

Bonilla-Musoles F, Machado LE, Osborne NE: Two- and three-dimensional ultrasound in malformations of the medullary canal: Report of four cases. Prenat Diagn 2001;20:622–626.

Bruner JP, Tulipan N, Paschall RL, et al: Fetal surgery for myelomeningocele and the incidence of shunt dependent hydrocephalus. JAMA 1999;282:1819–1825.

Dennis MA, Drose JA, Pretorius DH, Manco-Johnson ML: Normal fetal sacrum simulating spina bifida: "Pseudodysraphism." Radiology 1985;155:751–754.

Goldstein RB, Podrasky AE, Filly RA, Callen PW: Effacement of the fetal cisterna magna in association with myelomeningocele. Radiology 1989;172:409–413.

Hall JG, Friedman JM, Kenna BA, et al: Clinical, genetic, and epidemiological factors in neural tube defects. Am J Hum Genet 1988;43:827–837.

Jindal R, Mahapatr AK, Kamal R: Spinal dysraphism. Indian J Pediatr 1999;66:697–705.

Kollias SS, Goldstein RB, Cogen PH, Filly RA: Prenatally detected myelomeningoceles: Sonographic accuracy in estimation of the spinal level. Radiology 1992;185:109–112.

Lennon CA, Gray DL: Sensitivity and specificity of ultrasound for the detection of neural tube and ventral wall defects in a high risk population. Obstet Gynecol 1999;4:562–565.

Lirette M, Filly RA: Relationship of fetal hydronephrosis to spinal dysraphism. J Ultrasound Med 1983;2:495–497.

McDonnel GV, Mcann JP: Issues of medical management in adults with spina bifida. Childs Nerv Sust 2000;16:222–227.

Morrow RJ, McNay MB, Whittle MJ: Ultrasound detection of neural tube defects in patients with elevated maternal serum alpha-fetoprotein. Obstet Gynecol 1991;78:1055–1057.

Neutzel MJ: Myelomeningocele: Current concepts of management. Clin Perinatol 1989;16:311.

Nyberg DA, Mack LA, Hirsch J, Mahony BS: Abnormalities of fetal cranial contour in sonographic detection of spina bifida: Evaluation of the lemon sign. Radiology 1988;167:387–392.

Pilu G, Romero R, Reece EA, et al: Subnormal cerebellum in fetuses with spina bifida. Am J Obstet Gynecol 1988;158:1052–1056.

Riegel D, Rotenstein D: Pediatric Neurosurgery, 3rd ed. Philadelphia, WB Saunders, 1994, p 51.

Sauerbrei EE, Grant P: Prenatal diagnosis of myelocystoceles: Report of two cases. J Ultrasound Med 1999;18:247–252.

Sutton LN, Adzick NS, Bilaniuk LT, et al: Improvement in hindbrain herniation demonstrated by serial magnetic resonance imaging following fetal surgery for myelomeningocele. JAMA 1999;282:1826–1831.

Van Allen MI, Kalousek DK, Chernoff GF, et al: Evidence for multi-site closure of the neural tube in humans. Am J Med Genet 1993;47:723–743.

Van den Hof MC, Nicolaides KH, Campbell J, Campbell S: Evaluation of the lemon and banana signs in one hundred thirty fetuses with open spina bifida. Am J Obstet Gynecol 1990;162:322–327.

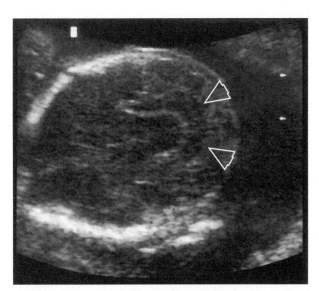

Spinal dysraphism. Cranial changes of Arnold-Chiari malformation; the cerebellum (*arrows*) forms a "banana" shape and there is no visible cisterna magna. The anterior aspect of the skull is flattened, so the skull assumes a lemon shape.

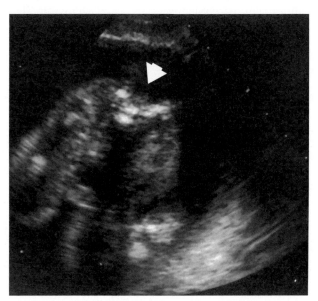

Transverse view of myeloschisis. The lumbar spine lateral ossification centers are separated and there is a dip between them (*arrow*).

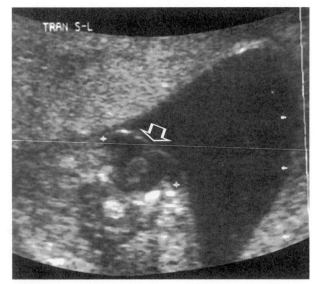

Myelomeningocele. There is a similar appearance, but a membrane covers the defect (*arrow*, between +'s). Some nerves can be seen within the meningocele.

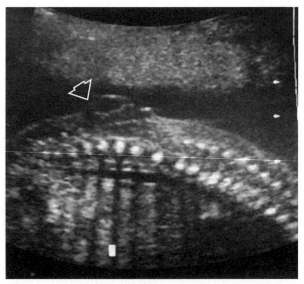

Sagittal view. The septated cystic mass (*arrow*) can be seen in the L4/L5 area.

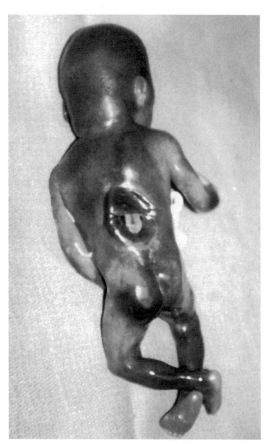

A 20-week fetus with lower thoracic–upper lumbar meningomyelocele.
Neural elements are visible below the ruptured sac.

2.19 Vein of Galen Malformation

Epidemiology/Genetics

Definition Aneurysms of the vein of Galen are dilations of the vein ranging from a large single arteriovenous malformation to multiple smaller communications.

Epidemiology Rare (M2:F1).

Embryology The cerebral vessels derive from a primitive plexus that differentiates into arteries and veins. It is not clear how, when, or why cerebral or other arteriovenous malformations arise. Pathologically, the vein of Galen appears dilated and communicates with normal-appearing arteries. Most cases occur as isolated abnormalities. Congenital heart defects, cystic hygromas, and hydrops are associated with vein of Galen malformations.

Inheritance Patterns Sporadic.

Teratogens None suspected.

Prognosis Infants presenting with heart failure or hydrops usually die. Later childhood presentation is associated with a 20% surgical mortality rate. Successfully repaired survivors are often normal.

Sonography

FINDINGS

1. **Fetus:**
   a. CNS
      1. There is a large irregularly shaped, ovoid, cystic space—the aneurysm—in the posterior aspect of the brain in the midline. The aneurysm lies posterosuperior to the third ventricle. Multiple small feeder arteries can be seen with real-time and color flow Doppler. A large tubular vein flows toward the occipital region. Careful color flow Doppler analysis of feeder arteries to the aneurysm helps surgical planning. Three-dimensional color power angiography aids in seeing the feeder vessels. Poor prognostic factors include the numerous feeder vessels, a wide draining vein (the straight sinus), the existence of "steal" retrograde aortic flow, and evidence of a high output state (e.g., ascites).
      2. Secondary third and lateral ventriculomegaly may be present.
   b. Thorax—The cardiac size may be increased, with large neck arteries and superior vena cava.
   c. Abdomen
      1. Hepatosplenomegaly may be seen.
      2. Secondary hydrops, due to congenital heart failure arteriovenous shunting, may be the presenting feature. There may be ascites, pleural effusion, pericardial effusion, and skin thickening.
2. **Amniotic Fluid:** Normal.
3. **Placenta:** Normal unless hydrops is present.
4. **Measurement Data:** Normal.
5. **When Detectable:** About 14 weeks.

Pitfalls

1. Confusion with a quadrigeminal cistern, a normal cystic structure posterior to the third ventricle, may occur. Doppler ultrasonography will show no flow in the normal cistern.
2. The cavum vergi and septum pellucidum usually extend anteriorly but may persist only posteriorly.

Differential Diagnosis

1. Quadrigeminal cistern.
2. Centrally placed arachnoid cyst.

Where Else to Look Any central intracranial cystic structure of uncertain origin should be examined with Doppler ultrasonography, and the heart and abdomen should be examined for cardiomegaly and hydrops. Hydrops and cardiomegaly should precipitate a look for a vein of Galen malformation.

Pregnancy Management

Investigations or Consultations Required No further diagnostic evaluation is necessary if Doppler confirms the vascular nature of the lesion. Fetal echocardiography may be helpful in detecting early signs of congestive heart failure. A pediatric neurosurgeon should be consulted to assist with prenatal management and to discuss the postnatal treatment options with the family.

Fetal Intervention In utero therapy is not indicated.

Monitoring Because of the high risk of fetal hydrops and subsequent development of preeclampsia in some of these cases, careful follow-up by a perinatologist is appropriate. Frequent ultrasonographic studies should be performed (e.g., every 2 weeks), since more severe hydrops may precipitate early delivery.

Pregnancy Course The high risk of fetal hydrops and subsequent preeclampsia or the development of obstructive hydrocephalus makes this fetal malformation one with significant risk for obstetric complications.

Pregnancy Termination Issues   As with all brain malformations, termination of pregnancy and subsequent fetal autopsy must be performed in institutions with special expertise in neuropathology.

Delivery   In severe cases, nonaggressive management may be the best approach. In those cases without complications, elective delivery, when fetal lung maturity is attained, might improve prognosis. However, there is little information available on which to base recommendations regarding timing or mode of delivery.

Neonatology

Resuscitation   The approach to resuscitation is based on the extent of congestive heart failure and hydrops present prior to delivery in addition to the anatomic characteristics and thus surgical correctability of the lesion. Planned delivery after fetal lung maturity is achieved, and avoidance of fetal distress followed by immediate and atraumatic resuscitation offers the best opportunity for favorable outcome. Consideration should be given to early institution of inotropic agents to improve myocardial function and paralysis to reduce oxygen consumption and fluctuations in cerebral vascular pressures. Drainage of serous fluid collections (pleural, pericardial, and peritoneal), if present, may be needed to facilitate cardiorespiratory adaptation.

As with any abnormality in which there is a strong chance of neonatal death and of a poor long-term prognosis, a discussion with the parents regarding nonintervention is appropriate.

Transport   Referral to a tertiary center with pediatric cardiology and pediatric neurosurgery capabilities is imperative. Support of oxygenation and perfusion during transport is critical.

Testing and Confirmation   Vein of Galen aneurysms present in the newborn period with heart failure and/or hydrops. Later childhood presentations include headache or other central nervous system symptoms and are associated with a better prognosis. Occasionally, vein of Galen malformations are associated with hydrocephalus or porencephaly. Postnatal CT or MRI scans and arteriograms can define this abnormality.

Nursery Management   The priority issues are maintenance of adequate gas exchange and tissue perfusion and avoidance of wide fluctuations in cerebral intravascular pressure. Myocardial ischemia and intracranial hemorrhage are the reported causes of death. Measures to control congestive heart failure include inotropic agents, diuretics and fluid restriction, and correction of metabolic abnormalities such as acidosis, hypoglycemia, and electrolyte imbalances.

Timing and techniques for closure of the feeding vessels to the aneurysm are determined both by the infant's clinical status and by the vascular anatomy of the lesion. Magnetic resonance imaging is the preferable study to determine the latter.

Surgery

Preoperative Assessment   Vein of Galen malformations can be divided into two distinct types.
1. True aneurysmal dilation of the vein of Galen as a consequence of a true arteriovenous fistula with shunting of arterial blood into an embryologic venous precursor, the median vein of the prosencephalon.
2. Secondary enlargement of the vein of Galen as a consequence of an adjacent parenchymal arteriovenous malformation.

Assessment of cardiac status as well as associated intracranial vascular or structural anomalies, hydrocephalus, or hemorrhages is required.

Post-natal assessment involves MRI evaluation and cerebral angiography. Management in children who are asymptomatic, i.e., without cardiac failure or hydrocephalus, is observation alone with follow-up ultrasonogram at 3 or 6 months of age.

Operative Indications   If the malformation persists, then angiography and treatment are performed at 6 to 8 months of age. In children who present with cardiac failure or progressive hydrocephalus, immediate diagnostic angiography is indicated.

Types of Procedures   Treatment of vein of Galen malformations is either transarterial or transvenous endovascular embolization with obliteration of the arteriovenous fistula. In some situations, direct surgical obliteration may be necessary, but this is associated with significant morbidity and mortality. Vein of Galen dilations are treated by addressing the primary arteriovenous malformation.

Surgical Results/Prognosis   In general, excellent outcomes are obtained with modern endovascular treatment, with two-thirds of children having an excellent outcome with minimal mortality and morbidity. Neonates who present with cardiac failure that cannot be managed medically fair poorly. This group includes almost all vein of Galen aneurysms diagnosed in utero.

REFERENCES

Dan U, Shalev E, Greif M, Weiner E: Prenatal diagnosis of fetal brain arteriovenous malformation: The use of color Doppler imaging. J Clin Ultrasound 1992;20:149–151.

Garcia-Monaco R, Lasjaunias P, Berenstein A: Therapeutic management of vein of Galen aneurysmal malformations. In Vinuela F, et al (eds): Interventional Neuroradiology: Endovascular Therapy of the Central Nervous System. New York, Raven Press, 1992, p 113.

Heling KS, Chaoui R, Bollman R: Prenatal diagnosis of an aneurysm of the vein of Galen with three-dimensional color power angiography. Ultrasound Obstet Gynecol 2000;15:333–336.

Hoffman HJ, Chuang S, Hendrick EB, Humphreys RP: Aneurysms of the vein of Galen: Experience at the Hospital for Sick Children, Toronto. J Neurosurg 1982;57:316–322.

Jeanty P, Kepple D, Roussis P, Shah D: In utero detection of cardiac failure from an aneurysm of the vein of Galen. Am J Obstet Gynecol 1990;163:50–51.

Sepulveda W, Platt CC, Fisk NM: Prenatal diagnosis of cerebral arteriovenous malformation using color Doppler ultrasonography: Case report and review of the literature. Ultrasound Obstet Gynecol 1995; 6:182–186.

Vintzileos AM, Eisenfeld LI, Campbell WA, et al: Prenatal ultrasonic diagnosis of arteriovenous malformation of the vein of Galen. Am J Perinatol 1986;3:209–211.

Yuval Y, Lerner A, Lipitz Z, et al: Prenatal diagnosis of vein of Galen aneurysmal malformation: Report of two cases with proposal for prognostic indices. Prenatal Diag 1997;17:972–977.

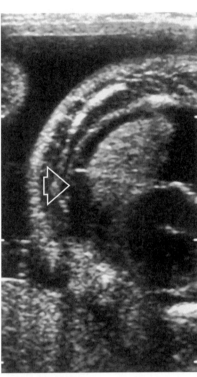

Vein of Galen aneurysm, transverse view through the chest. There is a pleural effusion and skin thickening.

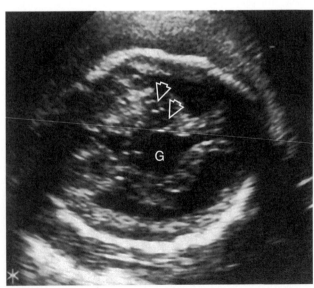

Axial view at the level of the third ventricle. The large black area (G) is the vein of Galen aneurysm. The small cystic areas (*arrows*) adjacent to the big cystic area represent feeder arteries.

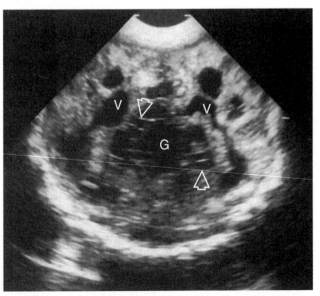

Coronal view shows the aneurysm (G) with feeder vessels (*arrows*). There is a mild lateral ventriculomegaly (V).

Cardiac Entities 3

3.1 Transposition of the Great Arteries (D-Transposition of the Great Arteries)

Epidemiology/Genetics

Definition The aorta connects with the right ventricle, and the main pulmonary artery connects with the left ventricle. The most common form of transposition is D-transposition, sometimes referred to as complete transposition. Patients are cyanotic, since deoxygenated blood (i.e., systemic venous blood) is pumped by the right ventricle to the body and oxygenated blood (i.e., pulmonary venous blood) is pumped by the left ventricle to the lungs. In D-transposition of the great arteries, the heart tube loops during development to the right (D-looping), resulting in normal ventricular orientation. D-transposition of the great arteries is the focus of this section.

Complete transposition should be distinguished from congenitally corrected transposition of the great arteries, sometimes referred to as physiologically corrected or L-transposition. Usually in physiologically corrected transposition, the heart tube loops to the left (L-looping), resulting in ventricular inversion. Anatomically, transposition is present because the right ventricle connects with the aorta and the left ventricle connects with the main pulmonary artery. Physiologically, the baby is not cyanotic. Systemic venous blood is pumped by the left ventricle to the pulmonary artery, and pulmonary venous blood is pumped by the right ventricle to the aorta.

Epidemiology Prevalence per 1000 live births: 0.201 to 0.432. Accounts for 4% to 6% of children with cardiac disease.

Embryology Transposition of the great arteries is probably caused by an abnormality in conotruncal development at 4 to 5 weeks' gestation.

Inheritance Pattern Recurrence risk is 1.5% when one sibling is affected and 5% when two siblings are affected. Rarely associated with chromosomal abnormalities or other syndromes.

Teratogens Retinoic acid has induced transposition in mouse embryo models. Maternal diabetes mellitus.

Prognosis Operative mortality is 3 to 5% with corrective surgery, and midterm results are good. Long-term results are unknown at this time.

Early data suggest that prenatal diagnosis may improve the preoperative condition of the neonate. Data are mixed as to whether prenatal diagnosis lowers the operative mortality rate.

Sonography

FINDINGS

1. **Fetus:**
   a. The diagnosis is made by identifying the origin of the aorta from the right ventricle and the origin of the main pulmonary artery from the left ventricle. Establishing the origins of the branch pulmonary arteries identifies the main pulmonary artery. Demonstrating the vessel supplying the head and neck vessels identifies the aorta.
   b. The aortic valve is most commonly to the right of and anterior to the pulmonary valve, but the aorta can be side-by-side with, straight anterior to, or even left of and anterior to the pulmonary valve.
   c. Ventricular septal defect is present in 30 to 50% of patients.
   d. Restrictive patent foramen ovale can be associated with worse postnatal cyanosis.
   e. Small or restrictive ductus arteriosus may also be associated with worse postnatal outcome.
   f. The ascending aorta and main pulmonary artery should be measured and compared with normative data. Ascending aortic hypoplasia occurs in association with coarctation, interrupted aortic arch, and subvalvular aortic stenosis. Marked main pulmonary artery hypoplasia is associated with subvalvular and valvular pulmonary stenosis.
   g. Less common associated abnormalities include hypoplastic tricuspid valve or right ventricle, pulmonary stenosis, subaortic stenosis, coarctation or interrupted arch, and coronary abnormalities.
2. **Amniotic Fluid:** Normal.

3. **Placenta:** Normal.
4. **Measurement Data:** Normal.
5. **When Detectable:** Transabdominal imaging at 16 to 18 weeks. Although the fetal heart can be examined by transvaginal echocardiography at 13 to 15 weeks, the diagnosis of transposition of the great arteries has not yet been reported at this stage.

Pitfalls

1. Transposition can be missed if the main pulmonary artery is not distinguished from the ascending aorta. Identification of the branch pulmonary arteries is crucial in reliably establishing which great vessel is the main pulmonary artery. Other methods to exclude transposition, such as the crossing of the great vessels, are not consistently reliable.
2. Transposition can be confused with double-outlet right ventricle or tetralogy of Fallot.

Differential Diagnosis   When one great vessel overrides a ventricular septal defect, transposition can be confused with either double-outlet right ventricle or tetralogy of Fallot. In double-outlet right ventricle, one great vessel and the majority of the other arise from the right ventricle. It may be confusing when the aorta arises from the right ventricle and the pulmonary artery straddles the ventricular septal defect. When the pulmonary artery is more than 50% above the right ventricle, the diagnosis is double-outlet right ventricle. When the pulmonary artery is more than 50% above the left ventricle, the diagnosis is transposition with ventricular septal defect.

In tetralogy of Fallot, the aorta overrides a ventricular septal defect and the main pulmonary artery arises from the right ventricle. If the great vessels are inaccurately identified (i.e., the main pulmonary artery and the aorta are confused for one another), then transposition of the great arteries with ventricular septal defect could be confused with tetralogy of Fallot.

Where Else to Look

1. It is unusual for complete transposition of the great arteries to be associated with other noncardiac abnormalities.
2. Look for evidence of hydrops—ascites, pleural and pericardial effusion, and skin thickening.

Pregnancy Management

Investigations and Consultations Required   Chromosomal studies should be done, including in situ hybridization for chromosome 22q deletion.

Pediatric cardiology consultation should be obtained for confirmation of and/or definitive diagnosis and to coordinate the prenatal and postnatal cardiac plans.

Fetal Intervention   None.

Monitoring   Repeat echocardiography is indicated at 28 to 30 weeks, primarily to assess the outflow tracts, ductus arteriosus, and foramen ovale.

Pregnancy Course   Generally well tolerated.

Pregnancy Termination Issues   Given the probability of a favorable outcome, termination is unusual for this lesion. If chosen, an intact fetus should be delivered for confirmation of diagnosis.

Delivery   Delivery should be performed at a tertiary center where pediatric cardiology consultation is immediately available and where balloon atrial septostomy can be performed on an emergency basis.

Neonatology

Resuscitation   Spontaneous respirations are generally present, and immediate mechanical ventilation is usually not necessary. Secure venous access is needed, and, depending on the oxygen saturation and clinical condition, an arterial catheter may be indicated as well. Prostaglandin E is sometimes started to improve mixing by maintaining ductal patency.

Transport   The neonate should be transported to a center with expertise in echocardiographic diagnosis, interventional catheterization, and pediatric cardiac surgery. Equipment should be immediately available for endotracheal intubation and mechanical ventilation.

Testing and Confirmation   A complete and accurate diagnosis can generally be obtained using echocardiography alone.

Nursery Management   Oxygen saturations between 70% and 85% without metabolic acidosis are desirable. When oxygen saturations are inadequate, supplemental oxygen can be administered to increase pulmonary venous saturation. If the oxygen saturation is still inadequate, prostaglandin E and balloon atrial septostomy can be helpful. Maintaining systemic blood pressure will often facilitate mixing as well.

Surgery

Preoperative Assessment   Echocardiographic diagnosis is generally definitive.

Operative Indications   All patients with transposition require surgery. This generally should be performed after the pulmonary resistance falls and is usually within the first week of life. In some cases, associated lesions such as pulmonary stenosis or ventricular septal defect may change the timing of surgery.

Types of Procedures   The arterial switch operation is most commonly used to repair D-transposition of the great arteries. The great vessels are transected and reconnected to the appropriate ventricles. The coronary arteries are removed from the aortic root and translocated to the neoaortic root (i.e., the great vessel arising from the left ventricle).

A Rastelli operation is performed when transposition of the great arteries is associated with ventricular septal defect and subvalvular pulmonary stenosis. In such cases, the pulmonary stenosis does not allow an arterial switch procedure, since postoperatively there would be aortic stenosis. In a Rastelli operation, the pulmonary venous blood is baffled from the left ventricle through the ventricular septal defect to the aorta, and a homograft or conduit is placed from the right ventricle to the pulmonary artery. This allows physiologic correction, and the left ventricle becomes the systemic ventricle (in contrast to the atrial switches).

In rare cases, in which there is severe ventricular hypoplasia or straddling of atrioventricular valves that does not allow ventricular septal defect closure, single ventricle operation is required.

Surgical Results/Prognosis The operative mortality rate for the arterial switch procedure is between 3 and 5%. Subsequent reoperation or interventional catheterization procedures are required in 10% of patients. Late complications of the arterial switch operation include supravalvular pulmonary stenosis, neoaortic root enlargement, aortic regurgitation, left ventricular dysfunction, branch pulmonary artery stenosis, aortic anastomotic stenosis, and coronary artery stenosis or distortion. Long-term survival appears to be excellent.

Patients who have undergone the arterial switch have a 10 to 15% probability of significant right ventricular dysfunction or tricuspid regurgitation.

REFERENCES

Bonnet D, Coltri A, Butera G, et al: Prenatal diagnosis of transposition of great vessels reduces neonatal morbidity and mortality. Arch Mal Coeur Vaiss 1999;92:637–640.

Frohn-Mulder IM, Wesby SE, Bouwhuis C, et al: Chromosome 22q11 deletions in patients with selected outflow tract malformations. Genet Couns 1999;10:35–41.

Fyler DC: Trends. In Fyler DC (ed): Nadas' Pediatric Cardiology. Philadelphia, Hanley & Belfus, 1992, pp 273–284.

Goldmuntz E, Clark BJ, Mitchell LE, et al: Frequency of 22q11 deletions in patients with conotruncal defects [see comments]. J Am Coll Cardiol 1998;32:492–498.

Johnson BL, Fyfe DA, Gillette PC, et al: In utero diagnosis of interrupted aortic arch with transposition of the great arteries and tricuspid atresia. Am Heart J 1989;117:690–692.

Kumar RK, Newburger JW, Gauvreau K, et al: Comparison of outcome when hypoplastic left heart syndrome and transposition of the great arteries are diagnosed prenatally versus when diagnosis of these two conditions is made only postnatally. Am J Cardiol 1999;83:1649–1653.

Maeno YV, Kamenir SA, Sinclair B, et al: Prenatal features of ductus arteriosus constriction and restrictive foramen ovale in D-transposition of the great arteries. Circulation 1999;99:1209–1214.

Melchionda S, Digilio MC, Mingarelli R, et al: Transposition of the great arteries associated with deletion of chromosome 22q11. Am J Cardiol 1995;75:95–98.

Nakajima Y, Morishima M, Nakazawa M, et al: Distribution of fibronectin, type I collagen, type IV collagen, and laminin in the cardiac jelly of the mouse embryonic heart with retinoic acid-induced complete transposition of the great arteries. Anat Rec 1997;249:478–485.

Nora JJ, Nora AH: Update on counseling the family with a first-degree relative with a congenital heart defect. Am J Med Genet 1988;29:137–142.

Yasui H, Morishima M, Nakazawa M, et al: Developmental spectrum of cardiac outflow tract anomalies encompassing transposition of the great arteries and dextroposition of the aorta: Pathogenic effect of extrinsic retinoic acid in the mouse embryo. Anat Rec 1999;254:253–260.

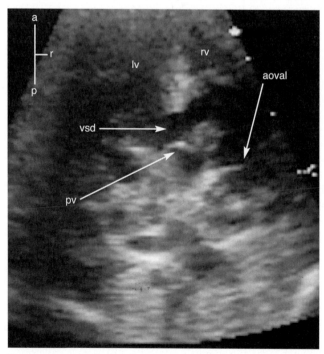

Transposition of the great arteries. Visualization of the origin of the left pulmonary artery (lpa) establishes that the vessel arising from the left ventricle (lv) is the main pulmonary artery (mpa). The absence of branching of the vessel arising from the right ventricle (rv) establishes that the other vessel is the aorta (ao). Visualization of the branch pulmonary arteries is the easiest way to accurately identify the great vessels.

Transposition of the great arteries with ventricular septal defect. The aortic valve (aoval) receives blood from the right ventricle (rv). While the pulmonary valve (pv) straddles the ventricular septum above a malalignment type ventricular septal defect (vsd), the pulmonary valve is more than 50% related to the left ventricle (lv). Therefore, this is transposition of the great arteries rather than double-outlet right ventricle. Also, note that if the aorta and main pulmonary artery were misidentified, one might incorrectly believe that it is the aorta that is overriding and that the diagnosis is tetralogy of Fallot.

3.2 Tetralogy of Fallot

Epidemiology/Genetics

Definition   A conoventricular abnormality involving (1) an anterior malalignment type of ventricular septal defect, (2) subvalvular and often valvular pulmonary stenosis, (3) overriding of the aorta above the ventricular septal defect, and (4) right ventricular hypertrophy. The ventricular septal defect is located below the aortic valve.

Epidemiology   Prevalence per 1000 livebirths: 0.2 to 0.3. Accounts for 6 to 8% of children with cardiac disease.

Embryology   The conus or infundibulum is muscular tissue derived from the bulbus cordis, forming a "collar" of muscle below a semilunar valve and separating it from direct continuity with the atrioventricular valves. Normally, the conus develops below the pulmonary valve and there is absence of the subaortic conus. Hypoplasia of the subpulmonary conus is hypothesized to be the primary abnormality resulting in the four features of tetralogy of Fallot.

Inheritance Pattern   Recurrence of congenital heart disease in siblings of patients with tetralogy of Fallot is 2.5% if one sibling is affected and 8% if two siblings are affected. The recurrence risk for congenital heart defects in offspring when a parent is affected with tetralogy of Fallot is 2.5% when the mother is affected and 1.5% when the father is affected.

Among patients with tetralogy of Fallot, the prevalence of the chromosome 22q microdeletion is 11 to 34%. When there is a right aortic arch, associated dysplastic pulmonary valve syndrome, or associated pulmonary valve atresia, the risk of chromosome 22q microdeletion is greater. Tetralogy of Fallot can occur in trisomy 21, Melnick-Needles syndrome, Adams-Oliver syndrome, prune belly syndrome, and CHARGE syndrome.

Teratogens   Associations include valproate, amantadine, coumadin, and maternal diabetes mellitus.

Prognosis   The prognosis is worse in the subset with pulmonary atresia and/or with severely hypoplastic branch pulmonary arteries. These patients may require multiple operations and interventional catheterization procedures to recruit an adequate pulmonary bed to allow repair.

Sonography

FINDINGS

1. **Fetus:**
   a. The anterior malalignment type of ventricular septal defect is clear in long-axis views of the heart by recognizing the overriding aorta above the ventricular septal defect. The ascending aorta is often dilated, but not always so.
   b. Short-axis views of the heart at a level just apical to the aortic valve are also helpful in appreciating the ventricular septal defect, the anterior deviation of conal septum, and the severity of outflow obstruction. The pulmonary valve, main pulmonary artery, and branch pulmonary arteries should be measured and compared with normative data, since with more severe obstruction there is a greater degree of hypoplasia.
   c. The direction of ductal flow should be assessed. With more severe pulmonary obstruction, ductal flow will reverse and course from aorta to pulmonary artery. Reversed ductal flow suggests that postnatally the fetuses will be ductus dependent.
   d. Tetralogy of Fallot can occur with pulmonary valve atresia. The main pulmonary artery may or may not be absent. Recognition of the absence of antegrade pulmonary blood flow across the pulmonary valve is important. In such cases, pulmonary blood flow may be supplied by aorta to pulmonary artery collaterals or a patent ductus arteriosus. These collaterals have continuous flow and can sometimes be identified prenatally.
   e. An unusual variant of tetralogy is that in which the pulmonary valve is quite dysplastic (sometimes incorrectly referred to as absent pulmonary valve syndrome). There is considerable pulmonary regurgitation and the pulmonary stenosis is usually only moderate. Typically, the main and branch pulmonary arteries are quite dilated and the ductus arteriosus is absent.
   f. A left superior vena cava is present in 15% of patients with tetralogy of Fallot.
   g. Levorotation of the heart is more frequent in tetralogy of Fallot.
2. **Amniotic Fluid:** Usually normal. Polyhydramnios and hydrops can develop when there is pulmonary and tricuspid regurgitation, especially when there is dysplastic pulmonary valve syndrome.
3. **Placenta:** Normal.
4. **Measurement Data:** Normal.
5. **When Detectable:** Identified at 16 to 18 weeks with transabdominal imaging. Tetralogy of Fallot has been diagnosed at 13 to 14 weeks with transvaginal imaging, but the sensitivity and specificity at this gestational age are unknown.

Pitfalls

1. An overriding great vessel above a ventricular septal defect is a nonspecific finding in tetralogy of Fallot and

can also be seen in double-outlet right ventricle, transposition of the great arteries with ventricular septal defect, or truncus arteriosus. One must not assume that the overriding great vessel is the aorta.

2. Tetralogy of Fallot is distinguished from double-outlet right ventricle by the degree of aortic overriding and the presence of subaortic conus. In tetralogy, the aorta is committed to the left ventricle (i.e., is less than 50% above the right ventricle), and in double-outlet right ventricle the aorta will be more than 50% above the right ventricle. In tetralogy of Fallot, the aortic valve is in continuity with the anterior leaflet of the mitral valve whereas in double-outlet right ventricle, there usually is subaortic conus.

3. Tetralogy of Fallot can also be confused with truncus arteriosus. In truncus arteriosus, there is a single semilunar root from which both the branch pulmonary arteries and the ascending aorta arise.

4. Tetralogy of Fallot can be confused with transposition of the great arteries with ventricular septal defect.

5. The severity of pulmonary stenosis in tetralogy can progress in utero and pulmonary atresia can even develop. Sometimes it is difficult to identify antegrade flow across the pulmonary valve. Detection of even a small amount of pulmonary regurgitation is a clue that the pulmonary valve is patent.

Differential Diagnosis   As discussed earlier, tetralogy of Fallot can be confused with double-outlet right ventricle, transposition with ventricular septal defect, or truncus arteriosus. These lesions are distinguished by careful identification of the ascending aorta and main pulmonary artery and their relationships to the ventricles.

Where Else to Look   A complete fetal survey should be performed because of the association with trisomy 21, 18, and 13. There is a 16% association with noncardiac anomalies. Although tetralogy of Fallot is not an essential component of any syndrome, it is frequently associated with malformation groups (e.g., cardiofacial, CHARGE, VACTERL) and has been described in the Lange, Goldenhar, and Klippel-Feil syndromes. Look for (1) facial and orbital asymmetry and hypotelorism; (2) hemivertebrae, caudal regression, and short cervical spine; (3) gut obstruction; (4) intrauterine growth retardation; and (5) genital hypoplasia in males.

Pregnancy Management

Investigations and Consultations Required   Chromosomal analysis and complete fetal survey indicated. Chromosome studies are essential, including fluorescent in situ hybridization for the 22q11 deletion. Up to 27% of prenatally diagnosed cases will have a chromosome abnormality. Fluorescent in situ hybridization assay is indicated, since the chromosome 22q microdeletion occurs in 11 to 34% of patients with tetralogy of Fallot. The family should meet with a pediatric cardiologist to discuss the cardiac findings and to coordinate a prenatal and postnatal management plan.

Fetal Intervention   None.

Monitoring   A fetal echocardiogram should be repeated at 28 and 34 weeks to assess the growth of the pulmonary valve, main pulmonary artery, and branch pulmonary arteries. One should also exclude the development of pulmonary atresia.

Pregnancy Course   Generally well tolerated.

Pregnancy Termination Issues   Given the generally favorable prognosis after surgical treatment of tetralogy of Fallot (without pulmonary atresia or dysplastic pulmonary valve syndrome), most families continue to term unless associated syndromes or chromosomal abnormalities are identified. If termination is chosen, an intact fetus should be delivered for confirmation of diagnosis and exclusion of noncardiac abnormalities.

Delivery   Delivery should be performed at a regional center where pediatric cardiology consultation is immediately available, given the potential for a ductus-dependent lesion.

Neonatology

Resuscitation   Spontaneous respirations are usually present and mechanical ventilation is not necessary. Secure venous access may be needed, depending on the oxygen saturation and the clinical condition. Prostaglandin E is not started unless ductal patency is required to achieve adequate pulmonary blood flow.

Transport   Transport to a center with pediatric cardiology and cardiac surgery capability should be arranged. If the infant becomes symptomatic, with worsening cyanosis or perfusion, transport should occur immediately. Consultation with a pediatric cardiologist prior to transport to consider the need for prostglandin E_1 infusion to maintain ductal flow is necessary.

Testing and Confirmation   A definitive diagnosis of tetralogy of Fallot and identification of associated findings should be made with echocardiography.

Nursery Management   The ductus arteriosus is allowed to close and the baby observed to ensure that there is adequate pulmonary blood flow. If the oxygen saturation exceeds 85% after the ductus is closed, there generally is sufficient antegrade pulmonary blood flow to allow the baby to be discharged home.

Surgery

Preoperative Assessment   In most cases, echocardiography is sufficient for preoperative diagnosis. Cardiac catheterization is rarely needed to exclude coronary artery abnormalities, additional ventricular septal defects, or branch pulmonary artery distortion. In tetralogy of Fallot with pulmonary atresia, cardiac catheterization is required, since associated aorta to pulmonary artery collaterals and distal branch pulmonary artery distortion are not well seen with echocardiography.

Operative Indications   All patients require surgical repair. Most patients are electively repaired between 2 and 6 months of age or earlier, if cyanosis worsens or tetralogy of Fallot spells occur.

When there is pulmonary atresia with an unreliable source of pulmonary blood flow, surgery will be needed in the newborn period.

Centers that do not do repairs in infancy may perform a Blalock-Taussig shunt to achieve a reliable source of pulmonary blood flow. Repair is then performed at 2 to 5 years of age.

Types of Procedures   Surgical repair involves closure of the ventricular septal defect either through a right ventriculotomy or via a transtricuspid valve approach. The subpulmonary obstruction is resected and frequently an outflow patch is placed to enlarge the subpulmonary area. If the pulmonary annulus is hypoplastic, the patch may need to extend across the annulus and into the main pulmonary artery. Branch pulmonary artery stenoses are addressed at surgery as well.

Some centers do not advise early infant repair of tetralogy of Fallot and, if cyanosis worsens, may perform a Blalock-Taussig shunt. Surgery is then electively performed at 2 to 3 years of age. Alternatively, others may attempt to increase pulmonary blood flow to delay surgery by performing balloon dilation of valvular pulmonary stenosis.

Surgical Results/Prognosis   Operative mortality for tetralogy of Fallot is less than 5%. Approximately 5 to 10% of patients may require intervention for peripheral pulmonary artery stenosis postoperatively, but these stenoses can often be addressed with interventional catheterization. Balloon dilation and/or placement of intravascular stents is used to relieve the branch pulmonary artery distortion.

REFERENCES

Achiron R, Rotstein Z, Lipitz S, et al: First-trimester diagnosis of fetal congenital heart disease by transvaginal ultrasonography. Obstet Gynecol 1994;84:69–72.

Allan LD, Sharland GK, Milburn A, et al: Prospective diagnosis of 1006 consecutive cases of congenital heart disease in the fetus. J Am Coll Cardiol 1994;23:1452–1458.

Balde MD, Breitbach OP, Wettstein A, et al: [Tetralogy of Fallot following coumarin administration in early pregnancy: An embryopathy?] Geburtshilfe Frauenheilkd 1988;48:182–183.

DeVore GR, Siassi B, Platt LD: Fetal echocardiography. VIII. Aortic root dilatation: A marker for tetralogy of Fallot. Am J Obstet Gynecol 1988;159:129–136.

Donnenfeld AE, Conard KA, Roberts NS, et al: Melnick-Needles syndrome in males: A lethal multiple congenital anomalies syndrome. Am J Med Genet 1987;27:159–173.

Espinasse M, Manouvrier S, Boute O, Farriaux JP: [Embryofetopathy due to valproate: A pathology only little known. Apropos of 4 cases (see comments)]. Arch Pediatr 1996;3:896–899.

Fouron JC, Sahn DJ, Bender R, et al: Prenatal diagnosis and circulatory characteristics in tetralogy of Fallot with absent pulmonary valve. Am J Cardiol 1989;64:547–549.

Frohn-Mulder IM, Wesby SE, Bouwhuis C, et al: Chromosome 22q11 deletions in patients with selected outflow tract malformations. Genet Couns 1999;10:35–41.

Fyler DC: Trends. In Fyler DC (ed): Nadas' Pediatric Cardiology. Philadelphia, Hanley & Belfus, 1992, pp 273–284.

Goldmuntz E, Clark BJ, Mitchell LE, et al: Frequency of 22q11 deletions in patients with conotruncal defects. J Am Coll Cardiol 1998;32:492–498.

Hornberger LK, Sanders SP, Sahn DJ, et al: In utero pulmonary artery and aortic growth and potential for progression of pulmonary outflow tract obstruction in tetralogy of Fallot. J Am Coll Cardiol 1995;25:739–745.

Iserin L, de Lonlay P, Viot G, et al: Prevalence of the microdeletion 22q11 in newborn infants with congenital conotruncal cardiac anomalies. Eur J Pediatr 1998;157:881–884.

Kim WG, Suh JW, Chi JG: Nitrofen-induced congenital malformations of the heart and great vessels in rats: An animal model. J Pediatr Surg 1999;34:1782–1786.

Kuribayashi T, Roberts WC: Tetralogy of Fallot, truncus arteriosus, abnormal myocardial architecture and anomalies of the aortic arch system induced by bis-diamine in rat fetuses. J Am Coll Cardiol 1993;21:768–776.

Lee W, Smith RS, Comstock CH, et al: Tetralogy of Fallot: Prenatal diagnosis and postnatal survival. Obstet Gynecol 1995;86:583–588.

Nora JJ, Nora AH: Maternal transmission of congenital heart diseases: New recurrence risk figures and the questions of cytoplasmic inheritance and vulnerability to teratogens. Am J Cardiol 1987;59:459–463.

Nora JJ, Nora AH: Update on counseling the family with a first-degree relative with a congenital heart defect. Am J Med Genet 1988;29:137–142.

Pandit PB, Chitayat D, Jefferies AL, et al: Tibial hemimelia and tetralogy of Fallot associated with first trimester exposure to amantadine [see comments]. Reprod Toxicol 1994;8:89–92.

Sameshima H, Nishibatake M, Ninomiya Y, Tokudome T: Antenatal diagnosis of tetralogy of Fallot with absent pulmonary valve accompanied by hydrops fetalis and polyhydramnios. Fetal Diagn Ther 1993;8:305–308.

Shipp TD, Bromley B, Hornberger LK, et al: Levorotation of the fetal cardiac axis: A clue for the presence of congenital heart disease. Obstet Gynecol 1995;85:97–102.

Tasaka H, Takenaka H, Okamoto N, et al: Abnormal development of cardiovascular systems in rat embryos treated with bisdiamine. Teratology 1991;43:191–200.

Yoshida M, Matsumura M, Shintaku Y, et al: Prenatally diagnosed female prune belly syndrome associated with tetralogy of Fallot. Gynecol Obstet Invest 1995;39:141–144.

Zapata HH, Sletten LJ, Pierpont ME: Congenital cardiac malformations in Adams-Oliver syndrome. Clin Genet 1995;47:80–84.

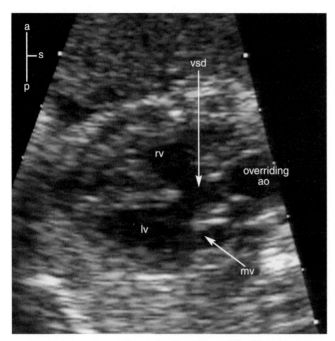

Aortic overriding in tetralogy of Fallot. The mildly dilated aorta (ao) straddles an anterior malalignment type of ventricular septal defect (vsd). The aortic valve is in fibrous continuity with the anterior leaflet of the mitral valve (mv) (i.e., there is no subaortic conus). lv, left ventricle; rv, right ventricle.

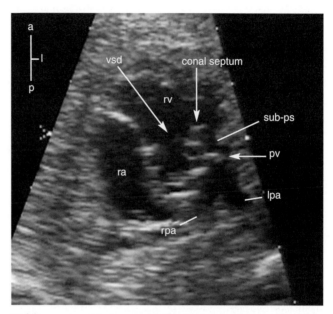

Malalignment ventricular septal defect (vsd) and pulmonary stenosis in tetralogy of Fallot. Short-axis view of the heart demonstrating anterior malalignment of conal septum resulting in the ventricular septal defect and subvalvular pulmonary stenosis (sub-ps). The pulmonary valve (pv) annulus as well as the main pulmonary artery is hypoplastic. lpa, left pulmonary artery; ra, right atrium; rpa, right pulmonary artery; rv, right ventricle.

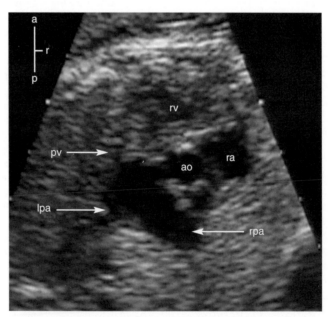

Tetralogy of Fallot with dysplastic pulmonary valve syndrome. The main and right pulmonary artery (rpa) are quite dilated and the right pulmonary artery is twice the size of the ascending aorta (ao). The pulmonary valve (pv) is thickened and dysplastic. lpa, left pulmonary artery; ra, right atrium; rv, right ventricle.

3.3 Ebstein's Anomaly

Epidemiology/Genetics

Definition Ebstein's anomaly refers to an abnormal tricuspid valve with apical displacement of the attachment of the septal leaflet. This commonly results in tricuspid regurgitation and, much less commonly, tricuspid stenosis. The right heart is frequently dilated, and there is often an associated atrial septal defect and, sometimes, pulmonary stenosis. Approximately 30% of patients with Ebstein's anomaly have Wolff-Parkinson-White syndrome.

Epidemiology Prevalence per 1000 live births is approximately 0.012 (M1:F1). It accounts for 0.3% of children with congenital cardiac disease.

Inheritance Pattern The majority of cases are sporadic. Recurrence risk is 1% when one sibling is affected and 3% when two siblings are affected. Familial cases have been documented. A kindred with an autosomal dominant inheritance pattern for Ebstein's anomaly associated with mild skeletal abnormalities has been reported.

Teratogens Older reports suggested an increased risk for Ebstein's anomaly with maternal lithium exposure. More recent data suggest that this risk is much lower and even that lithium may not be a teratogen for Ebstein's anomaly. Four case-control studies did not demonstrate a connection between lithium exposure and Ebstein's anomaly. Two more recent cohort studies showed a relative risk for cardiac anomalies to be 1.2 (95% CI, 0.1–18.3) in one study and 7.7 (95% CI, 0.4–6.8) in the other study. Maternal diabetes mellitus.

Prognosis There is a wide spectrum in severity and therefore also in prognosis. Among patients diagnosed during fetal life or immediately after birth, death by 3 months of age was associated with tethered distal attachments of the anterior leaflet, right ventricular dysplasia, interference of left ventricular filling by right-sided volume overload, and the magnitude of functional right ventricular dilation. Some practitioners have reported worse prognosis with severity of tricuspid regurgitation, fetal presentation, and right ventricular outflow tract obstruction. Others have reported worse prognosis with more marked cardiomegaly and right atrial dilation. Those with less severe findings are likely to do well and may be asymptomatic.

Among fetuses with severe tricuspid regurgitation and marked right atrial dilation, the prognosis is very poor. One study reported that among 20 fetuses with severe tricuspid regurgitation, 48% died in utero and 35% of the liveborn died despite vigorous medical and, as indicated, surgical treatment.

Sonography

FINDINGS

1. **Fetus:**
   a. The displacement of the hingepoint of the tricuspid valve (i.e., the septal leaflet and sometimes the posterior leaflet) into the right ventricle is quantified by measuring the distance from the crux (from which the mitral valve hinges) to the hingepoint of the septal leaflet of the tricuspid valve. This distance should be less than 5 mm at term.
   b. Cardiomegaly due to right atrial and ventricular dilation.
   c. Most commonly tricuspid regurgitation and rarely tricuspid stenosis.
   d. Right ventricular dysfunction or dysplasia.
   Associated findings may include:
   a. Valvular pulmonary stenosis or pulmonary atresia.
   b. Branch pulmonary artery hypoplasia.
   c. Atrial septal defect or patent foramen ovale.
   d. Limitation of left ventricular filling when there is severe right ventricular volume overload with diastolic bowing of the interventricular septum.
   e. Reversed ductal flow from aorta to pulmonary artery occurs when there is pulmonary atresia.
2. **Amniotic Fluid:** With severe tricuspid regurgitation and/or severe right ventricular outflow tract obstruction, polyhydramnios and hydrops may develop.
3. **Placenta:** Normal unless hydrops develops.
4. **Measurement Data:** Normal unless hydrops develops.
5. **When Detectable:** Transabdominal imaging at 16 to 18 weeks. Although the fetal heart can be examined by transvaginal echocardiography at 11 to 13 weeks, the diagnosis of Ebstein's anomaly has not yet been reported. In one study, the tricuspid valve was visualized at 11 weeks in approximately 60% of fetuses.

Pitfalls

1. With severe tricuspid regurgitation, the right ventricle may be unable to generate sufficient pressure to open the pulmonary valve, even though the valve is patent. This is termed functional pulmonary atresia, in contrast to anatomic pulmonary atresia in which the valve leaflets may actually be fused closed. Both functional and anatomic pulmonary valve atresia can occur in Ebstein's anomaly. Functional pulmonary atresia can be distinguished from anatomic atresia if even a small amount of pulmonary regurgitation is noted. The pulmonary regurgitation is evidence that the leaflets are patent even if no antegrade flow is present. Postnatally, when the pulmonary vascular resistance falls, antegrade pulmonary flow may be possible.

2. The dilated right heart may be mistakenly interpreted as hypoplastic left heart syndrome. This mistake should easily be avoided if measurements of the mitral and tricuspid valve annuli are made and identification of the morphologic and functional abnormality of the tricuspid valve is determined.

3. The severity of tricuspid regurgitation may be overestimated by reducing the color Doppler scale so that the Nyquist limit occurs at lower velocities.

Differential Diagnosis   Mild tricuspid regurgitation can occur in 6 to 7% of normal fetuses. In such cases, the tricuspid valve morphology and annulus size are normal and should be easily distinguishable from Ebstein's anomaly. There is no right heart dilation.

Tricuspid regurgitation can also be present with critical right heart obstruction such as pulmonary stenosis or atresia. This can be distinguished from Ebstein's anomaly by recognizing the absence of septal displacement of the tricuspid valve and the presence of obstruction at the pulmonary valve.

Tricuspid valve dysplasia can result in significant and even severe tricuspid regurgitation. Generally the leaflet tips are thickened, but there is no septal displacement of the tricuspid valve as in Ebstein's anomaly.

Giant right atrium as an isolated finding can occur without tricuspid valve disease.

Where Else to Look   Pulmonary hypoplasia can occur when there is severe cardiomegaly. Supraventricular tachycardia can occur, especially when there is Wolff-Parkinson-White syndrome.

Outside the heart, look for these associated problems: low-set ears, micrognathia, cleft lip and palate, absent kidney, megacolon, and undescended testes.

Pregnancy Management

Investigations and Consultations Required   Pediatric cardiology consultation should be obtained for confirmation of and/or definitive diagnosis and to coordinate the prenatal and postnatal cardiac plans.

Fetal Intervention   None.

Monitoring   With significant tricuspid regurgitation, particularly in the presence of pulmonary stenosis or atresia, hydrops may develop. As discussed, there is the potential for supraventricular tachycardia.

Pregnancy Course   Unless severe tricuspid regurgitation develops, fetuses are generally delivered at term.

Pregnancy Termination Issues   Termination should be presented as an option in the case of fetuses with associated anatomic pulmonary atresia and/or in the presence of severe tricuspid regurgitation with marked right heart dilation. If termination is chosen, an intact fetus should be delivered for confirmation of diagnosis.

Delivery   Unless the lesion is quite mild, delivery should be performed where immediate pediatric cardiac consul-

tation is available and where nitric oxide therapy can be administered.

Neonatology

Resuscitation   In the absence of fetal hydrops or cardiac dysrhythmia, assistance with the onset of breathing is usually not required. Neonates with Ebstein's anomaly who are asymptomatic may exhibit intense cyanosis early after birth. Initial measures are directed toward lowering pulmonary vascular resistance and maintaining cardiac output.

Transport   If the newborn is asymptomatic at birth except for cardiomegaly, referral for evaluation can be done at nursery discharge. If there is cyanosis, congestive failure, or rhythm disturbance, immediate referral to a tertiary perinatal center with full pediatric cardiac diagnostic capabilities is necessary. Consultation with a pediatric cardiologist prior to transport to determine management requirements during transport is recommended.

Testing and Confirmation   Echocardiography will confirm anatomic and functional abnormalities. A 12-lead electrocardiogram is necessary to exclude or diagnose dysrhythmia or potential for a conduction defect. Assessment of oxygenation by arterial P_{O_2} or pulse oximetry is indicated.

Nursery Management   In most cases, the ductus arteriosus should be allowed to close. One hopes that with the fall in pulmonary vascular resistance, the systemic oxygen saturation will increase as the right-to-left shunt decreases. In some cases, in which there is markedly diminished pulmonary blood flow due to elevated pulmonary vascular resistance, nitric oxide may be efficacious. In cases in which there is critical right heart obstruction, prostaglandin E may be required to maintain ductal patency.

Surgery

Preoperative Assessment   In the majority of cases, echocardiography provides definitive anatomic and physiologic information. In rare cases, however, single-ventricle management may be necessary. In such cases, cardiac catheterization may be needed to assess pulmonary artery anatomy and physiology.

Operative Indications   In general, one wishes to avoid surgery in a newborn when the oxygen saturation exceeds 75%. As noted, the saturation will usually increase as pulmonary resistance falls. However, when the oxygen saturation is less than 75% or when there is anatomic right heart obstruction, surgery is necessary to achieve adequate oxygenation.

Beyond infancy, patients are referred for surgery when the tricuspid regurgitation results in significant right ventricular volume load or when there is disadvantageous shunting at the atrial level.

Types of Procedures   Two-ventricle management is possible in most patients but requires adequate right ventricular and tricuspid valve function. In such cases, tricuspid valve surgery is directed toward decreasing tricuspid regurgitation with annuloplasty or, later in childhood, tricuspid valve replacement. In general, the atrial septal defect is also closed.

When there is severe right heart obstruction, the surgical options are more complicated and the results are less favorable. With anatomic pulmonary valve atresia, a systematic shunt is indicated to establish a reliable source of pulmonary blood flow. The volume load of tricuspid regurgitation may compromise left ventricular filling.

Surgical Results/Prognosis   With mild-to-moderate Ebstein's anomaly without critical right heart obstruction, the results are generally good. Infants requiring neonatal surgery because of severe Ebstein's anomaly have a guarded prognosis.

REFERENCES

Balaji S, Dennis NR, Keeton BR: Familial Ebstein's anomaly: A report of six cases in two generations associated with mild skeletal abnormalities. Br Heart J 1991;66:26–28.

Celermajer DS, Bull C, Till JA, et al: Ebstein's anomaly: Presentation and outcome from fetus to adult. J Am Coll Cardiol 1994;23:170–176.

Cohen LS, Friedman JM, Jefferson JW, et al: A reevaluation of risk of in utero exposure to lithium [published erratum appears in JAMA 1994;271(19):1485]. JAMA 1994;271:146–150.

Dolkart LA, Reimers FT: Transvaginal fetal echocardiography in early pregnancy: Normative data. Am J Obstet Gynecol 1991;165:688–691.

Fyler DC: Trends. In Fyler DC (ed): Nadas' Pediatric Cardiology. Philadelphia, Hanley & Belfus, 1992, pp 273–284.

Gembruch U, Smrcek JM: The prevalence and clinical significance of tricuspid valve regurgitation in normally grown fetuses and those with intrauterine growth retardation. Ultrasound Obstet Gynecol 1997;9:374–382.

Homberger LK, Sahn DJ, Kleinman CS, et al: Tricuspid valve disease with significant tricuspid insufficiency in the fetus: Diagnosis and outcome. J Am Coll Cardiol 1991;17:167–173.

McIntosh N, Chitayat D, Bardanis M, Fouron JC: Ebstein anomaly: Report of a familial occurrence and prenatal diagnosis. Am J Med Genet 1992;42:307–309.

Nora JJ, Nora AH: Update on counseling the family with a first-degree relative with a congenital heart defect. Am J Med Genet 1988;29:137–142.

Paladini D, Chita SK, Allan LD: Prenatal measurement of cardiothoracic ratio in evaluation of heart disease. Arch Dis Child 1990;65:20–23.

Pavlova M, Fouron JC, Drblik SP, et al: Factors affecting the prognosis of Ebstein's anomaly during fetal life. Am Heart J 1998;135:1081–1085.

Reinhardt-Owlya L, Sekarski N, Hurni M, et al: [Idiopathic dilatation of the right atrium simulating Ebstein's anomaly. Apropos of a case diagnosed in utero]. Arch Mal Coeur Vaiss 1998;91:645–649.

Roberson DA, Silverman NH: Ebstein's anomaly: Echocardiographic and clinical features in the fetus and neonate. J Am Coll Cardiol 1989;14:1300–1307.

Silva SR, Bruner JP, Moore CA: Prenatal diagnosis of Down's syndrome in the presence of isolated Ebstein's anomaly. Fetal Diagn Ther 1999;14:149–151.

Weinstein MR, Goldfield M: Cardiovascular malformations with lithium use during pregnancy. Am J Psychiatry 1975;132:529–531.

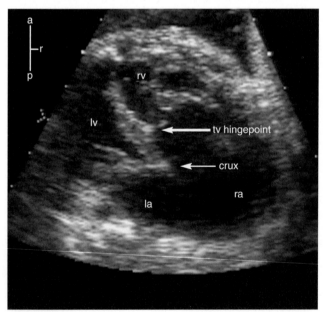

Marked tricuspid valve displacement in Ebstein's anomaly. The hingepoint of the septal leaflet of tricuspid valve (tv) is displaced from the crux by 11 mm. This results in an atrialized portion of the right ventricle (rv) (i.e., that portion above the tricuspid valve that is functionally within the right atrium). As this area and that of the true right atrium (ra) increases (in proportion to the rest of the heart), the abnormality is more severe. The right heart dilation results in marked cardiomegaly. la, left atrium; lv, left ventricle.

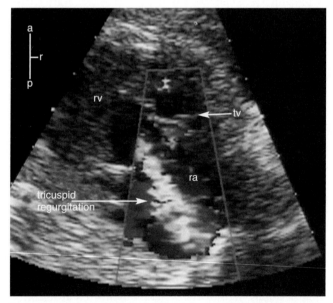

Severe tricuspid regurgitation in Ebstein's anomaly. A broad jet of tricuspid regurgitation is seen into the markedly dilated right atrium (ra). Machine settings are optimized to increase temporal and spatial resolution. rv, right ventricle; tv, tricuspid valve. (See color figure following p. x.)

3.4 Tricuspid Valve Atresia

Epidemiology/Genetics

Definition Most commonly the tricuspid valve is absent, but less commonly there can be a tiny tricuspid valve apparatus that is imperforate. Often, there is right ventricular hypoplasia. The great vessels may be normally related or transposed.

Epidemiology Prevalance per 1000 live births: 0.039 to 0.185. Accounts for approximately 0.6% of children with cardiac disease.

Embryology Some investigators have suggested that a failure of the right-sided venous valves to regress may be causative in the development of diseases with right heart hypoplasia such as tricuspid atresia.

Inheritance Pattern The inheritance pattern is unknown in most cases. In one family, tricuspid atresia recurred in siblings, suggesting an autosomal recessive inheritance. The recurrence risk for all congenital heart disease is 1% when one sibling with tricuspid atresia is affected and 3% when two siblings are affected. Rare chromosomal and syndromic associations have been reported.

Teratogens In a mouse model, sodium valproate administration was associated with the development of cardiovascular abnormalities, including tricuspid atresia. Maternal diabetes mellitus.

Prognosis Tricuspid valve atresia requires single ventricle management. In general, two and sometimes three operations are required before the age of 6 years. During the past decade, the survival rate at 6 years of age has improved to between 80 and 90%. Among survivors, approximately 90% of patients who have had multiple operations are in New York Heart Association class I or II. Long-term follow-up suggests that there may be a decrease in functional status in some patients.

Sonography

FINDINGS

1. **Fetus:**
   a. Lack of an outlet from the right atrium to the right ventricle (or the atria related to the right ventricle if there is ventricular inversion). This can be easily appreciated through a four-chamber view. Visualization of a single flow stream from atria to ventricle using color Doppler mapping may be helpful as well.
   b. In most cases, there is right ventricular hypoplasia.

An atrial septal defect or patent foramen ovale must be present to allow egress from the right atrium.
   c. The great vessels are normally related in approximately 70 to 80% of newborns with tricuspid atresia and therefore the pulmonary valve arises from the hypoplastic right ventricle. There is frequently pulmonary stenosis or, sometimes, pulmonary atresia. Since the blood only gets to the right ventricle and pulmonary valve across the ventricular septal defect from the left ventricle, restriction at the ventricular septal defect results in subvalvular pulmonary stenosis. The ventricular septal defect shown in the figure is of a relatively good size for tricuspid valve atresia with normally related great arteries. A small ventricular septal defect or pulmonary valve with normally related great arteries suggests that pulmonary stenosis will be severe. When severe pulmonary stenosis is present, ductal flow may be "reversed" (i.e., from aorta to pulmonary artery). This strongly suggests that, postnatally, the lesion will be ductus dependent.
   d. Between 12 and 28% of patients with tricuspid atresia have D-transposition of the great arteries. In these patients, subaortic obstruction is frequent, as is aortic coarctation or interruption of the aortic arch. A small aortic valve, ascending aorta, and/or transverse arch suggests that the aortic stenosis will be more severe and that there is an increased probability for aortic arch obstruction. When there is severe aortic stenosis, the transverse arch aortic flow may be retrograde. This also suggests that the lesion will be ductus dependent postnatally.
   e. Tricuspid valve atresia occurs with ventricular inversion and transposition of the great arteries (so-called L-transposition of the great arteries) in approximately 5% of patients with tricuspid valve atresia. In this case, the atretic valve and hypoplastic right ventricle are on the left side of the heart, and the mitral valve and left ventricle are on the right.
   f. Left ventricular dysfunction with associated abnormal myocardial architecture has been seen in tricuspid atresia. Abnormal histology and ultrastructure have been described within the left ventricle of patients with tricuspid atresia. Mitral valve abnormalities have been reported in as many as 45% of patients with tricuspid atresia.
   g. Tricuspid atresia has occurred with aortopulmonary window and in truncus arteriosus.
2. **Amniotic Fluid:** Usually normal. Complete heart block with hydrops and polyhydramnios has been described in a fetus with tricuspid atresia and ventricular inversion.
3. **Placenta:** Normal.
4. **Measurement Data:** Normal.

5. **When Detectable:** Transabdominal imaging at 16 to 18 weeks. Although the fetal heart can be examined by transvaginal echocardiography at 11 to 13 weeks, the diagnosis of tricuspid atresia has not yet been reported at that stage. The mitral and tricuspid valves were resolved in 60% of fetuses at 11 weeks.

Pitfalls

Since only a single atrioventricular valve is patent, tricuspid atresia can be confused with a complete common atrioventricular canal defect. Noting the origin of the atrioventricular valve hinges makes it easy to recognize the distinction. In tricuspid atresia, the mitral valve hinges from the atrial septum and the lateral left atrial wall. With a common atrioventricular valve, the valve hinges from both atrial free walls and not from the atrial septum. Also, in a canal defect, there is nearly always a primum type of atrial septal defect. This type of atrial defect would be unusual with tricuspid atresia.

It is crucial to recognize abnormal great vessel connections in tricuspid valve atresia. The presence of outflow obstruction is what influences the severity of this heart lesion.

Right/left orientation is crucial to maintain. The inexperienced echocardiographer could confuse tricuspid valve atresia with mitral atresia and hypoplastic left heart syndrome. The prognosis and management are quite different.

Differential Diagnosis   As discussed, tricuspid atresia should be differentiated from atrioventricular canal defects and mitral atresia.

Where Else to Look   Screen for rare associated syndromes described earlier.

Pregnancy Management

Investigations and Consultations Required   Chromosomal studies should be done, including analysis with in situ hybridization for chromosome 22q deletion. The prevalence of 22q deletion is 7 to 8%.

Pediatric cardiology consultation should be obtained for confirmation of and/or definitive diagnosis and to coordinate the prenatal and postnatal cardiac plans.

Fetal Intervention   None indicated.

Monitoring   Follow-up echocardiography at 28 to 32 weeks should be performed to assess fetal cardiac status.

Pregnancy Course   Usually normal.

Pregnancy Termination Issues   Because of the necessity of multiple operations and the necessity for single ventricle management, families are offered the option of termination. If termination is chosen, an intact fetus should be delivered for confirmation of diagnosis.

Delivery   Delivery should be performed in an institution where immediate pediatric cardiology and cardiac

surgery consultation is available, since the lesion may be ductus dependent.

Neonatology

Resuscitation   Babies generally breathe spontaneously but are cyanotic. Initial measures should be directed toward establishing venous and, if necessary, arterial access. If the lesion is ductus dependent, then prostaglandin E therapy should be initiated (after consultation with a pediatric cardiologist).

Transport   Babies should be transported to regional cardiac centers for definitive management.

Testing and Confirmation   In the majority of cases, echocardiography is adequate for delineating the anatomy and necessary physiology prior to surgical intervention.

Nursery Management   With normally related great vessels, a reliable route for pulmonary blood flow must be established. If there is no significant pulmonary stenosis, the infant will develop congestive heart failure due to pulmonary overcirculation, and measures are necessary to treat congestive heart failure. Alternatively, if severe pulmonary stenosis occurs, ductal patency is necessary to provide adequate pulmonary blood flow.

With associated transposition of the great arteries, there is the possibility for obstruction of systemic or pulmonary blood flow. In such cases, prostaglandin E therapy may be necessary.

Surgery

Preoperative Assessment   During infancy, echocardiography is generally adequate for preoperative evaluation. In rare situations in which there is inadequate visualization of the aortic arch, cardiac catheterization might be needed. At times of later operations, preoperative catheterization is required to assess the branch pulmonary arteries and to measure the pulmonary resistance.

Operative Indications   Surgery is generally needed in infancy to achieve an appropriate balance of systemic and pulmonary blood flow. Longer term, since there is only one functional ventricle, the systemic and pulmonary venous circulations must be separated to achieve normal oxygen saturations.

Types of Procedures   Often a surgical procedure is necessary in the newborn period. When there is inadequate pulmonary blood flow, a Blalock-Taussig shunt is placed, which is a connection between the right subclavian artery or innominate artery and the right pulmonary artery. When there is no significant pulmonary stenosis, excessive pulmonary blood flow may be controlled with a pulmonary artery band. When there is obstruction to systemic blood flow, surgery often involves repair of aortic coarctation but sometimes requires a more extensive operation if there is associated severe subaortic obstruction.

To separate the systemic and pulmonary venous circulations, the Glenn and Fontan operations are performed. In the Glenn operation, blood returning to the heart in the superior vena cava is directed to the branch pulmonary arteries, thereby bypassing the heart. In the Fontan operation, blood returning from both the superior vena cava and inferior vena cava is directed to the branch pulmonary arteries.

Surgical Results/Prognosis Tricuspid atresia with normally related great vessels generally requires two or three operations before the age of 6 years. After the Fontan operation, the oxygen saturation is 90% or higher. Operative mortality rates for the Glenn and Fontan operations are between 2 and 10%.

When tricuspid atresia is present with significant subaortic obstruction or aortic arch obstruction, the operations are more complicated. The combined operative mortality rate probably ranges between 10 and 40%, depending on the need for aortic arch reconstruction.

REFERENCES

Chiba Y, Kanzaki T, Kobayashi H, et al: Evaluation of fetal structural heart disease using color flow mapping. Ultrasound Med Biol 1990;16:221–229.

Dolkart LA, Reimers FT: Transvaginal fetal echocardiography in early pregnancy: Normative data. Am J Obstet Gynecol 1991;165:688–691.

Fyler DC: Trends. In Fyler DC (ed): Nadas' Pediatric Cardiology. Philadelphia, Hanley & Belfus, 1992, pp 273–284.

Gembruch U, Hansmann M, Redel DA, et al: [Non-immunologically-induced hydrops fetalis in complete atrioventricular block of the fetus. A summary of 11 prenatally diagnosed cases]. Geburtshilfe Frauenheilkd 1988;48:494–499.

Gentles TL, Gauvreau K, Mayer JE Jr, et al: Functional outcome after the Fontan operation: Factors influencing late morbidity. J Thorac Cardiovasc Surg 1997;114:392–403.

Geva T, Ott DA, Ludomirsky A, et al: Tricuspid atresia associated with aortopulmonary window: Controlling pulmonary blood flow with a fenestrated patch. Am Heart J 1992;123:260–262.

Grant JW: Congenital malformations of the tricuspid valve in siblings. Pediatr Cardiol 1996;17:327–329.

Johnson BL, Fyfe DA, Gillette PC, et al: In utero diagnosis of interrupted aortic arch with transposition of the great arteries and tricuspid atresia. Am Heart J 1989;117:690–692.

Kaneko H, Tsukahara M, Tachibana H, et al: Congenital heart defects in Sotos sequence. Am J Med Genet 1987;26:569–576.

Kumar A, Victorica BE, Gessner IH, Alexander JA: Tricuspid atresia and annular hypoplasia: Report of a familial occurrence. Pediatr Cardiol 1994;15:201–203.

Mair DD, Hagler DJ, Puga FJ, et al: Fontan operation in 176 patients with tricuspid atresia. Results and a proposed new index for patient selection. Circulation 1990;82:IV164–IV169.

Marino B, Digilio MC, Novelli G, et al: Tricuspid atresia and 22q11 deletion. Am J Med Genet 1997;72:40–42.

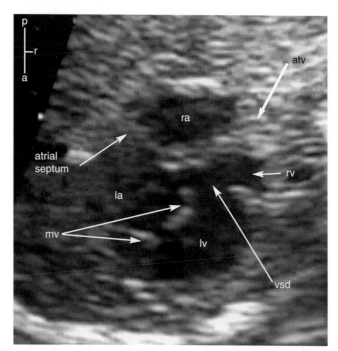

Tricuspid valve atresia. The *broader arrow* points to the atretic tricuspid valve (atv). The only outlet from the right atrium (ra) is across the foramen ovale to the left atrium (la). There is severe right ventricular hypoplasia. A ventricular septal defect (vsd) is typical in tricuspid valve atresia and is seen in this figure. The mitral valve (mv) hinges from the atrial septum and the lateral left atrial wall. If this were a common atrioventricular valve, the valve would hinge from the lateral wall of each atrium and not from the atrial septum (see discussion under Pitfalls). la, left atrium; lv, left ventricle; rv, right ventricle.

3.5 Critical Valvular Pulmonary Stenosis and Pulmonary Atresia

Epidemiology/Genetics

Definition In valvular pulmonary stenosis, leaflet motion is restricted and frequently there is pulmonary annular hypoplasia. With valvular pulmonary atresia, no antegrade flow is present across the pulmonary valve. Valve leaflets are often still present but completely fused.

Epidemiology Prevalence per 1000 live births: 0.07 to 0.66 for valvular pulmonary stenosis and 0.04 to 0.08 for pulmonary atresia. Valvular pulmonary stenosis accounts for 5 to 7% and pulmonary atresia for 0.3% of all patients with congenital heart disease.

Embryology The pulmonary valve forms from the truncus arteriosus. Although normal pulmonary valve formation is largely completed by 7 to 8 weeks' gestation, in utero progression of pulmonary valve disease has been reported from mild to more severe stenosis and even from pulmonary stenosis to pulmonary atresia.

Inheritance Pattern Most often sporadic. Recurrence risks for all congenital heart disease in siblings in whom the proband has pulmonary stenosis are 2% when one sibling is affected and 6% when two are affected. When the proband has valvular pulmonary atresia, the recurrence risk for all congenital heart disease is 1% when one sibling is affected and 3% when two siblings are affected. The recurrence risk for all congenital heart defects in offspring is 4 to 6.5% when the mother has pulmonary stenosis and 2% when the father is affected. Chromosome abnormalities and Noonan and William syndromes have been reported with pulmonary stenosis.

Teratogens Rubella.

Prognosis The prognosis for the neonate with pulmonary stenosis is more favorable than for the neonate with pulmonary atresia. In most cases, balloon dilation can attain effective relief of obstruction in 90% of patients. The remainder may require redilation or a surgical valvuloplasty. Approximately 97% of patients are in New York Heart Association functional class I. Long-term survival is good.

With pulmonary atresia and intact ventricular septum, the right heart size may be adequate to allow two-ventricle management. In such cases, multiple operations culminating in the Fontan operation may be necessary, resulting in 1- and 5-year survival rates of approximately 82% and 76%, respectively. A subset of patients with pulmonary atresia and intact ventricular septum can achieve a two-ventricle physiology with effective relief of the right ventricular outflow tract obstruction. Long-term survival may be similar to that with single-ventricle management.

The fetus with critical right ventricular outflow tract obstruction and severe tricuspid regurgitation is at risk for the development of hydrops and fetal demise.

Sonography

FINDINGS

1. **Fetus:**
   a. The pulmonary valve leaflets are thickened and dome-shaped. With pulmonary stenosis, significant acceleration in flow can be detected with pulse and continuous wave Doppler echocardiography. Sometimes, small amounts of pulmonary regurgitation can be appreciated with color Doppler interrogation and give a clue that the pulmonary valve is patent.
   b. With valvular pulmonary atresia, no antegrade flow is present across the pulmonary valve.
   c. With critical pulmonary stenosis or atresia, reverse ductal flow is present (i.e., from aorta to pulmonary artery).
   d. With both pulmonary stenosis and atresia, tricuspid valve and right ventricular hypoplasia are common. This may be the initial clue to critical right ventricular outflow tract obstruction. The tricuspid valve annulus size should be compared with normative data and the long-axis length of the right ventricle compared with that of the left ventricle.
   e. Right ventricular hypertension develops with increasing obstruction. The right ventricle pressure can be ascertained by measuring the velocity of tricuspid valve regurgitation. The pressure gradient between right ventricle and right atrium can be estimated from the Bernoulli equation. In addition, the ventricular septum may bow into the left ventricle when the right ventricular pressure exceeds the left ventricular pressure.
   f. With pulmonary atresia and intact ventricular septum, sinusoids can develop between the right ventricle and the coronary arteries when there is severe right ventricular hypertension. Flow occurs into the sinusoids from the right ventricle during systole. These connections have been visualized with transvaginal imaging, and visualization is improved by reducing the color Doppler scale to accentuate low velocity flow. The recognition of retrograde systolic flow in the coronary arteries is a clue to these abnormal connections. Visualization of these coronary connections is quite difficult prenatally and is imprecise at this time.
2. **Amniotic Fluid:** Generally normal unless hydrops develops, in which case polyhydramnios may occur. Hydrops is more likely to develop if severe tricuspid regurgitation occurs.

3. **Placenta:** Generally normal.
4. **Measurement Data:** Generally normal.
5. **When Detectable:** Transabdominal imaging at 16 to 18 weeks' gestation. The right ventricular to coronary communications discussed earlier have been recognized by transvaginal imaging at 17 weeks.

Pitfalls

1. Distinguishing critical valvular pulmonary stenosis from pulmonary atresia can be difficult. Detection of a small amount of pulmonary regurgitation or of a high-velocity antegrade jet in the main pulmonary artery establishes that the pulmonary valve is patent. In addition, pulmonary stenosis can progress in utero to pulmonary valve atresia. Serial studies are helpful in recognizing this evolution.
2. If right-left orientation is reversed, one could misdiagnose hypoplastic right heart (in pulmonary atresia) as hypoplastic left heart syndrome. This should be easily avoidable.
3. Right ventricular hypoplasia can rarely occur as an isolated cardiac anomaly without pulmonary valve disease.
4. Severe tricuspid regurgitation in tricuspid valve dysplasia or Ebstein's anomaly can result in functional pulmonary atresia.

Differential Diagnosis The main differential diagnosis is between pulmonary stenosis and pulmonary atresia. Pulmonary atresia can occur with tetralogy of Fallot. This echocardiographic appearance, prognosis, and treatment are markedly different in pulmonary atresia with intact ventricular septum and in tetralogy of Fallot with pulmonary atresia.

Where Else to Look

1. Pulmonary stenosis and pulmonary atresia can occur as a component of other serious forms of congenital heart disease, including double-outlet right ventricle, transposition of the great arteries, and complete atrioventricular canal defects.
2. Extracardiac features of Noonan syndrome include cystic hygroma, micropenis, and hemivertebrae.

Pregnancy Management

Investigations and Consultations Required Chromosome studies should be performed. Because it can be a conotruncal malformation, appropriate fluorescent in situ hybridization should be done, looking for 22q deletion. Pediatric cardiac consultation should be obtained in all cases of valvular pulmonary stenosis or atresia. The lesion may be ductus dependent and/or early delivery may be indicated if hydrops develops.

Fetal Intervention Relief of obstruction prenatally has been attempted but with poor results to date.

Monitoring The fetus with right ventricular outflow tract obstruction should be reimaged at the end of the second trimester because of the potential for worsening obstruction and for the development of tricuspid regurgitation and hydrops.

Pregnancy Course Development of severe tricuspid regurgitation, right heart dilation, or cardiomegaly may predict fetuses at risk for the development of hydrops.

Pregnancy Termination Issues Because of favorable results in critical valvular pulmonary stenosis, most families continue to term when this diagnosis is made prenatally. When there is severe hypoplasia of the right heart, particularly when there is valvular pulmonary atresia, some families may consider termination when single-ventricle management seems likely. Decision-making is complicated by the potential for disease progression in utero and the inability to predict with certainty whether the heart will allow biventricular management. Given the prognosis in pulmonary atresia with intact ventricular septum, some families will choose to terminate the pregnancy. If so, an intact fetus should be delivered for confirmation of diagnosis.

Delivery Except in cases of mild right heart obstruction, fetuses with more severe obstruction should be delivered in a facility where immediate pediatric cardiac consultation is available. The presence of reversed ductal flow is an important clue to a ductus-dependent lesion.

Neonatology

Resuscitation Patients with severe stenosis or atresia generally breathe spontaneously and resuscitation is unnecessary. In those with pulmonary atresia with intact ventricular septum or critical valvular pulmonary stenosis, prostaglandin E_1 should be administered to maintain ductal patency.

Transport The baby should be transported to a regional center where interventional cardiac catheterization and pediatric cardiac surgery can be performed.

Testing and Confirmation The diagnosis of valvular pulmonary stenosis and pulmonary atresia is reliably made by echocardiography. Cardiac catheterization is indicated for valvular pulmonary stenosis to perform balloon dilation and in patients with pulmonary atresia with intact ventricular septum, to exclude associated coronary artery abnormalities. Coronary stenoses sometimes occur in addition to the right ventricular-coronary connections, and the stenoses are not well seen with echocardiography.

Nursery Management Adequate venous and arterial access is indicated when there is critical right heart obstruction. Prostaglandin E should be initiated in such cases.

Intervention

Preintervention Assessment Echocardiography should be definitive for establishing the diagnosis of valvular pulmonary stenosis or atresia. No further testing is required in valvular pulmonary stenosis. In pulmonary atresia, catheterization is required to define coronary abnormalities already discussed earlier.

Indications for Therapeutic Catheterization or Surgery in the Newborn   In valvular pulmonary stenosis, patients are referred for interventional catheterization when the obstruction is severe and results in cyanosis or systemic right ventricular pressure.

In pulmonary atresia, all patients require surgery or interventional catheterization.

Types of Procedures   Interventional catheterization with balloon valvuloplasty is the treatment of choice for the neonate with valvular pulmonary stenosis.

Patients with pulmonary atresia are usually referred for surgery to relieve the right ventricular outflow tract obstruction and to place a Blalock-Taussig shunt. Rarely, coronary abnormalities make it unwise to relieve the right ventricular outflow tract obstruction, since in these cases, decompression of the hypertensive right ventricle could compromise coronary blood flow.

Some centers open the atretic pulmonary outflow tract with interventional catheterization.

In pulmonary atresia, one hopes that, with relief of the right ventricular outflow tract obstruction, the right ventricle and tricuspid valve will grow. If not, single-ventricle management may be necessary.

Interventional Catheterization and Surgical Results/ Prognosis   Balloon dilation in valvular pulmonary stenosis results in a significant reduction in gradient in more than 90% of patients. Repeat dilation is subsequently required in a small subset, generally within the first 2 years of life. Balloon dilation may fail when the pulmonary annulus is very hypoplastic or the pulmonary valve very dysplastic. When balloon dilation fails, surgery is generally successful in nearly all patients.

The results in pulmonary atresia with intact ventricular septum are less favorable and depend on the ability to open the right ventricular outflow tract and subsequent growth of the tricuspid valve and right ventricle. When two-ventricle physiology can be achieved, good results can be achieved in the majority of patients. When single-ventricle management is necessary, multiple operations are required, with a 5-year survival rate of approximately 75%.

REFERENCES

Berning RA, Silverman NH, Villegas M, et al: Reversed shunting across the ductus arteriosus or atrial septum in utero heralds severe congenital heart disease. J Am Coll Cardiol 1996;27:481–486.

Chaoui R, Tennstedt C, Goldner B, Bollmann R: Prenatal diagnosis of ventriculo-coronary communications in a second-trimester fetus using transvaginal and transabdominal color Doppler sonography. Ultrasound Obstet Gynecol 1997;9:194–197.

Chitayat D, McIntosh N, Fouron JC: Pulmonary atresia with intact ventricular septum and hypoplastic right heart in sibs: A single gene disorder? Am J Med Genet 1992;42:304–306.

Colli AM, Perry SB, Lock JE, Keane JF: Balloon dilation of critical valvar pulmonary stenosis in the first month of life. Cathet Cardiovasc Diagn 1995;34:23–28.

Daubeney PE, Sharland GK, Cook AC, et al: Pulmonary atresia with intact ventricular septum: Impact of fetal echocardiography on incidence at birth and postnatal outcome. UK and Eire Collaborative Study of Pulmonary Atresia with Intact Ventricular Septum. Circulation 1998;98:562–566.

Davies J, Jaffe A, Bush A: Distal 10q trisomy syndrome with unusual cardiac and pulmonary abnormalities. J Med Genet 1998;35:72–74.

De Wolf D, Naeff MS, Losekoot G: Right ventricular hypoplasia: Outcome alter conservative perinatal management. Acta Cardiol 1994;49: 267–273.

Fyler DC: Trends. In Fyler DC (ed): Nadas' Pediatric Cardiology. Philadelphia, Hanley & Belfus, 1992, pp 273–284.

Hayes CJ, Gersony WM, Driscoll DJ, et al: Second natural history study of congenital heart defects. Results of treatment of patients with pulmonary valvar stenosis. Circulation 1993;87:I28–I37.

Hordnes K, Engebretsen LF, Knudtzon J: De novo balanced 5;21 translocation in a child with acrobrachycephaly, ventriculomegaly, pulmonary stenosis, ectopic anus and mental retardation. Clin Genet 1995;48:321–323.

Kaneko H, Tsukahara M, Tachibana H, et al: Congenital heart defects in Sotos sequence. Am J Med Genet 1987;26:569–576.

Pulmonary stenosis/atresia. In this patient with valvular pulmonary stenosis, the image is at the level of the great vessels. The pulmonary valve is quite thickened. Valve motion is markedly reduced when the valve is seen in real time. Proximal to the right ventricular outflow tract (rvot), one can appreciate the right ventricular hypertrophy (rvh). Although the pulmonary annulus is often hypoplastic, it is of normal size in this patient. The branch pulmonary arteries are typically of normal size, as they are here. ao, aorta; lpa, left pulmonary artery; rpa, right pulmonary artery.

Pulmonary stenosis. This continuous wave Doppler tracing demonstrates a high-velocity jet across the pulmonary valve and establishes that the valve is stenotic and not atretic. Using the Bernoulli equation, the gradient is calculated to be 50 mm Hg. The wall filter is increased to optimize the signal-to-noise ratio.

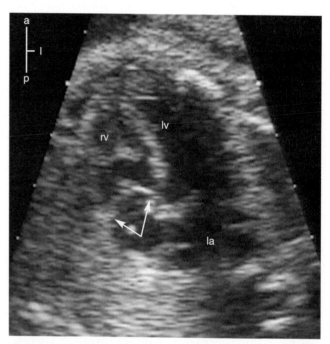

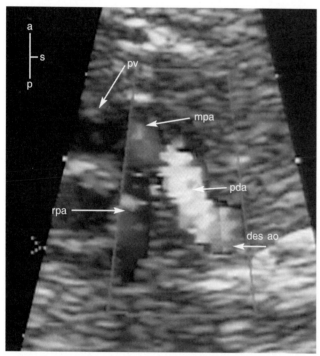

Retrograde flow in the patent ductus arteriosus in pulmonary atresia. With severe pulmonary stenosis or with pulmonary atresia, ductal flow is reversed. Here, one sees retrograde flow in the patent ductus arteriosus (pda) representing flow from the descending aorta (des ao) to the main pulmonary artery (mpa). Normal antegrade flow is seen in the right pulmonary artery (rpa). pv, pulmonary vein. (See color figure following p. x.)

Hypoplastic and hypertensive right heart in pulmonary atresia. The right ventricle (rv) and tricuspid valve are hypoplastic in this patient with pulmonary atresia. The right ventricle is not apex forming. The ventricular septum bows into the left ventricle (lv) because the right ventricular pressure is elevated because of the right-sided outflow obstruction. la, left atrium. Arrows point to the hypoplastic tricuspid valve annulus.

3.6 Critical Valvular Aortic Stenosis

Epidemiology/Genetics

Definition Critical valvular aortic stenosis almost always occurs because of fusion of one or both of the aortic commissures, resulting in decreased leaflet mobility. Frequently there is hypoplasia of left heart structures such as the mitral valve, aortic valve, and/or left ventricle.

Epidemiology Prevalence per 1000 live births: 0.05 to 0.34. Accounts for 5 to 7% of children with cardiac disease and for 2% of those with critical heart disease during infancy. A bicommissural aortic valve is present in as many as 3% of the population but does not necessarily result in significant stenosis in infancy.

Embryology The aortic valve forms from the truncus arteriosus, and valve formation is nearly complete by 8 weeks' gestation. The valve is formed at this point, but aortic stenosis can develop and progress during all trimesters.

Inheritance Pattern Recurrence risk for congenital heart disease is 2% when one sibling is affected and 6% when two siblings are affected. The recurrence risk for all congenital heart defects in offspring given one affected parent is 13 to 18% when the mother is affected and 3% when the father is affected. Aortic stenosis occurs in Adams-Oliver, Williams, and Turner syndromes.

Teratogens Maternal diabetes mellitus.

Prognosis The prognosis for valvular aortic stenosis is quite dependent on the severity of stenosis and the presence of associated lesions. Among neonates with critical valvular aortic stenosis, the 8-year survival rate is 88%. Among children older than 1 month of age undergoing intervention, 8-year survival is 95%. When severe obstruction results in hydrops, the prognosis is often poor. The left heart may be critically small in a subset of patients with valvular aortic stenosis, and patients are best managed like those with hypoplastic left heart syndrome. Five-year survival among patients with hypoplastic left heart syndrome who are at standard risk is 70%.

Sonography

FINDINGS

1. **Fetus:**
   a. With severe stenosis, the left ventricle is hypokinetic. The left ventricular size may be quite dilated or hypoplastic. When dilated, there may be significant mitral regurgitation. When critically hypoplastic, counseling and management are the same as for hypoplastic left heart syndrome. The endocardium is often hyperechoic due to endocardial fibroelastosis.
   b. The leaflets are thickened with reduced motion. The annulus is frequently hypoplastic.
   c. Pulse Doppler interrogation of the aortic valve often shows increased antegrade flow velocities. In the presence of severe left ventricular dysfunction, however, the gradient may be trivial because of decreased forward flow across the aortic valve.
   d. Mitral regurgitation can be detected with color Doppler echocardiography and is a poor prognostic sign.
   e. With severe stenosis, there can be hypoplasia of the mitral valve, left ventricle, and aortic arch. There may be mitral stenosis or coarctation.
   f. With severe aortic or associated mitral stenosis and/or left ventricular dysfunction, flow across the atrial septum may be reversed (i.e., from left to right atrium) and/or there may be retrograde flow in the transverse aortic arch.
   g. Sometimes an early clue when the aortic valve is only mildly stenotic is dilation of the ascending aorta.
   h. Aortic stenosis can occur with ventricular septal defect.
   i. Hydrops can develop when there is severe left ventricular dysfunction, particularly when there is severe mitral regurgitation.
2. **Amniotic Fluid:** Normal except if hydrops develops.
3. **Placenta:** Normal unless hydrops develops.
4. **Measurement Data:** None.
5. **When Detectable:** Transabdominal imaging at 17 to 18 weeks. Valvular aortic stenosis has been diagnosed with transvaginal imaging at 13 to 16 weeks. It is important to remember that aortic stenosis can develop or the severity can increase during the second and third trimesters.

Pitfalls

1. Severe aortic stenosis must be distinguished from aortic atresia, as the management and outcome for the two conditions are dramatically different. Aortic stenosis is managed in a similar manner to hypoplastic left heart syndrome. The absence of antegrade flow across the aortic valve establishes that aortic atresia is present.
2. Associated left heart hypoplasia, which, if sufficiently severe, will alter management as in hypoplastic left heart syndrome. Left heart structures should be measured and compared with normative data.
3. Low gradients across the aortic valve in patients with severe obstruction in the presence of severe left ventricular dysfunction may fool some practitioners into

underestimating the severity of left heart obstruction. One needs to recognize clues such as left ventricular dysfunction, retrograde flow in the transverse arch, or reversed flow at the atrial level to avoid this mistake.

Differential Diagnosis   As discussed above, the differential diagnosis includes hypoplastic left heart syndrome.

Where Else to Look   Aortic stenosis is not usually associated with other noncardiac findings.

Pregnancy Management

Investigations and Consultations Required   Chromosome studies should be performed. Pediatric cardiac consultation should be obtained to confirm the diagnosis, to discuss the significance of the prenatal findings, and to coordinate the postnatal management plan.

Fetal Intervention   Interventional catheterization has been attempted in the fetus, with mixed but usually poor results. At this time, prenatal intervention is not indicated.

Monitoring   In cases with significant aortic stenosis, the fetal heart should be re-examined at 28 weeks, and then as often as every 2 weeks thereafter to check for the development of hydrops.

Pregnancy Course   The pregnancy will most commonly continue to term unless hydrops develops. Hydrops is more likely to develop when there is significant mitral regurgitation and/or severe left ventricular dysfunction. Polyhydramnios may also complicate cases with hydrops.

Pregnancy Termination Issues   In cases in which the prognosis is similar to hypoplastic left heart syndrome, some families may elect to terminate the pregnancy. If termination is chosen, an intact fetus should be delivered for confirmation of diagnosis.

Delivery   Delivery should occur where immediate pediatric cardiology and cardiac surgery support are available.

Neonatology

Resuscitation   Respiratory distress can develop soon after delivery if there is pulmonary venous congestion and poor cardiac output. This more commonly occurs when the ductus arteriosus closes. Babies will generally breathe spontaneously. Venous and arterial access should be achieved in cases of severe obstruction to allow administration of prostaglandin E_1 and inotropic agents when indicated and to allow appropriate monitoring.

Transport   When aortic stenosis is suspected or confirmed as the diagnosis, the baby should be transported to a center with pediatric surgery and cardiothoracic surgery capability. Consultation with a pediatric cardiologist should occur before transport to determine whether the lesion is ductus dependent.

Testing and Confirmation   The diagnosis of aortic stenosis is definitively made with echocardiography.

Nursery Management   When the stenosis is sufficiently severe that the left ventricle cannot supply sufficient cardiac output, prostaglandin E_1 therapy should be initiated. When the ventricular function is normal and the lesion is not ductus dependent, the ductus arteriosus is allowed to close and the infant carefully observed. The decision is made during the first few days of life as to whether intervention is indicated. Intervention is nearly always indicated in the presence of ventricular dysfunction.

Intervention

Preintervention Assessment   Echocardiography is definitive for assessment prior to intervention.

Interventional Indications   The patient is referred for balloon angioplasty of the aortic valve when the stenosis is sufficiently severe to result in ventricular dysfunction or when the infant is symptomatic. In addition, the patient is referred for balloon angioplasty when the gradient is greater than 70 to 80 mm Hg in the absence of ventricular dysfunction.

Types of Procedures   Balloon angioplasty is now the procedure of choice for valvular aortic stenosis in infancy and childhood. In the small minority of cases in which balloon angioplasty is unsuccessful, surgery may be needed. It is unusual for the aortic valve to require replacement in infancy. When surgery is needed, it is generally because relief of aortic stenosis has produced significant aortic regurgitation. In these patients, surgical options include the Ross procedure (use of pulmonary autograft to replace the aortic valve with replacement of the pulmonary valve with homograft), or homograft valve replacement of the aortic valve. In both of these procedures, long-term anticoagulation is not necessary.

Intervention Results/Prognosis   In cases of critical valvular stenoses treated during infancy, balloon angioplasty is effective in reducing the gradient on average 50 to 60%. Procedure mortality rate is between 5 and 15%. Redilation later in infancy or early childhood is needed in approximately 40% of patients. It is common for mild aortic regurgitation to be present after the procedure. Long-term follow-up of patients treated surgically between 1958 and 1969 shows good quality of life. Nearly 50% of patients have aortic regurgitation. Approximately 40% of patients of that era required reoperation.

REFERENCES

Achiron R, Malinger G, Zaidel L, Zakut H: Prenatal sonographic diagnosis of endocardial fibroelastosis secondary to aortic stenosis. Prenat Diagn 1988;8:73–77.

Allan LD, Maxwell DJ, Carminati M, Tynan MJ: Survival after fetal aortic balloon valvoplasty. Ultrasound Obstet Gynecol 1995;5:90–91.

Berning RA, Silverman NH, Villegas M, et al: Reversed shunting across the ductus arteriosus or atrial septum in utero heralds severe congenital heart disease. J Am Coll Cardiol 1996;27:481–486.

Bitar FF, Byrum CJ, Kveselis DA, et al: In utero management of hydrops fetalis caused by critical aortic stenosis. Am J Perinatol 1997;14:389–391.

Bove EL: Current status of staged reconstruction for hypoplastic left heart syndrome. Pediatr Cardiol 1998;19:308–315.

Egito ES, Moore P, O'Sullivan J, et al: Transvascular balloon dilation for neonatal critical aortic stenosis: Early and midterm results. J Am Coll Cardiol 1997;29:442–447.

Fyler DC: Aortic outflow abnormalities. In Fyler DC (ed): Nadas' Pediatric Cardiology. Philadelphia, Hanley & Belfus, 1992, pp 493–512.

Fyler DC: Trends. In Fyler DC (ed): Nadas' Pediatric Cardiology. Philadelphia, Hanley & Belfus, 1992, pp 273–284.

Gersony WM, Hayes CJ, Driscoll DJ, et al: Second natural history study of congenital heart defects. Quality of life of patients with aortic stenosis, pulmonary stenosis, or ventricular septal defect. Circulation 1993;87:152–165.

Homberger LK, Bromley H, Lichter E, Benacerraf BR: Development of severe aortic stenosis and left ventricular dysfunction with endocardial fibroelastosis in a second trimester fetus. J Ultrasound Med 1996;15:651–654.

Keane JF, Driscoll DJ, Gersony WM, et al: Second natural history study of congenital heart defects. Results of treatment of patients with aortic valvar stenosis. Circulation 1993;87:I16–I27.

Lin AE, Westgate MN, van der Velde ME, et al: Adams-Oliver syndrome associated with cardiovascular malformations. Clin Dysmorphol 1998;7:235–241.

Lopes LM, Cha SC, Kajita LJ, et al: Balloon dilatation of the aortic valve in the fetus: A case report. Fetal Diagn Ther 1996;11:296–300.

Moore P, Egito E, Mowrey H, et al: Midterm results of balloon dilation of congenital aortic stenosis: predictors of success. J Am Coll Cardiol 1996;27:1257–1263.

Nora JJ, Nora AH: Update on counseling the family with a first-degree relative with a congenital heart defect. Am J Med Genet 1988;29:137–142.

Rustico MA, Benettoni A, Bussani R, et al: Early fetal endocardial fibroelastosis and critical aortic stenosis: A case report. Ultrasound Obstet Gynecol 1995;5:202–205.

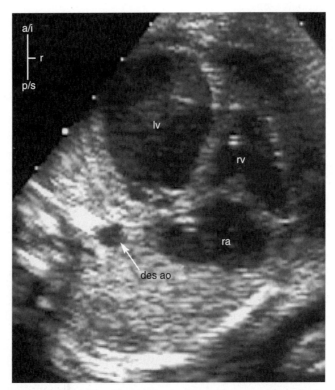

Dilated left ventricle with critical valvular aortic stenosis. Markedly dilated left ventricle (and overall heart size) in a patient with critical valvular aortic stenosis. The *arrow* points to the descending aorta (des ao). Real-time views show markedly depressed left ventricular function. lv, left ventricle; ra, right atrium; rv, right ventricle.

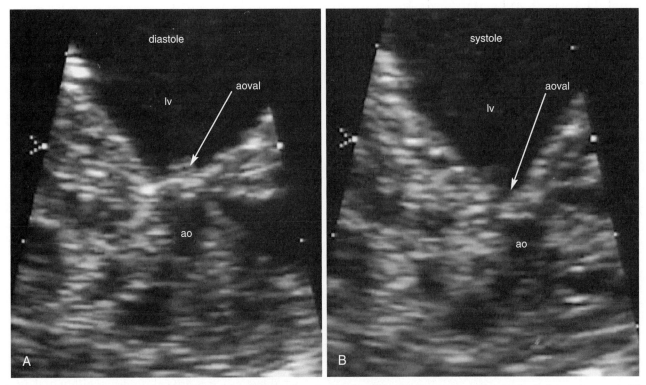

Diastolic and systolic views of an abnormal aortic valve. Thickened aortic valve (aoval) in the same patient with critical valvular aortic stenosis. The aortic valve barely opens from the diastolic frame to the systolic frame. ao, aorta; lv, left ventricle.

Aortic Doppler in patient with critical valvular aortic stenosis. The flow velocities are only minimally increased from normal even though the aortic valve is markedly stenotic. The low gradient reflects the markedly depressed left ventricular function and the poor cardiac output. The ejection time is reduced, also a reflection of poor left ventricular function.

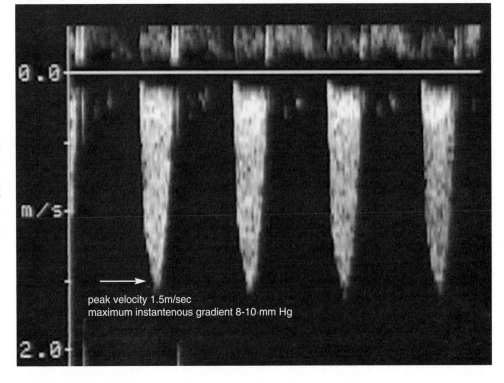

3.7 Hypoplastic Left Heart Syndrome

Epidemiology/Genetics

Definition Left ventricular hypoplasia with mitral stenosis or atresia and valvular aortic stenosis or atresia. There is usually hypoplasia of the ascending aorta. The left ventricle is considered critically hypoplastic when it is so small that it is not able to supply an adequate systemic output.

Epidemiology Prevalence per 1000 live births: 0.103 to 0.267. Accounts for 3 to 4% of children with congenital cardiac disease. In one series, approximately 8% of infants with hypoplastic left heart syndrome had trisomy 18. In another report, chromosomal abnormalities occurred in 16% of infants and chromosomal abnormalities or one or more extracardiac abnormalities in 28%.

Embryology The left ventricle forms from the primitive left ventricle, the mitral valve forms from the endocardial cushions, and the aortic valve forms from the truncus arteriosus.

Inheritance Pattern Recurrence risk for hypoplastic left heart syndrome is reported to be 2% when one sibling is affected and 6% when two siblings are affected. The recurrence risk for any left-sided abnormality could be 10 to 15% among siblings of a proband with hypoplastic left heart syndrome. Hypoplastic left heart syndrome has been reported in three siblings. There are inadequate data to estimate recurrence risk for congenital heart defects in offspring given an affected parent with hypoplastic left heart syndrome. Hypoplastic left heart syndrome has been reported in X;16 translocation, trisomy 9, trisomy 18, Adams-Oliver syndrome, Rubinstein-Taybi syndrome, and Turner syndrome.

Teratogens None reported in humans. In a mouse model, sodium valproate exposure resulted in an increased frequency of hypoplastic left heart syndrome.

Prognosis Untreated hypoplastic left heart syndrome is lethal. The syndrome may be associated with other abnormalities such as chromosomal abnormalities, which would exclude surgery. Palliative surgery generally involves the Norwood operation and subsequently the Glenn and then the Fontan procedure. Among centers with favorable results with this management strategy, the operative survival rate for the Norwood procedure is 76% for all patients and 86% among those at standard risk. Five-year survival rate including all patients is 70%. Results do vary between centers, with survival at 2 years closer to 50% at some centers.

Sonography

FINDINGS

1. **Fetus:**
   a. Critical left ventricular hypoplasia is generally present when the long-axis length of the left ventricle is less than 80% of the long-axis length of the heart. Early during the second trimester, the degree of left ventricular hypoplasia may be subtle. Simply assessing the short-axis dimension of the left ventricle at a basal level may underestimate the degree of left ventricular hypoplasia. Often the left ventricular endocardium is hyperechoic because of endocardial fibroelastosis.
   b. With mitral stenosis or atresia, the mitral valve annulus is hypoplastic and leaflet motion is restricted. Sometimes it is difficult to distinguish mitral atresia from critical mitral stenosis. Color Doppler interrogation with the color scale reduced may accentuate a small amount of antegrade flow or regurgitation.
   c. With critical aortic stenosis or atresia, the annulus is hypoplastic and leaflet motion is restricted. Again, color Doppler interrogation may demonstrate a small amount of antegrade flow when the valve is patent.
   d. The ascending aorta is frequently hypoplastic.
   e. Retrograde flow in the transverse aortic arch is a critical finding and strongly suggests that the left heart is inadequate to supply systemic output and that the lesion will be ductal dependent after delivery.
   f. Reversed flow across the atrial septum (i.e., from left atrium to right atrium) also suggests that the left heart is inadequate to supply the systemic output postnatally.
   g. Tricuspid valve and right ventricular function should be assessed, since the right heart is providing most, if not all, of the cardiac output. Tricuspid regurgitation increases the chance for the development of hydrops.
   h. Increased nuchal translucency may be detected at 11 to 14 weeks.
2. **Amniotic Fluid:** Normal except in the presence of hydrops.
3. **Placenta:** Normal except in the presence of hydrops.
4. **Measurement Data:** May be abnormal in fetuses with abnormal karyotype or extracardiac abnormalities.
5. **When Detectable:** By transabdominal imaging at 17 to 18 weeks. Although transvaginal imaging can achieve appropriate imaging planes at 12 to 14 weeks, the reliability of diagnosis is not clear. Furthermore, in cases with a family history of left-sided obstructive

disease, the fetus should be reimaged at 28 to 32 weeks, since the findings of hypoplastic left heart syndrome can be subtle or absent in the early second trimester.

Pitfalls

1. The left heart can be close to normal size in the early second trimester and become severely hypoplastic later during pregnancy. One can avoid being fooled in such cases by carefully measuring the mitral and aortic valves to exclude hypoplasia, by examining for "reversed" flow at the atrial septum and transverse arch, and by demonstrating antegrade flow with color Doppler interrogation at the mitral and aortic valves.
2. One should assess the adequacy of the atrial septal defect. With critical left atrial outflow obstruction, such as with mitral atresia, an inadequate atrial septal defect will not allow left atrial decompression. In such cases, the pulmonary veins are dilated and there is prominent flow reversal with atrial systole. In addition, pulse Doppler interrogation shows restrictive flow from left to right atrium. A restrictive atrial septal defect is associated with a very poor outcome.

Differential Diagnosis   Mild left heart hypoplasia occurs with aortic coarctation. Left heart hypoplasia occurs in association with diaphragmatic hernia and omphalocele.

Extracardiac anomalies (12%) include duodenal atresia, imperforate anus, vertebral anomalies, and single umbilical artery.

Where Else to Look

1. There are occasional reports of associated omphalocele, diaphragmatic hernia, or hypospadias. Twenty-nine percent of cases have been found to have minor or major central nervous system malformations at autopsy, including microcephaly, immature cortical mantle formation, holoprosencephaly, and agenesis of the corpus callosum.
2. Look for trisomy 18.
3. Look for hydrops—pleural effusion, ascites, and pericardial effusion.

Pregnancy Management

Investigations and Consultations Required   Prenatal consultation with a pediatric cardiologist should occur for confirmation of diagnosis, discussion of options, and coordination of a postnatal management plan when appropriate.

Fetal Intervention   None available at this time.

Monitoring   Fetuses with left heart obstructive disease should be re-examined at 28 and 32 weeks. This will allow assessment for any progression in the severity of left heart hypoplasia and obstruction. Hydrops can develop and is more likely to occur when there is severe tricuspid regurgitation or right ventricular dysfunction.

Pregnancy Course   Unless hydrops develops, fetuses will generally go to term and can be delivered vaginally.

Pregnancy Termination Issues   Given the complex management and guarded prognosis, some families choose not to continue pregnancy. If termination is chosen, an intact fetus should be delivered for confirmation of diagnosis.

Delivery   Delivery should occur in the center where immediate pediatric cardiology and cardiac surgery consultation are available. This lesion will be ductus dependent, and even more urgent management is necessary if there is a restrictive atrial septal defect. Vaginal delivery is generally possible and safe.

Neonatalogy

Resuscitation   Such infants will generally breathe spontaneously and not immediately require assisted ventilation. Adequate venous and arterial access should be obtained and prostaglandin E_1 therapy begun.

Transport   In most cases, infants should be transported to regional centers skilled in taking care of infants with hypoplastic left heart syndrome. Rarely, in cases in which an accurate prenatal diagnosis of hypoplastic left heart syndrome is made and in which the family has chosen compassionate care, transport may not be required.

Testing and Confirmation   The diagnosis of hypoplastic left heart syndrome is definitively made by echocardiography.

Nursery Management   Institution of prostaglandin E therapy often stabilizes the infant with hypoplastic left heart syndrome and allows adequate systemic blood flow. As the pulmonary vascular resistance drops, there may be a tendency for excessive pulmonary blood flow and diminished systemic blood flow. In such situations, measures to reduce excessive pulmonary blood flow include avoidance of supplemental oxygen, administration of nitrogen or carbon dioxide to reduce inspired oxygen concentration, and positive pressure ventilation.

Surgery

Preoperative Assessment   Echocardiography is adequate for preoperative diagnosis whether one pursues the Norwood procedure or heart transplantation.

A fetus with a definitive prenatal diagnosis of hypoplastic left heart syndrome should be listed for heart transplantation prenatally and fetal blood samples obtained to allow for typing. If a donor heart becomes available during the late third trimester, induction or cesarean section may be performed to allow heart transplantation.

Operative Indications   Hypoplastic left heart syndrome is fatal without surgical intervention and therefore the diagnosis itself represents an indication for surgery unless the family chooses compassionate care.

Types of Procedures   Palliative surgery involves three operations. The Norwood procedure is performed soon after birth. The main pulmonary artery is transected proximal to the branch pulmonary arteries and anastomosed to the ascending aorta and transverse arch. The atrial septum is resected to allow unobstructed flow from left to right atrium. A Blalock-Taussig shunt is placed to supply pulmonary blood flow.

A Glenn procedure is performed between 3 and 6 months of age. The superior vena cava is anastomosed to the right pulmonary artery and the Blalock-Taussig shunt removed. This allows systemic venous blood from the head and neck vessels to travel directly to the branch pulmonary arteries.

A Fontan operation is performed between 1 and 6 years of age. The blood from the inferior vena cava and hepatic veins is baffled directly to the lungs. Therefore, the only blood returning to the atria is pulmonary venous blood, which is routed directly to the aorta.

Some centers have chosen to pursue infant heart transplantation. Securing an adequate number of donor hearts for infant transplantation is problematic.

Surgical Results/Prognosis   Among centers with favorable results pursuing the Norwood procedure and later Fontan operation, 5-year survival is 70%. Results are less favorable at other centers, with 2-year survival closer to 50%.

There is significant attrition in infants waiting for a donor heart. Among infants receiving hearts, the actuarial survival rate after transplantation is 84% at 1 month, 70% at 1 year, and 69% at 2 years.

There are some families who do not wish to pursue surgical management and ask for the prostaglandin therapy to be discontinued. This results in fetal death usually within days, sometimes within weeks.

REFERENCES

Allan LD, Apfel HD, Printz BF: Outcome after prenatal diagnosis of the hypoplastic left heart syndrome. Heart 1998;79:371–373.

Bacino CA, Lee B, Spikes AS, Shaffer LG: Trisomy 16q in a female newborn with a de novo X;16 translocation and hypoplastic left heart. Am J Med Genet 1999;82:128–131.

Bartsch O, Wagner A, Hinkel GK, et al: FISH studies in 45 patients with Rubinstein-Taybi syndrome: Deletions associated with polysplenia, hypoplastic left heart and death in infancy. Eur J Hum Genet 1999; 7:748–756.

Berning RA, Silverman NH, Villegas M, et al: Reversed shunting across the ductus arteriosus or atrial septum in utero heralds severe congenital heart disease. J Am Coll Cardiol 1996;27:481–486.

Better DJ, Apfel HD, Zidere V, Allan LD: Pattern of pulmonary venous blood flow in the hypoplastic left heart syndrome in the fetus. Heart 1999;81:646–649.

Blake DM, Copel JA, Kleinman CS: Hypoplastic left heart syndrome: Prenatal diagnosis, clinical profile, and management. Am J Obstet Gynecol 1991;165:529–534.

Bove EL: Surgical treatment for hypoplastic left heart syndrome. Jpn J Thorac Cardiovasc Surg 1999;47:47–56.

Canter C, Naftel D, Caldwell R, et al: Survival and risk factors for death after cardiac transplantation in infants. A multi-institutional study. The Pediatric Heart Transplant Study. Circulation 1997;96:227–231.

Fyler DC: Trends. In Fyler DC (ed): Nadas' Pediatric Cardiology. Philadelphia, Hanley & Belfus, 1992, pp 273–284.

Grobman W, Pergament E: Isolated hypoplastic left heart syndrome in three siblings. Obstet Gynecol 1996;88:673–675.

Hajdu J, Marton T, Toth-Pal E, et al: [Prenatal diagnosis of left cardiac abnormality]. Orv Hetil 1995;136:2333–2337.

Ishino K, Stumper O, De Giovanni JJ, et al: The modified Norwood procedure for hypoplastic left heart syndrome: Early to intermediate results of 120 patients with particular reference to aortic arch repair. J Thorac Cardiovasc Surg 1999;117:920–930.

Lin AE, Westgate MN, van der Velde ME, et al: Adams-Oliver syndrome associated with cardiovascular malformations. Clin Dysmorphol 1998;7:235–241.

Munn MB, Brumfield CG, Lau Y, Colvin EV: Prenatally diagnosed hypoplastic left heart syndrome: Outcomes after postnatal surgery. J Matern Fetal Med 1999;8:147–150.

Natowicz M, Chatten J, Clancy R, et al: Genetic disorders and major extracardiac anomalies associated with the hypoplastic left heart syndrome. Pediatrics 1988;82:698–706.

Nora JJ, Nora AH: Update on counseling the family with a first-degree relative with a congenital heart defect. Am J Med Genet 1988;29:137–142.

Norwood WI, Kirklin JK, Sanders SP: Hypoplastic left heart syndrome: Experience with palliative surgery. Am J Cardiol 1980;45:87–91.

Reis PM, Punch MR, Bove EL, van de Ven CJ: Outcome of infants with hypoplastic left heart and Turner syndromes. Obstet Gynecol 1999;93:532–535.

Rychik J, Rome JJ, Collins MH, et al: The hypoplastic left heart syndrome with intact atrial septum: Atrial morphology, pulmonary vascular histopathology and outcome. J Am Coll Cardiol 1999;34:554–560.

Saneto RP, Applegate KE, Frankel DG: Atypical manifestations of two cases of trisomy 9 syndrome: Rethinking development delay. Am J Med Genet 1998;80:42–45.

Sonoda T, Ohdo S, Ohba K, et al: Sodium valproate-induced cardiovascular abnormalities in the Jcl:ICR mouse fetus: Peak sensitivity of gestational day and dose-dependent effect. Teratology 1993;48:127–132.

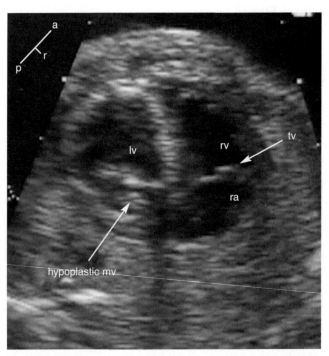

Hypoplastic left heart syndrome. Although there is aortic atresia (not demonstrated in this image), the left ventricle (lv) is still of good size. The left ventricle forms the apex of the heart and its short-axis dimension is comparable to that of the right ventricle (rv). Over the next 6 weeks, the left ventricular cavity dramatically contracts as left ventricular hypertrophy develops. Although in this image the left ventricle is of normal size, the mitral valve (mv) annulus is hypoplastic in absolute terms and in comparison to the tricuspid valve (tv). ra, right atrium.

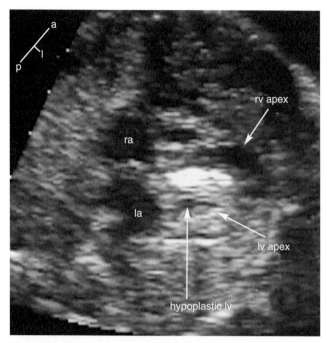

Hypoplastic left heart syndrome with tiny left ventricle. This image is from the same fetus but 6 weeks later. Now the left ventricular cavity is tiny (particularly in the long-axis dimension) and there is marked hypertrophy of left ventricular free wall. The apex of the heart is formed by the right ventricle. la, left atrium; lv, left ventricle; ra, right atrium; rv, right ventricle.

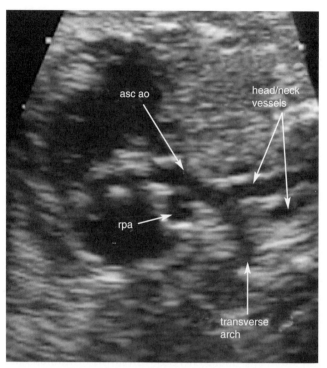

Hypoplastic left heart syndrome with hypoplastic ascending aorta and arch. In the same fetus, the ascending aorta (asc ao) is hypoplastic and is even slightly smaller than the normal size right pulmonary artery (rpa).

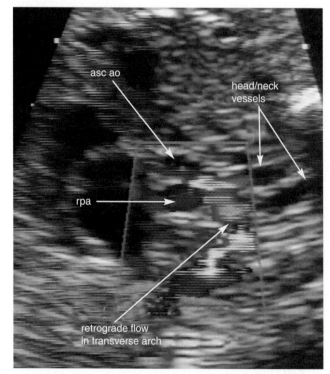

Hypoplastic left heart syndrome with retrograde flow in the transverse aortic arch. Same image but with color Doppler interrogation showing retrograde flow in the transverse arch. This is an ominous finding and strongly suggests a ductus dependent lesion postnatally. asc ao, ascending aorta; rpa, right pulmonary artery. (See color figure following p. x.)

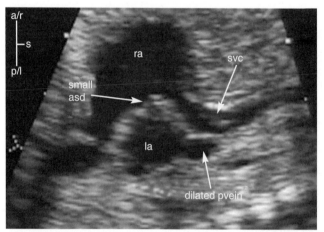

Restrictive atrial septal defect in patient with hypoplastic left heart syndrome. In the same patient, the atrial septal defect (asd) is quite small. Since there is also critical mitral stenosis, the lack of an effective atrial septal defect results in left atrial hypertension as evidenced by a dilated upper lobe pulmonary vein. Left atrial hypertension in utero adversely affects postnatal outcome and frequently is associated with pulmonary lymphangiectasia. Pulse Doppler interrogation shows accelerated flow across the atrial septal defect from left (la) to right atrium (ra). Reversed shunting (i.e., from left to right atrium) is seen in severe left-sided structural or functional disease. svc, superior vena cava.

3.8 Aortic Coarctation

Epidemiology/Genetics

Definition Coarctation is a narrowing of the aorta and most commonly occurs just distal to the origin of the left subclavian artery. Often coarctation is associated with hypoplasia of the transverse arch and other left heart structures such as the mitral and aortic valves.

Epidemiology Prevalence per 1000 live births: 0.2 to 0.6 (M2:F1). Accounts for 3 to 4% of children with congenital cardiac disease. Forty percent have associated cardiac anomalies.

Embryology In the primitive embryo, there are six paired arches. The distal arch forms from the distal dorsal aorta, the ductus arteriosus from the sixth arch, and the distal transverse arch from the fourth arch. Coarctation clinically presents after the first few days of life when the ductus closes. Ductal tissue is present around the posterior aspect of the proximal descending aorta and this tissue constricts along with the ductus itself.

Inheritance Pattern Recurrence risk is 2% when one sibling is affected and 6% when two siblings are affected. The recurrence risk for congenital heart defects in offspring given one affected parent is 4% when the mother is affected and 2% when the father is affected. Coarctation occurs in mosaic trisomy 16, DiGeorge syndrome (deletion 22q), Turner syndrome, and in about 25 other syndromes.

Teratogens Maternal diabetes mellitus. No others clearly identified. There is a report of cousins with coarctation whose mothers had comparable exposure to insecticide.

Prognosis With isolated coarctation of the aorta, surgical management generally results in a good long-term outcome. When coarctation occurs along with other, more complex intracardiac disease, it is often the associated disease that more strongly influences the prognosis.

Sonography

FINDINGS

1. **Fetus:**
   a. It is difficult to identify a discrete narrowing of the arch on a fetal echocardiogram, as one sees postnatally once the ductus arteriosus begins to close. A helpful predictor of aortic coarctation is recognition of significant transverse arch hypoplasia. Normative data are available for these measurements. In relative terms, the transverse arch to ascending aorta ratio in a normal fetus is on average 0.94 and the ratio of left common carotid artery to transverse arch diameter is on average 0.48 ($\pm$0.08). In five fetuses with coarctation, the ratio of left common carotid artery to transverse arch was 0.77 $\pm$ 0.05.
   b. Frequently, there is absolute hypoplasia of other left heart structures, including the mitral valve, aortic valve, and left ventricle. The annuli should be measured and compared with normative data. These structures should be compared with their respective right-sided structures as well. The ratio of the diameter of the ascending aorta to the diameter of the main pulmonary artery is a helpful clue to aortic coarctation but is less specific during the third trimester. When ascending aorta to main pulmonary artery mismatch is recognized before 25 weeks, arch abnormalities may be present in as many as 70% of infants postnatally. At 14 to 16 weeks, a significant discrepancy between a large ductus arteriosus and a smaller aorta may be seen. However, if fetuses at all stages are considered (i.e., including those from the third trimester), coarctation may be falsely predicted on the basis of left heart hypoplasia in as many as 55 to 60% of patients.
   c. Left-to-right flow across the atrial septum occurs in coarctation when the left heart is significantly hypoplastic and may be a marker of a ductus-dependent lesion.
   d. Ventricular septal defects are present in approximately 50% of patients. When there is a posterior malalignment type of defect, there is often critical arch obstruction or even interrupted aortic arch. In a posterior malalignment type of defect, the conal septum is deviated posteriorly under the aortic valve, resulting in a ventricular septal defect with subaortic stenosis.
   e. Other morphologic abnormalities of the left heart are common in coarctation. The aortic valve is abnormal in approximately 60% of infants with coarctation and most commonly the valves are bicommissural. Color and pulse Doppler interrogation of the aortic valve may show accelerated flow if there is significant stenosis. The mitral valve may have closely spaced papillary muscles or even a single left ventricular papillary muscle (termed a parachute mitral valve). This is recognized in short-axis scans of the left ventricle.
   f. A left superior vena cava is present in approximately 18% of patients with coarctation.
   g. Increased nuchal translucency is often present at 11 to 14 weeks.
2. **Amniotic Fluid:** Generally normal.
3. **Placenta:** Generally normal.
4. **Measurement Data:** Generally normal.
5. **When Detectable:** Fetal echocardiography can diagnose aortic coarctation when it is severe, but the test is incompletely sensitive, particularly with mild coarc-

tation. As discussed earlier, one can rely on inferential clues of left heart or arch hypoplasia.

Pitfalls

1. One needs to realize the inadequacy of prenatal echocardiography in reliably predicting all cases of aortic coarctation. When families are counseled after any fetal echocardiogram, the examiner should explain this important limitation.
2. The severity of left heart hypoplasia can progress during the second and third trimester. Where one is screening because of a family history of left-sided disease such as hypoplastic left heart syndrome, valvular aortic stenosis, or coarctation, it is wise to re-examine the fetus at 28 weeks even if the initial study results are normal.

Differential Diagnosis   Aortic coarctation needs to be distinguished from interrupted aortic arch. Most commonly, interruptions occur between the left carotid and left subclavian arteries.

Where Else to Look

1. Coarctation may be associated with other congenital heart defects, most commonly ventricular septal defect or transposition of the great arteries.
2. Look for the stigmata of Turner syndrome such as abnormal renal position, cystic hygroma, isolated pleural effusion, or ascites.
3. Additional features of DiGeorge syndrome, apart from cardiac anomalies, are cleft lip and palate and renal anomalies.

Pregnancy Management

Investigations and Consultations Required   Karyotype analysis (with fluorescent in situ hybridization assay for the chromosome 22q deletion) should be considered when coarctation or interrupted aortic arch is strongly suspected due to the association of Turner syndrome and DiGeorge syndrome. With interrupted aortic arch, chromosome 22q deletion may be present in more than 50% of patients. In this situation, the interruption is most often between the left common carotid artery and left subclavian artery. A complete fetal survey and chromosomal analysis are indicated. The family should meet with a pediatric cardiologist to discuss the cardiac findings and to coordinate a prenatal and postnatal management plan.

Fetal Intervention   None.

Monitoring   A fetal echocardiogram should be repeated at 28 weeks and at 34 weeks because of the potential for worsening of left heart hypoplasia.

Pregnancy Course   Generally well tolerated.

Pregnancy Termination Issues   Given the prognosis after surgical treatment of isolated aortic coarctation, most families continue the pregnancy to term unless associated syndromes or chromosomal abnormalities are identified.

Delivery   Delivery should occur at centers where prostaglandin therapy can be administered if the lesion is ductus dependent.

Neonatology

Resuscitation   Assistance with respiration is usually not required. However, if there is delay in the spontaneous onset of breathing, oxygen supplementation should be limited to 40 to 60% maximum and only for the time needed to establish adequate color to avoid closing the ductus. Infants should be immediately transported to the neonatal intensive care unit and prostaglandin E_1 infusion begun.

Transport   Immediate transport to a tertiary center with full pediatric cardiac diagnostic and surgical capabilities is essential for infants with coarctation with congestive heart failure, low cardiac output, or evidence of ductus-dependent systemic perfusion. Consultation with a pediatric cardiologist prior to transport to determine appropriate supportive measures is indicated. Management during transport should be by personnel experienced in neonatal transport with capability for mechanical ventilation and delivery of cardiotonic infusions.

Testing and Confirmation   Coarctation should be considered when lower extremity pulses are decreased or when there is a gradient between upper and lower extremity systolic blood pressures of more than 10 mm Hg. Oxygen saturation in the lower extremity of 94% or less is suggestive of right-to-left shunting at the ductal level, which can occur in severe arch obstruction. Echocardiography should be definitive in making the diagnosis of coarctation.

Nursery Management   The goal of initial neonatal management is to achieve and sustain a balance between pulmonary and systemic blood flow by maintaining patency of the ductus and a pulmonary-to-systemic shunt across the ductus to provide adequate perfusion to the lower body, particularly the liver and kidneys. Hyperventilation and supplemental oxygen decrease pulmonary resistance and thereby alter the direction and magnitude of ductal or intracardiac shunting through associated lesions. Both should be avoided. Acidosis should be treated aggressively with buffer. Dopamine infusion may be needed to improve cardiac output and renal perfusion. Recovery from surgical repair is enhanced by limiting organ damage from inadequate perfusion prior to surgery.

Surgery

Preoperative Assessment   Echocardiography is sufficient for preoperative diagnosis in most cases of aortic coarctation during the newborn period. In older children or adolescents, magnetic resonance imaging may be helpful when echocardiography does not achieve adequate visualization.

Operative Indications   Surgery is indicated during the newborn period when the lesion is ductal dependent or when the coarctation is severe. In less severe cases of coarctation, surgery is usually performed after 2 months of age or when the diagnosis is made if not recognized during infancy.

Types of Procedures Most centers recommend surgical repair of aortic coarctation. One of two procedures can be performed. The coarctation can be resected and an end-to-end anastomosis performed. An alternative approach is the left subclavian flap plasty procedure in which the proximal left subclavian artery is used to augment the area of coarctation. A few centers recommend balloon dilation for native coarctation, but the long-term results are probably not as good as for surgical treatment.

Surgical Results/Prognosis Operative mortality for aortic coarctation is less than 5%. Longer term, recurrent coarctation can develop in approximately 10% of patients. Recurrent coarctation is usually successfully treated with balloon angioplasty.

REFERENCES

Allan LD, Chita SK, Anderson RH, et al: Coarctation of the aorta in prenatal life: An echocardiographic, anatomical, and functional study. Br Heart J 1988;59:356–360.

Benacerraf BR, Saltzman DH, Sanders SP: Sonographic sign suggesting the prenatal diagnosis of coarctation of the aorta. J Ultrasound Med 1989;8:65–69.

Blagowidow N, Page DC, Huff D, Mennuti MT: Ullrich-Turner syndrome in an XY female fetus with deletion of the sex-determining portion of the Y chromosome. Am J Med Genet 1989;34:159–162.

Bronshtein M, Zimmer EZ: Sonographic diagnosis of fetal coarctation of the aorta at 14–16 weeks of gestation. Ultrasound Obstet Gynecol 1998;11:254–257.

Daebritz SH, Nollert GD, Zurakowski D, et al: Results of Norwood stage I operation: Comparison of hypoplastic left heart syndrome with other malformations. J Thorac Cardiovasc Surg 2000;119:358–367.

David N, Iselin M, Blaysat G, et al: [Disproportion in diameter of the cardiac chambers and great arteries in the fetus. Contribution to the prenatal diagnosis of coarctation of the aorta]. Arch Mal Coeur Vaiss 1997;90:673–678.

Fyler DC: Trends. In Fyler DC (ed): Nadas' Pediatric Cardiology. Philadelphia, Hanley & Belfus, 1992, pp 273–284.

Ghi T, Higgin IC, Zasmer N , et al: Incidences of major structural cardiac defects associated with increased nuchal translucency but normal karyotype. Ultrasound Obstet Gynecol 2001;18:610–614.

Greally JM, Neiswanger K, Cummins JH, et al: A molecular anatomical analysis of mosaic trisomy 16. Hum Genet 1996;98:86–90.

Hornberger LK, Weintraub RG, Pesonen E, et al: Echocardiographic study of the morphology and growth of the aortic arch in the human fetus. Observations related to the prenatal diagnosis of coarctation. Circulation 1992;86:741–747.

Lewin MB, Lindsay EA, Jurecic V, et al: A genetic etiology for interruption of the aortic arch type B. Am J Cardiol 1997;80:493–497.

Momma K, Matsuoka R, Takao A: Aortic arch anomalies associated with chromosome 22q11 deletion (CATCH 22). Pediatr Cardiol 1999;20:97–102.

Nora JJ, Nora AH: Update on counseling the family with a first-degree relative with a congenital heart defect. Am J Med Genet 1988;29:137–142.

Sharland OK, Chan KY, Allan LD: Coarctation of the aorta: Difficulties in prenatal diagnosis. Br Heart J 1994;71:70–75.

Trost D, Engels H, Bauriedel G, et al: [Congenital cardiovascular malformations and chromosome microdeletions in 22q11.2]. Dtsch Med Wochenschr 1999;124:3–7.

Wilson DI, Cross IE, Goodship JA, et al: DiGeorge syndrome with isolated aortic coarctation and isolated ventricular septal defect in three sibs with a 22q11 deletion of maternal origin. Br Heart J 1991;66:308–312.

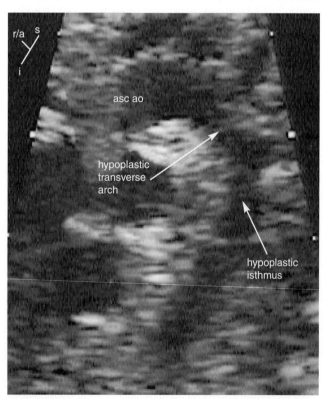

Hypoplastic transverse and distal aortic arch. In this 37-week fetus, the transverse arch measures 4 mm (5 standard deviations below the mean) and the isthmus (the segment distal to the left subclavian artery and before the ductal insertion) is hypoplastic as well. In utero, it is unusual to image the actual coarctation unless the narrowing is extremely severe or the arch is interrupted. Arch hypoplasia represents a clue that coarctation may develop postnatally. asc ao, ascending aorta.

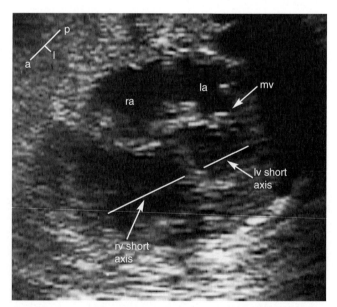

Ventricular mismatch with aortic coarctation. In the same fetus, the left ventricular (lv) short-axis dimension is reduced compared with normative data, but even more striking is the relative hypoplasia in comparison to the right ventricular (rv) short-axis dimension. As is common in aortic coarctation, the mitral valve (mv) is also hypoplastic. Postnatally, this patient developed coarctation and required surgery. The left heart hypoplasia is another clue of postnatal arch obstruction. la, left atrium; ra, right atrium.

3.9 Ventricular Septal Defect

Epidemiology/Genetics

Definition   Refers to incomplete septation between the left and right ventricles. Ventricular septal defects are classified into four major types: conoventricular, muscular, inlet (also called atrioventricular canal or posterior), and conal septal or intraconal (also called subpulmonary and, less accurately, supracristal).

Epidemiology   Prevalance per 1000 live births: 0.4 to 2.7. Ventricular septal defect is the most common congenital heart lesion diagnosed during the first year of life and accounts for 20 to 30% of congenital heart disease.

Embryology   The embryology varies depending on the location of the sepal defect. Malalignment defects, a subtype of conoventricular defects, represent an abnormality of the conotruncus and are frequently associated with abnormalities of either the pulmonary or the systemic outflow. Muscular defects are thought to be due to excessive excavation during ventricular growth. Inlet, outlet, and membranous defects are thought to be due to a failure of fusion.

Inheritance Pattern   Recurrence risk is 3% when one sibling is affected and 10% when two siblings are affected. The recurrence risk when a parent has a ventricular septal defect is approximately 3%. The majority of ventricular septal defects are sporadic; however, more than 100 genetic and chromosomal syndromes have been described with ventricular septal defect as an abnormality.

Teratogens   Many reported teratogens, including fetal alcohol syndrome, maternal anticonvulsants, maternal diabetes, maternal phenylketonuria, and fetal infections.

Prognosis   Isolated ventricular septal defects usually have an excellent prognosis, with a quality of life for the patient similar to that of the general population. Muscular and sometimes membranous defects can undergo sufficient spontaneous closure to avoid a need for surgery. Spontaneous closure can occur in utero. Inlet and intraconal defects usually do require surgery. Malalignment defects nearly always require surgery and carry the prognosis of the associated lesion such as tetralogy of Fallot or interrupted aortic arch with ventricular septal defect. Prognosis is frequently dependent on associated abnormalities or syndrome diagnosis.

Sonography

FINDINGS

1. **Fetus:**
   a. Conoventricular septal defects are defects between the conal and muscular septum. They can be of two types.

1. Membranous defects are anatomically located beneath the septal leaflet of the tricuspid valve on the right ventricular septal surface and below the aortic valve along the left ventricular septal surface. These defects are best imaged when the scan plane is perpendicular to this portion of the septum. False dropout can occur in this portion of the septum when viewed from the standard four-chamber view.
2. Malalignment defects occur when the conal septum is malaligned in relation to the muscular septum. There are two types of malalignment defects.
   - Anterior malalignment: Malalignment of the conal septum is often best seen when one or both outflows are profiled from a high parasagittal imaging or apical view. Short-axis views at the level of great vessels will also demonstrate malalignment of conal septum. An anterior malalignment type of defect in a fetus with normally related great vessels may result in subvalvular pulmonary stenosis and most commonly occurs in tetralogy of Fallot. An anterior malalignment type of defect in a fetus with transposition of the great arteries may result in subvalvular aortic stenosis and is frequently associated with arch obstruction. Details concerning the imaging of these defects are reviewed in the relevant sections on tetralogy of Fallot and transposition of the great arteries with ventricular septal defect.
   - Posterior malalignment: A posterior malalignment defect in a fetus with normally related great vessels may result in subvalvular aortic stenosis and is frequently associated with valvular aortic stenosis and aortic arch obstruction. The posteriorly malaligned conal septum is best profiled from an apical four-chamber view or a high parasagittal view. A posterior malalignment defect in a fetus with transposition of the great arteries may result in subvalvular pulmonary stenosis and is frequently associated with pulmonary valve stenosis and annular hypoplasia.
   b. Muscular septal defects are further subcategorized based on their location within the muscular septum as anterior, middle, posterior, or apical muscular defects. Muscular defects are difficult to see prenatally when they are small and even sometimes when they are moderately sized. Frequently muscular defects are multiple. Color Doppler echocardiography with appropriate optimization can sometimes show biphasic flow across the defects.
   c. Inlet defects involve the atrioventricular canal septum and are immediately adjacent to the atrioven-

tricular valves and confluent with the crux of the heart. These defects can be seen in isolation but are more commonly seen in a complete atrioventricular canal defect. Discussion of these lesions occurs in the section on complete atrioventricular canal defects.

   d. Conal septal defects occur when there is a deficiency of conal septum and are located immediately below the pulmonary and aortic valves. These defects do not involve malalignment of the conal septum. These defects are very rare in North America but are more common among Asian populations.

2. **Amniotic Fluid:** Generally normal. High-grade atrioventricular block can occur in some patients with atrioventricular canal defects and heterotaxy syndrome and, if so, may result in hydrops.
3. **Placenta:** Normal unless there is hydrops.
4. **Measurement Data:** Normal.
5. **When Detectable:** Transabdominal imaging can detect defects between 16 to 18 weeks, and transvaginal imaging has detected malalignment defects at 14 weeks.

Pitfalls

1. It may be difficult to distinguish false dropout of the ventricular septum from a true septal defect. This is most easily avoided by imaging in a plane perpendicular to the suspected defect and imaging the defect from multiple views. False dropout is most likely to occur when the beam is parallel to the suspected defect.
2. Color Doppler flow mapping is also most reliable when the angle of flow interrogation is perpendicular to the suspected defect and when machine settings are optimized. Using low persistence and achieving a color Doppler frame rate in excess of 20 Hz is important.

Differential Diagnosis   When a septal defect is recognized, the examiner must exclude other associated heart disease, particularly when the septal defect is one of the conoventricular types.

Where Else to Look   Particularly when malalignment defects are detected, other complex heart disease must be excluded and the chromosome 22q microdeletion syndrome should be considered. Chromosomal abnormalities are present in 40 to 50% of fetuses with atrioventricular canal defects, with Down syndrome accounting for the majority. Conoventricular defects occur in 70 to 80% of infants with trisomy 13 and 18. In trisomy 18, the ventricular septal defect is frequently associated with tricuspid (80%), pulmonary (70%), and aortic (68%) valve abnormalities. Look throughout the rest of the fetus for the sonographic findings of chromosomal anomalies.

Pregnancy Management

Investigations and Consultations Required   Pediatric cardiology consultation should be obtained when a septal defect is recognized, to allow prenatal counseling and also to help exclude the association of more complex congenital heart disease. Karyotyping and deletion 22q fluorescent in situ hybridization should be performed in cases of conoventricular and atrioventricular canal ventricular septal defects due to associated chromosomal abnormalities.

Fetal Intervention   None relevant.

Monitoring   Conoventricular septal defect should be re-imaged between 28 and 30 weeks' gestation to ensure that the outflow tracts are not obstructed.

Pregnancy Course   Generally uneventful.

Pregnancy Termination Issues   Termination is not generally relevant with an isolated ventricular septal defect given the favorable prognosis.

Delivery   If the septal defect is isolated and not associated with outflow obstruction, it would be acceptable for the baby to be delivered and pediatric cardiology consultation obtained during the first week of life. However, with a conoventricular defect with outflow obstruction, in which there is the potential for a ductus dependent lesion, more urgent cardiology consultation may be needed and the baby should be delivered where these resources are available.

Neonatology

Resuscitation   Infants will generally breathe spontaneously and not require resuscitation.

Transport   An infant with a ventricular septal defect without outflow tract obstruction can be discharged with a pediatric cardiology follow-up within the first week of life.

Testing and Confirmation   The urgency of postnatal testing is determined by the presence of associated cardiac defects and the type of septal defect. If the defect is located in the muscular or membranous septum and is in isolation, pediatric cardiology follow-up can be obtained electively within the first week of life. When conotruncal abnormalities are present, an echocardiogram should be performed before discharge.

Nursery Management   Small muscular ventricular septal defects usually remain asymptomatic, whereas moderate to large and membranous defects become progressively more symptomatic as pulmonary vascular resistance falls in the first 4 to 6 weeks of life. Sodium and fluid restriction and diuretic therapy are used to control congestive heart failure. High-calorie formulas and tube feedings may be needed to sustain adequate growth.

Surgery

Preoperative Assessment   Noninvasive diagnosis using echocardiography is generally adequate. If it is uncertain whether the ventricular septal defect is significant or whether there is irreversible pulmonary vascular disease, cardiac catheterization will also be required preoperatively.

Operative Indications   During infancy, isolated ventricular septal defects are closed if congestive heart failure results in failure to thrive despite maximum medical management or if there is pulmonary artery hypertension. Longstanding pulmonary artery hypertension can result

in the development of pulmonary vascular obstructive disease.

A large left ventricular volume overload may represent an indication for surgery during childhood even if the patient is thriving and the pulmonary artery pressures are normal.

When the ventricular septal defect is part of other more complicated congenital heart disease, the indications for the other diseases are generally relevant.

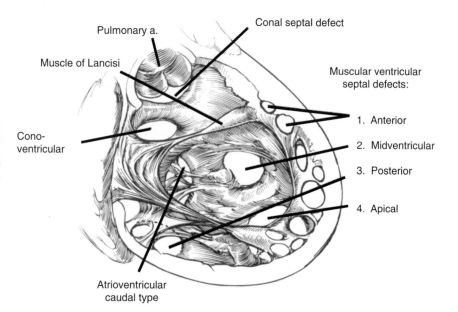

Locations of ventricular septal defects as viewed from the right ventricle. (From ventricular septal defect. In Castaneda AC, Jonas RA, Mayer JE, Hanley F (eds): Cardiac Surgery of the Neonate and Infant. Philadelphia, WB Saunders, 1994, p 188.)

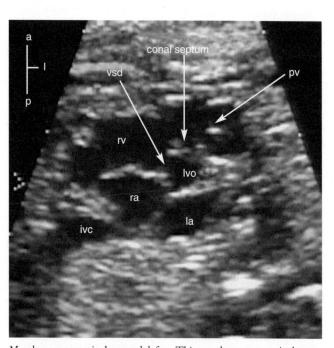

Membranous ventricular septal defect. This membranous ventricular septal defect (vsd) is seen just anterior to the tricuspid valve along the right septal surface and just below the aortic annulus along the left septal surface. The conal septum is intact and there is no malalignment as in tetralogy of Fallot. Compared with a malalignment ventricular septal defect as in tetralogy of Fallot, a membranous defect is more rightward and posterior. ivc, inferior vena cava; la, left atrium; lvo, left ventricular outflow tract; pv, pulmonary valve; ra, right atrium; rv, right ventricle.

3.10 Atrioventricular Canal Defects (Endocardial Cushion Defect)

Epidemiology/Genetics

Definition Atrioventricular canal defects include a spectrum of lesions ranging from a complete common atrioventricular canal to an isolated primum type of atrial septal defect. A complete canal defect consists of good-sized ventricular and atrial defects associated with a common atrioventricular valve. Canal defects with smaller ventricular septal defects are referred to as incomplete, partial, or transitional canal defects. In even more mild cases, there may be no ventricular defect at all but only a primum type of atrial septal defect. In such cases, there is always an abnormality of the formation of the mitral valve such that the anterior leaflet is divided, or cleft.

Epidemiology Prevalence per 1000 live births: 0.1 to 0.4. Accounts for approximately 5% of patients followed with congenital heart disease postnatally. There is a 60% association with chromosomal anomalies.

Embryology Abnormalities of the atrioventricular canal result from malformation in the development of the endocardial cushion. The endocardial cushions are involved in the closure of both the atrial and the ventricular septum and in the development of both atrioventricular valves.

Inheritance Pattern The recurrence risk for congenital heart disease is 3% when one sibling is affected with an endocardial cushion defect and 10% when two siblings are affected. When a parent is affected, the recurrence risk is 14% when the mother is affected and only 1% when the father is affected. When complete atrioventricular canal defects occur as isolated lesions, Down syndrome is present in 57 to 72% of fetuses. Atrioventricular canal defects also occur, but less commonly, in trisomy 13 and 18, short arm deletion of chromosome 8, and trisomy 22.

Teratogens Maternal diabetes mellitus.

Prognosis Atrioventricular canal defects occurring in isolation generally have a good prognosis in terms of the cardiac disease, but surgery is required. When occurrence is associated with chromosomal abnormalities or as a part of a heterotaxy syndrome, the prognosis is worsened.

Sonography

FINDINGS

1. **Fetus:**
   a. A common atrioventricular valve is easily recognized from a four-chamber view and, frequently, so are the atrial and ventricular septal defects. The inlet ventricular septal defect is confluent with the crux, and the primum type of atrial defect involves the most inferior, leftward, and anterior portion of the atrial septum. False dropout can occur from the apical four-chamber view, and it is important to image these defects in a scan plane perpendicular to the septum.
   b. Valve abnormalities are nearly always present with endocardial cushion defects, with the exception being an isolated atrioventricular type of ventricular septal defect. A common atrioventricular valve is well demonstrated in short-axis imaging of the ventricles. Isolated primum atrial septal defects are always associated with a cleft of the mitral valve. The cleft of the anterior leaflet refers to the division of the anterior leaflet with attachments to the left ventricular surface of the septum.
   c. Color Doppler interrogation for atrioventricular valve regurgitation is important, since outcome is adversely affected when the atrioventricular valve (or valves) is regurgitant.
   d. Increased nuchal translucency is often present at 11 to 16 weeks.
2. **Amniotic Fluid:** Generally normal, although hydrops can develop when high-grade atrioventricular block occurs in heterotaxy syndrome or when there is severe atrioventricular valve regurgitation.
3. **Placenta:** Normal unless there is hydrops.
4. **Measurement Data:** May be helpful in estimating the likelihood of associated Down syndrome.
5. **When Detectable:** Transabdominal imaging reveals canal defects at 16 to 18 weeks and transvaginal imaging between 10 and 14 weeks.

Pitfalls

1. False dropout can mimic atrial and ventricular septal defects. Imaging in a scan plane perpendicular to the suspected defect and identification of the abnormalities of the atrioventricular valve (which are nearly always present in true atrioventricular canal defects) is important.
2. A dilated coronary sinus may be confused for a primum type of atrial septal defect, since both are located near the level of the atrioventricular valve. The dilated coronary sinus is more posterior (along the posterior atrioventricular valve groove) than the primum atrial septal defect that is located just posterior to the aortic root. Atrioventricular valve abnormalities are also nearly always present in primum defects and are not present with isolated coronary sinus dilation. The most common reason for a dilated coronary sinus is a left superior vena cava.

Differential Diagnosis   Atrioventricular canal defects occur in the heterotaxy syndrome. Abnormalities of the outflow tracts and venous return should be excluded. Conotruncal abnormalities such as double-outlet right ventricle are frequent in heterotaxy.

Where Else to Look

1. Look for associated cardiac defects such as left ventricular hypoplasia or outflow tract obstruction.
2. Look for the features of the chromosomal abnormalities, particularly Down syndrome.
3. Look for a spleen to exclude heterotaxy syndrome.

Pregnancy Management

Investigations and Consultations Required   Pediatric cardiology consultation should be obtained for confirmation of prenatal diagnosis and initiation of a management plan. Chromosomal analysis should be obtained in all cases.

Fetal Intervention   None available except for pacing, which has been attempted in complete heart block.

Monitoring   Fetuses should be re-examined at 28 to 32 weeks to assess for development or progression of atrioventricular valve regurgitation and hydrops.

Pregnancy Course   When there is severe atrioventricular valve regurgitation and/or complete heart block, hydrops can develop and fetal demise may occur.

Pregnancy Termination Issues   If termination is chosen, an intact fetus should be delivered for confirmation of diagnosis and exclusion of noncardiac abnormalities.

Delivery   Isolated atrioventricular canal defects without significant atrioventricular valve regurgitation do not necessarily need to be delivered in a regional center, but pediatric cardiology consultation should be obtained within the first few days after delivery.

Neonatology

Resuscitation   Assistance with the onset of respiration is usually not required for infants with an isolated defect. In the presence of other defects, particularly those involving the central nervous system or the respiratory tract, spontaneous breathing may be affected and assistance required.

Transport   Infants with isolated canal defects do not require referral in the immediate neonatal period.

Testing and Confirmation   Postnatal diagnosis is confirmed with echocardiography.

Nursery Management   Mild oxygen desaturation is typical while the pulmonary vascular resistance remains elevated. As the pulmonary resistance falls, the oxygen sat-

uration will gradually increase, and symptoms of congestive heart disease may develop. Heart failure generally develops within the first 1 to 3 weeks of life.

Surgery

Preoperative Assessment   Echocardiography is usually definitive in assessing atrioventricular canal defects.

Operative Indications   Nearly all atrioventricular canal defects require surgery. Infants with complete canal defects should undergo elective repair by 4 months of age, or earlier if congestive heart failure limits growth. Primum atrial septal defects should be closed between 6 and 18 months of age. When there is pulmonary artery hypertension, surgery should take place earlier.

Types of Procedures   Canal defects are generally approached through a right atriotomy and septal defects closed with either a single- or a double-patch technique. The common atrioventricular valve is divided at repair.

A pulmonary artery band is sometimes used as a palliative procedure instead of performing a complete repair to control pulmonary blood flow where repair cannot be performed at acceptable risk (i.e., with other more complex lesions or if the patient is too small).

Surgical Results/Prognosis   Repair of isolated complete atrioventricular canal defects carries a good prognosis, with operative survival in excess of 97%. A minority of patients will have significant atrioventricular canal regurgitation postoperatively, and some may require mitral valve replacement or reoperation. There is a less than 5% incidence of postoperative complete heart block, which would require a pacemaker.

REFERENCES

Allan LD: Atrioventricular septal defect in the fetus. Am J Obstet Gynecol 1999;181:1250–1253.

Cesko I, Hajdu J, Marton T, et al: [Fetal atrioventricular septal defect associated with Patau and Edwards syndromes, as well as trisomy 22]. Orv Hetil 1998;139:1087–1089.

Delisle MF, Sandor GG, Tessier F, Farquharson DF: Outcome of fetuses diagnosed with atrioventricular septal defect. Obstet Gynecol 1999;94:763–767.

Devriendt K, Van Schoubroeck D, Eyskens B, et al: Prenatal diagnosis of a terminal short arm deletion of chromosome 8 in a fetus with an atrioventricular septal defect. Prenat Diagn 1998;18:65–67.

Fyler DC: Trends. In Fyler DC (ed): Nadas' Pediatric Cardiology. Philadelphia, Hanley & Belfus, 1992, pp 273–284.

Gembruch U, Knopfle G, Chatterjee M, et al: First-trimester diagnosis of fetal congenital heart disease by transvaginal two-dimensional and Doppler echocardiography. Obstet Gynecol 1990;75:496–498.

Ghi T, Higgin IC, Zasmer N, et al: Incidence of major structural cardiac defects associated with increased nuchal translucency but normal karyotype. Ultrasound Obstet Gynecol 2001;18:610–614.

Grech V, Vella C: Atrioventricular septal defect with separate right and left atrioventricular valvar orifices in a patient with foetal hydantoin syndrome. Cardiol Young 1999;9:73–74.

Hajdu J, Marton T, Papp C, et al: [Prenatal diagnosis of atrioventricular septal defect and its prognostic significance]. Orv Hetil 1998;139:23–26.

Nora JJ, Nora AH: Update on counseling the family with a first-degree relative with a congenital heart defect. Am J Med Genet 1988;29:137–142.

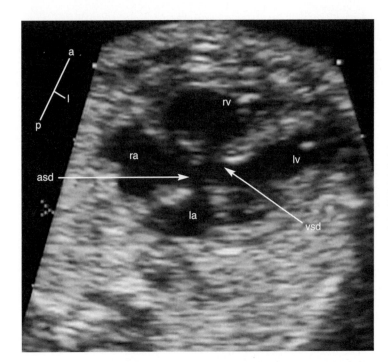

Apical four chamber view in a fetus with complete common atrioventricular canal defect. The atrial (asd) and ventricular (vsd) septal defects are seen above and below the common atrioventricular valve. Note that the primum atrial septal defect is in the most inferior portion of the atrial septum. False dropout is avoided by imaging in a scan plane not completely parallel to the septum. la, left atrium; lv, left ventricle; ra, right atrium; rv, right ventricle.

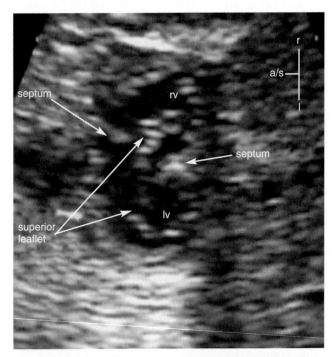

Cross-sectional view of the common atrioventricular valve. The ventricles are displayed in short axis and the superior leaflet of the common atrioventricular valve extends across the septum. This view is helpful in demonstrating that there is a single atrioventricular valve. In this patient, the valve is mildly malaligned toward the left ventricle (lv) with approximately 60% of the valve directed to the left ventricle. Severe malalignment of more than 70% complicates repair, particularly if malalignment is toward the right ventricle (rv).

3.11 Truncus Arteriosus

Epidemiology/Genetics

Definition A single great vessel arises from the heart and supplies the systemic, pulmonary, and coronary blood flow. The single vessel usually arises above a malalignment type of ventricular septal defect and straddles the ventricular septum.

There is variability in the origins of the branch pulmonary arteries and whether or not the aortic arch is interrupted. Van Praagh has suggested classifying truncus arteriosus with ventricular septal defect into four types. In type I, a main pulmonary artery arises from the truncal root and bifurcates into the branch pulmonary arteries. In type II, the branch pulmonary arteries arise separately from the truncal root. In type III, the left pulmonary artery is supplied by collaterals from the aortic arch and does not arise from the truncal root. In type IV, the aortic arch is interrupted. Truncus arteriosus may rarely occur without a ventricular septal defect.

Epidemiology Prevalence per 1000 live births: 0.03 to 0.21 cases. Accounts for 0.4% of children with congenital cardiac disease.

Embryology The bulbus cordis differentiates into the right ventricle, conus cordis, and truncus arteriosus. The truncus arteriosus should septate into the aortic and pulmonary valves and the ascending aorta and main pulmonary artery. Failure of septation results in persistence of the truncus arteriosus.

Inheritance Pattern The recurrence risk for congenital heart disease in siblings of a patient with nonsyndromic truncus arteriosus is 1% when one sibling is affected and 3% when two are affected. The recurrence risk in offspring of parents affected with truncus arteriosus is unknown. Rare familial cases have been reported, showing an autosomal dominant inheritance pattern. A microdeletion of chromosome 22 occurs in 12 to 35% of infants with truncus arteriosus.

Teratogens Apart from maternal diabetes mellitus, none reported in humans.

Prognosis There is an operative mortality rate of approximately 5% at the initial operation. Replacement of the conduit placed during the repair between the right ventricle and pulmonary arteries is needed in the future. The operative mortality rate for conduit replacement is approximately 1 to 3%. The frequent association of the chromosome 22q deletion may significantly impact the prognosis.

Sonography

FINDINGS

1. **Fetus:**
   a. A single great vessel arises from the heart and supplies both the branch pulmonary arteries and the ascending aorta. The ascending aorta continues to supply the head and neck vessels. Identification of the right and left pulmonary arteries and their origins is crucial.
   b. Usually the truncal root will straddle the muscular septum above a malalignment type of ventricular septal defect. Therefore, the truncal root will receive blood from both the right and left ventricles. If the root is predominantly above the right ventricle, the repair is more difficult.
   c. The truncal valve is frequently abnormal. Color and pulse Doppler interrogation should identify truncal stenosis and/or regurgitation.
   d. Interrupted aortic arch occurs in 10 to 15% of patients with truncus arteriosus. The ascending aorta supplies the head and neck vessels, but the descending aorta is supplied by the ductus arteriosus and not by continuation of the aortic arch. In truncus arteriosus without interrupted aortic arch, a ductus arteriosus is usually not present.
   e. A right aortic arch is present in 20 to 30% of patients. The probability of the chromosome 22q deletion is increased when the arch is right-sided.
2. **Amniotic Fluid:** Normal.
3. **Placenta:** Normal.
4. **Measurement Data:** Normal.
5. **When Detectable:** By transabdominal imaging at 16 to 18 weeks. Malalignment ventricular septal defects have been diagnosed with transvaginal echocardiography at 14 weeks.

Pitfalls

1. A single great vessel arises above a malalignment ventricular septal defect in other diseases besides truncus arteriosus. Teratology of Fallot with pulmonary artery atresia is the most common example. In this case, the aorta straddles the septum and the main pulmonary artery is absent. Another heart disease that may mimic truncus arteriosus is aortic atresia with ventricular septal defect, in which the main pulmonary artery straddles the septum and the ascending aorta is tiny. Careful identification of the branch pulmonary arteries and the origins of the head and neck vessels distinguishes truncus arteriosus from these diseases.
2. In truncus arteriosus with interrupted aortic arch, the ductus arteriosus can mimic the transverse arch and

might confuse the sonographer into believing that the arch is not interrupted. One will not make this mistake if the origins of the head and neck vessels are identified. They will arise from the transverse arch, not from the ductus arteriosus.

Differential Diagnosis   As mentioned, truncus arteriosus should be distinguished from other diseases such as tetralogy of Fallot or aortic atresia with ventricular septal defect.

Where Else To Look   Truncus arteriosus is associated with the DiGeorge syndrome or velocardiofacial syndrome (deletion 22q) in approximately 12 to 35% of cases. The microdeletion is more common in type III truncus and when the arch is right-sided. Look for cleft lip and palate, micrognathia, and renal problems.

Pregnancy Management

Investigations and Consultations Required   Pediatric cardiology consultation should be obtained for confirmation of diagnosis and coordination of prenatal and potential postnatal management. Karyotype analysis and fluorescent in situ hybridization assay for the 22 deletion syndrome are recommended in all patients with truncus arteriosus.

Fetal Intervention   None available.

Monitoring   The fetus should be re-examined at 28 and 32 weeks to assess truncal valve function and growth of the branch pulmonary arteries.

Pregnancy Termination Issues   Truncus arteriosus may be associated with other noncardiac malformations and an intact fetus should be delivered for complete examination.

Delivery   Delivery should occur in a tertiary center with full pediatric cardiac diagnostic and surgical capabilities.

Neonatology

Resuscitation   Assistance with the onset of respiration is usually not required. Early-onset cyanosis may occur and be confusing in the transition immediately following delivery.

Transport   Immediate referral to a tertiary center with full pediatric cardiac diagnostic and surgical capability is imperative once a diagnosis of cyanotic congenital heart disease is suspected. Consultation with a pediatric cardiologist prior to transport is recommended to determine the need for initiation of a prostaglandin E_1 infusion. Management in transport should be by personnel experienced in neonatal transport and with the capability of mechanical ventilation.

Testing and Confirmation   Postnatal echocardiography is generally sufficient for preoperative assessment.

Nursery Management   The critical issues that determine early management are (1) the anatomy of pulmonary blood flow, thus the potential for early-onset congestive heart failure; and (2) the anatomy of the aortic arch and the integrity of systemic flow to the distal body. Infants with the former may require measures to limit pulmonary flow such as limited fluid intake, decreased inspired oxygen concentration, and diuretics. Infants with an interrupted aortic arch require the administration of prostaglandin E to maintain ductal flow and thus blood to the descending aorta.

Surgery

Preoperative Assessment   Postnatal echocardiography is generally sufficient for preoperative assessment.

Operative Indications   All infants with truncus arteriosus require surgical treatment.

Types of Procedures   In most cases, definitive repair is performed within the first 10 days of life or at the time of diagnosis if not recognized as a newborn. The septal defect is patched such that the truncal root receives blood only from the left ventricle. The branch pulmonary arteries are removed from the truncal root and are connected to the right ventricle, generally using a homograft. The donor pulmonary artery sites are carefully patched so as to not distort the coronary arteries that are in close proximity. When the aortic arch is interrupted, complete repair is still performed within the newborn period. The interrupted segments are directly anastomosed.

It is not advisable to palliate infants with truncus arteriosus by banding the branch pulmonary arteries. This has been performed historically and generally results in long-term problems with branch pulmonary artery distortion and/or pulmonary vascular disease.

Surgical Results/Prognosis   With infant reparative surgery, the operative mortality rate is approximately 5%. The mortality rate is higher when the truncal valve is more abnormal. In rare cases, the truncal valve must be replaced, and this considerably elevates the operative mortality rate.

Because a homograft is generally used to establish continuity between the right ventricle and the branch pulmonary arteries, the homograft needs to be replaced as the child grows. In general, two replacements are necessary before adulthood. Homograft replacement carries an operative mortality rate of 1 to 3%.

The postoperative outcome is directly related to the presence or absence of the DiGeorge syndrome. When present, the syndrome includes important developmental abnormalities, hypocalcemia due to hypoparathyroidism, and immune deficiencies from T-cell lymphocyte abnormalities.

REFERENCES

Bronshtein M, Siegler E, Yoffe N, Zimmer EZ: Prenatal diagnosis of ventricular septal defect and overriding aorta at 14 weeks' gestation, using transvaginal sonography. Prenat Diagn 1990;10:697–702.

Edwards JE, McGoon DC: Absence of anatomic origin from heart of pulmonary arterial supply. Circulation 1973;47:393–398.

Frohn-Mulder IM, Wesby SE, Bouwhuis C, et al: Chromosome 22q11 deletions in patients with selected outflow tract malformations. Genet Couns 1999;10:35–41.

Fyler DC: Trends. In Fyler DC (ed): Nadas' Pediatric Cardiology. Philadelphia, Hanley & Belfus, 1992, pp 273–284.

Goldmuntz E, Clark BJ, Mitchell LE, et al: Frequency of 22q11 deletions in patients with conotruncal defects [see comments]. J Am Coll Cardiol 1998;32:492–498.

Han XY, Wu SS, Conway DH, et al: Truncus arteriosus and other lethal internal anomalies in Goltz syndrome. Am J Med Genet 2000;90: 45–48.

Hopkin RJ, Schorry E, Bofinger M, et al: New insights into the phenotypes of 6q deletions. Am J Med Genet 1997;70:377–386.

Johnson MC, Hing A, Wood MK, Watson MS: Chromosome abnormalities in congenital heart disease. Am J Med Genet 1997;70:292–298.

Miyagawa S, Kirby ML: Pathogenesis of persistent truncus arteriosus induced by nimustine hydrochloride in chick embryos. Teratology 1989;39:287–294.

Momma K, Matsuoka R, Takao A: Aortic arch anomalies associated with chromosome 22q11 deletion (CATCH 22). Pediatr Cardiol 1999;20: 97–102.

Nora JJ, Nora AH: Update on counseling the family with a first-degree relative with a congenital heart defect. Am J Med Genet 1988;29: 137–142.

Okishima T, Takamura K, Matsuoka Y, et al: Cardiovascular anomalies in chick embryos produced bis-diamine in dimethylsulfoxide. Teratology 1992;45:155–162.

Rohn RD, Leffell MS, Leadem P, et al: Familial third-fourth pharyngeal pouch syndrome with apparent autosomal dominant transmission. J Pediatr 1984;105:47–51.

Van Praagh R, Van Praagh S: The anatomy of common aorticopulmonary trunk (truncus arteriosus communis) and its embryologic implications. A study of 57 necropsy cases. Am J Cardiol 1965;16:406–425.

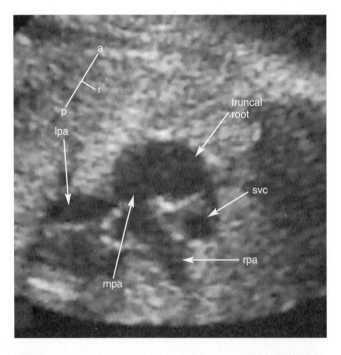

Short axis of single semilunar root in truncus arteriosus. A single great vessel is imaged in short axis from which both branch pulmonary arteries arise. The right superior vena cava (svc) is seen anterior to the right pulmonary artery. The absence of another great vessel is a necessary but nonspecific finding of truncus arteriosus. lpa, left pulmonary artery; mpa, main pulmonary artery; rpa, right pulmonary artery.

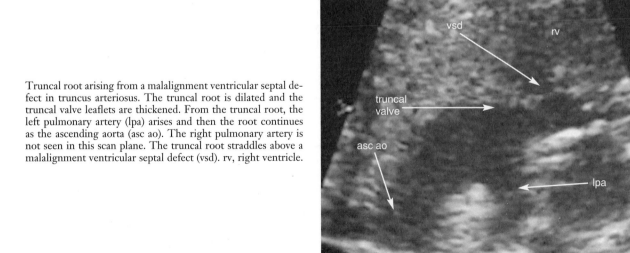

Truncal root arising from a malalignment ventricular septal defect in truncus arteriosus. The truncal root is dilated and the truncal valve leaflets are thickened. From the truncal root, the left pulmonary artery (lpa) arises and then the root continues as the ascending aorta (asc ao). The right pulmonary artery is not seen in this scan plane. The truncal root straddles above a malalignment ventricular septal defect (vsd). rv, right ventricle.

3.12 Double-Inlet Ventricle (Single Ventricle)

Epidemiology/Genetics

Definition Both atrioventricular valves relate to a dominant or single ventricle. Double-inlet ventricles can be of either left or right ventricular morphology. The term "single ventricle" is less accurate than double-inlet ventricle, since another small chamber may be present, particularly in cases of double-inlet left ventricle. Double-inlet ventricle can occur with atresia of one of the atrioventricular valves, but even in such cases, the atretic valve is positioned above the dominant ventricle.

Epidemiology Prevalence per 1000 live births: 0.05 to 0.1. Accounts for 0.8% of children with congenital cardiac disease.

Embryology The left ventricle forms from the primitive ventricle and the right ventricle is derived from a component of the bulbus cordis.

Inheritance Pattern The inheritance pattern and recurrence risks are not defined.

Teratogens None identified.

Prognosis The patient with double-inlet ventricle requires multiple operations culminating in the Fontan procedure. Generally two, or more likely, three operations are required before the age of 6 years. Long-term prognosis with the Fontan procedure is described within the prognosis section for tricuspid atresia.

Sonography

FINDINGS

1. **Fetus:**
   a. From an apical four-chamber view, one can usually appreciate that one ventricle is dominant and receives the inflow of both atrioventricular valves and atria. The fact that both atrioventricular valves are related to the same ventricle is also clear when the ventricle is imaged in short-axis. The open atrioventricular valves appear as "spectacles."
   b. One should identify the morphology of the dominant ventricle. Typical morphologic features of a left ventricle are an ellipsoid shape and a less heavily trabeculated myocardium than the right ventricle. A right ventricle has a more triangular shape. Also, in double-inlet left ventricle, an anterior right ventricular outflow chamber from which one of the great vessels arises is very typical. In double-inlet right ventricle, a small chamber posterior to the dominant right ventricle is sometimes seen.
   c. The origins of both great vessels must be identified. In most cases, one of the great vessels will arise directly from the dominant ventricle and the other from an outlet chamber or infundibulum.
   d. Commonly, there is obstruction either at the subvalvular or valvular level to one of the great vessels. When there is subvalvular or valvular aortic stenosis, the ascending aorta is often hypoplastic and there is an increased chance of aortic coarctation or interrupted aortic arch. When there is subvalvular or valvular pulmonary stenosis, the branch pulmonary arteries may be hypoplastic. Both great vessels and the aortic arch should be measured and compared to normative data. With outflow obstruction, the distal vessel will typically be hypoplastic.
   e. Transposition can occur as part of double-inlet ventricle.
   f. Pulse and color Doppler interrogation should be performed for both atrioventricular valves. Recognition of atrioventricular valve regurgitation is quite important, because severe regurgitation is associated with the development of hydrops fetalis. Even when one of the atrioventricular valves is stenotic by imaging, minimal or no significant inflow gradient is expected with pulse Doppler interrogation in the presence of a patent foramen ovale. With atrioventricular valve stenosis, flow is redistributed to the normal atrioventricular valve. The atrioventricular valve diameter should be measured and compared with normative data.
   g. Complete heart block can occur in double-inlet ventricle, particularly when there is ventricular inversion (i.e., L-looped ventricles). The mechanism and rate of the rhythm need to be identified.
2. **Amniotic Fluid:** Normal unless hydrops develops.
3. **Placenta:** Normal in the absence of hydrops.
4. **Measurement Data:** Normal.
5. **When Detectable:** Double-inlet ventricle can be detected at 16 to 18 weeks.

Pitfalls/Differential Diagnosis

1. Double-inlet ventricle with atrioventricular valve atresia should be distinguished from typical tricuspid valve atresia and mitral atresia such as in hypoplastic left heart syndrome. In all of these different diseases, there is only one functional ventricle, but the management and prognosis for each are different.
2. In some forms of complete common atrioventricular canal, the common valve may be severely malaligned over one ventricle while the other ventricle is quite hypoplastic. Such a heart could be confused with double-inlet ventricle with atresia of one of the valves. The distinction is important, since atrioventricular canal defects are commonly associated with karyotype ab-

normalities and heterotaxy syndrome, whereas double-inlet ventricles are not.

3. Recognition of outflow obstruction is crucial, as this strongly determines the postnatal clinical course and prognosis. When there is severe obstruction to either outflow, the lesion will be ductus dependent and prostaglandin E therapy will be required. Prenatal prediction of the severity of outflow obstruction postnatally can be difficult.

Pregnancy Management

Investigations and Consultations Required A pediatric cardiologist should be consulted for confirmation of diagnosis and development of prenatal and postnatal management plans. Chromosomal analysis is desirable, as with other cardiac malformations.

Fetal Intervention None available.

Monitoring The heart should be re-examined at 28 and 32 weeks' gestation to assess for competence of the atrioventricular valves and to determine the degree of outflow obstruction to the systemic or pulmonary circulation.

Pregnancy Course Atrioventricular valve regurgitation can progress in utero and can result in hydrops. The degree of outflow tract obstruction can also progress during pregnancy.

Pregnancy Termination Issues If termination is chosen, an intact fetus should be delivered for confirmation of diagnosis.

Delivery A fetus with double-inlet ventricle should be delivered in a facility where immediate pediatric cardiology and cardiac surgery consultation are available.

Neonatology

Resuscitation Spontaneous respirations are expected, and resuscitation is generally not necessary. When there is significant obstruction to pulmonary outflow, persistent cyanosis may be present from birth, which may be confusing in the immediate transition following delivery. If obstruction to pulmonary outflow is suspected, venous access should be established for prostaglandin E_1 infusion, as indicated.

Transport Transport to a tertiary center with full pediatric cardiac diagnostic and surgical capability is essential. If the infant presents with cyanosis, consultation with a pediatric cardiologist prior to transport is recommended to determine the need for prostaglandin E_1 infusion during the transport.

Testing and Confirmation Echocardiography is usually definitive for diagnosis. Rarely, cardiac catheterization is required for delineation of distal branch pulmonary arteries.

Nursery Management Symptomatology depends on the balance of systemic and pulmonary blood flow. When there is obstruction to systemic blood flow, there will be pulmonary overcirculation, with development of congestive heart failure, poor systemic perfusion, and metabolic acidosis. In contrast, with obstruction to pulmonary blood flow, there will be cyanosis.

Nursery management is directed toward establishing the proper balance of systemic and pulmonary blood flow. When there is severe obstruction to either outflow, prostaglandin E_1 therapy is useful in maintaining ductal patency. Measures to reduce pulmonary overcirculation include avoidance of supplemental oxygen and, in some cases, administration of diuretic or inotropic drugs.

Surgery

Preoperative Assessment Echocardiography is usually definitive for preoperative assessment.

Operative Indications All forms of double-inlet ventricle require surgery. The goal is to achieve an appropriate balance of systemic and pulmonary blood flow and to achieve normal pulmonary artery pressure. If the appropriate balance is present, no surgery may be required as a newborn, and the infant is discharged home. When the balance is inappropriate, surgery is required.

Types of Procedures If there is obstruction to systemic blood flow, the main pulmonary artery may be transected and anastomosed to the ascending aorta to provide an unobstructed route for systemic blood flow. Arch obstruction is repaired if present. Pulmonary blood flow is established using an arterial shunt such as the Blalock-Taussig shunt (right subclavian artery or innominate artery to right pulmonary artery connection). Different surgery is performed if the problem is with pulmonary flow. If there is diminished pulmonary blood flow due to pulmonary stenosis, a Blalock-Taussig shunt may be indicated. If there is pulmonary overcirculation but sufficient systemic flow, the main pulmonary artery may be banded.

Subsequent surgical management out of the newborn period is directed toward separating the desaturated and saturated blood. The Glenn operation is generally performed at 6 to 12 months of age, and the Fontan operation some time before the age of 6 years. In some cases, the Glenn operation can be incorporated at the time of the Fontan procedure. The Glenn operation and Fontan operation are discussed in detail in the surgical section of tricuspid atresia.

Surgical Results/Prognosis The operative mortality rate for surgery performed during the newborn period varies between 5 and 25%. Higher operative mortality rates occur when aortic arch reconstruction is required.

The operative mortality rates for the Glenn and Fontan procedures are each around 5%.

REFERENCES

Fyler DC: Trends. In: Fyler DC (ed): Nadas' Pediatric Cardiology. Philadelphia, Hanley & Belfus, 1992, pp 273–284.

Rychik J, Tian ZY, Fogel MA, et al: The single ventricle heart in the fetus: Accuracy of prenatal diagnosis and outcome. J Perinatol 1997;17(3):183–188.

Williams RG: Echocardiography in the management of single ventricle: Fetal through adult life. Echocardiography 1993;10(3):331–342.

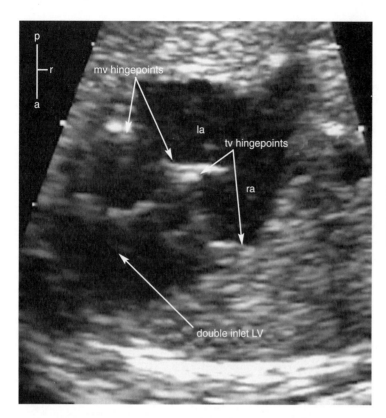

Double-inlet left ventricle (LV). In this "four"-chamber view, both atrioventricular valves drain to a single ventricle of left ventricular morphology. The *arrows* point to the hingepoints of the mitral (mv) and tricuspid (tv) valves. Features of the ventricle that illustrate left ventricular morphology are its ellipsoid shape and its paucity of trabeculations. la, left atrium; ra, right atrium.

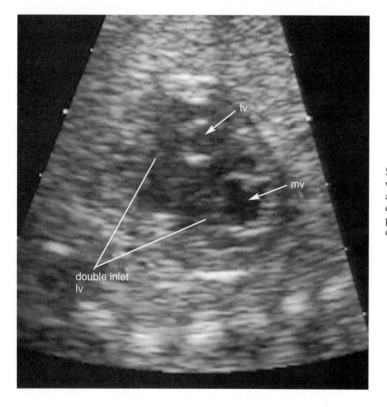

Short-axis view of double-inlet left ventricle (lv). In this diastolic view, the left ventricle is imaged in its short axis. One appreciates that both atrioventricular valves enter this ventricle. The tricuspid valve (tv) is smaller. Atrioventricular valve stenosis is suspected if annular hypoplasia and leaflet opening limitation are demonstrated. mv, mitral valve.

3.13 Double-Outlet Right Ventricle

Epidemiology/Genetics

Definition Both the aorta and the pulmonary artery arise from the right ventricle.

Epidemiology Prevalence per 1000 live births: 0.03 to 0.07. Accounts for 0.9% of children with congenital cardiac disease.

Embryology The embryology of double-outlet right ventricle is quite complicated, since the disease may occur as an element of widely varying disorders ranging from complete atrioventricular canal to double-inlet ventricle. The normal connections of the great vessels are related to appropriate differentiation and growth of components of the bulbus cordis. The bulbus cordis differentiates into the right ventricle, the conus cordis becomes the conal or infundibular septum, and the truncus arteriosus forms the great vessels.

Inheritance Patterns The sibling recurrence rate has not been reliably reported but is probably low. Karyotype abnormalities are present in approximately 5% of fetuses with double-outlet right ventricle. Double-outlet right ventricle has been reported in trisomy 13 and 18 and in duplication 3p. Chromosome 22q deletion occurs in approximately 5% of patients with double-outlet right ventricle.

Teratogens Apart from maternal diabetes mellitus none reported.

Prognosis Double-outlet right ventricle requires surgical treatment. The prognosis varies considerably depending on the complexity of the heart defect and the presence or absence of associated abnormalities.

Sonography

FINDINGS

1. **Fetus:**
   a. The necessary feature is demonstration of the connection of the aorta and the pulmonary artery to the right ventricle.
   b. The ventricular septal defect present in double-outlet right ventricle is a malalignment defect.
   c. The manner by which both vessels connect with the right ventricle is variable and important for definitive counseling and discussion of prognosis. The ventricular septal defect can be subaortic, subpulmonary, doubly committed, or uncommitted.
   d. A common feature is subvalvular or valvular obstruction of either outflow tract. With aortic stenosis, there is frequently hypoplasia of the ascending aorta and the association of aortic coarctation or interrupted aortic arch. With pulmonary stenosis, there may be hypoplasia of the branch pulmonary arteries.
   e. Double-outlet right ventricle sometimes occurs with abnormalities of the atrioventricular valves, including atresia, straddling (in which the atrioventricular valve attaches into the contralateral ventricles), or overriding (in which the annulus overrides both ventricles but does not necessarily attach to both ventricles). Double-outlet right ventricle can occur with complete common atrioventricular canal defects, particularly in heterotaxy syndrome.
   f. One should consider heterotaxy syndrome and determine abdominal and atrial situs as well as pulmonary and systemic venous return.
2. **Amniotic Fluid:** Normal unless hydrops develops.
3. **Placenta:** Normal.
4. **Measurement Data:** Normal.
5. **When Detectable:** At 16 to 18 weeks by transabdominal imaging and potentially at 12 to 14 weeks with transvaginal imaging.

Pitfalls/Differential Diagnosis

1. Double-outlet right ventricle should be distinguished from transposition, as they are mutually exclusive. In transposition, the aorta arises from the right ventricle and the pulmonary artery arises from the left ventricle. It is inaccurate to say that transposition of the great arteries and double-outlet right ventricle are present in the same heart. When one vessel arises from the right ventricle and the other straddles the septum, the convention is to label the heart as double outlet if more than one and a half great vessels connect with the right ventricle.
2. Tetralogy of Fallot with considerable aortic overriding may appear similar to double-outlet right ventricle with subaortic ventricular septal defect. In tetralogy, the aorta arises predominantly from the left ventricle (i.e., is more than 50% above the left ventricle), and the aortic valve is typically in direct continuity with the anterior leaflet of the mitral valve. In double-outlet ventricle with subaortic ventricular septal defect, more than one and a half great vessels arise from the right ventricle, and usually there is discontinuity between the aortic and mitral valves due to subaortic conal muscle.
3. As discussed, double-outlet right ventricle is frequently associated with outflow obstruction. The severity of outflow obstruction is an important determinant of the severity of presentation and whether or not the lesion is ductus dependent. With severe pulmonary stenosis,

newborns will be cyanotic. With severe subvalvular or valvular aortic stenosis, there frequently is associated coarctation and the lesion may require prostaglandin E therapy to maintain adequate systemic perfusion.

Where Else to Look

1. There is a strong association with chromosomal anomalies, particularly DiGeorge syndrome, so a detailed examination of the remainder of the fetus, especially the palate and kidneys, should be performed.
2. Anomalies elsewhere, such as situs inversus or single umbilical artery, are found in the majority of cases, even when the chromosomes are normal.

Pregnancy Management

Investigations and Consultations Required Pediatric cardiology consultation should be obtained to confirm management and establish appropriate prenatal and postnatal management. Karyotyping and the appropriate assays for the chromosome 22q deletion should be performed because of the frequent association with velocardiofacial syndrome.

Pregnancy Monitoring Fetal echocardiography should be repeated at 28 weeks' and sometimes at 32 weeks' gestation to assess for outflow obstruction and ascertain whether the lesion is likely to be ductus dependent.

Pregnancy Course Unless there is the development of severe atrioventricular valve regurgitation, particularly in the context of outflow obstruction, pregnancy will generally continue to term. With severe atrioventricular valve regurgitation, hydrops may develop.

Pregnancy Termination Issues An intact fetus should be delivered for a confirmation of cardiac diagnosis and to exclude potential associated noncardiac abnormalities.

Delivery Most cases of double-outlet right ventricle, particularly in those situations in which outflow obstruction is suspected, should be delivered in a center where immediate pediatric cardiac consultation is available. With outflow obstruction, the lesion may be ductus dependent.

Neonatology

Resuscitation Initial resuscitation is generally not required. When there is significant pulmonary outflow tract obstruction, persistent cyanosis may be present from birth, which may be confusing in the immediate transition following delivery. If significant outflow tract obstruction is suspected, venous access should be established to allow administration of prostaglandin E_1 as required.

Transport Transport to a tertiary center with full pediatric cardiac diagnostic and surgical capability is essential. If the infant presents with cyanosis, consultation with a pediatric cardiologist prior to transport is recommended

to determine the need for prostaglandin E_1 infusion during the transport.

Testing and Confirmation Echocardiography provides definitive diagnosis, and preoperative catheterization is generally not required.

Nursery Management Management depends on establishing an appropriate balance of systemic and pulmonary blood flow. In cases in which there is severe obstruction to pulmonary blood flow, prostaglandin E_1 therapy may be indicated to maintain ductal patency and ensure adequate pulmonary blood flow. When there is severe obstruction to systemic blood flow, prostaglandin E_1 therapy is necessary to maintain adequate systemic perfusion. When there is no significant obstruction to either outflow tract, congestive heart failure may develop with the normal fall in pulmonary vascular resistance. In these cases, anticongestive medications are used to control congestive heart failure.

Surgery

Preoperative Assessment Echocardiography provides definitive diagnosis, and preoperative catheterization is generally not required.

Operative Indications All forms of double-outlet right ventricle require surgical treatment. The purpose of all operations is to establish unobstructed blood flow of saturated blood to the aorta, preferably from the left ventricle, closure of the ventricular septal defect, and establishment of unobstructed effective pulmonary blood flow, preferably from the right ventricle. In some cases, a homograft is required to connect the right ventricle with the branch pulmonary arteries.

Types of Procedures Because of the spectrum of double-outlet right ventricle, the methods of surgical correction vary considerably. When the ventricular septal defect is subaortic, the surgical treatment resembles that used for treatment of tetralogy of Fallot. When the ventricular septal defect is subpulmonary and there is no pulmonary stenosis, the treatment is similar to that used in transposition of the great arteries with ventricular septal defect. In cases with an uncommitted ventricular septal defect, it may be impossible to connect the left ventricle with either great vessel. In these unusual cases, single ventricle management may be necessary.

Baffling the left ventricle to the aorta is relatively straightforward in double-outlet right ventricle with a subaortic ventricular septal defect. Double-outlet right ventricle with a subpulmonary ventricular septal defect may still allow treatment with a relatively low rate of operative mortality, but the surgery often involves an arterial switch operation as with transposition of the great arteries.

Surgical Results/Prognosis The operative mortality rate varies based on the complexity of the form of double-outlet right ventricle and the presence of associated lesions. In general, the operative mortality rate ranges between 3 and 10%. More complex operations are required in the cases in which there is an obstruction to systemic blood flow, such as with interrupted aortic arch or coarctation.

REFERENCES

Braga S, Schmidt A: Clinical and cytogenetic spectrum of duplication 3p. Eur J Pediatr 1982;138:195–197.

Fyler DC: Trends. In Fyler DC (ed): Nadas' Pediatric Cardiology. Philadelphia, Hanley & Belfus, 1992, pp 273–284.

Goldmuntz E, Clark BJ, Mitchell LE, et al: Frequency of 22q11 deletions in patients with conotruncal defects. J Am Coll Cardiol 1998; 32:492–498.

Johnson MC, Hing A, Wood MK, Watson MS: Chromosome abnormalities in congenital heart disease. Am J Med Genet 1997;70:292–298.

Smith RS, Comstock CH, Kirk JS, et al: Double-outlet right ventricle: An antenatal diagnostic dilemma. Ultrasound Obstet Gynecol 1999; 14:315–319.

Wladimiroff JW, Stewart PA, Reuss A, Sachs ES: Cardiac and extracardiac anomalies as indicators for trisomies 13 and 18: A prenatal ultrasound study. Prenat Diagn 1989;9:515–520.

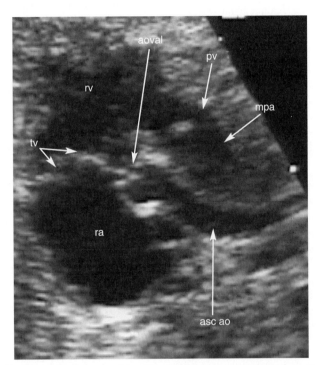

Double-outlet right ventricle with subpulmonary conus. Both the aorta and the pulmonary artery arise from the right ventricle (rv). The aortic valve (aoval) is in continuity with the tricuspid valve (tv), so there is no subaortic conus. The left ventricle is not seen in this image. The ascending aorta (asc ao) is relatively hypoplastic in comparison to the main pulmonary artery (mpa). This suggests that arch hypoplasia or obstruction may be present. pv, pulmonary valve; ra, right atrium.

3.14 Cardiac Arrhythmias: Tachycardia and Extrasystoles

Epidemiology/Genetics

Definition The normal fetal heart rate usually ranges from 120 to 160 beats per minute. Tachycardia refers to a rate faster than 160 beats per minute.

In *sinus tachycardia*, the rate typically ranges between 170 and 220 beats per minute, the impulse originates at the sinus node, and there is one-to-one conduction between the atrium and the ventricle. Atrial contraction precedes ventricular contraction by 60 to 150 msec with an interval that is constant from beat to beat. The onset and offset of sinus tachycardia are gradual and are frequently due to changes in autonomic tone.

Supraventricular tachycardia is usually a re-entry tachycardia involving an accessory pathway between the atrium and the ventricle. A re-entry tachycardia requires two electrical pathways between atrium and ventricle (the pathway through the atrioventricular node can be and is usually one of the pathways). The two pathways must have different conduction properties. The ventricular rate during supraventricular tachycardia is fairly constant at rates between 220 and 280 beats per minute. There is usually one-to-one conduction between atria and ventricles. Supraventricular tachycardia is typically initiated by an atrial premature beat and the tachycardia has an abrupt onset and offset. In newborns with supraventricular tachycardia due to a re-entry pathway, the interval from ventricular contraction to the following atrial contraction usually exceeds 70 msec.

Atrial flutter results from a single re-entry circuit within the atria. Typically, the atrial rate ranges from 300 to 600 beats per minute. There are varying degrees of block at the atrioventricular node. The block may be up to and even exceeding four to one (i.e., the atrial rate is four times the ventricular rate), but there may be one-to-one conduction between atria and ventricles (in which case, the atrial and ventricular rates are identical).

Atrial fibrillation results from multiple small intra-atrial re-entry circuits. Organized atrial contraction is absent, so distinct contraction of the atrial wall on echocardiogram is not seen. The ventricular rate usually ranges between 100 and 200 beats per minute and is irregularly irregular, since there is variable block at the atrioventricular node.

Ventricular tachycardia is a rare arrhythmia in the fetus and is most commonly due to a re-entry mechanism (although other mechanisms can produce ventricular tachycardia). During ventricular tachycardia, the ventricular rate usually ranges between 150 and 250 beats per minute and often there is dissociation between the ventricles and atria. Less commonly, there can be retrograde conduction from ventricle to atrium and there will be a one-to-one atrial-ventricular relationship. Ventricular tachycardia will not be further discussed in this section.

Extrasystoles or premature beats may originate in the atria, the atrioventricular node, or the ventricles. In the fetus, atrial premature beats account for the majority of extrasystoles.

Not discussed here are two very rare automatic rhythms, *ectopic atrial tachycardia* and *junctional ectopic tachycardia*.

Epidemiology Arrhythmia (including premature atrial beats) represents the referral indication and/or is present on fetal scans in approximately 10 to 20% of fetuses. Extrasystoles account for 70 to 88% of fetal arrhythmia, tachycardia for 10 to 15%, and bradycardia for 8 to 12%. Among fetuses with tachycardia, the mechanism is supraventricular tachycardia with a re-entry pathway in 65 to 93%, atrial flutter in 7 to 29%, and ventricular tachycardia in 4%.

Inheritance Pattern In most cases sporadic. There is a small subgroup of patients with familial preexcitation syndromes. In one large study, the prevalence of an accessory pathway was identified within a first-degree relative in 1.06% of patients, compared with the prevalence in the general population for accessory pathways of 0.15%.

Teratogens None reported.

Prognosis Survival and prognosis are most highly correlated with the development of hydrops. Hydrops develops in 25 to 50% of fetuses with sustained tachycardia. In a group with tachycardia treated pharmacologically, sinus rhythm was restored in 73% of those without hydrops, compared with 30% with hydrops. No fetus without hydrops died, compared with 45% of those with hydrops.

Risk factors for the development of hydrops include sustained tachycardia greater than 12 hours and lower gestational age at presentation. Some investigators have reported that the mechanism of tachycardia and the heart rate do not correlate with the risk for developing hydrops, although the number fetuses in this study may have left the study with insufficient power. Others have reported an association of severe hydrops during supraventricular tachycardia with severe atrioventricular valve regurgitation.

Atrial premature beats are usually benign but can precede the development of supraventricular tachycardia.

Sonography

FINDINGS

1. **Fetus:**
   a. Of fundamental importance in determining the mechanism of fetal arrhythmia is the identification of atrial and ventricular contraction and the rela-

tionship between them. There are four ways of assessing the timing.

1. Simultaneous M-mode echocardiography of the atrial wall and a ventricular event (either ventricular free wall motion or semilunar valve motion) is a reliable way of determining timing. It is sometimes difficult and time-consuming to achieve an appropriate angle for simultaneous M-mode assessment, although this method of analysis is most accurate. The motion of the atrial wall is often easiest to see within the atrial appendage.
2. Spectral pulse Doppler can be performed within the left ventricular outflow tract so that mitral inflow (for atrial timing) and aortic outflow (for ventricular timing) are recorded. Doppler echocardiography is not more sensitive than M-mode echocardiography in the interpretation of arrhythmia, but Doppler tracings of a quality to analyze rate and rhythm may be easier to obtain in some cases. If the force of atrial contraction is inadequate to open the mitral valve (which may be the case in very rapid atrial rhythms) or if atrial contraction occurs simultaneously with ventricular contraction, mitral inflow may not occur, and the timing of atrial contraction is unclear using this method.
3. Similar to the pulsed Doppler technique, color Doppler M-mode echocardiography across the left ventricular outflow tract and mitral valve inflow can be performed. It may be quicker to obtain color Doppler M-mode images than to achieve a suitable angle for pulsed Doppler interrogation or pure M-mode analysis. The same limitation discussed for the pulsed Doppler technique applies.
4. Finally, some have suggested using simultaneous pulsed Doppler velocimetry of the fetal abdominal aorta and inferior vena cava to assess timing.
   b. Analysis of the onset and offset of tachycardia is quite helpful. Re-entry tachycardia, like supraventricular tachycardia and atrial flutter, has an abrupt onset and offset. Automatic rhythms such as sinus tachycardia or ectopic atrial tachycardia have a gradual "warm-up" and "cool-down." Supraventricular tachycardia typically is initiated by an atrial premature beat.
   c. Ventricular function should be assessed and pulsed and color Doppler echocardiography performed to exclude atrioventricular valve regurgitation.
2. **Amniotic Fluid:** Normal unless hydrops develops.
3. **Placenta:** Normal.
4. **Measurement Data:** Normal.
5. **When Detectable:** By transabdominal imaging at 16 to 18 weeks. With transvaginal imaging, arrhythmias have been examined during the first trimester.

Pitfalls Supraventricular tachycardia is frequently intermittent, and during the echocardiogram no tachycardia may be noted, even though at other times there are periods of sustained tachycardia. Continuous fetal heart rate monitoring may be useful to confirm and determine the frequency and duration of tachycardia episodes.

Differential Diagnosis Based on the criteria discussed, arrhythmias are distinguished by the atrial and ventricular rates, the presence and degree of atrioventricular block, and the pattern of onset and offset.

Where Else to Look

1. Sinus tachycardia occurs with sepsis and fetal anemia. Atrial premature beats and sustained supraventricular tachycardia have been noticed in fetuses with intracardiac tumors.
2. Look for the signs of hydrops.
3. Rule out underlying cardiac structural abnormality.
4. Structural heart disease must be excluded, although in the majority of fetuses with tachycardia, the anatomy is normal. Among 90 patients with Wolff-Parkinson-White syndrome who presented with supraventricular tachycardia in the first 4 months of life, structural heart

Rhythm	Mechanism	Atrial Rate	Ventricular Rate	Atrioventricular Block	Onset/Offset	Atrioventricular Dissociation
Sinus tachycardia	Automatic	170–220	170–220	No	Gradual	No
Supraventricular tachycardia	Re-entry between atrium and ventricle	220–280	220–280	Usually no	Abrupt	No
Atrial flutter	Intra-atrial re-entry	300–600	Variable depending on atrioventricular block	Variable	Abrupt	No
Atrial fibrillation	Small intra-atrial re-entry	Contraction indistinct	Irregularly irregular, usually 100–200	Variable	Abrupt	No
Ventricular tachycardia	Usually re-entry	120–160 unless retrograde conduction	150–250	Not relevant	Abrupt	Usually, but not if retrograde conduction

disease was present in 20%, most commonly Ebstein's anomaly.

Pregnancy Management

Investigations and Consultations Required   Fetuses with frequent arrhythmia are usually best managed in consultation with a perinatologist and a pediatric cardiologist skilled in the analysis and treatment of fetal arrhythmia.

Fetal Intervention   With sinus tachycardia, attention is directed toward the primary disorder causing the tachycardia, and specific treatment for the tachycardia is not usually indicated. In fetuses with sustained arrhythmia, such as supraventricular tachycardia, atrial flutter, or atrial fibrillation, treatment is indicated in most cases. The one exception is the fetus during the late third trimester who is tolerating the tachycardia without evidence of hydrops. Careful follow-up and/or early delivery is reasonable if one wishes to avoid pharmacologic treatment.

Alternative therapies include digoxin, digoxin with a second agent such as flecainide or procainamide, or sotalol (alone or as part of multidrug treatment). Less commonly used because of the increased frequency of side effects is amiodarone.

Among nonhydropic fetuses, digoxin has been efficacious in restoring sinus rhythm in approximately 50% of fetuses. When hydrops is present, however, maternal-placental transmission of the digoxin is unreliable and conversion to sinus rhythm may occur in less than 10% of patients. Among fetuses with successful cardioversion using maternal intravenous administration of digoxin, it may take 5 to 7 days from initiation of therapy to achieve sinus rhythm. Direct fetal intramuscular injection of digoxin can shorten the time of conversion but at some increased risk.

When pharmacologic therapy is unsuccessful, one should consider early delivery. When early delivery is contemplated, a brief course of corticosteroids may be useful to facilitate lung maturity.

Monitoring   Until effective rate control is achieved, the fetus with sustained tachycardia should be re-examined daily. In most cases, the mother should be hospitalized until effective rate control is achieved. Maternal drug levels should be drawn to ensure adequacy of dosing.

Pregnancy Termination Issues   Generally not relevant.

Delivery   The fetus is generally carried to term unless the fetus is in sustained tachycardia and unresponsive to pharmacologic treatment or if there are signs of hydrops and the fetus is in the late third trimester.

Neonatology

Resuscitation   Infants generally breathe spontaneously and do not require resuscitation.

Transport   The neonate should be transferred to a center where pediatric cardiology consultation is available.

Testing and Confirmation   The mechanism of the arrhythmia can generally be confirmed with a surface electrocardiogram. Sometimes transesophageal electrocardiography helps to identify the mechanism of the arrhythmia. Invasive electrophysiologic studies in infants are not generally indicated during infancy.

Nursery Management   Hemodynamically unstable infants may require electrical cardioversion. Re-entry tachycardia is frequently terminated with adenosine. The same agents used to control the arrhythmia prenatally are often used postnatally as well.

Surgery/Intervention   In the majority of patients, supraventricular tachycardia can be controlled with pharmacologic therapy, or the rhythm does not recur after the age of 1 year without treatment. In patients requiring long-term antiarrhythmic therapy, radiofrequency ablation is quite successful in extinguishing the accessory pathway. The long-term prognosis is excellent.

REFERENCES

Achiron R, Rotstein Z, Lipitz S, et al: First-trimester diagnosis of fetal congenital heart disease by transvaginal ultrasonography. Obstet Gynecol 1994;84:69–72.

Azancot-Benisty A, Jacqz-Aigrain E, Guirgis NM, et al: Clinical and pharmacologic study of fetal supraventricular tachyarrhythmias. J Pediatr 1992;121:608–613.

Birnbaum SE, McGahan JP, Janos GO, Meyers M: Fetal tachycardia and intramyocardial tumors. J Am Coll Cardiol 1985;6:1358–1361.

Chan FY, Woo SK, Ghosh A, et al: Prenatal diagnosis of congenital fetal arrhythmias by simultaneous pulsed Doppler velocimetry of the fetal abdominal aorta and inferior vena cava. Obstet Gynecol 1990;76:200–205.

Deal BJ, Keane JF, Gillette PC, Garson A Jr: Wolff-Parkinson-White syndrome and supraventricular tachycardia during infancy: Management and follow-up. J Am Coll Cardiol 1985;5:130–135.

De Catte L, De Wolf D, Smitz J, et al: Fetal hypothyroidism as a complication of amiodarone treatment for persistent fetal supraventricular tachycardia. Prenat Diagn 1994;14:762–765.

Eronen M: Outcome of fetuses with heart disease diagnosed in utero Arch Dis Child Fetal Neonatal Ed 1997;77:F41–F46.

Frohn-Mulder IM, Stewart PA, Witsenburg M, et al: The efficacy of flecainide versus digoxin in the management of fetal supraventricular tachycardia [see comments]. Prenat Diagn 1995;15:1297–1302.

Gembruch U, Bald R, Hansmann M: [Color-coded M-mode Doppler echocardiography in the diagnosis of fetal arrhythmia]. Geburtshilfe Frauenheilkd 1990;50:286–290.

Gembruch U, Hansmann M, Bald R, Redel BA: [Supraventricular tachycardia of the fetus in the 3d trimester of pregnancy following persistent supraventricular extrasystole]. Geburtshilfe Frauenheilkd 1987;47:656–659.

Gembruch U, Manz M, Bald R, et al: Repeated intravascular treatment with amiodarone in a fetus with refractory supraventricular tachycardia and hydrops fetalis. Am Heart J 1989;118:1335–1338.

Gembruch U, Redel DA, Bald R, Hansmann M: Longitudinal study in 18 cases of fetal supraventricular tachycardia: Doppler echocardiographic findings and pathophysiologic implications. Am Heart J 1993;125:1290–1301.

Gutierrez RA, Iturralde TP, Colin LL, et al: [The familial incidence of accessory atrioventricular pathways (the pre-excitation syndrome)]. Arch Inst Cardiol Mex 1999;69:228–234.

Hamel P, Febbraro W, Barjot P, et al: [Fetal supraventricular tachycardia with anasarca complicating benign extrasystole: treatment with flecainide. Apropos of a case]. Arch Mal Coeur Vaiss 1997;90:407–410.

Knudson JM, Kleinman CS, Copel JA, Rosenfeld LE: Ectopic atrial tachycardia in utero. Obstet Gynecol 1994;84:686–689.

Kohl T, Kirchhof PF, Gogarten W, et al: Fetoscopic transesophageal electrocardiography and stimulation in fetal sheep: a minimally invasive approach aimed at diagnosis and termination of therapy-refractory supraventricular tachycardias in human fetuses. Circulation 1999; 100:772–776.

Lisowski LA, Verheijen PM, Benatar AA, et al: Atrial flutter in the perinatal age group: Diagnosis, management and outcome. J Am Coll Cardiol 2000;35:771–777.

Lopes LM, Kahhale S, Barbato A, et al: [Prenatal diagnosis of congenital heart diseases and cardiac arrhythmias by Doppler echocardiography]. Arq Bras Cardiol 1990;54:121–125.

Lupoglazoff JM, Denjoy I, Luton D, et al: Prenatal diagnosis of a familial form of junctional ectopic tachycardia. Prenat Diagn 1999;19: 767–770.

Macedo AJ, Ferreira M, Borges A, et al: [Fetal echocardiography. The results of a 3-year study]. Acta Med Port 1993;6:(Suppl 1):I9–13.

Maragnes P, Fournier A, Lessard M, Fouron JC: [Evaluation and prognosis of fetal arrhythmia]. Pediatrie (Bucur) 1991;46:481–488.

Meden H, Neeb U: [Transplacental cardioversion of fetal supraventricular tachycardia using sotalol]. Z Geburtshilfe Perinatol 1990;194: 182–184.

Naheed ZJ, Strasburger JF, Deal BJ, et al: Fetal tachycardia: Mechanisms and predictors of hydrops fetalis. J Am Coll Cardiol 1996;27: 1736–1740.

Parilla BV, Strasburger JF, Socol ML: Fetal supraventricular tachycardia complicated by hydrops fetalis: A role for direct fetal intramuscular therapy. Am J Perinatol 1996;13:483–486.

Reed KL, Sahn DJ, Marx GR, et al: Cardiac Doppler flows during fetal arrhythmias: physiologic consequences. Obstet Gynecol 1987;70:1–6.

Strasburger JF, Huhta JC, Carpenter RJ Jr, et al: Doppler echocardiography in the diagnosis and management of persistent fetal arrhythmias. J Am Coll Cardiol 1986;7:1386–1391.

van Engelen AD, Weijtens O, Brenner JI, et al: Management outcome and follow-up of fetal tachycardia. J Am Coll Cardiol 1994;24:1371–1375.

Wang LW, Wu JM, Lin CS, et al: Refractory fetal supraventricular tachycardia with hydrops: Report of one case. Chung Hua Min Kuo Hsiao Erh Ko I Hsueh Hui Tsa Chih 1995;36:300–303.

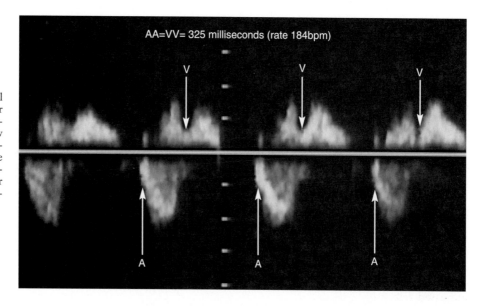

Sinus rhythm determined using spectral pulse Doppler within the left ventricular outflow tract. Atrial contraction is recognized by atrioventricular valve inflow (flow below the baseline) and ventricular contraction by aortic outflow (flow above the baseline). In this fetus with sinus tachycardia, the ventricular rate is 184 beats per minute and there is a one-to-one relationship between atria (A) and ventricle (V).

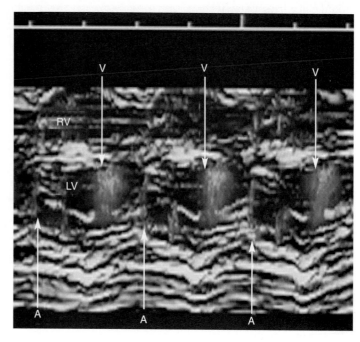

Sinus rhythm determined by M-mode color Doppler across the left ventricular outflow tract. One can easily see the one-to-one relationship between each atrial (A) and ventricular (V) contraction and that ventricular rate is 142 beats per minute. One can also time ventricular contraction by noting the motion of the right ventricular free wall on the M-mode recording. In this fetus, the atrioventricular interval is increased. (See color figure following p. x.)

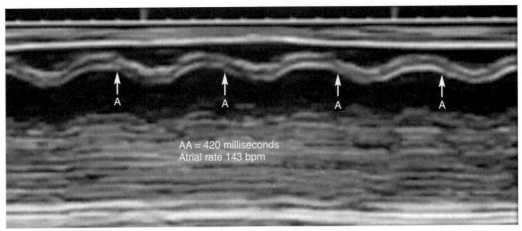

Sinus rhythm before initiation of supraventricular tachycardia analyzed using M-mode of atrial free wall. Atrial contraction is well seen in this M-mode recording of the lateral atrial wall. The atrial rate is regular at a rate of 143 beats per minute.

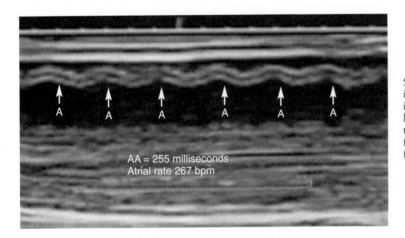

Supraventricular tachycardia analyzed using M-mode recording of atrial free wall. After a single atrial premature beat (not illustrated in this M-mode recording), the atrial rate is regular at 267 beats per minute. There is one-to-one conduction to the ventricle, also not illustrated here. This rate is too fast for sinus tachycardia and slower than that seen with atrial flutter.

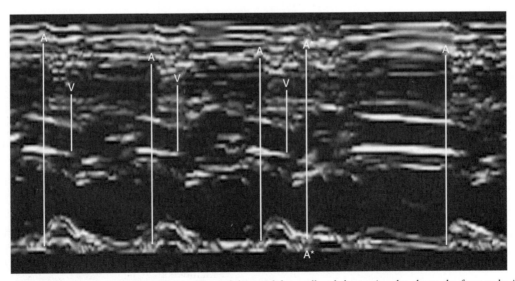

Blocked atrial premature beat. Simultaneous M-mode recording of the atrial free wall and the aortic valve shows the fetus to be in sinus rhythm. The aortic valve M-mode recording is used to time ventricular contraction, and there is a one-to-one relationship between atrial (A) and ventricular (V) systole. After the third sinus beat, a premature atrial contraction occurs (A*) but is not conducted to the ventricle due to block at the atrioventricular node. Sinus rhythm returns with the next (normal) atrial systole. Atrial premature beats, while usually benign, are usually what initiates supraventricular tachycardia.

3.15 Cardiac Arrhythmias: Bradycardia (Including Blocked Premature Beats)

Epidemiology/Genetics

Definition The normal fetal heart rate usually ranges from 120 to 160 beats per minute. Bradycardia, defined as a ventricular rate less than 120 beats per minute, has multiple causes.

In *sinus bradycardia*, the ventricular rate typically ranges between 70 and 120 beats per minute, the impulse originates at the sinus node, and there is one-to-one conduction between the atrium and the ventricle. Atrial contraction precedes ventricular contraction by 60 to 150 msec. The onset and offset of sinus bradycardia are gradual and are frequently caused by changes in autonomic tone.

Complete heart block (also termed third-degree atrioventricular block) occurs when there is complete dissociation between atrial and ventricular contraction due to dysfunction of the atrioventricular node and/or bundle of His. The atrium contracts but the electrical impulse from the atrium cannot penetrate to the ventricle and the ventricle beats independently as an escape rhythm.

Second-degree atrioventricular block allows some but not all atrial impulses to penetrate the atrioventricular node and bundle of His. Second-degree block is of two types. In *Mobitz type I second-degree atrioventricular block* (also termed Wenckebach block), the time to travel through the atrioventricular node gradually increases over consecutive beats until, finally, the impulse does not penetrate the atrioventricular node at all. This is recognized on fetal echocardiogram by a gradually increasing atrioventricular conduction time until finally there is no conduction through the atrioventricular node. In *Mobitz type II second-degree block*, the atrioventricular conduction time is constant, but intermittently the atrioventricular node and bundle of His fail to conduct the atrial impulse. Mobitz type II second-degree atrioventricular block represents disease of the bundle of His and may progress to third-degree block (i.e., complete heart block). Mobitz type I second-degree block is due to a conduction abnormality of the atrioventricular node, is generally benign, and does not progress to complete heart block.

Other abnormalities of the sinus node can result in bradycardia but are quite rare. In *sinoatrial exit block*, the electrical impulse of the sinus node cannot propagate beyond the perimeter of the sinus node. In *sinus arrest*, the sinus node fails to generate an electrical impulse at all. These arrhythmias will not be discussed further.

Blocked atrial premature contractions can cause bradycardia, since not all atrial contractions are conducted through the atrioventricular node. The ventricular rate at the time of block will slow.

Epidemiology The frequency of fetal bradycardia is not clear. Among fetuses with bradycardia, complete heart block probably accounts for in excess of 80% of cases. Complete heart block occurs in the context of structural heart disease in 30 to 60% of patients. Associated structural heart disease, if present, is most commonly heterotaxy syndrome or corrected transposition. When structural heart disease is absent, complete heart block most often occurs in the fetus of a mother with systemic lupus erythematosus.

In a fetus with maternal lupus, complete heart block occurs in approximately 5% of patients. Complete heart block generally presents between 18 and 38 weeks' gestation. In cases of complete heart block related to maternal lupus, the arrhythmia was identified between 16 and 24 weeks in 53%, between 25 and 30 weeks in 24%, between 31 and 37 weeks in 11%, and between 38 and 40 weeks in 7% of cases.

Complete heart block during the first trimester raises the likelihood that structural heart disease is present. In four fetuses presenting during that period all had structural heart disease, most commonly heterotaxy syndrome.

Embryology In complete heart block secondary to maternal lupus, transmission of maternal immunoglobulin G antibodies across the placenta appears to be causative. The antibodies are either anti-SSA/Ro or anti-SSB/La. In a rat heart experimental model, perfusion of myocytes with autoantibodies induced conduction abnormalities related to inhibition of L-type calcium channels.

Inheritance Pattern Complete heart block related to structural heart disease is less likely to recur in subsequent pregnancies. Recurrence in the context of maternal lupus does occur, although the frequency has not been reported.

Teratogens None.

Prognosis Among 36 fetuses and infants with complete heart block reviewed retrospectively, 12 died. Of those fetuses that died, two were electively aborted, seven died in utero related to congestive heart failure and hydrops, two died immediately in the postnatal period also related to heart failure, and one died from unrelated causes. Risk factors for mortality included bradycardia at a ventricular rate less than 55 beats per minute during early pregnancy, rapid decrease in ventricular rate during pregnancy, and the development of hydrops. Among 12 fetuses who developed hydrops, the mortality rate was in excess of 80%. The presence of structural heart disease has also been described as a risk factor for fetal demise. Other risk factors have included an atrial rate less than or equal to 120 beats per minute, although this particular risk factor was highly correlated with the presence of polysplenia. While quite unusual, one case has been reported of spontaneous in utero resolution of complete heart block.

Sonography

FINDINGS

1. **Fetus:**
   a. The same methods used to determine the timing and relationship of atrial and ventricular contraction discussed in the section on tachycardia are applied to the analysis of fetal bradycardia. Atrial timing can be established by M-mode echocardiography of the atrial wall, particularly the atrial appendage, whereas ventricular contraction is identified from the M-mode echocardiography of the ventricular wall or a semilunar valve. Alternatively, pulsed Doppler or color M-mode echocardiography in the left ventricular outflow tract can be used.
   b. Sinus bradycardia is present when there is one-to-one conduction between the atrium, and the ventricle and the atrial rate is less than 120 beats per minute.
   c. Atrioventricular block is diagnosed when atrial contraction does not result in ventricular capture. In cases in which the atrial contraction is premature, the lack of ventricular contraction reflects refractoriness of the atrioventricular node and does not reflect disease of the atrioventricular node. In contrast, in complete heart block, atrial depolarization that would be expected to conduct to the ventricle does not penetrate the atrioventricular node and bundle of His. In complete heart block, the ventricular rate is unrelated to the atrial rate, and none of the atrial contractions reach and capture the ventricle.
   d. The fetus should be examined for structural heart disease. In particular, one should exclude heterotaxy syndrome and corrected transposition. It is important to examine the continuity of the inferior vena cava, since an interrupted inferior vena cava is a frequent feature of polysplenia syndrome. Noting ventricular inversion is a clue to the diagnosis of corrected transposition.
   e. The fetus should be examined for signs of hydrops, including increased skin-fold thickness, pleural and/or pericardial effusion, and fetal ascites.
   f. Ventricular function should be assessed and the ventricular dimensions and heart size should be measured. Increasing heart size reflects, to some degree, a normal response to bradycardia so as to increase stroke volume; however, with ventricular decompensation, excessive cardiomegaly and decreased function alert the examiner to an increased risk of fetal demise.
2. **Amniotic Fluid:** Normal unless hydrops develops.
3. **Placenta:** Normal unless hydrops develops when the placenta is enlarged.
4. **Measurement Data:** Normal.
5. **When Detectable:** Arrhythmias are relatively easily diagnosed with transabdominal imaging from 16 to 17 weeks and later. Transvaginal imaging has diagnosed complete heart block in a fetus as young as 11 weeks. Pulsed Doppler interrogation in the fetal abdominal aorta and inferior vena cava has been used in a 13-week fetus to diagnose fetal arrhythmias.

Differential Diagnosis   When some atrial contractions fail to result in ventricular depolarization, the differential diagnosis includes complete heart block, second-degree atrioventricular block (Mobitz type I and Mobitz type II), and blocked atrial premature beats. Blocked atrial premature beats are easily distinguished by the fact that the atrial contraction occurs earlier than normal and the atrial contractions occurring at the normal time are conducted through the atrioventricular node.

In Mobitz type I second-degree block, some of the atrial contractions are conducted through the atrioventricular node; however, gradually the atrioventricular conduction time increases until finally one atrial contraction will not result in ventricular capture. This form of second-degree block is also termed Wenckebach block and generally does not reflect serious pathology.

In type II second-degree block, some atrial contractions result in ventricular capture. Intermittently, some impulses do not penetrate the bundle of His and/or the atrioventricular node. This is an ominous finding, as second-degree block can progress to complete heart block, particularly in fetuses of mothers with systemic lupus erythematosus.

Where Else to Look

1. Look for the findings of hydrops—pericardial and pleural effusions, ascites, skin thickening, polyhydramnios, and placentomegaly.
2. Look for structural cardiac anomalies.
3. Make sure the bradycardia is not preterminal and related to a central nervous system anomaly.
4. Check for intrauterine growth retardation.

Pregnancy Management

Investigations and Consultations Required   In all cases of complete heart block, autoantibodies to anti-SS-A/Ro and/or anti-B/La related to lupus should be measured in the mother. In cases in which maternal lupus is present, management should be coordinated with a rheumatologist with experience in lupus, a perinatologist, and a pediatric cardiologist with experience in the management of fetal arrhythmias. Karyotype analysis should be performed in cases of suspected heterotaxy syndrome.

Fetal Intervention   In the fetus greater than 32 weeks' gestational age, early delivery and postnatal pacing is appropriate if hydrops develops. In fetuses of mothers with systemic lupus, the administration of fluorinated steroids should be strongly considered with the diagnosis of second- or third-degree block (and even in cases in which the atrioventricular conduction time exceeds 150 msec). The data are not clear that corticosteroids are efficacious and prospective trials are underway. Fetuses with complete heart block secondary to maternal lupus who received corticosteroids had no significant difference compared with the group that did not receive steroids in terms of the duration of pregnancy, the number of fetal deaths, the final degree of heart block, or the requirement for a pacemaker. The efficacy of steroid therapy was more apparent in terms of the resolution of pleural effusions, ascites, and the signs of hydrops. Since an element of myocarditis has been hypothesized in the fetal hearts of mothers with lupus, it is possible that the improvement in fluid collections is related to a decrease in myocardial inflammation. A trial of sympathomimetics has been reported in complete heart block secondary to maternal lupus, although the data are very preliminary. Prenatal pacing for complete hydrops has been performed in a fetal ewe model. In humans, early delivery of a premature infant with subsequent staged epicardial pacing has been described.

Monitoring Pregnancy/Course   Once atrioventricular node disease has been recognized, the fetus should be examined weekly for progression of the disease or the development of hydrops or ventricular dysfunction.

With blocked atrial bigeminy and no evidence of atrioventricular node disease, the fetus should be examined weekly with fetal Doppler echocardiography and biweekly with fetal echocardiography for evidence of development of supraventricular tachycardia or sequelae of this arrhythmia.

Sinus bradycardia should result in evaluation of overall fetal well-being. Maternal thyroid status should be screened. One should explore for a family history of long QT syndrome, since Romano-Ward syndrome has been recognized prenatally. Sinus bradycardia is one feature of the long QT syndrome.

Pregnancy Termination Issues   Termination may be considered in those cases of complete heart block associated with serious structural heart disease, particularly in the presence of hydrops. An intact fetus should be delivered and a complete examination performed because of the potential presence of associated abnormalities. Termination is generally not considered in the case of complete heart block secondary to maternal lupus.

Delivery   A fetus with complete heart block or high-grade second-degree block should be delivered in a center where immediate pediatric cardiac consultation is available and where there is the potential for ventricular pacing. Early delivery should be considered during the third trimester when hydrops develops if the fetus is of sufficient size that epicardial pacing is feasible postnatally.

Neonatology

Resuscitation   Spontaneous breathing is generally present, and resuscitation is not required. In cases in which hydrops is present secondary to complete heart block, isoproterenol at very low doses may be helpful by increasing the ventricular rate. The appropriate equipment should be prearranged for ventricular pacing.

Transport   Immediate referral to a tertiary center with pediatric cardiology is indicated. Consultation prior to transfer with a pediatric cardiologist should be obtained to determine if measures to increase the heart rate or improve peripheral transfusion are needed during transport.

Nursery Management   The mechanism of rhythm disorder can generally be established with a surface electrocardiogram. Indications for ventricular pacing generally include a ventricular rate less than 55 beats per minute in neonates, ventricular dysfunction thought to be related to low heart rate, or ventricular ectopy and/or increased QT interval. (For mangement of hydrops, refer to Chapter 13.2.)

Surgery/Intervention

Preoperative Assessment   Indications for epicardial pacing have been described.

Types of Procedures/Prognosis   Temporary transvenous ventricular pacing is used to achieve an adequate ventricular rate for the short term. When long-term pacing is required, epicardial pacing leads are placed surgically and the results are usually satisfactory unless the newborn is premature or small for birth weight. When children are older, dual-chamber pacing is often instituted.

REFERENCES

Assad RS, Jatene MB, Moreira LF, et al: Fetal heart block: A new experimental model to assess fetal pacing. Pacing Clin Electrophysiol 1994;17:1256–1263.

Baschat AA, Gembruch U, Knopfle G, Hansmann M: First-trimester fetal heart block: A marker for cardiac anomaly. Ultrasound Obstet Gynecol 1999;14:311–314.

Boris JR, Drose JA, Schaffer MS, Shaffer EM: Spontaneous resolution of atrioventricular dissociation in utero. Pediatr Cardiol 1998;19:487–489.

Boutjdir M, Chen L, Zhang ZH, et al: Serum and immunoglobulin G from the mother of a child with congenital heart block induce conduction abnormalities and inhibit L-type calcium channels in a rat heart model. Pediatr Res 1998;44:11–19.

Buyon JP, Waltuck J, Klienman C, Copel J: In utero identification and therapy of congenital heart block. Lupus 1995;4:116–121.

Crawford D, Chapman M, Allan L: The assessment of persistent bradycardia in prenatal life. Br J Obstet Gynaecol 1985;92:941–944.

Fukushige J, Takahashi N, Igarashi H, et al: Perinatal management of congenital complete atrioventricular block: Report of nine cases. Acta Paediatr Jpn 1998;40:337–340.

Gembruch U, Knopfle G, Chatterjee M, et al: First-trimester diagnosis of fetal congenital heart disease by transvaginal two-dimensional and Doppler echocardiography. Obstet Gynecol 1990;75:496–498.

Groves AM, Allan LD, Rosenthal E: Outcome of isolated congenital complete heart block diagnosed in utero [see comments]. Heart 1996;75:190–194.

Groves AM, Allan LD, Rosenthal E: Therapeutic trial of sympathomimetics in three cases of complete heart block in the fetus. Circulation 1995;92:3394–3396.

Machado MV, Tynan MJ, Curry PV, Allan LD: Fetal complete heart block. Br Heart J 1988;60:512–515.

Rosenthal D, Druzin M, Chin C, Dubin A: A new therapeutic approach to the fetus with congenital complete heart block: Preemptive, targeted therapy with dexamethasone. Obstet Gynecol 1998;92:689–691.

Saleeb S, Copel J, Friedman D, Buyon JP: Comparison of treatment with fluorinated glucocorticoids to the natural history of autoantibody-associated congenital heart block: retrospective review of the research registry for neonatal lupus. Arthritis Rheum 1999;42:2335–2345.

Schmidt KG, Ulmer HE, Silverman NH, et al: Perinatal outcome of fetal complete atrioventricular block: A multicenter experience. J Am Coll Cardiol 1991;17:1360–1366.

Weindling SN, Saul JP, Triedman JK, et al: Staged pacing therapy for congenital complete heart block in premature infants. Am J Cardiol 1994;74:412–413.

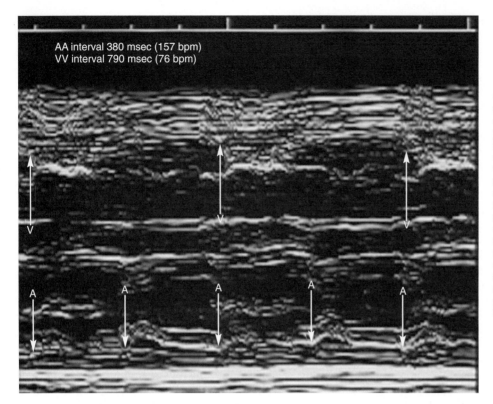

AA interval 380 msec (157 bpm)
VV interval 790 msec (76 bpm)

Complete heart block. In this fetus of a mother with lupus erythematosus, atrial contraction occurs at a rate of 157 beats per minute while ventricular contraction is at a rate of 76 beats per minute. None of the atrial contractions result in ventricular contraction. This rhythm should not be confused with second-degree block with two-to-one atrioventricular conduction, in which every other atrial contraction results in ventricular contraction. In this illustration, the first atrial contraction occurs nearly simultaneously with ventricular contraction and certainly has not resulted in ventricular systole. The second atrial systole also fails to conduct to the ventricle. There is no pericardial effusion or signs of hydrops in this fetus.

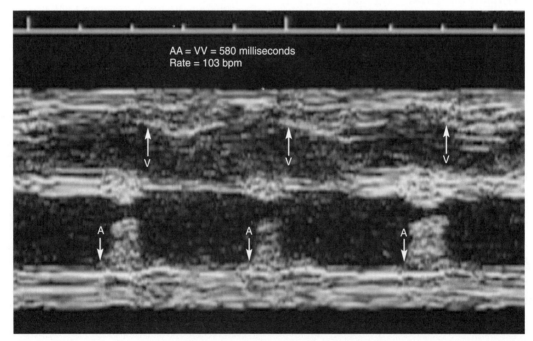

AA = VV = 580 milliseconds
Rate = 103 bpm

Sinus rhythm with sinus bradycardia determined by simultaneous M-mode of atrial and ventricular contraction. In this fetus with sinus bradycardia, the atrial contraction precedes ventricular contraction by 100 msec, and there is a one-to-one relationship between atrial (A) and ventricular (V) contraction. In this case, there is sinus bradycardia, as the rate is less than 120 beats per minute.

3.16 Hypertrophic Cardiomyopathy

Epidemiology/Genetics

Definition Hypertrophy of the left ventricle and sometimes the right ventricle not in response to an increased pressure or volume load. The systolic function is usually normal but the diastolic function is frequently abnormal because of decreased ventricular compliance.

Epidemiology Prevalence has not been defined. Approximately 10% of cases are secondary to genetic disorders. Infants of insulin-dependent diabetes mothers account for almost all of the remainder. Cardiomegaly and septal hypertrophy identified by fetal echocardiography have been reported in 20% to 30% of pregnancies in insulin-dependent women with current glycemia management approaches. Of that group, approximately 10% of the fetuses progress to a true cardiopathy that is symptomatic before or following delivery. Both the incidence and severity have been correlated with glycemia management during pregnancy.

Embryology Unknown.

Inheritance Pattern Familial idiopathic hypertrophic cardiomyopathy is inherited in an autosomal dominant pattern; however, new mutations are present in approximately 50% of cases recognized postnatally. Hypertrophic cardiomyopathy may sometimes be secondary to mutations in the cardiac beta myosin heavy chain (14q11-q12), alpha-tropomyosin (15q22), troponin T (1q32), or protein C gene (11p11-q13). In the fetus, however, hypertrophic cardiomyopathy occurs much more commonly in maternal diabetes mellitus than as familial hypertrophic cardiomyopathy. Hypertrophic cardiomyopathy has also occurred in monosomy 14 and in Noonan syndrome.

Teratogens Ritodrine exposure has been associated with hypertrophic cardiomyopathy. The hypertrophy generally regresses within 3 months postnatally. With maternal diabetes, the degree of septal hypertrophy correlates with the level of fetal hyperinsulinism.

Prognosis Hypertrophic cardiomyopathy in the context of maternal diabetes generally carries a good prognosis. Usually the hypertrophy resolves spontaneously by 3 to 6 months of age. With marked hypertrophy, particularly with associated obstruction, stroke volume is reduced secondary to reduced diastolic filling. Hypertrophic cardiomyopathy that is idiopathic has a more guarded prognosis, as there is an annual risk of death of approximately 1%.

Sonography

FINDINGS

1. **Fetus:**
   a. When ventricular hypertrophy is detected, one should exclude diseases resulting in anatomic obstruction such as aortic stenosis. In most cases of severe aortic stenosis detected prenatally, however, the left ventricular dimension is increased more than the left ventricular wall thickness is (i.e., the thickness to dimension ratio is typically decreased, even though left ventricular mass is increased).
   b. The distribution of hypertrophy should be assessed. With hypertrophic cardiomyopathy secondary to maternal diabetes mellitus and in familial hypertrophic cardiomyopathy, the septum is typically but not always disproportionately hypertrophied. One should measure ventricular dimensions, left ventricular posterior wall thickness, and septal thickness.
   c. Dynamic left- or right-sided obstruction can occur when septal hypertrophy is severe. In addition, the anterior leaflet of the mitral valve can be distorted by the septal hypertrophy and mitral regurgitation can occur.
2. **Amniotic Fluid:** Normal.
3. **Placenta:** Normal.
4. **Measurement Data:** Macrosomia is common with maternal diabetes mellitus.
5. **When Detectable:** Hypertrophic cardiomyopathy secondary to maternal diabetes can present in the second trimester but more commonly presents in the third trimester. Idiopathic hypertrophic subaortic stenosis can also present in the second or the third trimester.

Pitfalls/Differential Diagnosis When the hypertrophy primarily involves the ventricular septum, one might mistakenly diagnose a myocardial tumor. Rhabdomyomas are the most common fetal cardiac tumor. (See Chapter 14.7.) In most cases of fetal rhabdomyomas, the masses are multiple. In twin-twin transfusion, volume contraction can result in increased wall thickness to ventricular cavity dimension, even though the actual myocardial mass is not increased. This mistake is avoided by recognizing the reduced ventricular dimensions and understanding the clinical contexts in which volume contraction can occur.

Where Else To Look One needs to screen for maternal diabetes with a hemoglobin A_{1c} and establish whether there is a family history of cardiomyopathy. Hypertrophic cardiomyopathy can occur with Noonan syndrome. One should therefore exclude cystic hygroma and associated cardiac disease such as pulmonary stenosis. Look for the findings of the VACTERL syndrome, which occurs often in diabetic patients.

Pregnancy Management

Investigations and Consultations Required   Maternal hemoglobin A_{1c}.

Fetal Intervention   None indicated.

Monitoring   The fetal heart should be re-examined at the beginning of the third trimester to determine whether there is outflow tract obstruction or mitral regurgitation.

Pregnancy Course   In most cases, fetuses will survive to term unless there is serious outflow obstruction and/or the presence of significant atrioventricular valve regurgitation.

Pregnancy Termination Issues   Usually not relevant.

Delivery   If there is obstruction or the hypertrophy is moderate to severe, delivery should occur in a facility where pediatric cardiology consultation can be obtained.

Neonatology

Resuscitation   In general, resuscitation is not necessary. Volume contraction should be avoided in the infant, as dynamic outflow obstruction can result.

Transport   If no obstruction is present, transport is not generally required as long as the diagnosis can be confirmed and symptoms such as tachypnea, hypotension, metabolic acidosis, arrhythmia, and desaturation are absent.

Testing and Confirmation   Echocardiography is sufficient for establishing the diagnosis of hypertrophic cardiomyopathy and excluding outflow obstruction and mitral regurgitation.

Nursery Management   One should avoid maneuvers that could increase outflow tract obstruction such as hypovolemia or administration of inotropic or afterload reduction agents. In particular, digoxin is contraindicated in most cases. In cases in which there is significant outflow tract obstruction, beta blocker therapy may be indicated, but this is a minority of cases.

Extracorporeal membrane oxygenation (ECMO) support has been reported to be successful in severe cases of cardiac failure from hypertrophic cardiomyopathy of infants of diabetic mothers.

Surgical Results/Prognosis   Surgery for hypertrophic cardiomyopathy is almost never indicated in the newborn period. In some cases of hypertrophic cardiomyopathy, beta blocker therapy may be administered. Calcium channel blockers are used after infancy. The prognosis with hypertrophic cardiomyopathy secondary to maternal diabetes mellitus is usually good.

REFERENCES

Chen CP, Chern SR, Lee CC, et al: De novo unbalanced translocation resulting in monosomy for proximal 14q and distal 4p in a fetus with intrauterine growth retardation, Wolf-Hirschhorn syndrome, hypertrophic cardiomyopathy, and partial hemihypoplasia. J Med Genet 1998;35:1050–1053.

Coates TL, McGahan JP: Fetal cardiac rhabdomyomas presenting as diffuse myocardial thickening. J Ultrasound Med 1994;13:813–816.

Debrus S, de Meeus A, Jean MK, Bouvagnet P: [Genetics of hereditary cardiopathies]. Arch Mal Coeur Vaiss 1996;89:619–627.

Hagemann LL, Zielinsky P: [Prenatal study of hypertrophic cardiomyopathy and its association with insulin levels in fetuses of diabetic mothers]. Arq Bras Cardiol 1996;66:193–198.

Lusson JR, Gaulme J, Raynaud EJ, Cheynel J: [Asymmetrical hypertrophic cardiomyopathy in neonates of diabetic mothers]. Arch Fr Pediatr 1982;39:433–436.

Medvenskaia VV: Characteristics of hemodynamics in cardiomyopathies of newborn infants of diabetic mothers Akush Ginekol (Mosk) 1995;4:32–34.

Nuchpuckdee P, Brodsky N, Porat R, Hurt H: Ventricular septal thickness and cardiac function in neonates after in utero ritodrine exposure. J Pediatr 1986;109:687–691.

Reller MD, Kaplan S: Hypertrophic cardiomyopathy in diabetic mothers: An update. Am J Perinatol 1988;5:353–358.

Sonesson SE, Fouron JC, Lessard M: Intrauterine diagnosis and evolution of a cardiomyopathy in a fetus with Noonan's syndrome. Acta Paediatr 1992;81:368–370.

Tyrala EE: The infant of the diabetic mother. Obstet Gynecol Clin North Am 1996;23:221–241.

Weber HS, Botti JJ, Bayler BG: Sequential longitudinal evaluation of cardiac growth and ventricular diastolic findings in fetuses of well controlled diabetic mothers. Pediatric Cardiol 1994;15:184–189.

Zielinsky P: Role of prenatal echocardiography in the study of hypertrophic cardiomyopathy in the fetus. Echocardiography 1991;8:661–668.

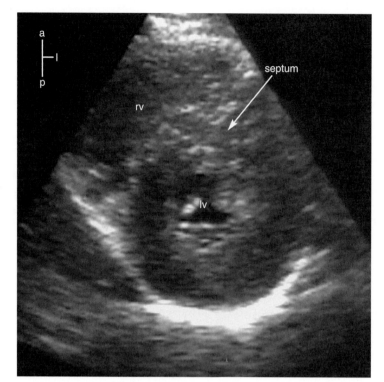

Hypertrophic cardiomyopathy. Marked anteroseptal, lateral wall, and posterior wall hypertrophy in a newborn with familial hypertrophic cardiomyopathy. The middle and posterior muscular septum is less hypertrophied. The father of the infant also had hypertrophic cardiomyopathy. Note that the left ventricular cavity size is reduced. lv, left ventricle; rv, right ventricle.

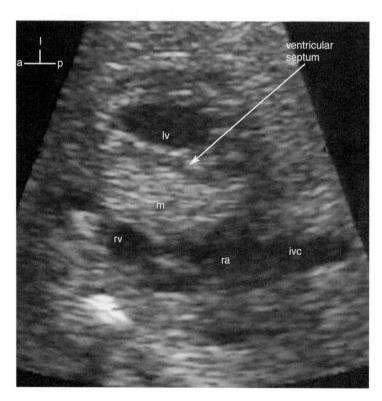

Large rhabdomyoma in tuberous sclerosis. This large mass (m) is broadly adherent to the right ventricular septal surface and mimics the septal hypertrophy seen in hypertrophic cardiomyopathy. Rhabdomyomas are typically multiple and are consistently hyperechoic in relation to normal myocardium (which is apparent here). Recognition of multiple hyperechoic masses is very helpful in differentiating tuberous sclerosis with a large septal mass from hypertrophic cardiomyopathy. The septum in hypertrophic cardiomyopathy can also be relatively hyperechoic and may be confused with a mass such as a rhabdomyoma or fibroma. ivc, inferior vena cava; lv, left ventricle; ra, right atrium; rv, right ventricle.

3.17 Heterotaxy Syndrome (Asplenia and Polysplenia) (Ivemark Syndrome)

Epidemiology/Genetics

Definition   Heterotaxy is from the Greek words "heteros," or other, and "taxis," meaning order or arrangement (i.e., other than normal order or arrangement of the heart and abdominal viscera). The spleen is almost always affected, and heterotaxy syndrome is subdivided into the asplenia and polysplenia syndromes. Frequently there is associated complex congenital heart disease.

Epidemiology   Prevalence per 1000 live births: unknown. Accounts for approximately 0.8% of children with congenital heart disease (53% with asplenia, 42% with polysplenia, and 5% with a single, normal-sized spleen).

Embryology   The primitive cardiac tube normally loops to the right (termed D-looping) at approximately 21 days of gestation and results in normal ventricular orientation (the right ventricle to the right of and anterior to the left ventricle). When looping is reversed (termed L-looping), ventricular inversion usually occurs and most commonly the right ventricle is posterior and left-sided. Abnormalities in looping occur in 30 to 40% of patients with heterotaxy syndrome.

In heterotaxy syndrome, there is frequently abnormal symmetry of organs that normally have some degree of asymmetry. For example, the lung is bilaterally trilobed in 81% of patients with asplenia and bilaterally bilobed in 72% of patients with polysplenia syndrome. The liver is symmetrical in 76% of patients with asplenia and 67% of patients with polysplenia.

Inheritance Patterns   The recurrence risk for congenital heart disease in siblings of a patient with heterotaxy syndrome is unknown, as is the recurrence risk in offspring of affected parents. Heterotaxy syndrome has reoccurred within families. Some investigators have described heterotaxy syndrome within Cumming syndrome (campomelia, multicystic dysplastic kidneys, and cervical lymphocele). Three types of mendelian inheritance have been described with heterotaxy syndrome.

Teratogens   Maternal diabetes mellitus.

Prognosis   Heterotaxy includes a large spectrum of cardiac diseases from extremely mild to extremely complex groups of lesions. The prognosis is dependent on the severity of the disease but is particularly poor when there is complete heart block prenatally.

Sonography

FINDINGS

1. **Fetus:**
   a. Characteristic findings of asplenia syndrome (and their frequency of occurrence within a group of patients with asplenia syndrome) include the following: intact inferior vena cava (100%), bilateral superior vena cava (71%), absent coronary sinus septum (97%), totally anomalous pulmonary venous connection to a systemic vein (58%), common atrioventricular canal defect (69%), double-outlet right ventricle (82%), bilateral subarterial conus (82%), subvalvular or valvular pulmonary stenosis (88–96%), and dextrocardia (36%). The stomach is right-sided and the liver is in the midline.
   b. Characteristic features of polysplenia syndrome (and their frequency of occurrence within a group of patients with polysplenia syndrome) include the following: interrupted inferior vena cava with azygous extension (80%), bilateral superior vena cava (50%), absent coronary sinus septum (26%), totally anomalous pulmonary venous connection to a systemic vein (2%), common atrioventricular canal (33%), normally related great arteries (61%), double-outlet right ventricle (37%), subvalvular pulmonary stenosis (43%), subvalvular aortic stenosis (22%), and dextrocardia (33%). The stomach is on the right and the liver is midline.
   c. The position of the gastric bubble and the cardiac mass should be identified on all fetal echocardiograms. Abnormalities of situs are a necessary but nonspecific feature of heterotaxy syndrome. For example, dextrocardia with abdominal situs inversus can occur without heterotaxy syndrome.
   d. The inferior vena cava and abdominal aorta should be identified at the level of the diaphragm. Normally, the inferior vena cava is right-sided and anterior to the left-sided aorta. With abdominal situs inversus, the relationship of the inferior vena cava to aorta is a mirror image of normal. This pattern is most typical of asplenia syndrome. When the inferior vena cava is interrupted (i.e., the renal to hepatic segment of the inferior vena cava is absent), the infrahepatic portion of the inferior vena cava continues as either a right-sided or a left-sided azygous vein. The azygous vein is posterior to the aorta and can be on the ipsilateral or contralateral side to the aorta. The azygous vein should be followed to its connection above the diaphragm, which will be to either a right-sided or a left-sided superior vena cava. An interrupted inferior vena cava with azy-

gous extension is frequently present in polysplenia syndrome. One should examine anterior to the central branch pulmonary arteries to exclude bilateral cavae, which are present in 50 to 70% of patients with heterotaxy syndrome.

   e. Reducing the color Doppler scale to accentuate low-velocity flow facilitates the identification of the pulmonary venous return.

   f. Atrioventricular canal lesions are obvious when there is a common atrioventricular valve, but more subtle defects are detected by identifying a primum atrial septal defect (a defect in the most inferior and anterior portion of the atrial septum and confluent with the atrioventricular valves).

   g. The connection of both great vessels and the exclusion of outflow obstruction are critical.

   h. Fetal bradycardia may be the referral indication and may be due to complete heart block, a not uncommon feature of polysplenia.

2. **Amniotic Fluid:** Polyhydramnios can occur when hydrops is present, particularly in patients with severe atrioventricular valve regurgitation and/or complete heart block.
3. **Placenta:** Generally normal.
4. **Measurement Data:** Generally normal.
5. **When Detectable:** Transabdominal imaging can detect defects between 16 and 18 weeks, and transvaginal imaging may detect these defects between 10 and 14 weeks.

Pitfalls

1. Some practitioners find it easier to remember associated abnormalities in heterotaxy syndrome by thinking of asplenia as "bilateral right-sidedness" and polysplenia as "bilateral left-sidedness." Although this may be a helpful pneumonic, it is not entirely accurate. For example, a symmetric liver is present in the majority of patients with asplenia and polysplenia syndromes.
2. One needs to consider heterotaxy syndrome on detecting "isolated" findings such as complete heart block, common atrioventricular canal defects, and interrupted inferior vena cava.
3. A dilated coronary sinus may mimic a primum type of atrial septal defect, as both are adjacent to the atrioventricular valves. However, the coronary sinus is a posterior structure whereas a primum defect is anterior.

Differential Diagnosis Many of the defects of heterotaxy syndrome can occur in isolation and not represent heterotaxy syndrome. Abnormalities in laterality must be present to diagnose heterotaxy syndrome.

Where Else to Look

1. One should attempt to identify the spleen in heterotaxy syndrome, which is usually absent in asplenia but multiple (and tiny) in polysplenia syndrome.
2. Renal anomalies such as multicystic kidney disease are seen in 25% of cases of asplenia.

Pregnancy Management

Investigations and Consultations Required Pediatric cardiology consultations should be obtained for confirmation of diagnosis and counseling. Karyotype should be obtained to exclude associated chromosomal abnormalities. Down syndrome is extremely unusual in heterotaxy syndrome.

Fetal Intervention Not relevant.

Monitoring Fetuses with heterotaxy syndrome should be reimaged at 28 weeks because of the potential for worsening of atrioventricular valve regurgitation and further progression of outflow tract obstruction. The fetal heart rate should be assessed on a weekly basis after 28 weeks, when the probability for complete heart block is increased (e.g., polysplenia syndrome).

Pregnancy Course Generally uneventful unless there is severe atrioventricular valve regurgitation or complete heart block. Complete heart block is poorly tolerated when associated with structural heart disease.

Pregnancy Termination Issues A complete postmortem examination should be performed for confirmation of cardiac diagnosis and because of the frequent association of abdominal abnormalities.

Delivery In general, the fetus with heterotaxy syndrome should be delivered at a center where immediate pediatric cardiology consultation can be obtained, as lesions can be ductus dependent when there is severe outflow obstruction.

Neonatology

Resuscitation Infants will generally breathe spontaneously and not require resuscitation.

Transport Infants should be transferred to a center with pediatric cardiology and multiple pediatric surgical specialities available.

Testing and Confirmation Echocardiography is definitive for an accurate anatomic diagnosis. An upper gastrointestinal examination should be performed in suspected heterotaxy syndrome to exclude malrotation. Abdominal ultrasonography and splenic function testing are indicated in cases of suspected asplenia or polysplenia syndrome. A labeled red blood cell scan may also be helpful in assessing splenic function.

Nursery Management Management is directed toward rapid identification of the extent of organ malformation and dysfunction present while maintaining adequate cardiorespiratory support. The management of the cardiac component of the malformation complex will be dictated by the lesion(s) identified and the consequent impact on adequate cardiac function. See the appropriate section for the management of the specific lesions in each organ system.

Surgery

Preoperative Assessment   Echocardiography is generally sufficient for preoperative testing.

Operative Indications   The indications are often similar to those discussed for individual lesions, such as complete common atrioventricular canal, double outlet, aortic stenosis, or pulmonary stenosis.

Types of Procedures   The spectrum of heterotaxy is so variable that the reader is referred to management of each lesion in the sections where they are discussed separately.

Surgical Results/Prognosis   The spectrum of disease and the prognosis are quite variable. Prognosis is poor in those infants with total anomalous pulmonary venous return, particularly in cases in which the return is mixed to multiple sites and in fetuses in whom there is severe systemic outflow tract obstruction. In cases in which there is severe ventricular hypoplasia, single-ventricle management is necessary and multiple operations are required.

REFERENCES

Cesko I, Hajdu J, Toth T, et al: Ivemark syndrome with asplenia in siblings. J Pediatr 1997;130:822–824.

Chitayat D, Lao A, Wilson RD, et al: Prenatal diagnosis of asplenia/polysplenia syndrome. Am J Obstet Gynecol 1988;158:1085–1087.

Crawford D, Chapman M, Allan L: The assessment of persistent bradycardia in prenatal life. Br J Obstet Gynaecol 1985;92:941–944.

Debrus S, de Meeus A, Jean MK, Bouvagnet P: [Genetics of hereditary cardiopathies]. Arch Mal Coeur Vaiss 1996;89:619–627.

Gembruch U, Hansmann M, Redel DA, et al: [Non-immunologically-induced hydrops fetalis in complete atrioventricular block of the fetus. A summary of 11 prenatally diagnosed cases]. Geburtshilfe Frauenheilkd 1988;48:494–499.

Gembruch U, Knopfle G, Chatterjee M, et al: First-trimester diagnosis of fetal congenital heart disease by transvaginal two-dimensional and Doppler echocardiography. Obstet Gynecol 1990;75:496–498.

Kim SH, Son CS, Lee JW, et al: Visceral heterotaxy syndrome induced by retinoids in mouse embryo. J Korean Med Sci 1995;10:250–257.

Machado MV, Crawford DC, Anderson RH, Allan LD: Atrioventricular septal defect in prenatal life. Br Heart J 1988;59:352–355.

Ming JE, McDonald-McGinn DM, Markowitz RI, et al: Heterotaxia in a fetus with campomelia, cervical lymphocele, polysplenia, and multicystic dysplastic kidneys: Expanding the phenotype of Cumming syndrome. Am J Med Genet 1997;73:419–424.

Rose V, Izukawa T, Moes CA: Syndromes of asplenia and polysplenia. A review of cardiac and non-cardiac malformations in 60 cases with special reference to diagnosis and prognosis. Br Heart J 1975;37:840–852.

Rubino M, Van Praagh S, Kadoba K, et al: Systemic and pulmonary venous connections in visceral heterotaxy with asplenia. Diagnostic and surgical considerations based on seventy-two autopsied cases. J Thorac Cardiovasc Surg 1995;110:641–650.

Sheley RC, Nyberg DA, Kapur R: Azygous continuation of the interrupted inferior vena cava: A clue to prenatal diagnosis of the cardiosplenic syndromes. J Ultrasound Med 1995;14:381–387.

Van Praagh S, Geva T, Friedberg DZ, et al: Aortic outflow obstruction in visceral heterotaxy: A study based on twenty postmortem cases. Am Heart J 1997;133:558–569.

Van Praagh S, Santini F, Sanders SP: Cardiac malpositions with special emphasis on visceral heterotaxy (asplenia and polysplenia syndromes). In Fyler DC (ed): Nadas' Pediatric Cardiology. Philadelphia, Hanley & Belfus, 1992, pp 589–608.

Yasui H, Morishima M, Nakazawa M, Aikawa E: Anomalous looping, atrioventricular cushion dysplasia, and unilateral ventricular hypoplasia in the mouse embryos with right isomerism induced by retinoic acid. Anat Rec 1998;250:210–219.

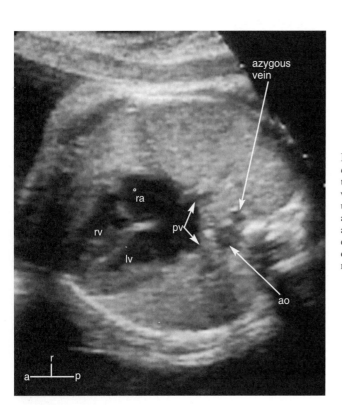

Heterotaxy syndrome: interrupted inferior vena cava in polysplenia syndrome. Cross section of fetus at the level of the diaphragm shows the anterior and left-sided aorta (ao) and the right-sided and posterior azygous vein. No inferior vena cava is seen because it is interrupted and continues via the right-sided azygous vein to the right superior vena cava. Right- and left-sided pulmonary veins (pv) are shown connecting with the left atrium. The azygous vein is posterior to the aorta, unlike the inferior vena cava, which is anterior. An interrupted inferior vena cava occurs in 80% of patients with polysplenia syndrome. lv, left ventricle; ra, right atrium; rv, right ventricle.

3.18 Ectopia Cordis/Pentalogy of Cantrell

Epidemiology/Genetics

Definition   The heart is partially or totally outside the thorax. Ectopia cordis can occur as part of other conditions such as limb-body wall complex and pentalogy of Cantrell. Pentalogy of Cantrell is composed of thoracoabdominal ectopia cordis, omphalocele-like supraumbilical wall defect, cleft sternum, pericardial defect, and other congenital heart defects.

Epidemiology   Very rare, less than 1 in 100,000 (M2:F1).

Embryology   The embryology and etiology of ectopia cordis are heterogeneous. Some cases are the result of early amnion rupture with other limb-body wall abnormalities. The pentalogy of Cantrell is thought to be due to a failure of ventral wall closure caused by defects in the mesodermal tissue elements. Failure of fusion of the sternal primordial bands occurs with a severity that varies from simple sternal cleft to true ectopia cordis.

Inheritance Patterns   Generally sporadic. Rare cases with trisomy 21 have been reported.

Teratogens   None known.

Prognosis   The prognosis is dependent on the severity of intracardiac abnormalities as well as associated defects. Generally, the pentalogy of Cantrell and most limb-body wall disruptions are lethal. Minor degrees of ectopia cordis resulting from failure of sternal closure may be surgically correctable.

Sonography

FINDINGS

1. **Fetus:** There are two forms, the thoracic and the thoracoabdominal.
   a. In the thoracic form (classic form), there is
      1. A sternal defect
      2. Absence of the parietal pericardium
      3. Cephalic orientation of cardiac apex (which often beats against the baby's chin)
      4. A small thoracic cavity
   b. In the thoracoabdominal form, there is partial absence or a cleft of the lower sternum and there is usually a defect of the diaphragmatic parietal pericardium. An omphalocele is frequently seen.
      In the absence of structural heart disease, Doppler flow patterns should be normal.
2. **Amniotic Fluid:** Normal.
3. **Placenta:** Normal.
4. **Measurement Data:** Normal.

When Detectable   The entity has been detected at 9 weeks with the vaginal probe.

Pitfalls   In some examples of the limb-body wall complex, the thoracic anatomy may be so distorted that the defect may be overlooked. It may be difficult to determine whether a portion of the heart is outside the chest with a large omphalocele.

Differential Diagnosis   This is a very distinct entity.

Where Else to Look   In the heart, there are numerous associated cardiac anomalies. Tetralogy of Fallot, ventricular septal defect, tricuspid atresia, Ebstein's anomaly, common atrium, atrioventricular canal, mitral atresia, total anomalous pulmonary venous return, single ventricle, pulmonary stenosis, pulmonary atresia, aortic stenosis, coarctation of the aorta, transposition of the great artery, left ventricular diverticulum, biventricular diverticulum, and persistent left superior vena cava have all been reported. Defects are common with the thoracoabdominal form. Omphalocele is common with both types. Ectopia cordis is a feature of the limb-body wall complex, so there may be gastroschisis, missing limbs, caudal regression, etc.

Pregnancy Management

Investigations and Consultations Required   Chromosome analysis is essential. Because of the association with neural tube defects, both amniotic fluid alpha-fetoprotein and acetylcholinesterase studies should be done. Fetal echocardiography must be performed to delineate the precise cardiac defects. Pediatric surgery and pediatric cardiology consultations should be obtained to assess prognosis and plan perinatal management.

Fetal Intervention   None is indicated.

Monitoring   The overall dismal prognosis for this disorder should preclude aggressive pregnancy intervention in most cases. If the structural cardiac malformation is relatively minor, then surgical correction may be successful, and standard obstetric management is appropriate.

Pregnancy Course   No specific obstetric complications are to be expected.

Pregnancy Termination Issues   Although examination of an intact fetus will establish what the associated malformations are, it is unlikely to alter recurrence risk information. Therefore, the method of termination can be a destructive one.

Delivery   A nonaggressive approach without fetal monitoring should be considered. The site for delivery should be a tertiary center where an immediate evaluation of the neonate can be undertaken to assess whether surgical correction should be attempted.

Neonatology

Resuscitation   Given the almost total lethality of this lesion, the decision to provide support following birth should be discussed with the family prior to delivery. When there is uncertainty regarding the prognosis, it is appropriate to provide at least assisted ventilation pending full evaluation and determination of the prognosis.

Transport   Immediate referral to a tertiary center with full pediatric cardiac diagnostic and surgical capabilities is essential, particularly for the infant with a minor or limited defect. The exposed viscera should be protected against trauma and contamination during transit with a warm, moist, sterile dressing.

Testing and Confirmation   Careful physical examination, postnatal echocardiography, and abdominal ultrasonography will confirm the nature and severity of the lesions. If not obtained prenatally, chromosomal karyotyping is important.

Nursery Management   Provision of respiratory support during the interval between birth and completion of the diagnostic evaluation is appropriate to allow time for parental adaptation and clarification of the feasibility of surgical correction.

Surgery

Preoperative Assessment   The initial goal of assessment is to determine the extent of the sternal defect and the severity of the associated anomalies, particularly cardiac, as the latter determines the survival prognosis. Ectopia cordia may also occur as a component of the limb-body wall complex.

Three categories of defects have been described:

1. Cleft sternum—either a partial or complete cleft beginning superiorly and without associated anomalies.
2. Ectopia cordis with the exposed heart presenting outside the chest wall through a cleft sternum and anterior chest wall of varying degrees.
3. Pentalogy of Cantrell—an association of defects, including cleft distal sternum, absent anterior crescent of the diaphragm, midline anterior abdominal wall defect above the umbilicus (omphalocele), defect of the apical pericardium with communication into the peritoneum, and a cardiac anomaly, most commonly a ventricular septal defect or left ventricular diverticulum.

Careful physical examination, echocardiography, chest radiography, and, if necessary, cardiac catheterization may be used to define the anatomic and functional defects.

Operative Indications   Experience has shown that surgical repair of the cleft sternum is best achieved in the newborn period while elasticity of the chest wall is such as to allow approximation of the separated sternal bands. The presence of an omphalocele mandates immediate surgical intervention to place an appropriate prosthetic covering for prevention of infection and fluid losses. Use of such a prosthetic covering to protect the exposed heart in a true ectopia cordis has been reported as a temporizing measure to facilitate completion of the evaluation of the associated cardiac lesion. Staging of cardiac repair may be necessary in both the true ectopia and the pentalogy because of severe and unusual anatomic abnormalities.

Types of Procedures   For the isolated cleft-sternal defect, usually a direct approximation of the sternal halves after appropriate excision or wedging to prevent buckling is done. If the thoracic volume is inadequate after approximation, sliding chondrotomy of several ribs on either side will provide further volume.

Return of the ectopic and exposed heart to the thoracic cavity and sternal closure, although technically possible, has not resulted in improved survival, usually because of the severity of the associated cardiac lesions. If a life-sustaining corrective or palliative procedure for the cardiac defect is possible in the newborn period, chest-wall closure, using prosthetic material to increase thoracic volume, is usually required.

Both primary and staged repair of the various defects present in the pentalogy of Cantrell have been reported. Small defects are more amenable to primary closure if the cardiac anomaly is limited to either a septal defect or ventricular diverticulum. The latter can be amputated during the primary procedure. For extensive defects, such as large omphaloceles, staged closure with an initial Silastic silo may be necessary.

Surgical Results/Prognosis   The prognosis is contingent primarily on the presence and severity of an accompanying cardiac defect. For an isolated cleft sternum repair, the prognosis for survival is very good although recurrence of the cleft has been reported. For the true ectopia cordis and for pentalogy of Cantrell, reported survival after surgical closure is poor, perhaps no more than 5% to 10%, with the underlying cardiac defect being the primary determinant of survival.

REFERENCES

Cantrell JR, Haller JA, Ravitch HH, et al: A syndrome of congenital defects involving the abdominal wall, sternum, diaphragm, pericardium and heart. Surg Gynecol Obstet 1958;107:602.

Carmi R, Boughman JA: Pentalogy of Cantrell and associated midline anomalies: A possible ventral midline developmental midline field. Am J Med Genet 1992;42:90–95.

Jones AF, McGrath RL, Edwards SM, et al: Immediate operation for ectopia cordis. Ann Thorac Surg 1979;28:484–486.

Khoury MJ, Cordero JF, Rasmussen S: Ectopia cordis, midline defects and chromosome abnormalities: An epidemiologic perspective. Am J Med Genet 1988;30:811–817.

Ravitch MM: The chest wall. In Welch KJ, Randolph JG, Ravitch MM, et al (eds): Pediatric Surgery, 4th ed. Chicago, Mosby-Year Book, 1986.

Ravitch MM: Congenital Deformities of the Chest Wall and their Operative Correction. Philadelphia, WB Saunders, 1977.

Sabiston DC: Disorders of the sternum and the thoracic wall. In Sabiston DC, Spencer FC (eds): Gibbon's Surgery of the Chest. Philadelphia, WB Saunders, 1990, pp 422–437.

Tongsong T, Wanapirak C, Sirivatanapa P, Wongtrangan S: Prenatal sonographic diagnosis of ectopia cordia. J Clin Ultrasound 1999;27:440–445.

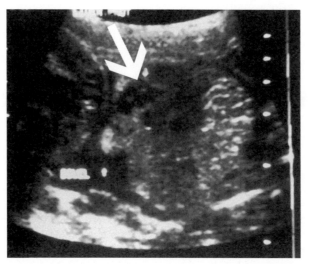

Cardiac chambers (*arrow*) are visualized here outside the thoracic cage. Bowel is also seen below the heart.

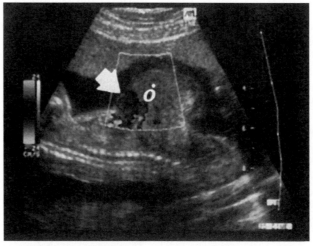

In addition to the omphalocele (O), the heart lies in the abdominal wall (*arrow*). Color flow Doppler shows flow in the heart.

4 The Genitourinary Tract

4.1 Adrenal Hematoma

Epidemiology/Genetics

Definition   An adrenal hematoma is the result of extravasation of blood from the vascular system into the tissue of the adrenal gland, resulting in an extravascular collection of blood. Large bleeds may result in fetal hypotension and death. Smaller bleeds may be asymptomatic and present as incidental calcification in the adrenal gland.

Epidemiology   Unknown, but rare.

Embryology   It has been suggested that ischemia, resulting from hypotension, vascular abnormalities, occlusion, emboli, or antenatal infection, is the most likely cause of adrenal hematomas.

Inheritance Patterns   Sporadic.

Teratogens   Antenatal infections.

Prognosis   Prognosis is dependent on the size of the bleed and ranges from lethal, for large bleeds, to asymptomatic, for smaller bleeds.

Sonography

FINDINGS

1. **Fetus:** A mass is present, superior to the kidney, involving all or part of the adrenal gland. The mass may be echogenic or cystic, with rapid changes in sonographic appearance on sequential studies. The process may be one-sided or bilateral. Color flow Doppler sonography will show no flow in the mass.
2. **Amniotic Fluid:** Normal.
3. **Placenta:** Normal.
4. **Measurement Data:** Usually large babies.
5. **When Detectable:** Although usually a third trimester finding, an adrenal hemorrhage has been detected at 21 weeks.

Pitfalls   The hematoma may be technically difficult to find because of fetal position.

Differential Diagnosis

1. Neuroblastoma may occur in the same location prior to delivery. Neuroblastoma does not change rapidly in appearance, unless there is associated hemorrhage. Color flow Doppler sonography may show flow within a neuroblastoma, unlike an adrenal hemorrhage.
2. A hydronephrotic second collecting system may be confused with an adrenal hematoma but will not change internal acoustic appearance with time.
3. Liver mass—Rare and should be visibly located in the liver.

Where Else to Look   Renal vein thrombosis is associated. Look for renal enlargement with prominent sinus echoes. The veins may become calcified.

Pregnancy Management

Investigations and Consultations Required   In the absence of other abnormalities on sonographic evaluation, no further diagnostic evaluation is necessary. A neonatology consultation should be obtained to plan perinatal management.

Monitoring   A sonogram should be performed every 2 weeks, since neuroblastoma is hard to exclude before birth.

Pregnancy Course   There are no obstetric complications associated with this fetal lesion.

Pregnancy Termination Issues   A diagnosis of fetal adrenal hematoma should not influence decisions about pregnancy termination.

Delivery   The rare occurrence of unexplained shock with large hemorrhages requires that delivery occur in a location where personnel and facilities are available to manage this complication.

Neonatology

Resuscitation If the diagnosis is made prior to onset of labor and the lesion is small, no resuscitation should be required on the basis of the hematoma. Acute adrenal hemorrhage occurs as a complication of a traumatic delivery or severe perinatal asphyxia. Rapid volume expansion, to support perfusion, may be needed in that situation.

Transport Referral to a tertiary care center on the basis of a prenatal diagnosis is probably not indicated, unless the hemorrhage was massive and there is concern for adrenal insufficiency.

Testing and Confirmation Postnatal radiographic studies may detect an acute hematoma or adrenal calcification from an earlier bleed.

Nursery Management No specific intervention is required for a prenatally diagnosed lesion. If the hematoma

was massive and/or bilateral, the infant should be monitored closely for evidence of adrenal insufficiency, that is, salt-wasting, hypoglycemia, hypotension, or failure to thrive.

REFERENCES

Chen CP, Chen SH, Chuang CY, et al: Clinical and perinatal sonographic features of congenital adrenal cystic neuroblastoma: A case report with review of the literature. Ultrasound Obstet Gynecol 1997;10:68–73.

Eklof O, Grotte G, Jorulf H, et al: Perinatal haemorrhagic necrosis of the adrenal gland. Pediatr Radiol 1975;24:31–36.

Fang SB, Lee HC, Sheu JC, et al: Prenatal sonographic detection of adrenal hemorrhage confirmed by postnatal surgery. J Clin Ultrasound 1999;27:206–209.

Hata K, Hata T, Kitao M: Ultrasonographic identification and measurement of the human fetal adrenal gland in utero: Clinical application. Gynecol Obstet Invest 1988;25:16–22.

Morganti VJ, Anderson NG: Simple adrenal cysts in fetus, resolving spontaneously in neonate. J Ultrasound Med 1991;10:521–524.

Romero R, Pilu G, Hobbins JC: Normal anatomy of the adrenal gland. In: Prenatal diagnosis of congenital anomalies. Norwalk, CT, Appleton and Lange, 1989, pp 295–296.

Schwarzler P, Bernard JP, Senat MV, Ville Y: Prenatal diagnosis of fetal adrenal masses: Differentiation between hemorrhage and solid tumor by color Doppler sonography. Ultrasound Obstet Gynecol 1999;13:351–355.

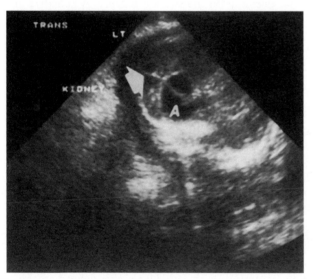

Transverse view of an adrenal hematoma (A). In this instance, the hematoma is cystic apart from a septum. Some adrenal hematomas can appear echogenic, and they change appearance rapidly, almost on a daily basis. The kidney (*arrow*) can be seen alongside the hematoma.

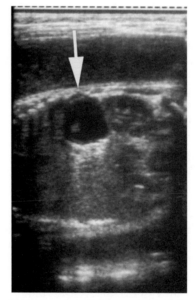

Cystic adrenal hematoma (*arrow*) lying superior to the right kidney.

4.2 Exstrophy of the Bladder

Epidemiology Genetics

Definition Bladder exstrophy is a failure of closure of the bladder, lower urinary tract, overlying symphysis pubis, rectus muscles, and skin.

Epidemiology Occurs in 1 in 30,000 births (M3:Fl).

Embryology Bladder exstrophy is thought to be caused by a defect in the development of the cloacal membrane, preventing medial migration of mesenchyme. Only rarely are there associated malformations outside of the genitourinary tract.

Inheritance Patterns Most cases are sporadic. There are rare familial case reports of affected siblings.

Teratogens None known.

Screening Maternal serum alpha-fetoprotein is elevated in most cases of bladder exstrophy.

Prognosis Surgical correction is difficult, but, in experienced hands, approximately 60% to 81% of patients will eventually have continence. Female sex assignment of 46,XY males is now discouraged, as these children identify themselves as males regardless of genital appearance. In unrepaired cases from the older literature, there was an 8% risk of malignancy, probably related to mucosal exposure and chronic infection.

Sonography

FINDINGS

1. **Fetus:**
   a. The bladder is absent. A sagittal anterior view will show a mound on the anterior aspect of the abdomen.
   b. Male genitalia will lie anterior and superior to the usual location. The umbilical cord insertion site is at a low level.
   c. Abnormal widening of the iliac crests may be detected with the iliac crests swung laterally.
2. **Amniotic Fluid:** Normal.
3. **Placenta:** Normal.
4. **Measurement Data:** Appropriate.
5. **When Detectable:** At about 16 weeks.

Pitfalls

1. A sagittal anterior view is the only view that will show the diagnostic mass on the anterior abdomen.

2. The fetal bladder occasionally empties completely when the fetus voids. Apparent absence of the bladder may be a transient normal finding. In patients with severe oligohydramnios, of renal origin, the bladder may be very small.

Differential Diagnosis

1. Sacrococcygeal teratoma—The mass will displace the bladder anteriorly and superiorly and will be in the posterior aspect of the pelvis.
2. Omphalocele—The cord exits through the center of an omphalocele and lies at a higher level.

Where Else to Look Occasionally, there is secondary hydroureter and hydronephrosis.

Pregnancy Management

Investigations and Consultations Required Associated abnormalities are rare in bladder exstrophy. In patients planning to continue the pregnancy, fetal echocardiography may be appropriate to exclude cardiac defects before deciding on the site for delivery. A pediatric urologist should be consulted to discuss management with the family. Although chromosome abnormalities are not associated with bladder exstrophy, confirmation of fetal sex may be useful in defining prognosis for surgical repair.

Monitoring No alteration in standard obstetric care is indicated.

Pregnancy Course No obstetric complications are associated with this disorder.

Pregnancy Termination Issues An intact fetus should be delivered to allow confirmation of the sonographic diagnosis.

Delivery There is no evidence that cesarean delivery improves prognosis. Delivery at a tertiary center is not required. It is more important that the infant be transferred to an institution with individuals experienced in the repair of this rare condition.

Neonatology

Resuscitation Respiratory difficulty is not expected with this lesion.

Transport Referral to a tertiary center with a pediatric urologist experienced in the repair of exstrophy is always indicated for early surgical intervention.

Testing and Confirmation The bladder and lower urinary tract are open anteriorly from the urethral meatus to the umbilicus. There is wide separation of the pubic symphysis and rectus muscles. In males, the scrotum is broad with frequent undescended testes and a short broad penis without canalization. In females, the clitoris and labia are widely separated with occasional vaginal stenosis. Upper tract anomalies are rare with this lesion, in contrast with hypospadius lesions. A screening abdominal sonogram is adequate to confirm upper tract anatomy.

Nursery Management The exposed viscera should be covered with plastic film (Saran wrap) to limit heat and water loss and contamination. Administration of antibiotics should be considered to reduce the risk of infection.

Surgery

Preoperative Assessment Imaging of the upper urinary tracts to make sure there are normal kidneys by ultrasonography or nuclear medicine is helpful.

Operative Indications Surgery is indicated if the bladder is opened to the surface of the abdomen. Surgery is not feasible if the bladder plate is too small to close.

Types of Procedures The bladder and posterior urethra are reapproximated to form a new bladder. A transverse innominate and ventral iliac osteotomy from an anterior approach is required so that the pubic symphysis can be reapproximated. An epispadias repair with the creation of a satisfactory penis is also needed.

Surgical Results/Prognosis The prognosis is dependent on any associated renal anomalies, but there is a survival rate of more than 90%. Secondary surgical procedures are frequently required at approximately 4 to 5 years of age to achieve urinary continence and functioning genitalia. An epispadias repair may be performed as early as 6 months to 1 year of age.

Possible surgical complications include wound dehiscence and infection.

REFERENCES

Barth RA, Filly RA, Sondheimer FK: Prenatal sonographic findings in bladder exstrophy. J Ultrasound Med 1990;9:359–361.

Ben-Chaim J, Docimo SG, Jeffs RD, Gearhart JP: Bladder exstrophy from childhood into adult life. J R Soc Med 1996;89:39P–46P.

Cacciari A, Pilu GL, Mordenti M, et al: Prenatal diagnosis of bladder exstrophy: What counseling? J Urol 1999;161:259–261.

Canning DA, Gearhart JP: Exstrophy of the bladder. In Ashcraft KM, Holder TM (eds): Pediatric Surgery. Philadelphia, WB Saunders, 1993, pp 678–693.

de la Hunt MN, O'Donnell B: Current management of bladder exstrophy: A BAPS collective review from eight centers of 81 patients born between 1975 and 1985. J Pediatr Surg 1989;24:584–585.

Gearhart JP: Bladder exstrophy: Staged reconstruction. Curr Opin Urol 1999;9:499–506.

Gearhart JP, Ben-Chaim J, Jeffs RD, Sanders RC: Criteria for the prenatal diagnosis of classic bladder exstrophy. Obstet Gynecol 1995;85:961–964.

Jaffee R, Schoenfeld A, Ovadia J: Sonographic findings in the prenatal diagnosis of bladder exstrophy. Am J Obstet Gynecol 1990;162:675–678.

Jeffs RD: Exstrophy, epispadias, and cloacal and urogenital sinus abnormalities. Pediatr Clin North Am 1987;34:1233–1257.

Mirk P, Calisti A, Fileni A: Prenatal sonographic diagnosis of bladder extrophy. J Ultrasound Med 1986;5:291–293.

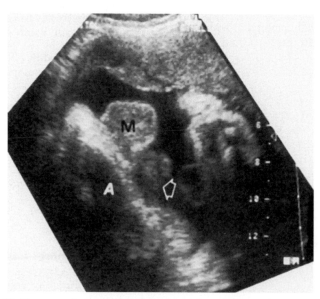

Bladder exstrophy, sagittal midline view. A large bulge can be seen related to the exstrophy (M). The cord insertion (*arrow*) is directly superior to the mass. A, abdomen.

4.3 Cloacal Exstrophy

Epidemiology/Genetics

Definition Cloacal exstrophy is an extensive lower abdominal wall defect that combines exstrophy of the bladder with intervening intestinal epithelium, imperforate anus, and wide separation of the anterior pubic arch.

Epidemiology One in 50,000 to 200,000 (M2:F1).

Embryology Exstrophies are thought to be caused by a defect in the development of the caudal embryonic fold and cloacal membrane, preventing medial migration of mesenchyme that occurs before 2 months' gestation. The bladder and lower urinary tract are open anteriorly from the urethral meatus to the umbilicus. There is wide separation of the pubic symphysis and rectus muscles. In males, the scrotum is broad with undescended testes, and there is a short, broad penis without canalization. In females, the clitoris and labia are widely separated with occasional vaginal stenosis. Only rarely are there associated malformations outside of the genitourinary system. Exstrophy of the cloaca is more severe and complex, and the bladder is widely separated with intervening intestinal mucosa. In females, the uterus is frequently bicornuate and the vagina is duplex, ending blindly near the bladder mucosa. Ninety percent of cloacal exstrophy patients have an omphalocele, and 40% have neural tube defects.

Inheritance Patterns Generally sporadic with presumed low recurrence risk. Only rare affected siblings have been described.

Teratogens None.

Additional Investigations Maternal serum alpha-fetoprotein is elevated in most cases. Karyotyping should be considered to aid in postnatal sex assignment.

Prognosis Surgical correction is difficult. Neonatal mortality in cloacal exstrophy is 50% to 100%. Survival beyond the immediate neonatal period is excellent. Urinary and fecal continence are only rarely established. Female sex assignment of 46XY males is now discouraged, as these children often identify themselves as males regardless of genital appearance. Intelligence in survivors is normal.

Sonography

FINDINGS

1. **Fetus:**
   a. Absent bladder with large midline infraumbilical anterior wall defect or wall mass. The mass may be cystic or solid. Bilateral bladder components may be present.
   b. An omphalocele is present. Much fetal bowel floating within ascites is usually seen.
   c. Lumbosacral anomalies, including myelomeningocele with secondary hydrocephalus and vertebral anomalies, are present in about 30% of patients.
   d. Renal anomalies such as renal agenesis, hydronephrosis, dysplasia, horseshoe kidney, and crossed renal ectopia are seen in about 50% of cases.
   e. Clubfeet and congenital dislocated hips are present in about 30% of cases.
   f. There is a narrow thorax.
2. **Amniotic Fluid:** Polyhydramnios is common. Oligohydramnios may be present if the kidneys are abnormal.
3. **Placenta:** Normal. A two-vessel cord is often seen.
4. **Measurement Data:** Intrauterine growth retardation is common.
5. **When Detectable:** At about 13 weeks, using the endovaginal probe.

Pitfalls Oligohydramnios may make the sonographic findings difficult to detect and analyze.

Differential Diagnosis

1. Body stalk anomaly and limb-body wall complex may have a similar combination of abdominal wall mass and spinal anomaly, but limbs will be missing in addition.
2. Bladder exstrophy has a similar infraumbilical mass but is not associated with spinal problems.

Where Else to Look Renal and gut anomalies such as duodenal and tracheoesophageal atresia may be associated.

Pregnancy Management

Investigations and Consultations Required Early presentation may be difficult to distinguish from urethral atresia. Chromosomal studies should be performed by amniocentesis (bladder tap) or chorionic villus sampling. Fetal echocardiography should be performed to exclude cardiac malformation. Consultation with a pediatric urologist should be obtained.

Fetal Intervention Cases with bladder obstruction and normal female karyotype may be candidates for catheter drainage if urine electrolytes indicate a good prognosis. However, it is essential to exclude other associated abnormalities, which are common, and to counsel the family extensively regarding the additional surgery required in these children.

Monitoring Serial ultrasonographic studies should be done to monitor the urinary tract, as enlargement of the vagina late in pregnancy has been associated with bladder outlet obstruction and late-onset oligohydramnios.

Pregnancy Course   No specific obstetric complications should be anticipated unless urinary tract obstruction results in oligohydramnios. There have been reports of associated intrauterine growth retardation, which should be detected by the serial sonograms.

Pregnancy Termination Issues   An intact fetus may be necessary to confirm the diagnosis and to exclude genetic syndromes that may have cloacal abnormalities as a component of the disorder.

Delivery   The timing of delivery will depend on the results of amniotic fluid assessment and fetal surveillance. Cesarean section may be necessary to prevent abdominal dystocia. Alternatively, decompression of the mass prior to labor induction may allow vaginal delivery.

Neonatology

Resuscitation   Both persistence of the cloaca and cloacal exstrophy have been diagnosed prenatally. Significant impairment of lung growth and thus impairment of respiratory adaptation at birth occurs only in the setting of urinary obstruction and oligohydramnios. The exact frequency of this condition is undetermined, having been reported only in sporadic case reports, principally with persistent cloaca. Thus, significant problems with the onset of respiration should not be anticipated except in the setting of oligohydramnios. Protection of exposed bowel and bladder mucosa, as well as the accompanying omphalocele present in 90% of cases with cloacal exstrophy, from surface contamination and trauma and limitation of evaporative heat and water loss can be achieved by encasing the lower body in a sterile plastic bag (bowel bag).

Transport   Transfer by an experienced neonatal transport team to a tertiary center with pediatric surgical subspecialists and diagnostic capabilities is indicated on an emergency basis.

Testing and Confirmation   The assessment and determination of the exact spectrum and aberrant anatomy in these conditions requires a coordinated multidisciplinary approach, often with the full range of imaging and endoscopic techniques used. In cloacal exstrophy, there is a high association with cardiac, skeletal, and neurologic anomalies necessitating diagnostic imaging of these organ systems as well. Chromosomal analysis for genetic gender identification is essential if such has not been done prenatally.

Nursery Management   Initial management is directed toward providing adequate fluid, electrolyte, and nutritional support and adequate decompression of both the urinary and the intestinal systems, as indicated, while progressing with the diagnostic evaluation in an expeditious manner. The choice and staging of surgical procedures for palliation and/or correction will vary with the results of the diagnostic evaluation.

Provision of social and emotional support and counseling for the parents is important in facilitating their adaptation to the long-term demands for the care of their child. Multiple surgeries ultimately will be required for complete management of all the abnormalities.

Surgery

Preoperative Assessment   The major areas that require preoperative evaluation are the upper urinary tract, the central nervous system, musculoskeletal deformities, and gender status. Ultrasonography is used to evaluate the spinal cord and genitourinary tract. Magnetic resonance imaging may be useful in assessing abdominal malformations.

Operative Indications   All children with this anomaly require bladder reconstruction and omphalocele repair. If a myelomeningocele is present, repair will be needed.

Types of Procedures   If the child is in excellent condition, a one-stage repair may be performed. The first operative stage consists of closure of the omphalocele, separation of the intestinal plate from the hemibladder with construction of a gastrointestinal stoma, and reapproximation of the separated bladder halves. Additional procedures may also be indicated related to the neurosurgical or orthopedic disorders. A second stage procedure is usually performed when the infant weighs about 20 to 25 pounds. The bladder and/or urethra and external genitalia are reconstructed.

Surgical Results/Prognosis   An excellent survival rate is expected, provided that lethal renal anomalies are not present.

REFERENCES

Austin PF, Homsy YL, Gearhart JP, et al: The prenatal diagnosis of cloacal exstrophy. J Urol 1998;160:1179–1181.

Cacciari A, Pilu GL, Mordenti M, et al: Prenatal diagnosis of bladder exstrophy: What counseling? J Urol 1999;161:259–261.

Geifman-Holtzman O, Crane SS, Winderl L, Holmes M: Persistent urogenital sinus: Prenatal diagnosis and pregnancy complications. Am J Obstet Gynecol 1997;176:709–711.

Lee DH, Cottrell JR, Sanders RC, et al: OEIS complex (omphalocele-exstrophy-imperforate anus-spinal defects) in monozygotic twins. Am J Med Genet 1999;84:29–33.

Meizner I, Levy A, Barnard Y: Cloacal exstrophy sequence: An exceptional ultrasound diagnosis. Obstet Gynecol 1995;86:446–450.

Petrikovsky BM, Walzal MP Jr, D'Addario PF: Fetal cloacal anomalies: Prenatal sonographic findings and differential diagnosis. Obstet Gynecol 1988;72:464.

Shalev E, Feldman E, Weiner E, Zuckerman H: Prenatal sonographic appearance of persistent cloaca. Acta Obstet Gynecol Scand 1986;65:517.

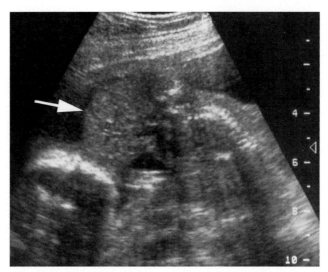

Cloacal exstrophy demonstrated on an 18-week sonogram. There was severe scoliosis, spinal dysraphism, and an omphalocele (*arrow*).

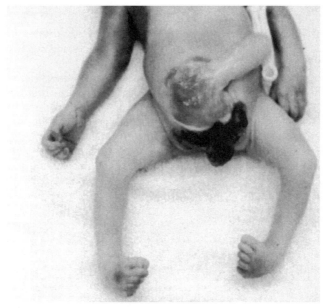

A 24-week stillborn female infant with OEIS (omphalocele–exstrophy of the bladder–imperforate anus–spinal defects) complex that combines omphalocele, cloacal exstrophy, and spinal dysraphism.

4.4 Hydronephrosis (Ureteropelvic Junction Obstruction and Reflux)

Epidemiology/Genetics

Definition Distention of the pelvis and calyces of the kidney with urine, as a result of ureteral obstruction.

Epidemiology One to 5 per 1000 births (ureteropelvic junction obstruction, M4:F1; ureterovesicular junction obstruction, M>F).

Embryology Hydronephrosis accounts for 75% of prenatally diagnosed fetal renal abnormalities. Many cases of unilateral and even bilateral hydronephrosis resolve spontaneously after birth. Ureteropelvic junction obstruction is the most common cause of hydronephrosis and is unilateral in 70% of cases. Vesicoureteric reflux is a common cause of renal pelvocalyceal dilation, particularly in males. Rare cases of hydronephrosis are due to ureteral stenosis or other lower urinary tract obstructions. Thirty percent of cases have associated urinary tract abnormalities and 20% of cases are part of a multiple malformation syndrome. More than 70 genetic, chromosomal, and sporadic multiple malformation syndromes have been described with hydronephrosis.

Inheritance Patterns Sporadic, unless part of a recognizable syndrome such as the urofacial syndrome (autosomal recessive), which combines a distinctive grimacing face with bilateral hydronephrosis.

Teratogens Thalidomide, maternal diabetes, cocaine, and benzodiazepine.

Prognosis The majority of antenatally diagnosed cases of prenatal hydronephrosis resolve spontaneously in the neonatal period, with only 3% to 4% requiring surgical treatment. Many patients with hydronephrosis will have good renal function because the ureters can absorb increased pressure by dilating. Oligohydramnios, however, suggests a poor prognosis. Untreated reflux, especially of infected urine, is thought to cause permanent renal damage that may lead to renal failure. Most cases can be treated either medically or surgically with excellent results.

Sonography

FINDINGS

1. **Fetus:** There is dilation of the pelvis and sometimes the calyces, which is graded by severity: grade 1, renal pelvis only; grade 2, renal pelvis and a few calyces; grade 3, renal pelvis and all calyces; and grade 4, renal pelvis, calyceal dilation, and parenchymal thinning.

   a. Ureteropelvic junction obstruction—One or both renal pelves and adjacent calyces are distended. The distension is asymmetrical if the condition is bilateral. No ureteric or bladder distension is seen if there is ureteropelvic junction obstruction. Dysplastic changes in the kidneys are very rare. Perinephric urinoma may develop; a fluid-filled sac will be seen, generally posterior to the obstructed kidney, which will be decompressed and not dilated. The decompressed kidney is usually dysplastic.
   b. Ureterovesical junction obstruction—In this rare entity, the kidney and ureter are dilated down to a normal bladder. The condition can be bilateral.
   c. Reflux—There is a dilated renal pelvis and ureter that may be unilateral or bilateral; both pelvis and ureter usually vary in size over the course of the examination. The dilated pelvis can usually be traced into the ureter. Peristalsis is often visible within the ureter. The bladder may be enlarged and empty ineffectively, since much of the urine returns up the ureter. The variant of reflux in which the bladder and ureters are persistently dilated, due to reflux, is termed the megacystis megaureter syndrome. Reflux is much more common in males in utero, although females are much more likely to suffer long-term complications.
   d. For ureterocele, see Chapter 4.15.
   e. For posterior urethral valves, see Chapter 4.11.
2. **Amniotic Fluid:** Oligohydramnios is unusual. Polyhydramnios occurs if the left renal pelvis is much enlarged due to ureteropelvic junction obstruction and compresses the stomach or small bowel.
3. **Placenta:** Normal.
4. **Measurement Data:** With severe unilateral or bilateral ureteropelvic junction obstructions, the abdomen may be enlarged to a size that raises concerns about delivery.
5. **When Detectable:** Renal obstruction may develop at any stage of pregnancy but is usually seen by 20 weeks. Lesser degrees of pelvic dilation carry more significance if they are seen before 18 weeks. Reflux is usually detectable by 22 weeks. It may become apparent that the cause of renal pelvic dilation is reflux only when marked variations in renal pelvic size are seen on follow-up examinations.

Pitfalls

1. An extrarenal pelvis, with measurements under 1.5 cm, may simulate a mild ureteropelvic junction obstruction. An extrarenal pelvis may be anteriorly located and simulate an intraperitoneal mass.
2. Renal pelvic measurements of greater than 4 mm up to 32 weeks' gestation may be a normal variant but require follow-up. Renal pelvis dilation of 7 mm or more

seen after 32 weeks likewise may be a normal variant but requires postnatal follow-up to exclude a renal pathologic condition. Other authors have suggested cut-offs of 5 mm at 15 to 20 weeks, 8 mm at 20 to 30 weeks, and 10 mm after 30 weeks.

3. Reflux may simulate other types of renal obstruction. There will be an inconsistent renal pelvic diameter. Reflux is easily confused with normal-variant renal pelvic dilation and ureteropelvic junction obstruction. Variability in pelvic and ureteric size is the diagnostic key.

4. Large renal veins can be mistaken for mild renal pelvic dilation. Color flow Doppler sonography will show the distinction.

5. Maternal overhydration may cause fetal renal pelves to be dilated. Re-examination when the patient is less hydrated may be worthwhile.

Where Else to Look Look for stigmata of trisomy 13, 18, and 21. A renal pelvis dilated to greater than 3 mm increases the risk of Down syndrome. Look at the other kidney for reflux. Reflux has no known associations.

Pregnancy Management

Investigations and Consultations Required Chromosomal evaluation is not indicated unless other sonographic markers of aneuploidy are seen. In cases of severe obstruction or renal pelvis dilation of 7 mm or greater seen after 32 weeks' gestation, consultation with a pediatric urologist is necessary to develop a prenatal and postnatal management plan.

Fetal Intervention Because of the significant risk of in utero catheter placement, fetal intervention for unilateral disease is not usually indicated. In the rare case in which obstruction is severe enough to cause bowel obstruction and polyhydramnios, intervention may be indicated. In cases with bilateral disease and normal amniotic fluid, intervention is not indicated. In cases with bilateral disease and decreasing amniotic fluid, early delivery should be performed if the gestational age is 32 weeks or greater. Prior to 32 weeks, assessment of renal function is by aspiration of urine from the renal pelvis (see Chapter 4.11). Intervention by catheter placement can be considered if renal function is normal and amniotic fluid is decreasing. However, the need for in utero intervention in ureteropelvic junction obstruction has been rare.

Monitoring Mild degrees of renal pelvis dilation should be assessed by a follow-up sonogram at 32 to 34 weeks' gestation. More significant dilation should be followed with sonographic evaluation every 3 to 4 weeks.

Pregnancy Course No specific obstetric complications should be expected for unilateral disease, although there have been rare reports of polyhydramnios resulting from bowel obstruction by a left-sided lesion.

Pregnancy Termination Issues The method of termination should provide an intact fetus for pathologic confirmation of the sonographic diagnosis. Isolated reflux would not be an indication for pregnancy termination.

Delivery When there is severe obstruction, the need for neonatal evaluation and treatment requires that delivery occur in a tertiary center with a pediatric urologist available. Even severe obstruction should not result in dystocia, and no change in standard obstetric care is necessary.

Neonatology

Resuscitation Usually not an issue. Onset of effective respiration may be impeded by abdominal distension secondary to renal enlargement. Intubation and ventilation may be required at least initially.

Transport Indicated with bilateral lesions for full confirmation of diagnosis and establishment of care plan, including surgical intervention. Infants with isolated unilateral lesions and normal renal function, as indicated by serum creatinine, can be referred for outpatient evaluation and management.

Testing and Confirmation Careful physical examination and abdominal ultrasonography will confirm the diagnosis. Diuretic renal nuclear scan is the best technique to assess renal function and drainage.

Nursery Management Support respiration as necessary to maintain adequate gas exchange.

Avoid fluid and protein loading initially until urinary tract patency and renal function have been determined.

Subsequent procedures will be contingent on the specific lesion suspected or discovered.

Surgery

Preoperative Assessment If the obstruction is considered, based on prenatal sonograms, to be of a severity that may warrant surgery, careful, staged evaluation of renal function and structure by urine production, urinalysis, blood and urine chemistries, and an abdominal sonogram is appropriate. If the infant is minimally symptomatic and immediate relief of obstruction is not necessary, imaging can be delayed for several days for better visualization. If the anatomy is not clearly defined prenatally, or immediate relief of obstruction is required, ultrasonographic imaging should be performed immediately. Subsequent procedures will be needed to further delineate the site of obstruction, status of reflux, and renal function, that is, cystogram, renal scan with diuretic stimulation, after 2 weeks of age when glomerular filtration rate has increased.

Operative Indications The surgical goal is to perform any needed decompression and/or pyeloplasty procedure prior to hypertrophy of the contralateral kidney. Poor renal function can frequently be improved by a decompression pyelostomy or ureterostomy. After 2 to 3 months of decompression, the renal scintigraphic study is repeated. If the kidney demonstrates at least 10% of total renal function, a pyeloplasty is indicated.

Types of Procedures Decompression versus primary repair is dependent on the amount of ipsilateral renal function. Early neonatal pyeloplasty is very successful, with a low recurrence rate.

Surgical Results/Prognosis Ultimate prognosis is dependent on the amount of remaining renal function and the degree of associated lung hypoplasia. It is excellent for unilateral or mild bilateral hydronephrosis. Repeat pyeloplasties are uncommon even when the initial procedure is done in early infancy (1.5%). Prognosis for infants treated with intrauterine decompression techniques has been poor.

REFERENCES

Anderson PA, Rickwood AM: Features of primary vesicoureteric reflux detected by prenatal sonography. Br J Urol 1991;67:267–271.

Arger PH, Coleman BG, Mintz MC, et al: Routine fetal genitourinary tract screening. Radiology 1985;156:485–489.

Babcook CJ, Silvera M, Drake C, Levine D: Effect of maternal hydration on mild fetal pyelectasis. J Ultrasound Med 1998;17:539–544.

Betz BW, Hertzberg BS, Carroll BA, Bowie JD: Mild fetal renal pelviectasis: Differentiation from hilar vascularity using color Doppler sonography. J Ultrasound Med 1991;10:243–245.

Brock WA, Kaplan G: Abnormalities of the lower tract. In Edelmann CM Jr (ed): Pediatric Kidney Disease. Boston, Little, Brown, 1992, p 2037.

Caione P, Zaccara A, Capozza N, De Gennaro M: How prenatal ultrasound can affect the treatment of ureterocele in neonates and children. Eur Urol 1989;16:195–199.

Chapman CJ, Bailey RR, Janus ED, et al: Vesicoureteric reflux: Segregation analysis. Am J Med Genet 1985;20:577–584.

Chevalier RL: Renal physiology and function In Kelalis PP, King LR, Belman AB (eds): Clinical Pediatric Urology. Philadelphia, WB Saunders, 1992, pp 1106–1120.

Dunn V, Glasier CM: Ultrasonographic antenatal demonstration of primary megaureters. J Ultrasound Med 1985;4:101–103.

Fernbach SK, Maizels M, Conway JJ: Ultrasound grading of hydronephrosis: Introduction to the system used by the Society for Fetal Urology. Pediatr Radiol 1993;23:478–480.

Flushner SC, King LR: Ureteropelvic obstruction. In Kelais PP, King LR, Belman AB (eds): Clinical Pediatric Urology. Philadelphia, WB Saunders, 1992, pp 693–725.

Grignon A, Filiatrault D, Homsy Y, et al: Ureteropelvic junction stenosis: Antenatal ultrasonographic diagnosis, postnatal investigation, and follow-up. Radiology 1986;160:649–651.

Grignon A, Filion R, Filiatrault D, et al: Urinary tract dilatation in utero: Classification and clinical applications. Radiology 1986;160:645–647.

Guys JM, Borella F, Monfort G: Ureteropelvic junction obstructions: Prenatal diagnosis and neonatal surgery in 47 cases. J Pediatr Surg 1988;23:156–158.

Herndon CD, McKenna PH, Kolon TF, et al: A multicenter outcomes analysis of patients with neonatal reflux presenting with prenatal hydronephrosis. J Urol 1999;162:1203–1208.

Hoddick WK, Filly RA, Mahony BS, Callen PW: Minimal fetal renal pyelectasis. J Ultrasound Med 1985;4:85–89.

Kass EJ, Bloom D: Anomalies of the upper urinary tract. In Edelmann CM Jr (ed): Pediatric Kidney Disease. Boston, Little, Brown, 1992, p 2023.

Kent A, Cox D, Downey P, James SL: A study of mild fetal pyelectosis: Outcome and proposed strategy of management. Prenat Diagn 2000;20:206–209.

King LR, Hatcher PA: Natural history of fetal and neonatal hydronephrosis. Pediatr Urol 1990;35:433–438.

Kitagawa H, Pringle KC, Stone P, et al: Postnatal follow-up of hydronephrosis detected by prenatal ultrasound: The natural history. Fetal Diagn Ther 1998;13:19–25.

Kleiner B, Callen PW, Filly RA: Sonographic analysis of the fetus with ureteropelvic junction obstruction. Am J Roentgenol 1987;148:359–363.

Koff SA, Campbell K: Non-operative management of unilateral neonatal hydronephrosis. J Urol 1992;148:525–531.

Lyon RP, Marshall SK, Scott MP: Treatment of vesicoureteral reflux: Point system based on twenty years of experience. Urology 1980;16:38–46.

Mandell J, Blyth BR, Peters CA, et al: Structural genitourinary defects detected in utero. Radiology 1991;178:193–196.

Mandell MD, Peters CA, Retik AB: Current concepts in the perinatal diagnosis and management of hydronephrosis. Urol Clin North Am 1990;17:247–261.

Mann CM Jr, Ellis DG: Ureteropelvic junction obstruction. In Ashcraft KW, Holder TM (eds): Pediatric Surgery. Philadelphia, WB Saunders, 1993, pp 582–587.

Misra D, Kempley ST, Hird MF: Are patients with antenatally diagnosed hydronephrosis being over-investigated and overtreated? Eur J Pediatr Surg 1999;9:303–306.

Oliveira EA, Diniz JS, Cabral AC, et al: Prognostic factors in fetal hydronephrosis: A multivariate analysis. Pediatr Nephrol 1999;13:859–864.

Patten RM, Mack LA, Wang KY, Cyr DR: The fetal genitourinary tract. Radiol Clin North Am 1990;28:115–130.

Persutte W, Lenke RR: Ultrasonographic standards for measuring renal collecting system dilation. Am J Obstet Gynecol 1992;167:858–860.

Wilson RD, Lynch S, Lessoway VA: Fetal pyelectosis: Comparison of post-natal renal pathology with unilateral and bilateral pyelectosis. Prenat Diagn 1997;17:451–455.

Severe renal pelvic dilation due to ureteropelvic junction obstruction (between +'s). The dilation is so severe that all calyces have been effaced. There was polyhydramnios. H, hydronephrotic pelvis; K, contralateral kidney; S, stomach.

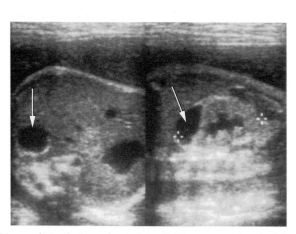

Urinoma due to hydronephrosis (*arrows*). Transverse and sagittal views. The adjacent kidney, which is more echogenic than usual suggesting early dysplasia, is mildly hydronephrotic.

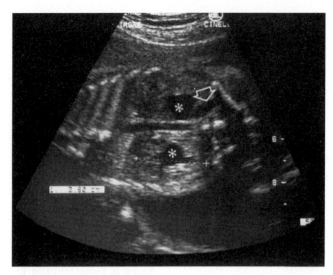

Renal pelvic dilation (∗) due to reflux. Calyces arising from the renal pelvis are dilated, consistent with grade 3, and both ureters can be seen (*arrow*). The ureters varied in size during the real-time study.

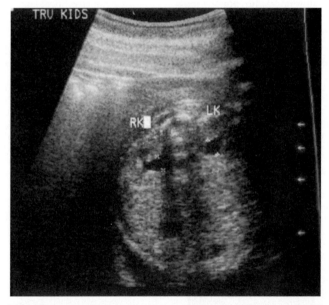

Mild bilateral renal pelvic dilatation to 6 mm (x's). This form of mild renal pelvic dilation has an excellent prognosis and is usually without long-term consequences. There is a low-grade association with Down syndrome.

4.5 Hydrocolpos

Epidemiology/Genetics

Definition   The accumulation of watery fluid in the uterus as a result of an imperforate hymen, vaginal atresia, or transverse vaginal septum resulting in a dilated uterus. This frequently presents as a pelvic cystic mass.

Epidemiology   Undetermined, but rare (M0:F1).

Embryology   Most cases probably result from a failure of the urogenital sinus derivatives that form the lower one third of the vagina to fuse and canalize properly with the müllerian duct derivatives that form the upper vagina, uterus, and fallopian tubes.

Inheritance Patterns   Generally sporadic. Rare recessive inheritance as well as rare genetic syndromes, such as the McKusick-Kaufman (polydactyly, congenital heart disease, and hydrometrocolpos) and short rib-polydactyly syndromes have been described.

Teratogens   None described.

Prognosis   Dependent on associated abnormalities and syndrome diagnosis. Uterine dilation may result in secondary hydronephrosis with renal damage and bowel obstruction. Normal function is generally possible with surgical treatment.

Sonography

FINDINGS

1. **Fetus:** A fluid-filled or echopenic mass is present, posterior to the bladder and anterior to the rectum. A small degree of vaginal fluid retention is a common normal variant in the third trimester. A large degree of vaginal dilation is rare. Echogenic material within the vagina may form a fluid level. In severe cases, fluid will leak through the fallopian tubes and cause "cysts." With cloacal exstrophy, the bladder and vagina drain into a common blocked organ, the cloaca. Dilation of the bladder, occasionally the ureters, and often the kidneys will also occur.
2. **Amniotic Fluid:** Decreased, if the urethra is obstructed.
3. **Placenta:** Normal.
4. **Measurement Data:** Usually appropriate.
5. **When Detectable:** Third trimester.

Pitfalls

1. Do not mistake a hydrocolpos for an intra-abdominal process such as ovarian cyst.

2. Rectal fluid is relatively common and may be mistaken for vaginal fluid.

Differential Diagnosis

1. Renal obstruction with dilated ureter.
2. Ovarian cyst.

Where Else to Look

1. Look at the genitourinary system for renal obstruction.
2. Imperforate anus is associated and there is occasionally dilated rectum and sigmoid colon visible.
3. Look at the stomach size, since there is an association with tracheoesophageal fistula.
4. Look for the features of McKusick-Kaufman syndrome—congenital heart disease, polydactyly, ovarian cysts, and hydrometrocolpos.

Pregnancy Management

Investigations and Consultations Required   If other abnormalities are present on ultrasonogram, chromosomal analysis should be done. Fetal echocardiography should be performed to exclude the McKusick-Kaufman syndrome. Consultation should be obtained from both a pediatric surgeon and a gynecologist because a precise diagnosis is rare prior to birth.

Monitoring   No change in standard obstetric care is warranted, unless there are associated abnormalities that could result in polyhydramnios. Serial ultrasonographic examinations to monitor the mass are appropriate.

Pregnancy Course   No obstetric complications are to be expected, unless there are associated malformations, such as esophageal atresia.

Pregnancy Termination Issues   An intact fetus should be delivered and a complete morphologic and pathologic examination performed.

Delivery   Because of the significant incidence of associated abnormalities and the need for surgical intervention, delivery should be in a tertiary center. The mode of delivery should be based on obstetric indications.

Neonatology

Resuscitation   Special measures in assisting the onset of respiration are rarely required, unless the enlargement of the uterine/vaginal mass is so great that there is concomitant urinary obstruction, leading to oligohydramnios and/or dystocia. In either circumstance, endotracheal intubation and positive-pressure ventilation may be required.

Transport   Transfer to a tertiary center with pediatric subspecialty and surgery capabilities is indicated for thorough diagnosis and management. Suspected urinary obstruction, respiratory distress, and suspected congenital heart defects are indications for emergency transfer by an experienced neonatal transport team.

Testing and Confirmation   The full spectrum of genitourinary diagnostic imaging may be needed for complete delineation of the pathologic anatomy and function. Echocardiography is indicated to exclude a congenital cardiac defect, particularly if polydactyly is present. High-resolution chromosome karyotyping is indicated if there are associated dysmorphic features or other malformations present.

Nursery Management   Maintenance of adequate fluid, electrolytes, and nutrition is essential, as is respiratory support if there is evidence of compromise of breathing. Priority should be given to early relief of urinary obstruction if such is present while the diagnostic evaluation is being completed.

The ultimate treatment is for surgical relief of the vaginal obstruction, with the exact approach dictated by the specific anatomic abnormality causing the obstruction.

Surgery

Preoperative Assessment   Hydrocolpos is synonymous with a common or persistent cloaca. The common cloaca is characterized as a fusion of rectum, vagina, and urethra into a single common channel. These newborn girls classically have very small genitalia and an imperforate anus. In cases of a common cloaca, the vagina is distended and full of secretions. This is referred to as a hydrocolpos. In some series, the incidence of hydrocolpos approaches 40%. The most significant problem that surgeons are faced with preoperatively is the presence of an obstructed bladder trigone and secondary ureteral obstruction, which are all the result of the hydrocolpos. Postnatal ultrasonography is used to evaluate the anatomy and possibility of obstruction. In addition, as in most cases of cloacal malformations, there can be associated anomalies including vaginal or urethral septations, hemivaginas, and hemiuteri. In general, urologic, neurologic, and bony abnormalities are commonly associated with a common cloacal malformation.

Operative Indications   Operative reconstruction of a common cloaca is one of the most complex and challenging malformations to perform. Typically the repair is staged. The initial procedure involves creation of a

colostomy at birth, but even more importantly, a full urologic evaluation must be performed to rule out the presence of urinary tract obstruction. If there is concomitant urinary tract obstruction, then both a colostomy and vesicostomy are created at the same operation. This double decompression generally alleviates the problem of the distended vagina or hydrocolpos. In rare cases it may be necessary to also decompress the vagina through the abdominal wall, using a procedure called vaginostomy.

The second stage repair of the cloaca is usually performed after 3 months of age. Longer intervals may be required if there are significant associated anomalies. As in many of the anomalies of the caudal region, there is a spectrum of cloacal defects but the two most frequent are distinguished by the presence of a long (greater than 3 cm) or short (less than 3 cm) common channel. This repair involves separation of the rectum and urogenital sinus (urethra and vagina) or separation of the rectum and vagina and simultaneous separation of the common wall between vagina and urethra. In some cases, vaginal replacement or advancement is necessary using intestine or skin, respectively. Ultimately the perineum is reconstructed with access of all three orifices in their normal anatomic positions.

Surgical Results/Prognosis   As in the case of any imperforate anus, the associated anomalies of muscle, bone, and nerve dictate the long-term outcome. The long common channel has a higher incidence of incontinence of both urine and feces. These girls all have sexual function and most can carry a pregnancy to term with a vaginal delivery.

REFERENCES

Banerjee AK, Clarke O, MacDonald LM: Sonographic detection of neonatal hydrometrocolpos. Br J Radiol 1992;65:268.

Baraiter M, Winter RM: Oxford Dysmorphology Database. Oxford, England, Oxford University Press, 1993.

Chen C-P, Liu F-F, Jan S-W, et al: Ultrasound-guided fluid aspiration and prenatal diagnosis of duplicated hydrometrocolpos with uterus didelphys and septate vagina. Prenat Diagn 1996;16:572.

Chitayat D, Hahm SYE, Marion RW, et al: Further delineation of the McKusick-Kaufman hydrometrocolpos-polydactyly syndrome. Am J Dis Child 1987;141:1133.

David A, Bitoun P, Lacombe D, et al: Hydrometrocolpos and polydactyly: A common neonatal presentation of Bardet-Biedl and McKusick-Kaufman syndromes. J Med Genet 1999;36:599.

Fryns J-P: Trichorhinophalangeal syndrome type 2: Another syndromic form of hydrometrocolpos. Am J Med Genet 1997;73:233.

Geipel A, Berg C, Germer U, et al: Diagnosis and therapeutic problems in a case of prenatally detected fetal hydrocolpos. Ultrasound Obstet Gynecol 2001;18:169–172.

Hahn-Pedersen J, Kvist N, Nielsen OH: Hydrometrocolpos: Current views on pathogenesis and management. J Urol 1984;132:537.

Mandell J, Stevens PS, Lucey DT: Diagnosis and management of hydrometrocolpos in infancy. J Urol 1978;120:262.

Mirk P, Pintus C, Speca S: Ultrasound diagnosis of hydrocolpos: Prenatal findings and postnatal follow-up. J Clin Ultrasound 1994;22:55.

Tran ATB, Arensman RM, Falterman KW: Diagnosis and management of hydrohematometrocolpos syndromes. Am J Dis Child 1987;141:632.

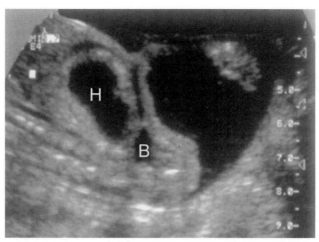

Sagittal view of an 18-week fetus showing large hydrometrocolpos (H) arising from the pelvis. The bladder (B) can be seen inferior to the hydrometrocolpos.

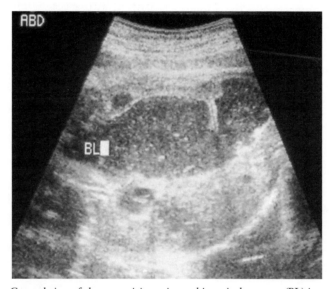

Coronal view of cloaca receiving urine and intestinal contents (BL) in a fetus with a cloacal anomaly.

4.6 Autosomal Recessive Polycystic Kidney Disease (Infantile Polycystic Kidney Disease)

Epidemiology/Genetics

Definition An autosomal recessive genetic disorder characterized by the replacement of normal renal tissue with dilated collecting tubules, resulting in symmetric renal enlargement and renal failure.

Epidemiology One in 20,000 to 50,000 births (M1:F1).

Embryology Autosomal recessive polycystic kidney disease causes both renal and hepatic cysts. The pathophysiology and genetic defect in this condition are unknown.

Inheritance Patterns Autosomal recessive. The gene for infantile polycystic kidney disease has been localized to chromosome 6p and genetic diagnosis is available in involved families. The current status of genetic testing should be investigated.

Teratogens None.

Prognosis Many fetuses with infantile polycystic kidney disease, diagnosed in utero, will be stillborn. Only a rare patient survives the first year of life when the condition is diagnosed in utero. Of these, about 50% will reach adolescence and all will ultimately need renal transplantation. Oligohydramnios suggests a lethal prognosis.

Sonography

FINDINGS

1. **Fetus:** Both kidneys are large and well above the 90th percentile for length and width. The renal parenchyma is very echogenic, particularly in the medullary areas. No cysts are visible in most cases. The cortex may be less echogenic. The bladder size is small, but some urine will be present. The liver appearances are normal, despite the presence of cysts and fibrosis.
2. **Amniotic Fluid:** Oligohydramnios is often severe, but fluid volume can be normal.
3. **Placenta:** Normal.
4. **Measurement Data:** A large abdominal circumference measurement is due to the massive kidney enlargement. Remaining fetal measurements are normal or small.
5. **When Detectable:** Oligohydramnios does not develop until 15 to 18 weeks' gestation at the earliest. Kidney findings may not develop until the late second or third trimester but have been seen at 18 weeks.

Differential Diagnosis

1. Meckel-Gruber syndrome (look for polydactyly and encephalocele). Renal cysts in this condition are usually visible. (See Chapter 11.4.)
2. Benign glomerulosclerosis—Large echogenic kidneys, but pyramids are echopenic and the amniotic fluid is normal or mildly increased.
3. Adult dominant polycystic kidney—Large kidneys that may not be symmetrically enlarged. Cysts may be visible and the kidneys are often echogenic. A positive family history can be obtained. An identical sonographic appearance to autosomal recessive polycystic kidney disease can be seen.
4. Trisomy 13—The kidneys may be slightly enlarged and are echogenic with cysts. Numerous other pathologic findings, such as holoprosencephaly, will be seen. (See Chapter 1.2.)
5. Beckwith-Wiedemann syndrome and Perlman syndrome—With both of these syndromes, the kidneys can be large and echogenic but there is also macrosomia, and amniotic fluid volumes are normal. In the case of Beckwith-Wiedemann syndrome, omphalocele and macroglossia are often present. (See Chapter 11.1.)

Where Else to Look

1. Look at paternal and maternal kidneys to exclude adult dominant polycystic kidney disease.
2. Look for congenital heart disease such as ventricular septal defect.
3. Look at the feet and hands for polydactyly and the skull for encephalocele (Meckel-Gruber).
4. Look for stigmata of trisomy 13.
5. Look at the cervix to exclude premature rupture of membranes as a cause of oligohydramnios.

Pregnancy Management

Investigations and Consultations Required If there is no family history of autosomal recessive polycystic kidney disease, the following investigations are appropriate:

1. Chromosomal evaluation.
2. Fetal echocardiography, to exclude other conditions that present with polycystic kidneys (trisomy 13 and Meckel-Gruber syndrome).
3. Consultation with a pediatric nephrologist should be arranged to develop a management plan and to discuss the implication of this diagnosis with the family.

Monitoring In recurrent cases or new cases with oligohydramnios, fetal assessment/monitoring is contraindicated. Electronic monitoring in labor should not be performed.

Pregnancy Course Most cases will develop oligohydramnios by the third trimester.

Pregnancy Termination Issues A precise pathologic diagnosis is essential for counseling the family regarding the risk of recurrence. An intact fetus should be delivered for complete external and internal examination.

Delivery Unless a precise diagnosis has been established prenatally (cases in a family with a previous affected child), delivery should occur at a tertiary center where an immediate evaluation can be performed to establish a diagnosis and to determine prognosis.

Dystocia from extremely large abdominal circumference may be an indication for elective cesarean section, in very rare cases.

Neonatology

Resuscitation A decision to withhold resuscitation is appropriate if, by reason of past family history or the prenatal diagnosis and course, a lethal prognosis is certain. If limited renal function is possible, but not certain, initial support is indicated until the prognosis can be determined.

Infants may present with respiratory distress at delivery, either from pulmonary hypoplasia as a result of longstanding oligohydramnios, or from severe abdominal distension from renal enlargement. Use positive pressure ventilation with caution, as pneumothorax occurs more frequently with pulmonary hypoplasia.

Transport Indicated for full confirmation of diagnosis and prognosis, if an infant demonstrates survival potential initially.

Testing and Confirmation Ninety percent of infantile polycystic kidney disease patients present with bilateral abdominal masses at birth.

Careful, staged evaluation of renal function and structure by urine production, urinalysis, blood and urine chemistries, and an abdominal sonogram is appropriate. If the infant is minimally symptomatic, imaging can be delayed for 24 to 36 hours for better visualization. If the anatomy is not clearly defined prenatally, ultrasonographic imaging should be obtained immediately. Subsequent procedures may be necessary to define renal function and, thus, survival potential, that is, renal scan without and with diuretic stimulation.

Nursery Management Support respiration as necessary to maintain adequate gas exchange.

Avoid fluid and protein loading initially until renal function has been determined.

REFERENCES

Bernstein J, Slovis TJ: Polycystic diseases of the kidney. In Edelmann CM Jr (ed): Pediatric Kidney Disease. Boston, Little, Brown, 1992, p 1139.

Chitty LS, Clark T, Maxwell D: Perlman syndrome: A cause of enlarged, hyperechogenic kidneys. Prenat Diagn 1998;18:1163–1168.

Fong KW, Rahmani MR, Rose TH, et al: Fetal renal cystic disease: Sonographic-pathologic correlation. Am J Roentgenol 1986;146:767–773.

Gillerot Y, Koulischer L: Major malformations of the urinary tract: Anatomic and genetic aspects. Biol Neonate 1988;53:186–196.

Kaplan BS, Fay J, Shah V, et al: Autosomal recessive polycystic kidney disease. Pediatr Nephrol 1989;3:43–49.

MacDermot KD, Saggar-Malik AK, Economides DL, Jeffery S: Prenatal diagnosis of autosomal dominant polycystic kidney disease (PKD1) presenting in utero and prognosis for very early onset disease. J Med Genet 1998;35:13–16.

Mahony BS, Callen PW, Filly RA, Golbus MS: Progression of infantile polycystic kidney disease in early pregnancy. J Ultrasound Med 1984;3:277–279.

Pretorius DH, Lee ME, Manco-Johnson ML, et al: Diagnosis of autosomal dominant polycystic kidney disease in utero and in the young infant. J Ultrasound Med 1987;6:249–255.

Reuss A, Wladimiroff JW, Niermeyer MF: Sonographic, clinical and genetic aspects of prenatal diagnosis of cystic kidney disease. Ultrasound Med Biol 1991;17:687–694.

Romero R, Cullen M, Jeanty P, et al: The diagnosis of congenital renal anomalies with ultrasound. II. Infantile polycystic disease. Am J Obstet Gynecol 1984;150:259–262.

Zerres K, Mucher G, Becker J, et al: Prenatal diagnosis of autosomal recessive polycystic kidney disease (ARPKD): Molecular genetics, clinical experience, and fetal morphology. Am J Med Genet 1998;76:137–144.

Zerres K, Volpel MC, Weiss H: Cystic kidneys: Genetics, pathologic anatomy, clinical picture and prenatal diagnosis. Hum Genet 1984;68:104–135.

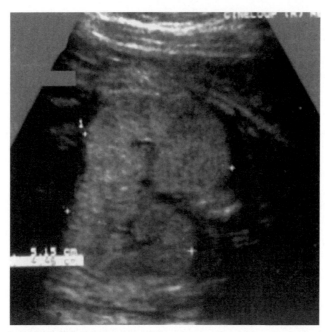

Infantile polycystic kidney, 30 week sonogram. Transverse view of fetal abdomen. The kidneys (between +'s) have almost the same echogenicity as the remainder of the abdomen. Notice that they have a longer length at 30 weeks than normal fetal kidneys at term. There is no amniotic fluid.

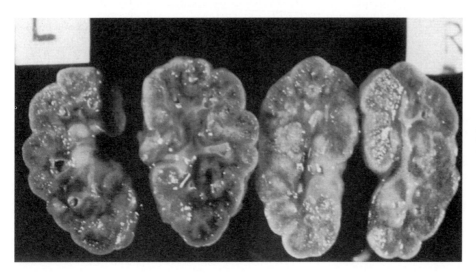

Massively enlarged newborn kidneys with multiple small cysts due to infantile polycystic kidney disease.

4.7 Mesoblastic Nephroma

Epidemiology/Genetics

Definition Congenital mesoblastic nephroma is a massive, firm, infiltrative, solitary renal tumor, grossly and microscopically resembling a leiomyoma or a low-grade leiomyosarcoma with trapped nephrons.

Epidemiology Rare (M>F). Congenital mesoblastic nephroma accounts for 3 to 6% of renal masses in childhood and 50% during the neonatal period.

Embryology Generally, this is a benign hamartomatous congenital renal tumor, although malignant degeneration has occasionally been reported.

Inheritance Patterns Sporadic. Recurrence risk is only the general population risk.

Teratogens None.

Prognosis The tumor is generally benign, but prognosis depends on histologic findings and on prematurity induced by the associated polyhydramnios.

Sonography

FINDINGS

1. **Fetus:** A moderately echogenic mass with an echogenic capsule is seen within the kidney. Cystic areas within the mass have been reported but are not usually seen. The mass distorts the renal sinus echoes but has not been reported to cause hydronephrosis. The kidney length is increased. Color flow sonography will show vascularity within the mass. The mass grows rapidly on sequential examinations. Nonimmune hydrops occasionally complicates large meso-blastic nephroma.
2. **Amniotic Fluid:** Moderate to severe polyhydramnios has been an almost invariable finding. It is unclear whether this is due to polyuria or intestinal obstruction.
3. **Placenta:** Normal
4. **Measurement Data:** The abdominal circumference is enlarged by the mass.
5. **When Detectable:** The earliest reported detection was at 26 weeks.

Pitfalls Massive polyhydramnios may make the mass difficult to see.

Where Else to Look

1. Make sure the mass is of renal rather than adrenal origin—identify the adrenal gland on the same side.
2. Although almost all renal masses in utero are benign,

malignant mesoblastic nephroma and Wilms tumor have been reported, so look for metastatic nodes and liver metastases.

Differential Diagnosis

1. Neuroblastoma—Usually echogenic or calcified and arises from the adrenal gland.
2. Wilms tumor—This mass has been identified in utero and has no distinguishing characteristics, allowing separation from mesoblastic nephroma.

Pregnancy Management

Investigations and Consultations Required Because of the similarity of ultrasonographic features between mesoblastic nephroma and Wilms tumor, an evaluation should be done to exclude other syndromes that are associated with Wilms tumor. Amniocentesis should be performed and fluorescent in situ hybridization done to exclude the chromosome 11 deletion seen in the WAGR syndrome (Wilms tumor, aniridia, genital abnormalities, mental retardation). A consultation with a pediatric urologist should be obtained.

Fetal Intervention None indicated.

Monitoring Pregnancies complicated by fetal mesoblastic nephroma usually have associated polyhydramnios. Serial ultrasonograms should be performed to assess fluid volume and growth of the mass.

Pregnancy Course As noted above, polyhydramnios with preterm labor may be a complication. Tocolytic agents may be required to prolong the pregnancy.

Pregnancy Termination Issues Not indicated, since the lesion is treatable postnatally.

Delivery Although immediate neonatal complications from mesoblastic nephroma are rare, delivery in a tertiary center allows for a thorough evaluation and confirmation of the diagnosis.

Neonatology

Resuscitation Infants with mesoblastic nephroma have a high incidence of polyhydramnios and preterm delivery. Hydrops fetalis has been reported, as has dystocia and rupture of the mass in the perinatal period. Respiratory distress secondary either to prematurity or to mechanical compromise from the abdominal distension is also possible. The approach to resuscitation is dictated by the presence of any of these complicating factors. Establishing adequate ventilation by the most gentle means possible with avoidance of undue pressure on the abdomen is essential.

Transport   Transfer to a tertiary center with pediatric surgical and diagnostic imaging capabilities, on an emergency basis if cardiorespiratory compromise is evident, is indicated. An experienced neonatal transport team is essential in the latter case.

Testing and Confirmation   Diagnostic imaging of the tumor mass with magnetic resonance imaging is indicated. Differentiation from other solid renal tumors requires histopathologic examination.

Nursery Management   The definitive treatment is surgical excision of the tumor.

Adjunctive antineoplastic therapy is recommended only for either tumor rupture with intraperitoneal spill or incomplete removal of the tumor. Preoperatively, careful fluid and electrolyte management may be critical, particularly if there has been polyhydramnios and/or hydrops. Polyuria sufficient to create hemodynamic and electrolyte abnormalities has been reported.

Surgery

Preoperative Assessment   Magnetic resonance imaging is used to assess the extent of the tumor and to ensure that local invasion has not taken place.

Operative Indications   Nephrectomy is performed as soon as the infant is stable. Chemotherapy and radiotherapy are not generally required, unless there is intraperitoneal tumor spill or incomplete tumor removal, even though atypical acellular tumors and tumors of

mixed histologic type are said to behave more aggressively.

Surgical Results/Prognosis   A 100% survival rate is reported, provided postoperative complications do not occur.

REFERENCES

Apuzzio JJ, Unwin W, Adhate A, Nichols R: Prenatal diagnosis of fetal renal mesoblastic nephromas. Am J Obstet Gynecol 1986;154:636–637.

DiMaggio Howey D, Farrell EE, Sholl J, et al: Congenital mesoblastic nephroma: Prenatal ultrasonic findings and surgical excision in a very-low-birth-weight infant. J Clin Ultrasound 1985;13:506–508.

Ehman RL, Nicholson SF, Machin GA: Prenatal sonographic detection of congenital mesoblastic nephroma in a monozygotic twin pregnancy. J Ultrasound Med 1983;2:555–557.

Fung TY, Hedy Fung YM, Ng PC, et al: Polyhydramnios and hypercalcemia associated with congenital mesoblastic nephroma: Case report and a new appraisal. Obstet Gynecol 1995;85:815–817.

Garble SH, Crombleholme TM, Semple JP, Bhan I: Prenatal diagnosis and management of fetal tumors. Semin Perinatol 1994;18:350–365.

Giulian BB: Prenatal ultrasonographic diagnosis of fetal renal tumors. Radiology 1984;152:69–70.

Haddad B, Haziza J, Touboul C, et al: The congenital mesoblastic nephroma: A case report of prenatal diagnosis. Fetal Diagn Ther 1996; 11:61–66.

Howell CG, Otherson HB, Kiviat NE, et al: Therapy and outcome in 51 children with mesoblastic congenital nephroma: A report of the National Wilms Tumor Study. J Pediatr Surg 1982;17:826.

Isaacs H Jr: Renal tumors. In Issacs H Jr (ed): Tumors of the Fetus and Newborn, Vol. 35, Major Problems in Pathology. Philadelphia, WB Saunders, 1997, pp 245–255.

Liu YC, Mai YL, Chang CC, et al: The presence of hydrops fetalis in a fetus with congenital mesoblastic nephroma. Prenat Diagn 1996;16: 363–365.

Schild RL, Plath H, Hofstaetter C, Hansmann M: Diagnosis of fetal mesoblastic nephroma by 3D-ultrasound. Ultrasound Obstet Gynecol 2000;15:533–536.

Suresh I, Suresh S, Arumugam R, et al: Antenatal diagnosis of Wilms tumor. J Ultrasound Med 1997;16:69–72.

Walter JP, McGahan JP: Mesoblastic nephroma: Prenatal sonographic detection. J Clin Ultrasound 1985;13:686.

Yazaki T, Akimoto M, Tsudoi N, et al: Congenital mesoblastic nephroma. Urology 1982;20:446.

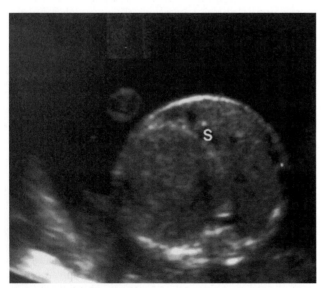

Transverse view showing large left mesoblastic nephroma compressing the stomach (S). Note the severe polyhydramnios.

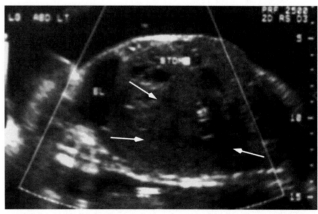

Sagittal left-side view showing the mesoblastic nephroma examined with color flow. Note the flow within the mass, which is outlined by *arrows*.

4.8 Multicystic Dysplastic Kidney

Epidemiology/Genetics

Definition Multicystic dysplastic kidney is a congenital dysplasia of the kidneys that is characterized by large non-homogeneous dilations of the collecting tubules. It may occur unilaterally or bilaterally.

Epidemiology One in 1000 to 5000 births (M>F). This is the most common cystic renal abnormality noted in the newborn.

Embryology Multicystic dysplastic kidney disease is a renal abnormality with severely disorganized tubules, glomeruli, ducts, and cortical cystic lesions of the collecting tubules. Although the pathogenesis is unknown, it is thought to be due to an early error in development of the mesonephric blastema or early obstructive uropathy. Ninety percent of cases are associated with urinary obstruction and/or other renal abnormalities. Eighty percent of cases are unilateral. Associated nonrenal malformations include anencephaly, hydrocephalus, spina bifida, cleft palate, microphthalmia, duodenal stenosis, tracheo-esophageal fistula, and imperforate anus. More than 35 genetic, chromosomal, and sporadic syndromes have been described with dysplastic kidneys.

Inheritance Patterns As an isolated abnormality, it is usually sporadic, but families with autosomal dominant inheritance have been described whose defects range from bilateral renal agenesis to double ureter, renal cysts, or hydronephrosis. It can occur as part of the Meckel syndrome (autosomal recessive), short rib polydactyly syndromes (autosomal recessive), Zellweger syndrome (autosomal recessive), Roberts syndrome (autosomal recessive), Fryns syndrome (autosomal recessive), Smith-Lemli-Opitz syndrome (autosomal recessive), Apert syndrome (autosomal dominant), and brachio-oto-renal syndrome (autosomal dominant).

Teratogens Maternal diabetes.

Prognosis Unilateral and isolated abnormalities may be asymptomatic and go undetected. Unilateral multicystic kidney disease spontaneously regresses with time and by age 2 the mass has often disappeared. Alternatively, a small bag of cysts with a calcified rim is seen at the site where the kidney lay. Bilateral severe defects are lethal. Partial dysplastic involvement of both kidneys leads eventually to renal function impairment.

Sonography

FINDINGS

1. **Fetus:**
   a. Cysts—There are multiple cysts of varied sizes that start at the periphery of the kidney. Initially, they are small, but they enlarge with time and may develop in the renal hilum. Eventually, the cysts will start to decrease in size, but this may not be until after birth.
   b. Parenchymal echogenicity—Echogenic renal parenchyma lies between the cysts. In early cases, echogenic parenchyma is the initial feature. Some normal, or partially normal, renal parenchyma may be interspersed with echogenic dysplastic areas.
   c. Kidney size—The overall kidney mass may be too small or too large. Large kidneys filled with large cysts occur when dysplastic kidney is due to a high (ureteropelvic junction) obstruction. More distal obstructions, such as posterior urethral valve, result in small dysplastic kidneys with few and small cysts.
   d. Bilateral—Bilateral multicystic kidneys may occur. The bladder may contain urine even if the condition is bilateral, since decreased renal function worsens progressively.
   e. Contralateral kidney—Compensatory hypertrophy and enlargement of the contralateral kidney will occur if the condition is unilateral. Renal abnormalities of the contralateral kidney such as hydronephrosis, ureterocele, or reflux are common (33%).
2. **Amniotic Fluid:** If bilateral, there will be no amniotic fluid after 15 to 18 weeks. If unilateral, amniotic fluid volume will be normal.
3. **Placenta:** Normal.
4. **Measurement Data:** There may be a large abdominal circumference because of the kidney mass, which can impede delivery in the case of very large multicystic kidneys.
5. **When Detectable:** Usually first detectable at 15 to 20 weeks. There is progressive enlargement of the cysts as pregnancy continues.

Pitfalls Echogenic parenchyma may occur normally. In the absence of cysts, distinguishing a dysplastic kidney from normal, on the basis of coarse texture and increased echogenicity, is difficult and dependent on the ultrasonographic system. This is particularly a problem with posterior urethral valve kidneys.

Differential Diagnosis:

1. Adult polycystic kidney—The cysts are randomly distributed, instead of being grouped at the periphery as they are in early multicystic dysplastic kidney.
2. Meckel-Gruber syndrome—The cysts are all the same size, are relatively small, and are scattered throughout the kidney.
3. Infantile polycystic kidney—As a rule, no cysts are visible and the kidneys are greatly enlarged.
4. Trisomy 13 kidneys—The kidneys are enlarged and echogenic. Randomly dispersed small cysts are present.
5. Severe hydronephrosis with no remaining parenchyma—

This entity may be indistinguishable from the hydronephrotic form of multicystic kidney.

Where Else to Look   Parents should have a renal ultrasonogram to look for unilateral renal agenesis or other renal abnormalities that may suggest autosomal dominant inheritance. Look for stigmata of chromosome disorders.

Pregnancy Management

Investigations and Consultations Required   The incidence of chromosome abnormalities is quite low in isolated unilateral multicystic dysplastic kidney, but amniocentesis should be performed to exclude this possibility before establishing a management plan. Fetal echocardiography should be performed to rule out an associated heart defect. A pediatric urologist should be consulted to discuss the neonatal evaluation and management of unilateral multicystic dysplastic kidney with the family. The presence of bilateral multicystic dysplastic kidney is a lethal condition, and a neonatologist should be consulted to assist in the development of a noninterventional perinatal management plan.

Fetal Intervention   There is an increased incidence of contralateral renal malformation when unilateral multicystic dysplastic kidney is present. If ureteropelvic junction obstruction is present in the opposite kidney, it is possible that either early delivery or in utero placement of a shunt may be necessary, in rare cases.

Monitoring   No changes in obstetric management should be necessary for unilateral multicystic dysplastic kidney. Monthly ultrasonographic examinations should be performed to monitor the status of the normal kidney. In bilateral multicystic dysplastic kidney, no intervention for fetal indications should be performed. Electronic fetal monitoring in labor is contraindicated once this diagnosis has been established.

Pregnancy Course   No specific obstetric complications are to be expected.

Pregnancy Termination Issues   Pathologic confirmation is essential because of the similar sonographic appearance of multicystic dysplastic kidney and other forms of renal dysplasia, especially the infantile presentation of adult polycystic kidney disease. Termination should be by a nondestructive procedure, unless performed in an institution with special expertise in suction evacuation and retrieval of the fetal organs.

Delivery   For unilateral disease, no special considerations for delivery are necessary. In cases of bilateral multicystic dysplastic kidney, the site should be one where the staff is comfortable with a noninterventional approach to labor management.

Neonatology

Resuscitation   With bilateral multicystic dysplastic kidney, respiratory distress is usually present from delivery secondary to pulmonary hypoplasia with significant oligohydramnios. Use positive-pressure ventilation cautiously when pulmonary hypoplasia is suspected because of the high risk for pneumothorax. Onset of effective respiration may be impeded by abdominal distension from renal enlargement, particularly with bilateral involvement.

A decision to withhold resuscitation should be considered when prenatal diagnosis of a lethal prognosis is certain, as with bilateral involvement and severe oligohydramnios. If limited renal function is possible, but not certain, initial support is indicated until the prognosis can be determined.

Transport   Indicated for bilateral lesions for full confirmation of diagnosis if the infant demonstrates survival potential after resuscitation. Infants with isolated unilateral lesions and normal renal function, as indicated by serum creatinine level, can be referred for outpatient evaluation and management.

Testing and Confirmation   Careful, staged evaluation of renal function and structure by urine production, urinalysis, blood and urine chemistries, and an abdominal sonogram is recommended. If the infant is minimally symptomatic, imaging can be delayed for 24 to 36 hours for better visualization. If the anatomy is not clearly defined prenatally, ultrasonographic imaging should be obtained immediately. Subsequent procedures may be needed to further delineate renal function, that is, renal scan without and with diuretic stimulation.

Nursery Management   Support respiration as necessary to maintain adequate gas exchange.

Avoid fluid and protein loading initially until renal function has been determined.

With adequate upper tract development (ureters), renal transplant may be possible in early childhood for bilateral lesions with limited function at birth.

REFERENCES

Avni EF, Thoua Y, Lalmand B, et al: Multicystic dysplastic kidney: Evolving concepts. In utero diagnosis and post-natal follow-up by ultrasound. Ann Radiol 1986;29:663–668.

Bernstein J: Renal hypoplasia and dysplasia. In Edelmann CM Jr (ed): Pediatric Kidney Disease. Boston, Little, Brown, 1992, p 1121.

D'Alton M, Romero R, Grannum P, et al: Antenatal diagnosis of renal anomalies with ultrasound. IV. Bilateral multicystic kidney disease. Am J Obstet Gynecol 1986;154:532–537.

Gillerot Y, Koulischer L: Major malformations of the urinary tract: Anatomic and genetic aspects. Biol Neonate 1988;53:186–196.

Hashimoto BE, Filly RA, Callen PW: Multicystic dysplastic kidney in utero: Changing appearance on ultrasound. Radiology 1986;159:107–109.

Hill LM, Nowak A, Hartle R, Tush B: Fetal compensatory renal hypertrophy with unilateral functioning kidney. Ultrasound Obstet Gynecol 2000;15:191–193.

Kim EK, Song TB: A study on fetal urinary tract anomaly: Antenatal ultrasonographic diagnosis and postnatal follow-up. J Obstet Gynaecol Res 1996;22:569–573.

Kleiner B, Filly RA, Mack L, Callen PW: Multicystic dysplastic kidney: Observations of the contralateral disease in the fetal population. Radiology 1986;161:27–29.

Lazelbnik N, Bellinger MF, Ferguson JE, et al: Insights into the pathogenesis and natural story of fetuses with multicystic dysplastic kidney disease. Prenat Diagn 1999;19:418–423.

Sanders RC, Nussbaum AR, Solez K: Renal dysplasia: Sonographic findings. Radiology 1988;167:623–626.

Wackman J, Phipps L: Report of multicystic kidney registry: Preliminary findings. J Urol 1993;150:1870–1872.

Zerres K, Volpel MC, Weiss H: Cystic kidneys. Genetics, pathologic anatomy, clinical picture and prenatal diagnosis. Hum Genet 1984;68:104–135.

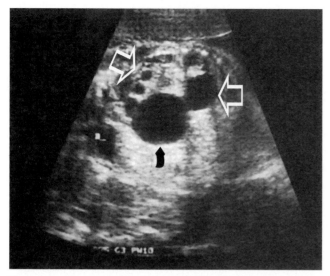

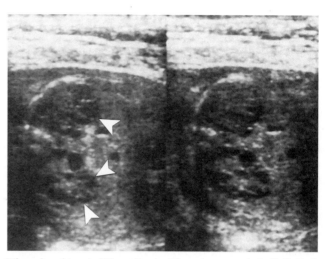

Unilateral multicystic dysplastic kidney disease. Some of the kidney mass (between the *arrows*) is occupied by cysts of varying sizes. The echogenic area elsewhere within the kidney is filled with tiny cysts. These cysts are too small for the ultrasonographic system to show them individually, but large enough to cause echoes.

Bilateral multicystic kidney disease. There is no amniotic fluid. Both kidneys (*arrows*) have multiple small cysts around the periphery in a typical location. As the disease progresses, these cysts will enlarge and appear to lie more in the center.

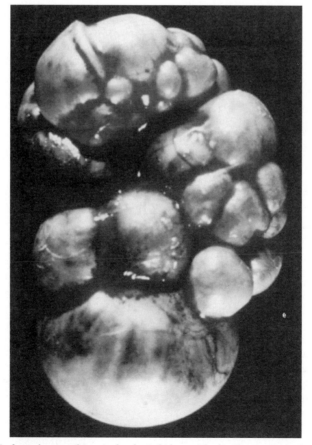

Left newborn multicystic dysplastic kidney with abundant cysts varying in size.

4.9 Neuroblastoma

Epidemiology/Genetics

Definition Neuroblastoma is the most frequently diagnosed neoplasm in infants and the most common extracranial solid tumor of childhood, accounting for 8% to 10% of all childhood cancers.

Epidemiology 8:7 (M>F). More common in whites. One in 40 incidence in autopsies but 1 in 100,000 clinical incidence.

Embryology The tumor originates in neural crest cells of the sympathetic nervous system and can develop anywhere from the posterior cranial fossa to the coccyx. About 70% of the tumors arise in the abdomen (50% in the adrenal gland), and another 20% arise in the posterior mediastinum. The familial form is thought to support the Knudson two-mutation model for a "tumor suppressor gene." This model presumes an inherited first mutation followed by a somatic second mutation resulting in the tumor. Sporadic cases presumably require two somatic mutations. Neuroblastoma in situ is a common autopsy finding in newborn adrenal glands. Most tumors presumably spontaneously regress.

Inheritance Patterns Both familial and sporadic cases occur. Familial cases may represent 20% of neuroblastomas and show complex genetic inheritance. A gene important for tumor suppression maps to chromosome 1p and may show autosomal recessive inheritance as well as follow the Knudson two-hit hypothesis of tumorgenesis with one inherited mutation and one acquired mutation.

Teratogens The condition has been reported in association with fetal Dilantin and fetal alcohol exposure, but this most likely is coincidental.

Differential Diagnosis Adrenal hemorrhage.

Additional Investigations Elevated catecholamine metabolites are seen in 95% of cases and may cause antenatal symptoms in the mother. Affected pregnancies may have maternal tachycardia and nausea and vomiting during the third trimester, sometimes in association with nonimmune hydrops fetalis. Postnatal radiographs, ultrasonograms, and computed tomography (CT) or magnetic resonance imaging (MRI) scans can demonstrate a suprarenal or posterior mediastinal mass with calcifications.

Prognosis Survival rates of infants with low-stage disease exceed 90%, and infants with metastatic disease have a long-term survival rate of 5 years or greater. Genomic amplification of the N-*myc* oncogene is an indicator of a poor prognosis.

Sonography

FINDINGS

1. **Fetus:**
   a. The normal adrenal gland appears as a disc-shaped hypoechoic structure superior to the kidneys. It has a hypoechoic border and a central hyperechoic line.
   b. With neuroblastoma in a typical location, a retroperitoneal mass is seen separate from the liver and superior to the kidney.
   c. The mass develops in the third trimester.
   d. Typically, the mass is cystic with solid components, but it may have an evenly echogenic appearance or a mixed echo texture with solid or even calcified components. Adrenal hemorrhage often complicates neuroblastoma and may be the predominant mass seen, in which case the mass has a complex appearance with cystic areas and changes from a cystic to a solid appearance over days.
   e. Color flow sonography will show internal vessels inside a neuroblastoma and not in a hematoma.
   f. Nonimmune hydrops very occasionally complicates neuroblastoma, thought to be related to catecholamine production.
2. **Amniotic Fluid:** If the mass enlarges enough to compress gut, polyhydramnios may develop.
3. **Placenta:** Normal unless hydrops develops, when the placenta will be enlarged.
4. **Measurement Data:** Usually normal.

Pitfalls Distinction between isolated adrenal hemorrhage and neuroblastoma is difficult, if not impossible.

Differential Diagnosis

1. Extralobar sequestration—An echogenic mass is seen superior to the kidney, usually on the left. The adrenal gland can be seen in addition to the mass. This mass is fluid-containing as seen on CT or MRI scans. (See Chapter 5.5.)
2. Dysplastic second collecting system—Usually small cysts can be seen in the mass, and the condition is often bilateral.
3. Adrenal hemorrhage may be initially indistinguishable from neuroblastoma, but follow-up sonograms will show rapid changes in adrenal hemorrhage appearance and not in neuroblastoma. Color flow sonography will show a rim of vessels around a hematoma but no internal vascularity. Hemorrhage is much more common on the right than the left kidney. (See Chapter 4.1.)
4. Mesoblastic nephroma develops in the kidney, but it may be difficult to determine the site of origin of the mass. (See Chapter 4.7.)

5. Hepatic tumor will lie anterior to the kidney and the adrenal gland. (See Chapter 6.5.)

Where Else to Look   Look for spread toward the midline and for evidence of metastases in the liver, lungs, and brain. Repeat scanning to make sure the mass is not a hematoma.

Pregnancy Management

Investigations and Consultations Required   No additional diagnostic evaluations are needed. A consultation should be obtained with a pediatric oncologist and a pediatric surgeon to discuss neonatal management.

Fetal Intervention   Early delivery may be indicated if there is evidence of fetal compromise.

Monitoring   Fetal hydrops and/or polyhydramnios may develop. Serial ultrasonograms may be helpful in the early detection of these findings. Regular fetal assessment using biophysical profiles also may be useful in determining compromised fetuses.

Pregnancy Course   May be uncomplicated, but in cases with metastatic disease in the liver, polyhydramnios and hydrops may complicate the pregnancy.

Pregnancy Termination Issues   If the pregnancy is terminated, careful histologic evaluation should be done to confirm the diagnosis. An intact fetus is essential to obtain appropriate organ samples.

Delivery   There is a significant risk of hemorrhage into the tumor, and cesarean section should be performed.

Neonatology

Resuscitation   Of the reported cases in the literature, most of the deaths have occurred early in the neonatal period. There were two stillbirths and two infants with hydrops who succumbed within the first several days; the remaining infants died later in the first month. Most had solid tumors with disseminated disease. Thus, the finding of hydrops prior to delivery or evidence of metastatic disease should serve as an alert for aggressive respiratory support from birth. Otherwise, the need for intervention for cardiorespiratory adaptation following delivery is unlikely.

Transport   Transfer to a tertiary center with pediatric oncology and surgery subspecialty capabilities is indicated on an emergency basis.

Testing and Confirmation   Careful diagnostic imaging with CT and/or MRI coupled with bone marrow aspiration, assay of catecholamine excretory by-products, and identification of tumor oncogenes are the key components for diagnosis and staging.

Nursery Management   Most infants require only general supportive care while the diagnostic evaluation is completed. The definitive treatment is surgical for most infants, with the timing of the surgery based on the tumor staging at diagnosis.

Surgery

Preoperative Assessment   MRI is considered the best method of assessing the extent of the mass. Many tumors in neonates regress spontaneously, so tumor resection may be deferred. Needle biopsy of the mass is helpful in confirming tumor.

Operative Indications   With stage 1 and 2 disease, complete tumor resection is performed once adrenal hemorrhage has been ruled out. With stage 3 (bilateral involvement), the tumor is biopsied and adequate amounts of tumor are obtained for histologic, immunologic, and genetic studies. Stage 4S tumors, in which there are skin, liver, and brain metastases, are biopsied only.

Surgical Results/Prognosis   The overall survival rate with tumors diagnosed at birth is approximately 80%. Tumors that would go undetected if it were not for prenatal ultrasonography or postnatal neuroblastoma screening characteristically undergo spontaneous regression or maturation and require little or no treatment. More bulky tumors require chemotherapy in addition to surgery. Even stage 4S tumors with liver, brain, and skin metastases usually regress spontaneously or respond to treatment. Short-term complications related to respiratory compromise or disseminated intravascular coagulation may prevent survival in infants with stage 4 or 4S disease.

REFERENCES

Acharya S, Jayabose S, Kogan SJ, et al: Prenatally diagnosed neuroblastoma. Cancer 1997;80:3044.

Brodeur GM, Pritchard J, Berthold F, et al: Revisions of the international criteria for neuroblastoma: Diagnosis, staging, and response to treatment. J Clin Oncol 1993;8:1466.

Chen CP, Chen SH, Chuang CY, et al: Clinical and perinatal sonographic features of congenital adrenal cystic neuroblastoma: A case report with review of the literature. Ultrasound Obstet Gynecol 1997;10:68–73.

Curtis MR, Mooney DP, Vaccaro TJ, et al: Prenatal ultrasound characterization of the suprarenal mass: Distinction between neuroblastoma and subdiaphragmatic extralobar pulmonary sequestration. J Ultrasound Med 1997;16:75–83.

Forman HP, Leonidas JC, Berdon WE, et al: Congenital neuroblastoma: Evaluation and multimodality imaging. Radiology 1990;175:365.

Goldstein I, Gomez K, Copel JA: The real-time and color Doppler appearance of adrenal neuroblastoma in a third-trimester fetus. Obstet Gynecol 1994;83:854–856.

Heling KS, Chaoui R, Hartung J, et al: Prenatal diagnosis of congenital neuroblastoma. Analysis of 4 cases and review of the literature. Fetal Diagn Ther 1999;14:47–52.

Ho PTG, Estroff JA, Kozakewich H, et al: Prenatal detection of neuroblastoma: A ten-year experience from the Dana-Farber Cancer Institute and Children's Hospital. Pediatrics 1993;92:358.

Hosoda Y, Miyano T, Kimura K, et al: Characteristics and management of patients with fetal neuroblastoma. J Pediatr Surg 1992;27:623.

Jennings RW, LaQuaglia MP, Leong K, et al: Fetal neuroblastoma: Prenatal diagnosis and natural history. J Pediatr Surg 1993;28:1168.

Kesrouani A, Duchatel F, Seilanian M, Muray JM: Prenatal diagnosis of adrenal neuroblastoma by ultrasound: A report of two cases and review of the literature. Ultrasound Obstet Gynecol 1999;13:446–449.

Knudson AG Jr, Strong LC: Mutation and cancer: Neuroblastoma and pheochromocytoma. Am J Med Genet 1972;24:514–532.

Lin JN, Lin GJ, Hung IJ, Hsueh C: Prenatally detected tumor mass in the adrenal gland. J Pediatr Surg 1999;34:1620–1623.

Moss TJ, Kaplan L: Association of hydrops fetalis with congenital neuroblastoma. Am J Obstet Gynecol 1978;132:905–908.

Rubenstein SC, Benacerraf BR, Retik AB, Mandell J: Fetal suprarenal masses: Sonographic appearance and differential diagnosis. Ultrasound Obstet Gynecol 1995;5:164–167.

Saylors RL, Cohn SL, Morgan ER, Brodeur GM: Prenatal detection of neuroblastoma by fetal ultrasonography. Am J Pediatr Hematol Oncol 1994;16:356.

Schwarzler P, Bernard JP, Senat MV, Ville Y: Prenatal diagnosis of fetal adrenal masses: Differentiation between hemorrhage and solid tumor by color Doppler sonography. Ultrasound Obstet Gynecol 1999;13:351–355.

Shen MR, Lin YS, Huang SC, Chou CY: Rapid growth of a fetal abdominal mass: A case report of congenital neuroblastoma. J Clin Ultrasound 1997;25:39–42.

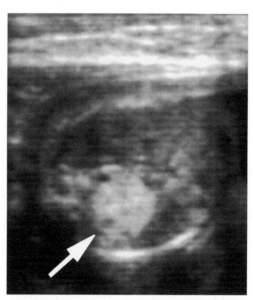

Transverse view showing a neuroblastoma adjacent to the spine. A few cystic areas can be seen within the echogenic mass (*arrow*).

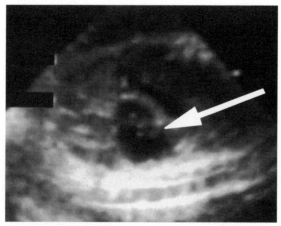

Cystic neuroblastoma, sagittal view (*arrow*).

4.10 Ovarian Cysts

Epidemiology/Genetics

Definition Ovarian cysts are fluid-filled ovarian tumors.

Epidemiology Unknown. Although ovarian cysts are rarely detected in infants, they are slightly more common on fetal ultrasonogram (M0:F1).

Embryology Almost all ovarian cysts are benign corpus luteal cysts of germinal or graafian tissue origin. The fetal ovaries respond to maternal hormonal stimulus.

Inheritance Patterns Most cases are sporadic, except for very rare genetic syndromes such as the McKusick-Kaufman syndrome (autosomal recessive) with congenital heart disease, polydactyly, and hydrometrocolpos.

Teratogens None.

Prognosis Generally excellent. Most spontaneously resolve without postnatal treatment. Large cysts (greater than 5 cm) can cause lethal complications such as ovarian torsion and bleeding.

Sonography

FINDINGS

1. **Fetus:** A cyst is present in the fetal abdomen in the mesentery, not related to the kidneys or gut. This entity occurs only in females. The cysts are usually echo-free but, if torsed, may contain internal echoes or a crescent-shaped mass. On rare occasions, very large cysts may cause gut obstruction. Since the broad ligament in utero is very stretchable, they can be located anywhere in the intraperitoneal abdomen.
2. **Amniotic Fluid:** Normal, unless there is gut obstruction, in which case polyhydramnios may develop.
3. **Placenta:** Normal.
4. **Measurement Data:** Normal.
5. **When Detectable:** Ovarian cysts do not develop before about 23 weeks' gestation, since they are related to maternal hormonal influence on the maturing fetal ovaries.

Pitfalls

1. An extrarenal pelvis with a ureteropelvic junction obstruction can appear intramesenteric.
2. Ovarian cysts can lie in the upper abdomen because all fetal ligaments are weak.

Differential Diagnosis

1. Duplication cysts are usually associated with gut dilation and may occur in males.
2. A mesenteric cyst may have a similar appearance to an ovarian cyst but is less common and may occur in males.
3. Liver cysts appear on the right and are related to the liver.
4. A choledochal cyst is related to, and partially within, the right lobe of the liver. A dilated bile duct entering a choledochal cyst is often seen.

Where Else to Look Make sure the fetus is female.

Pregnancy Management

Investigations and Consultations Required Because the diagnosis is often one of exclusion, chromosomal studies and fetal echocardiography may be appropriate before this presumptive diagnosis can be made. Pediatric surgical consultations should be obtained in the event that neonatal complications require surgical intervention.

Fetal Intervention None. Aspiration of the cysts is contraindicated because of the high incidence of spontaneous resolution, the significant risk of misdiagnosis, and the theoretical concerns of spillage of an irritant (contents of a dermoid cyst) or malignant cells into the peritoneal cavity.

Monitoring No alterations in obstetric care are necessary. Those cases complicated by polyhydramnios should be monitored for evidence of preterm labor. Follow-up at monthly intervals, with sonography, to check for ovarian cyst size, polyhydramnios, and gut dilation is helpful.

Pregnancy Course Polyhydramnios may develop secondary to extrinsic bowel obstruction.

Pregnancy Termination Issues Termination of pregnancy is not indicated if major associated malformations have been excluded.

Delivery In rare cases of large cysts that could result in dystocia, cesarean section may be indicated.

Neonatology

Resuscitation Rarely is there an issue with the onset of respiration. Giant-sized cysts may create such severe abdominal distension that they inhibit efficient breathing.

Transport   Neonatal transport to a tertiary facility with a pediatric surgeon is always indicated for an abdominal mass in the female infant.

Testing and Confirmation   Obtain an abdominal sonogram to confirm the prenatal diagnosis. Additional contrast studies of the gastrointestinal and urinary tracts may be necessary for a very large mass.

Nursery Management   Support respiration mechanically if abdominal distension is severe.

Surgery

Preoperative Assessment   Repeat postnatal sonography is indicated to determine whether the cyst is still present, as well as its characteristics.

Operative Indications

1. Cyst greater than 6 cm in diameter.
2. Evidence of hemorrhage or torsion.
3. Failure of regression after several months' observation or obstruction of alimentary or genitourinary tracts.

Types of Procedures   If the mass is uniformly echogenic, that is, no "layering" or loculations of cyst contents, and it is relatively small, less than 6 cm in a full-term infant, then it can be observed for spontaneous resolution. Repeat sonography at monthly intervals will allow appropriate monitoring. If the cyst enlarges or signs of gastrointestinal or urinary tract obstruction appear, then excision should be performed.

Careful dissection during surgical excision will frequently result in preservation of all or part of the ovary. Careful preservation of both ovary and fallopian tube vascularity is imperative. A multiloculated or layered ovarian cyst is a frequent finding with an intrauterine torsed ovary and/or ovarian necrosis and is an indication for abdominal exploration. Early removal of the dead tissue prevents subsequent sepsis. The fallopian tube can be involved and also requires excision. Pexis of the contralateral ovary is a controversial addition to the procedure.

Surgical Results/Prognosis   Excellent prognosis. Future reproduction is facilitated by retention of the involved ovary, but sterility is not a significant problem even if the ipsilateral ovary is removed.

REFERENCES

Adelman S, Benson CD, Hertzler JH: Surgical lesions of the ovary in infancy and childhood. Surg Gynecol Obstet 1975;141:219–226.

Ikeda K, Suita S, Nakano H: Management of ovarian cyst detected antenatally. J Pediatr Surg 1988;23:432–435.

Jafri SZ, Bree RL, Silver TM, Ouimette M: Fetal ovarian cysts: Sonographic detection and association with hypothyroidism. Radiology 1984;150:809–812.

Meizner I, Levy A, Katz M, et al: Fetal ovarian cysts: Prenatal ultrasonographic detection and postnatal evaluation and treatment. Am J Obstet Gynecol 1991;164:874–878.

Mizuno M, Kato T, Hebiguchi T, Yoshino H: Surgical indications for neonatal ovarian cysts. Tohoku J Exp Med 1998;186:27–32.

Nicolaides KH, Campbell S: Ultrasound diagnosis of congenital abnormalities. In Harrison MR, Golbus MS, Filly RA (eds): The Unborn Patient: Antenatal Diagnosis and Treatment. Philadelphia, WB Saunders, 1991, pp 595–648.

Nussbaum AR, Sanders RC, Benator RM, et al: Spontaneous resolution of neonatal ovarian cysts. Am J Roentgenol 1987;148:175–176.

Nussbaum AR, Sanders RC, Hartman DS, et al: Neonatal ovarian cysts: Sonographic-pathologic correlation. Radiology 1988;168:817–821.

Patten RM: The fetal genitourinary tract. Radiol Clin North Am 1990;28:115–130.

Rizzo N, Gabrielli S, Perolo A, et al: Prenatal diagnosis and management of fetal ovarian cysts. Prenat Diagn 1989;9:97–103.

Woo JS, Li DF, Wan MC, et al: Intrauterine cystocentesis: A simple procedure to relieve anatomic and physiologic dysfunction in the fetus. J Clin Ultrasound 1986;14:474–477.

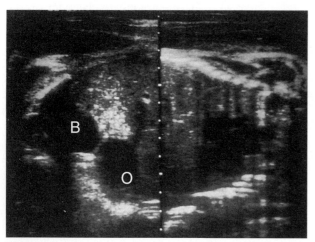

Coronal view of a female fetus with a cystic mass in the abdomen. Adjacent to the bladder (B) in a cyst (O). This echo-free cyst was treated conservatively after birth and disappeared spontaneously.

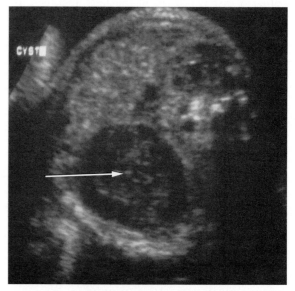

Transverse view of a fetus with a cyst anterior to the kidney. This cyst contains echogenic material. The fetus was a female, and long-term follow-up failed to show any resolution of the cyst, which at surgery proved to be a torsed ovarian cyst.

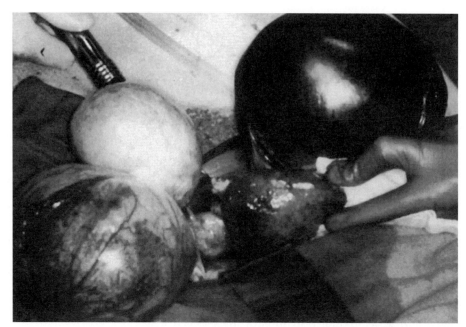

Newborn girl with massive ovarian bilateral cysts. The cyst on right side had torsion of the stalk and hemorrhagic necrosis.

4.11 Posterior Urethral Valves (PUV)

Epidemiology/Genetics

Definition Membrane-like valvular structures in the posterior urethra in a male infant that can result in urinary tract obstruction.

Epidemiology Undetermined, but rare. Unknown in females.

Embryology Posterior urethral valves are structures that normally develop in the prostatic urethra between 6 and 8 weeks of gestation. Hypertrophy of these valves causes proximal urethral distention, a thick-walled distended bladder, reflux, and hydronephrosis. Chromosome abnormalities, including trisomies 21, 13, and 18, have been reported in up to 20% of cases.

Inheritance Patterns Sporadic. Rare reports of familial recurrence.

Teratogens None.

Prognosis The prognosis is dependent on renal function. The overall mortality rate for antenatally diagnosed cases is 50%, but the mortality rate is 95% for those cases with oligohydramnios. Forty percent of neonatal survivors develop chronic renal failure.

Sonography

FINDINGS

1. **Fetus:** Only males are affected. There is a dilated, thick-walled bladder with "keyhole" posterior urethral expansion. There are three sonographic forms:
   a. The bladder occupies the entire abdomen and pushes up the diaphragm. The renal pelves may be only slightly distended. Signs of dysplastic kidney may be seen with echogenic parenchyma and possibly small cysts. No amniotic fluid is usual with this lethal form.
   b. Ascites may be present without other features of hydrops. With this form, the bladder may not be greatly enlarged, since it may have burst. There is usually moderate ureteropelvocalyceal dilation, sometimes with findings of dysplasia. No amniotic fluid is usual with this form.
   c. Moderately severe bladder dilation with dilated pelvocalyceal systems and tortuous ureters is the most common form. Obvious dysplastic changes (echogenic renal parenchyma with peripherally placed cysts) indicate a hopeless prognosis.
2. **Amniotic Fluid:** As the disease progresses, amniotic

fluid decreases. No fluid is almost always associated with pulmonary hypoplasia.
3. **Placenta:** Normal.
4. **Measurement Data:** A large abdomen, due to kidney enlargement and ascites, may be seen.
5. **When Detectable:** Posterior urethral valves have been detected as early as 11 weeks using the vaginal probe. Early presentations carry a stronger association with chromosome abnormalities and a worse prognosis. The disease usually presents at 18 to 22 weeks.

Pitfalls

1. Bilateral ureteropelvic junction obstruction or fullness with "full" bladder. The fetal bladder may not empty until the baby is born. This is a normal variant.
2. Be very cautious in the diagnosis of dysplasia if there are no cysts present. It is easy to overdiagnose echogenic parenchyma.
3. Dilated renal pelves and ureters and a thick-walled bladder with a "keyhole" notch may not relate to current obstruction. It is possible that urethral valves may have burst and left secondary obstructive consequences. This situation may be the origin of the Eagle-Barrett (prune belly) syndrome.

Differential Diagnosis

1. Megacystis megaureter syndrome—Also most often seen in males. This process is due to severe reflux. The bladder is enlarged but thin-walled with no keyhole urethra. The renal pelves vary in size, and the ureter shows much peristalsis.
2. Megacystis microcolon syndrome—Similar appearances to posterior urethral valves, but polyhydramnios may occur and this very rare entity is more frequent in females.

Where Else to Look

1. Look for signs of trisomy 21, 18, and 13.
2. Look for signs of dysplastic kidney—increased parenchymal echogenicity and peripherally placed small cysts—since dysplasia makes the prognosis hopeless.

Pregnancy Management

Investigations and Consultations Required Chromosome abnormalities are found in up to 20% of cases. Therefore, fetal karyotyping is essential. Fetal echocardiography should be performed to exclude associated heart defects. Pediatric urologic consultation is required to plan prenatal management.

Fetal Intervention Significant experience has been gained in this area. Generally, no intervention is appro-

164

priate if amniotic fluid volume remains normal. In pregnancies of 32 weeks' gestation or greater, decreasing amniotic fluid volume should prompt early delivery for ex utero drainage. In cases of less than 32 weeks' gestation, assessment of fetal renal function, by aspiration of bladder urine, should be performed. The analysis of urinary sodium, chloride, osmolality, and β_2-microglobulin should be done on "fresh" urine. An initial drainage of the fetal bladder should be followed in 3 to 7 days by a repeat aspiration. The criteria outlined by Crombleholme et al should be used to ascertain those fetuses with a good prognosis who may benefit from intervention, either by catheter drainage or by open fetal surgery. Fetuses with poor prognosis produce urine that is isotonic and subsequently become salt-wasters.

"Good" Prognostic Factors for Posterior Urethral Valves in Utero

Parameter	Finding
Sonography	No cortical cysts
	Normal echogenicity
Amniotic fluid analysis	
Na	<100 mEq/L
Cl	<90 mEq/L
Osm	<200 mEq/L
Ca	<8 mg/dL
Total protein	<20 mg/dL
β_2-microglobulin	<6 mg/L

Fetuses with a good prognosis treated with in utero decompression do not die of pulmonary hypoplasia at birth, but long-term prognosis for renal function is guarded. A significant proportion subsequently develop renal failure, and most children have had poor growth postnatally. Both catheter insertion and in utero vesicostomy carry a risk of chorioamnionitis and prematurity. Repeated shunt insertions may be required.

Monitoring   Ultrasonographic evaluation every 2 to 3 weeks should be performed to monitor amniotic fluid volume.

Pregnancy Course   Many examples of posterior urethral valves are recognizable as being so severe that the fetus cannot survive when the first sonogram is performed. In others, a steady reduction in amniotic fluid with the development of dysplastic kidneys makes it apparent that the condition is lethal. In still others, apparently normal kidneys with decreasing amniotic fluid compel drainage or early delivery. In some patients, the condition is mild and amniotic fluid volume is maintained.

No effect on the course of pregnancy is expected from the fetal condition. If the family chooses to continue a pregnancy in which the fetus has a poor prognosis, it is important to discuss with them that fetal assessment modalities are likely to produce abnormal results secondary to severe oligohydramnios. If the family requests ongoing fetal assessment, they must be informed of the high likelihood of operative delivery for a fetus that is unlikely to survive.

Pregnancy Termination Issues   Confirmation of the sonographic diagnosis should be done and requires pathologic examination of the intact fetus.

Delivery   The need for immediate neonatal evaluation and treatment and the potential for respiratory complications in cases with oligohydramnios require that delivery occur in a tertiary center.

Neonatology

Resuscitation   Respiratory distress is usually present secondary to pulmonary hypoplasia in infants with significant oligohydramnios. Use positive-pressure ventilation cautiously when pulmonary hypoplasia is suspected because of the high risk for pneumothorax. Onset of effective respiration may be impeded from abdominal distension secondary to bladder enlargement as well as renal enlargement.

Transport   Indicated for full confirmation of diagnosis and prognosis if the infant demonstrates survival potential.

Testing and Confirmation   Neonatal presentation depends on the severity and timing of the urethral obstruction. Very early and severe obstruction causes an oligohydramnios sequence with pulmonary hypoplasia and death. Severe early obstruction that is later relieved may cause a "prune belly." Milder or later obstruction is compatible with survival to birth. Presentations in the newborn period and early infancy include decreased urinary stream (25%), distended bladder (67%), urinary infection (50%), abdominal distention (30%), renal failure (33%), palpable kidneys (50%), and failure to thrive (50%).

Careful evaluation of renal function and structure by measurement of urine production, urinalysis, blood and urine chemistry studies, and an abdominal sonogram is appropriate. Voiding cystourethrogram, cystoscopy, and renal scan without and with diuretic stimulation may also be useful in confirming the diagnosis and assessing renal function.

Nursery Management   Support respiration, as necessary, to maintain adequate gas exchange.

Avoid fluid and protein loading initially until urinary tract patency and renal function have been determined.

Surgery

Preoperative Assessment   Dysplastic changes in the kidneys are assessed by a postdelivery sonogram and a DMSA (dimercaptosulfasuccinic acid) scan. A voiding cystourethrogram is obtained to be certain that the dilated bladder ureters and renal pelves are not caused by reflux.

Operative Indications   Surgical management is based on adequate resuscitation of the patient and decompression of the chronically obstructed bilateral upper urinary tracts and bladder. If the urethra is patent, early temporary catheter drainage is feasible.

Surgical repair is required to achieve bladder and upper tract decompression with prevention of further renal parenchymal damage.

Types of Procedures Drainage is best accomplished by vesicostomy, temporary loop cutaneous ureterostomies, or a pyelostomy. These procedures are usually planned dependent on the degree of lung hypoplasia and potential for pulmonary function. Milder forms of posterior urethral valve can be successfully treated by transurethral or open vesicostomy repair of the lesion with resection of the posterior urethral valves.

Surgical Results/Prognosis The degree of renal function is difficult to determine by radiographic contrast examination and is best assessed by nuclear renal scan technique. Potential renal function may appear to be insufficient, but early poor function can improve significantly after adequate decompression. Some patients have borderline renal function that becomes insufficient with subsequent skeletal growth and the need for dialysis and/or renal transplantation becomes apparent. Urethral bladder dysfunction, associated with posterior urethral valves, can have an adverse effect on the success of renal transplantation. Posterior urethral valves can be associated with prune belly syndrome with marginal early renal function. Incontinence occurs in approximately 14% to 38% of surviving patients. Over the long term, there is often impaired sexual function with a much higher incidence of undescended testes and impaired ejaculatory mechanism.

REFERENCES

Brock WA, Kaplan GW: Abnormalities of the lower tract. In Edelmann CM Jr (ed): Pediatric Kidney Disease. Boston, Little, Brown and Co, 1992, p 2037.

Crombleholme TM, Harrison MR, Golbus MS, et al: Fetal intervention in obstructive uropathy: Prognostic indicators and efficacy of intervention. Am J Obstet Gynecol 1990;162:1239–1244.

Favre R, Kohler M, Gasser B, et al: Early fetal megacystis between 11 and 15 weeks of gestation. Ultrasound Obstet Gynecol 1999;14:402–406.

Fitzsimmons RB, Keshane C, Gawin I: Prune belly syndrome with ultrasound demonstration of reduction of megacystis in utero. Br J Radiol 1985;58:374–376.

Freedman AL, Johnson MP, Smith CA, et al: Long-term outcome in children after antenatal intervention for obstructive uropathies. Lancet 1999;354:374–377.

Glazer GM, Filly RA, Callen PW: The varied sonographic appearance of the urinary tract in the fetus and newborn with urethral obstruction. Radiology 1982;144:563–568.

Henneberry MO, Stephens FD: Renal hypoplasia and dysplasia in infants with posterior urethral valves. J Urol 1980;123:912–915.

Hulbert WC, Duckett JW: Current views on posterior urethral valves. Pediatr Ann 1988;17:31–36.

Kaplan CW, Scherg HC: Intravesical obstruction in clinical pediatric urology. In Kelalis PP, King LR, Belman BA (eds): Clinical Pediatric Urology. Philadelphia, WB Saunders, 1992, pp 835–849.

Mahony BS: Fetal urethral obstruction: US evaluation. Radiology 1985;157:221–224.

Meizner I: Prenatal ultrasonic diagnosis of the extreme form of prune belly syndrome. J Clin Ultrasound 1985;13:581–583.

Paduano L, Giglio L, Bembi B, et al: Clinical outcome of fetal uropathy: I. Predictive value of prenatal echography positive for obstructive uropathy. J Urol 1991;146:1094–1096.

Paduano L, Giglio L, Bembi B, et al: Clinical outcome of fetal uropathy: II. Sensitivity of echography for prenatal detection of obstructive pathology. J Urol 1991;146:1097–1098.

Reinburg Y, Gongalez R, Fryd D, et al: The outcome of renal transplantation in children with posterior urethral valves. J Urol 1988;140:1491–1493.

Walsh DS, Johnson MP: Fetal intervention for obstructive urology. Semin Perinat 1999;23:484–495.

Washaw BL, Hymes LC, Trulack TS, et al: Prognostic features in infants with obstructive uropathy due to posterior urethral valves. J Urol 1985;133:240–242.

White SM, Chamberlain P, Hitchcock R, et al: Megacystis-microcolon-intestinal hypoperistalsis syndrome: The difficulties with antenatal diagnosis. Case report and review of the literature. Prenat Diagn 2000;20:697–700.

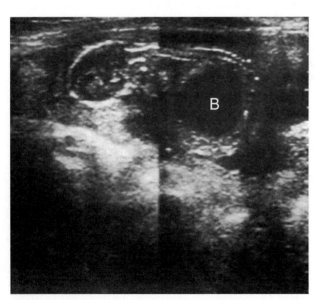

Sagittal view of a fetus with a huge bladder (B). The bladder is so large it compresses the chest. There is no amniotic fluid present. This type of posterior urethral valve is fatal.

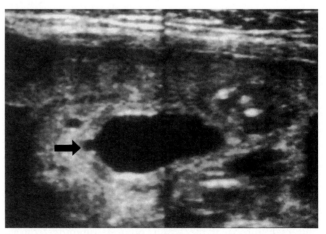

Sagittal view of lower fetal abdomen. There is a dilated bladder with a thick wall. A dilated proximal urethra can be seen, obstructed by posterior urethral valves (*arrow*). The kidneys and ureters were also dilated.

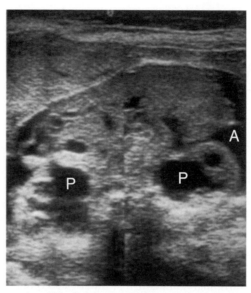

Transverse view of fetal abdomen. Both renal pelves (P) are markedly dilated, as are the calyces. The renal parenchyma is echogenic. There is fetal ascites (A) present within the fetal abdomen. No amniotic fluid is present between the fetal truck and the placenta. Posterior urethral valves were found at autopsy.

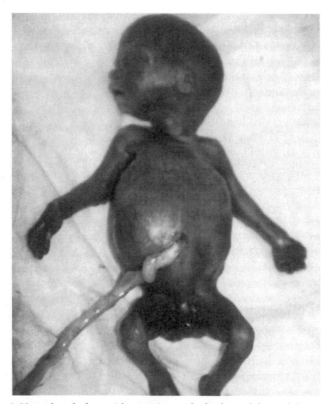

A 22-week male fetus with posterior urethral valves. Abdominal distention is due to massive hydronephrosis.

4.12 Renal Agenesis

Epidemiology/Genetics

Definition   Bilateral or unilateral absence of the kidneys.

Epidemiology   Unilateral renal agenesis occurs in 1 in 1000 births (M1:F1), and bilateral renal agenesis occurs in 12 in 100,000 births (M2.5:F1).

Embryology   The pathophysiology of this abnormality is unknown. Some cases of bilateral renal agenesis may represent the severe expression of an autosomal dominant gene whose effects include unilateral renal agenesis, double ureter, renal cysts, and hydronephrosis. Renal agenesis is associated with other genitourinary (50%), gastrointestinal, and cardiac abnormalities and is part of more that 50 multiple-malformation syndromes. Two birth defects associations, the VACTERL association and the MURCS association, have a high incidence of renal abnormalities, including renal agenesis.

Inheritance Patterns   Generally sporadic. Some cases may represent a highly variable autosomal dominant gene. Parents and siblings should have renal ultrasonograms looking for unilateral renal agenesis or other renal abnormalities that may suggest autosomal dominant inheritance.

Teratogens   Warfarin, cocaine, and maternal diabetes.

Prognosis   Forty percent of infants with bilateral renal agenesis are stillborn and the remainder die shortly after birth from respiratory or renal insufficiency. Unilateral renal agenesis may be asymptomatic and compatible with a normal life span. Girls with unilateral renal agenesis should have pelvic ultrasonograms looking for müllerian abnormalities.

Sonography

FINDINGS

1. **Fetus:**
   a. In bilateral renal agenesis, both kidneys are absent and the adrenal glands assume a discoid shape and move laterally and inferiorly. The bladder is apparently absent or is seen as an echopenic area.
   b. In unilateral renal agenesis, one kidney is absent. Other renal abnormalities such as reflux, vesicoureteric junction obstruction or ureteropelvic junction obstruction are found in 50% of patients with unilateral renal agenesis. Compensatory hypertrophy of the contralateral kidney develops.
2. **Amniotic Fluid:** There is no amniotic fluid after 15 to 18 weeks with bilateral renal agenesis.

3. **Placenta:** Normal.
4. **Measurement Data:** Since there are no kidneys with bilateral renal agenesis, there is a small trunk circumference. Limbs and head measurements are normal. There may be intrauterine growth retardation.
5. **When Detectable:** At 15 to 18 weeks.

Pitfalls

1. Absence of fluid makes the study difficult.
2. Confusion between adrenal glands and hypoplastic kidneys has often occurred, since, in utero, the adrenal glands are about one third the size of the kidneys and have an echogenic center.
3. With unilateral renal agenesis, make sure a pelvic kidney is not present.

Where Else to Look

1. Sirenomelia—Fused legs, with both femurs, tibia, and fibula alongside each other, is associated with renal agenesis. (See Chapter 4.16.)
2. Cardiac abnormalities may be found with unilateral renal agenesis.
3. Müllerian abnormalities such as hydrometrocolpos are associated with unilateral renal agenesis. (See Chapter 4.5.)
4. Renal agenesis is familial, so an examination of the parents' kidneys is recommended.

Pregnancy Management

Investigations and Consultations Required   Unilateral renal agenesis, if isolated, is not likely to be a marker for chromosome abnormalities. Fetal echocardiography should be performed to exclude associated congenital heart disease. Chromosomal analysis is appropriate for bilateral agenesis, since the condition is associated with trisomy 18, but may best be performed if termination is elected. In cases with either unilateral or bilateral renal agenesis, evaluation of parents' kidneys should be done to detect the families with autosomal dominant inheritance.

Fetal Intervention   An amnioinfusion procedure may be helpful in establishing the diagnosis. Injection of dextrose Ringer's solution (150 to 250 mL) into the amniotic space will improve fetal visualization and may show renal function. The fetus will start to drink, the stomach will fill, and bladder visualization with ultrasonography may be possible. Concomitant injection of indigo carmine may allow detection of premature rupture of membranes. A vaginal tampon will be stained blue. A false-positive diagnosis of premature rupture of membranes can occur if solution is placed in the extra-amniotic space.

Monitoring   No change in obstetric care is indicated for unilateral renal agenesis. For the pregnancy in which the fetus has bilateral renal agenesis, no further fetal assessment or monitoring is appropriate. Supportive care of the family should be provided.

Pregnancy Course   No specific obstetric complications are to be expected with unilateral lesions.

Pregnancy Termination Issues   Bilateral renal agenesis may be a component of multiple malformation syndromes. Therefore, a complete evaluation of an intact fetus should be done.

Delivery   No special precautions are necessary for the fetus with unilateral disease. For bilateral renal agenesis, vaginal delivery without electronic fetal monitoring in labor is appropriate.

Neonatology

Resuscitation   The majority of newborns with renal agenesis manifest severe respiratory distress from birth secondary to associated severe pulmonary hypoplasia. Use positive pressure cautiously, as the risk for pneumothorax is high. Early cessation of resuscitative efforts should be discussed with the parents prior to delivery, as this is a uniformly lethal condition.

Transport   Rarely an issue, as survival time is usually limited to hours, even with ventilatory support. In the occasional infant with mixed agenesis/dysplasia, the respiratory insufficiency may be adequately controlled with ventilatory assistance. In that circumstance, transport is indicated for confirmation of diagnosis and prognosis.

Testing and Confirmation   A postnatal renal sonogram will confirm the absence of kidneys.

Nursery Management   Continuing ventilatory support, even with severe respiratory failure, until diagnostic confirmation, determination of associated abnormalities, and parental counseling is completed, is appropriate. At present, there is no palliative or curative treatment for complete renal agenesis. Prolonged renal dialysis has not been successful.

REFERENCES

Bernstein J: Renal hypoplasias and dysplasia. In Edelmann CM Jr (ed): Pediatric Kidney Disease. Boston, Little, Brown, 1992, p 1121.

Cascio S, Paran S, Puri P: Associated urological anomalies in children with unilateral renal agenesis. J Urol 1999;162:1081–1083.

Dubbins PA, Kurtz AB, Wapner RJ, Goldberg BB: Renal agenesis: Spectrum of in utero findings. J Clin Ultrasound 1981;9:189–193.

Gillerot Y, Koulischer L: Major malformations of the urinary tract: Anatomic and genetic aspects. Biol Neonate 1988;53:186–196.

Hoffman CK, Filly RA, Callen PW: The lying down adrenal sign: A sonographic indicator of renal agenesis or ectopia in fetuses and neonates. J Ultrasound Med 1992;11:533–536.

Potter EL: Bilateral absence of ureters and kidneys: A report of 50 cases. Obstet Gynecol 1965;25:3–12.

Robson WL, Leung AK, Rogers RC: Unilateral renal agenesis. Adv Pediatr 1995;42:575–592.

Romero R, Cullen M, Grannum P, et al: Antenatal diagnosis of renal anomalies with ultrasound. III. Bilateral renal agenesis. Am J Obstet Gynecol 1985;151:38–43.

Roodhooft AM, Birnholz JC, Holmes LB: Familial nature of congenital absence and severe dysgenesis of both kidneys. N Engl J Med 1984;310:1341–1345.

Sepulveda W, Corral E, Sanchez J, et al: Sirenomelia sequence versus renal agenesis: Prenatal differentiation with power doppler ultrasound. Ultrasound Obstet Gynecol 1998;11:445–449.

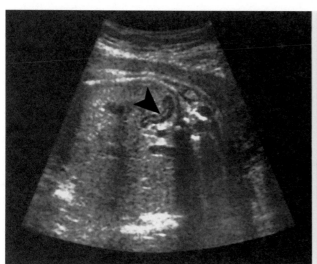
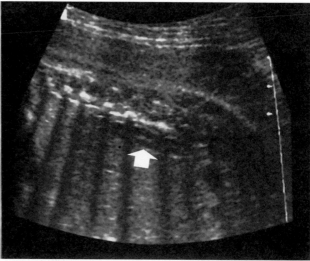

Sonogram of renal agenesis, transverse and longitudinal views. There is no amniotic fluid. The adrenal gland (*arrows*) has assumed a discoid shape and moved laterally. Since at this stage of life the adrenal gland has an echogenic center, it can be mistaken for a small kidney.

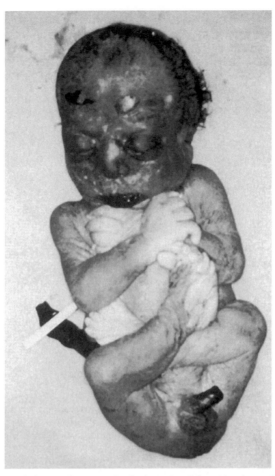

A 34-week fetus with severe oligohydramnios deformities due to bilateral renal agenesis.

4.13 Sacrococcygeal Teratoma

Epidemiology/Genetics

Definition Teratomas are tumors that are derived from totipotent cells and include embryonic ectodermal, endodermal, and mesodermal tissue derivatives. Commonly, gastrointestinal, respiratory, and nervous system tissue elements are present.

Epidemiology One in 40,000 births (M1:F3).

Embryology Teratomas occur most often in a para-axial, gonadal, or midline location from the brain to the sacral area. Primary sites in infants and children include sacrococcyx (60%), gonads (20%), and chest and abdomen (15%). Sacrococcygeal teratomas are the most common tumors presenting at birth. Forty-seven percent of the tumors are external, 34% are external with a significant presacral component, and 19% are predominantly, or completely, presacral.

Inheritance Patterns Generally sporadic. Rare families with autosomal dominant presacral teratomas and sacral dysgenesis have been reported.

Teratogens None.

Prognosis Diagnosis at an earlier gestational age, development of hydrops, and premature delivery predict a poor outcome with approximately 10% survival for cases diagnosed before 30 weeks' gestation. Cases diagnosed later have a reported 75% survival rate.

Sonography

FINDINGS

1. **Fetus:**
   a. There is a mass arising from the distal spine and rump area, which may be cystic or solid, or a mixture of both. Calcification is often present. There is almost always a large external component and there may be an intrapelvic component. The mass may grow to a huge size; it may be larger than the fetal trunk. MRI may be helpful in determining the extent of the mass and confirming mass presence when sonography is difficult to perform due to fetal position or maternal size.
   b. Secondary hydronephrosis and ureterectasis often develop if there is an intrapelvic component. The bladder is elevated by the intrapelvic component. Secondary gut dilation may also occur.
   c. Considerable atrioventricular shunting occurs through vascular solid masses, and there may be

secondary hydrops with ascites and skin thickening. A lethal outcome is more likely with this form. High output failure may be detected early by increased inferior vena cava diameter or increased descending aortic flow velocity.
2. **Amniotic Fluid:** Severe polyhydramnios is virtually always present and may be the presenting problem. Severe polyhydramnios almost always results in premature delivery.
3. **Placenta:** Frequently normal, but placentomegaly occurs if there is high output failure.
4. **Measurement Data:** Intrauterine growth retardation may develop.
5. **When Detectable:** The mass is usually visible by 18 weeks, but it may present later.

Pitfalls

1. The mass develops first between the legs, so it may be missed when it is small.
2. The teratoma may have a similar texture to a fibroid, with which it has been confused.

Differential Diagnosis

1. Anterior and posterior myelo-meningoceles widen the spine, whereas teratomas destroy the spine.
2. Fetus in fetu. A complex mass in which there is an echogenic complex surrounded by fluid may represent a fetus in fetu. In this variant form of monozygotic twinning, an aberrant symmetric twin becomes internalized within the other twin. Fetal heart motion may be seen.

Where Else to Look Secondary bladder and kidney dilation, due to obstruction, may occur and may result in renal dysplasia. Arteriovenous shunts within the teratoma may cause heart failure and fetal hydrops.

Pregnancy Management

Investigations and Consultations Required No specific associated abnormalities are known, but the high likelihood that intervention may be necessary mandates that other life-threatening abnormalities be excluded. Chromosomal analysis and fetal echocardiography should be performed. It should be noted that the amniotic fluid alpha-fetoprotein level may be elevated and acetylcholinesterase may be present in cases of sacrococcygeal teratoma. Amniotic fluid analysis will not help differentiate sacrococcygeal teratoma from myelomeningocele.

Fetal Intervention In cases diagnosed prior to 32 weeks' gestation in which polyhydramnios, placentomegaly, and/or fetal hydrops develop, prognosis is dismal. This small subset of fetuses (less than 20% of cases) should be referred to a center with expertise in in utero resection, which has been successful in a limited number of cases to date. Investigation is underway to treat the disorder by sonographically controlled interruption of the vascular supply to the mass, using radiofrequency ablation. In cases in which the disorder includes maternal preeclampsia in utero, treatment has failed to reverse the maternal condition, and these cases are not candidates for fetal surgery. Fetuses at 32 weeks who develop hydrops should be delivered for ex utero therapy.

Monitoring   Serial sonograms should be performed every 1 to 2 weeks to assess (1) size of the mass, which may grow rapidly; (2) kidneys and bladder for evidence of obstruction; (3) gastrointestinal tract for evidence of obstruction; (4) amniotic fluid volume for evidence of polyhydramnios; and (5) fetus for early signs of hydrops. The patient herself should be monitored for early signs of preeclampsia.

The presence of polyhydramnios may increase the risk of preterm labor, and regular assessment is necessary.

Pregnancy Course   Large lesions with predominantly solid components are associated with an increased risk for fetal hydrops, preeclampsia, and polyhydramnios.

Pregnancy Termination Issues   A precise diagnosis is essential for counseling regarding recurrence risk. Therefore, the method of termination should result in an intact fetus for a complete pathologic examination.

Delivery   The significant risk of maternal and neonatal complications necessitates delivery in a tertiary center. Because of the significant risk of hemorrhage, moderately sized (greater than 4.5 cm) and large lesions should prompt cesarean delivery to avoid dystocia. The section should be performed when fetal lung maturity is present or sooner if early evidence of hydrops is present. There appears to be no benefit from in utero decompression of cystic components of the mass to facilitate vaginal delivery.

Neonatology

Resuscitation   Assistance with onset of respiration is usually not required, unless the infant is premature and/or fetal hydrops is present.

Extreme care must be taken with the tumor mass, as tears of surface vessels can result in life-threatening hemorrhage. Support the mass to avoid torsion if there is a "stalk." Cover the mass with a warm, moist sterile dressing to minimize heat and water loss if the surface is thin and membranous.

Transport   Transfer to a tertiary care center is always indicated. Extreme care must be taken to avoid trauma to the mass, insensible water loss, and surface contamination. Reliable venous access should be established and adequate blood pressure documented before beginning transport.

Testing and Confirmation   Postnatally, an elevated serum alpha-fetoprotein level is highly correlated with malignancy.

Diagnostic evaluation should include imaging (CT or MRI scan) to determine, preoperatively, the extent of the lesion internally. Bedside sonography may be helpful in outlining the extent of the tumor, its relationship to other pelvic structures, and associated involvement of the genitourinary structures.

Nursery Management   Maintain thermal balance.

Maintain perfusion with volume expanders, packed red blood cells, and fluid and electrolytes. Parenteral nutrition may be required for protracted periods if the mass involves the distal alimentary tract or the course is complicated.

Systemic antibiotics may be indicated, preoperatively, and through the early recovery period, after surgical excision.

Surgery

Preoperative Assessment   Acute management includes evaluation of the extent of the intraperitoneal presacral portion of the tumor. Diagnostic studies should include serum levels of alpha-fetoprotein for a possible malignant component and sonography to determine the degree of presacral and intraperitoneal extension. A decision is then made about whether to use an abdominal approach to obtain control of the primary feeding vessels of the tumor, the middle sacral arteries, before attempting a perineal excision.

The acute preoperative complications of a large sacrococcygeal teratoma are cardiac failure due to atrioventricular shunting in the tumor, renal failure due to bilateral ureteral obstruction, and hemorrhage secondary to intraperitoneal, retroperitoneal, or surface necrotic tumor with bleeding.

If there is no high output state, then there is no urgency to resection of the tumor and attention should focus on the treatment of respiratory distress and correction of anemia. Delayed excision can predispose to sepsis because of the necrotic tumor, however. If a hyperdynamic state exists with elevated cardiac output, attention should focus on supporting the newborn heart with inotropic agents and urgent resection of the sacrococcygeal teratoma. The goal of this resection is reversal of the high output state, and this can usually be accomplished by resection of the exophytic portion of the tumor. Aortic occlusion by vessel loop may be used to minimize hemorrhage when resecting a sacrococcygeal teratoma in a severely premature infant. If residual pelvic extent of tumor remains, the urgency of resection can be guided by the pathologic lesion. The presence of yolk sac differentiation would necessitate earlier resection. In the absence of yolk sac differentiation, however, several months of growth of the infant can facilitate subsequent resection of the coccyx and the intrapelvic portion of the tumor.

Operative Indications   Surgical excision is always required but can be delayed to allow completion of the diagnostic evaluation, unless serious hemorrhaging is present.

Types of Procedures   Most tumors can be excised from the perineal approach, but blood loss can be great and preparations for adequate replacement are essential. Careful dissection and preservation of the thinned gluteal muscles over the tumor, excision of the coccyx, and reconstruction of the levator sling are very important to a good functional outcome. Extension into the dural space is rare but can occur.

Surgical Results/Prognosis   Survival after successful excision is excellent. Intraoperative mortality can approach 5% to 10% depending on tumor and patient size. A malignancy occurs in approximately 10% of the newborn infants with sacrococcygeal teratomas and can be totally excised in most patients. Secondary operations for retained benign teratoma are uncommon if a total coccygectomy is performed. The malignant germ cell tumors that commonly occur in sacrococcygeal teratomas are usually responsive to new chemotherapy modalities. A major long-term disability is stool and urinary incontinence in patients who have had neurologic impairment due to the pressure of very large sacrococcygeal teratomas. The incidence of this condition is as high as 25% in some series.

REFERENCES

Adzick NS, Crombleholme TM, Morgan MA, Quinn TM: A rapidly growing fetal teratoma. Lancet 1997;349:538.

Albanese CT, Harrison MR: Surgical treatment for fetal disease: The state of the art. Ann N Y Acad Sci 1998;847:74–85.

Altman RP, Randolph JG, Lilly JR: Sacrococcygeal teratoma: American Academy of Pediatrics Surgical Section Survey—1973. J Pediatr Surg 1974;9:389–398.

Billmire DF, Grosfeld JL: Teratomas in childhood: Analysis of 142 cases. J Pediatr Surg 1986;21:548–551.

Chervenak FA, Isaacson G, Touloukian R, et al: Diagnosis and management of fetal teratomas. Obstet Gynecol 1985;66:666–671.

Chisholm CA, Heider AL, Kuller JA, et al: Prenatal diagnosis and perinatal management of fetal sacrococcygeal teratoma. Am J Perinatol 1999;16:89–92.

Gross SJ, Benzie RJ, Sermer M, et al: Sacrococcygeal teratoma: Prenatal diagnosis and management. Am J Obstet Gynecol 1987;156:393–396.

Herrmann ME, Thompson K, Wojcik EM, et al: Congenital sacrococcygeal teratomas: Effect of gestational age on size, morphologic pattern, ploidy, p53, and ret expression. Pediatr Dev Pathol 2000;3:240–248.

Holterman AX, Filiatrault D, Lallier M, Youssef S: The natural history of sacrococcygeal teratomas diagnosed through routine obstetric sonogram: A single institution experience. J Pediatr Surg 1998;33:899–903.

Holzgreve W, Mahony BS, Glick PL, et al: Sonographic demonstration of fetal sacrococcygeal teratoma. Prenat Diagn 1985;5:245–257.

Irving IM: Sacrococcygeal teratoma. In Lister J, Irving IM (eds): Neonatal Surgery, 3rd ed. London, Butterworths, 1990, pp 142–151.

Kay S, Khalife S, Laberge JM, et al: Prenatal percutaneous needle drainage of cystic sacrococcygeal teratomas. J Pediatr Surg 1999;34:1148–1151.

Langer JC, Harrison MR, Schmidt KG, et al: Fetal hydrops and death from sacrococcygeal teratoma: Rationale for fetal surgery. Am J Obstet Gynecol 1989;160:1145–1150.

Lockwood C, Ghidini A, Romero R, Hobbins JC: Fetal bowel perforation simulating sacrococcygeal teratoma. J Ultrasound Med 1988;7:227–229.

Milan DF, Cartwright PC, Snow BW, et al: Urologic manifestations of sacrococcygeal teratoma. J Urol 1993;149:574–576.

Mintz MC, Mennuti M, Fishman M: Prenatal aspiration of sacrococcygeal teratoma. Am J Roentgenol 1983;141:367–368.

Nastanski F, Downey EC: Fetus in fetu: A rare cause of a neonatal mass. Ultrasound Obstet Gynecol 2001;18:72–75.

Sheth S, Nussbaum AR, Sanders RC, et al: Prenatal diagnosis of sacrococcygeal teratoma: Sonographic-pathologic correlation. Radiology 1988;169:131–136.

Teal LN, Angtuaco TL, Jimenez JF, Quirk JG Jr: Fetal teratomas: Antenatal diagnosis and clinical management. J Clin Ultrasound 1988;16:329–336.

Westerburg B, Feldstein VA, Sandberg PL, et al: Sonographic prognostic factors in fetuses with sacrococcygeal teratoma. J Pediatr Surg 2000;35:322–325.

Woolley MM: Teratomas. In Ashcraft K, Holder T (eds): Pediatric Surgery. Philadelphia, WB Saunders, 1993, pp 847–862.

Yates VD, Wilroy RS, Whitington GL, Simmons JC: Anterior sacral defects: An autosomal dominantly inherited condition. J Pediatr 1983;102:239–242.

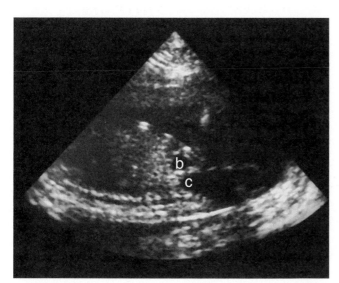

Small mostly cystic teratoma (c) elevating the bladder (b). Although the baby was premature, the mass was successfully removed. The child was left with fecal incontinence.

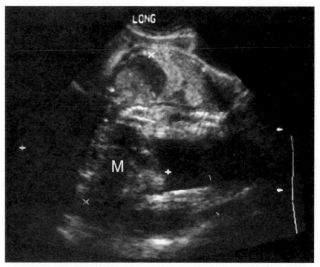

Large sacrococcygeal trauma teratoma with intrapelvic and extraabdominal compenents (between the x's). The entire mass (M) is solid. The fetus was stillborn and premature.

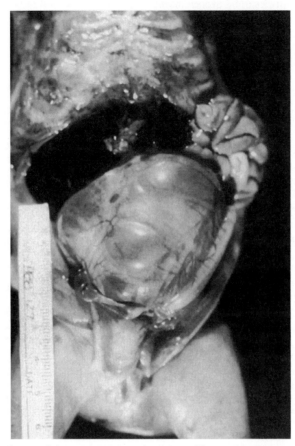

Newborn with large sacrococcygeal teratoma. Photograph shows massive intra-abdominal portion of the tumor.

4.14 Sirenomelia

Epidemiology/Genetics

Definition   Partial or complete fusion and/or severe deformity of the lower extremities frequently associated with renal agenesis, oligohydramnios, and anogenital anomalies.

Epidemiology   One to 4 in 100,000 (M3:F1).

Embryology   The pathogenesis is probably heterogeneous. Some cases may represent the severe end of the caudal regression spectrum, while a more recent theory has suggested a vascular pathogenesis resulting from a vitelline arterial steal, resulting in diversion of blood flow from caudal structures.

Inheritance Patterns   All cases have been sporadic. The incidence in monozygotic twins is increased 100 to 150 times.

Teratogens   Thalidomide.

Prognosis   Essentially lethal in all cases. Rare reports of mild cases in infants with good renal function who have survived the newborn period.

Sonography

FINDINGS

1. **Fetus:**
   a. There are fusion and severe deformities of the lower extremities (mermaid syndrome). The two legs may lie adjacent and be fused to each other with both feet present (sympus dipus), formed into one thicker than normal limb, or there may be a single leg which may be complete or incomplete (symelia, or sympus apus). In symelia unipus, up to 10 toes are derived from one foot. In symelia dipus, two distinct feet are seen arising from one lower limb.
   b. The spine is shortened and deformed with abnormal and absent vertebrae. A meningomyelocele may be present.
   c. The pelvic bones may be partially absent.
   d. There is either bilateral renal agenesis or bilateral dysplastic kidneys with small cysts. No bladder is present. Genitalia are either absent or ambiguous.
   e. Esophageal atresia, abdominal wall defects, and cardiac anomalies may be present.
   f. A two-vessel cord with a single large vitelline artery replacing the two umbilical arteries is usually present.
   g. There is an imperforate anus.
2. **Amniotic Fluid:** There is severe oligohydramnios or anhydramnios. If the diagnosis is made before about 18 weeks, some amniotic fluid will be present.
3. **Placenta:** Normal.
4. **Measurement Data:** Normal.
5. **When Detectable:** At about 19 weeks.

Pitfalls   Diagnosis is difficult because of the absence of amniotic fluid. The abnormal lower extremities are often overlooked. The two fused lower extremities never separate over prolonged observation. MRI may be a worthwhile follow-up procedure in confusing cases.

Differential Diagnosis

1. Renal agenesis—Since the limbs are so difficult to see, owing to the oligo/anhydramnios, the lower spine abnormalities and the arterial changes may be the clue to the presence of sirenomelia.
2. Caudal regression—There is a normal amount of amniotic fluid, both lower limbs are present, and both umbilical arteries are present (sirenomelia is considered by some practitioners to be the most severe form of caudal regression).

Where Else to Look   Look for the other features of the VACTERL syndrome to which this syndrome is related.

Pregnancy Management

Investigations and Consultations Required   Mother should have glucose tolerance testing to exclude diabetes mellitus, although it is considered to be a rare cause of true sirenomelia. Fetal echocardiography should be performed, as cardiac defects are common.

Fetal Intervention   Not appropriate in this lethal condition.

Monitoring   Maternal status should be monitored in standard fashion. Fetal evaluation is not appropriate because emergency intervention is not indicated.

Pregnancy Course   Oligohydramnios is seen in all cases.

Pregnancy Termination Issues   Oligohydramnios may make a precise diagnosis difficult. In many cases, delivery of an intact fetus may be necessary to ensure that correct counseling information can be given for subsequent pregnancies.

Delivery   Electronic fetal monitoring and cesarean section are contraindicated, given the lethal nature of this condition.

Neonatology

Resuscitation   Given a uniformly lethal prognosis, resuscitation is not indicated.

Transport   Not a consideration given the prognosis.

Testing and Confirmation   Careful physical examination complemented by detailed postmortem examination will confirm the spectrum of abnormalities.

Nursery Management   In the rare circumstance of fetal survival beyond delivery, warmth, hygiene, and comfort measures only are indicated. Support for parental grieving and genetic counseling for future pregnancies are essential.

REFERENCES

Brookshire-Quinn C, Jeanty P: Prenatal sonographic detection of symelic bipodia sirenomelia. J Diagn Med Sonogr 1990;2:103–105.

Chenoweth CK, Kellogg SJ, Abu-Yousef MM: Antenatal sonographic diagnosis of sirenomelia. J Clin Ultrasound 1991;19:167–171.

Fitzmorris-Glass R, Mattrey RF, Cantrell CJ: Magnetic resonance imaging as an adjunct to ultrasound in oligohydramnios: Detection of sirenomelia. J Ultrasound Med 1989;8:159–162.

Honda N, Shimokawa H, Yamaguchi Y, et al: Antenatal diagnosis of sirenomelia (sympus apus). J Clin Ultrasound 1988;16:675–677.

Raabe RD, Harnsberger HR, Lee TG, Mukuno DH: Ultrasonographic antenatal diagnosis of "mermaid syndrome": Fusion of fetal lower extremities. J Ultrasound Med 1983;2:463–464.

Sepulveda W, Corral E, Sanchez J, et al: Sirenomelia sequence versus renal agenesis: Prenatal differentiation with power Doppler ultrasound. Ultrasound Obstet Gynecol 1998;11:445–449.

Sepulveda W, Romero R, Pryde PG, et al: Prenatal diagnosis of sirenomelus with color Doppler ultrasonography. Am J Obstet Gynecol 1994;170:1377–1379.

Sirtori M, Ghidini A, Romero R, et al: Prenatal diagnosis of sirenomelia. J Ultrasound Med 1989;8:83–88.

Stocker JT, Heifetz SA: Sirenomelia: A morphological study of 33 cases and review of the literature. Perspect Pediat Pathol 1987;10:7.

Twickler D, Budorick N, Pretorius D, et al: Caudal regression versus sirenomelia: Sonographic clues. J Ultrasound Med 1993;12:323.

Valenzano M, Paoletti R, Rossi A, et al: Sirenomelia: Pathological features, antenatal ultrasonographic clues, and a review of current embryogenic theories. Hum Reprod Update 1999;5:82–86.

Van Zalen-Sprock MM, Van Vugt JMG, Van Der Harten J, et al: Early second-trimester diagnosis of sirenomelia. Prenat Diagn 1995;15:171–177.

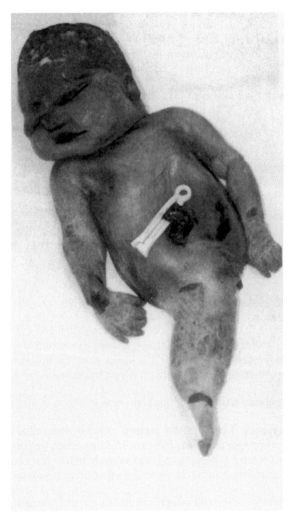

A 32-week stillborn with sirenomelia and the features of the oligohydramnios sequence.

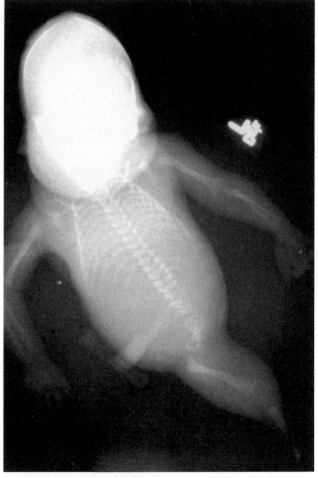

Radiograph of 32-week stillborn with sirenomelia showing abnormal pelvis and lower extremity.

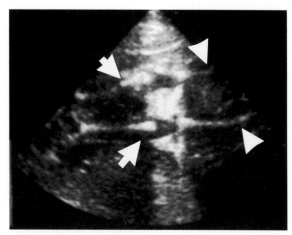

Fetus with sirenomelia. *Arrowheads* show the femur and *arrows* point to the tibia. The legs are too close together and did not change in position. Note the absent amniotic fluid. (Courtesy of Sheila Sheth, MD, Johns Hopkins Hospital.)

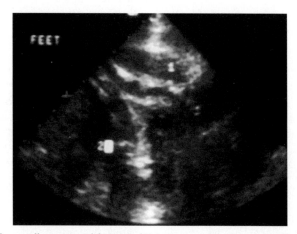

Abnormally positioned feet (1 and 2) in sirenomelia. (Courtesy of Sheila Sheth, MD, Johns Hopkins Hospital.)

4.15 Ureterocele

Epidemiology/Genetics

Definition   A ureterocele is a cystic dilation of the intravesicular portion of the ureter.

Epidemiology   One in 5000 births (M1:F5).

Embryology   Ureteroceles are most frequently associated with the upper pole ureter in a duplicated collecting system. The portion of the kidney served by the accessory ureter is usually small and dysplastic, possibly as a result of obstruction. Approximately 10% to 20% of cases are bilateral.

Inheritance Patterns   Sporadic, although rare families showing dominant inheritance have been reported.

Teratogens   None.

Screening   None.

Prognosis   If found as an isolated defect with good renal function, the prognosis for surgical correction is excellent.

Sonography

FINDINGS

1. **Fetus:**
   a. Kidney—If associated with a double collecting system (75% of cases), there will usually be a dilated upper pole collecting system. The lower pole of the kidneys may well be intermittently dilated due to reflux. With a simple ureterocele, there is unilateral hydronephrosis.
   b. Ureters—Ureteric dilation is usual. The ureter may well be very tortuous and is sometimes the most pronounced feature. The ureters may end alongside the bladder in an ectopic location rather than within the bladder as ureteroceles.
   c. Bladder—A crescent-shaped line will be seen at the base of the bladder. Two semicircles in the bladder are sometimes seen, since there are often bilateral ureteroceles. The bladder may be large if the ureterocele interferes with voiding (a "windsock ureterocele"), and the contralateral renal unit may be secondarily obstructed.
2. **Amniotic Fluid:** Normal, unless renal function is impaired, resulting in oligohydramnios.
3. **Placenta:** Normal.
4. **Measurement Data:** Normal.
5. **When Detectable:** At about 15 weeks.

Pitfalls   The umbilical arteries, as they pass alongside of the bladder, can be mistaken for ureteroceles. Color flow Doppler sonography will show the difference.

Differential Diagnosis

1. Posterior urethral valves—The typical "keyhole" dilated urethra, at the base of the bladder, will be seen. The bladder wall will be thick. The kidneys will probably show evidence of dysplasia.
2. Reflux—The ureters will vary in size. No ureterocele will be seen.

Where Else to Look   If a ureterocele is seen in the bladder, look for a second collecting system. Make sure there is no evidence of dysplasia in the obstructed segment.

Pregnancy Management

Investigations and Consultations Required   The diagnosis will be made most commonly because of hydronephrosis. Therefore, the evaluation should include chromosome analysis and fetal echocardiography. Pediatric urologic consultation should be obtained.

Fetal Intervention   In the rare case in which ureterocele mimics the picture of posterior urethral valves with oligohydramnios, bladder decompression may be indicated. A single needle aspiration may be both diagnostic and therapeutic.

Monitoring   No change in obstetric care is indicated. Serial ultrasonographic examinations monthly may be helpful in detecting the rare case in which the obstruction results in oligohydramnios.

Pregnancy Course   No obstetric complications should be expected.

Pregnancy Termination Issues   Ureterocele should not be an indication for pregnancy termination.

Delivery   In cases with significant obstruction, there is a need for immediate neonatal evaluation to establish a diagnosis and delivery should be in a tertiary center

Neonatology

Resuscitation   Usually not an issue. Onset of effective respiration may be impeded by abdominal distension secondary to renal enlargement. Intubation and ventilation may be required, at least initially.

Transport Transport is indicated if the condition is associated with renal enlargement, particularly bilateral, for confirmation of diagnosis and establishment of care plan, including surgical intervention. Isolated unilateral lesions and normal renal function, as indicated by serum creatinine level, can be referred for outpatient evaluation and management.

Testing and Confirmation Ureteroceles usually present with urinary infection in infants and children. Very large ureteroceles can cause bladder neck obstruction, and they are the most common cause of bladder obstruction in females. Large ureteroceles can also disrupt the anatomy of the contralateral ureter and cause reflux.

Careful staged evaluation of renal function and structure by measurement of urine production, urinalysis, blood and urine chemistry studies, and an abdominal sonogram is appropriate. If the infant is minimally symptomatic and immediate relief of obstruction is not required, imaging can be delayed for 24 to 36 hours for better visualization. If the anatomy is not clearly defined prenatally, or immediate relief of obstruction is required, sonographic imaging should be obtained immediately. Subsequent procedures will be contingent on the specific lesion suspected, that is, voiding cystourethrogram, cystoscopy, renal scan without and with diuretic stimulation, and/or abdominal CT.

Nursery Management Support respiration as necessary to maintain adequate gas exchange.

Avoid fluid and protein loading initially until urinary tract patency and renal function have been determined.

Surgery

Preoperative Assessment A sonographic assessment of the dilated upper pole and ureter serving the ureterocele is essential. Also, a functional scan showing the function of the upper pole is helpful to assess whether the upper pole can be saved.

Operative Indications A small ureterocele may not cause upper tract dilation, but all those discovered in utero so far have caused significant urinary back-up and have required drainage.

Type of Procedures An upper pole nephrectomy with partial ureterectomy is effective in over 60% of cases. Lately, there has been a resurgence in interest in transurethral incision of the ureterocele followed by an interval to see whether there is improvement in upper pole function.

Surgical Results/Prognosis The surgical prognosis is good. Damage to the lower pole of the kidney following an upper pole heminephrectomy can occur. The small size of the renal units increases the technical difficulty of the surgery.

Possible Surgical Complications

1. Incontinence secondary to sphincter damage if the ureterocele is excised from the bladder neck area.

2. Reflux secondary to transurethral incision of the ureterocele causing urinary tract infections may necessitate removal of the remaining renal unit.

REFERENCES

Austin PF, Cain MP, Casale AJ, et al: Prenatal bladder outlet obstruction secondary to ureterocele. Urology 1998;52:1132–1135.

Brock WA, Kaplan GW: Abnormalities of the lower tract. In Edelmann CM Jr (ed): Pediatric Kidney Disease. Boston, Little, Brown, 1992, p 2037.

Caione P, Zaccara A, Capozza N, De Gennaro M: How prenatal ultrasound can affect the treatment of ureterocele in neonates and children. Eur Urol 1989;16:195–199.

Garmel SH, Crombleholme TM, Cendron M, et al: The vanishing fetal ureterocele: A cause for concern? Prenat Diagn 1996;16:354–356.

Lefebvre O, Baumer H, Aubert J: Familial form of ureterocele with double ureter: 2 sisters and their father. Prog Urol 1999;9:747–749.

Patten RM: The fetal genitourinary tract. Radiol Clin North Am 1990; 28:115–130.

Vergani P, Ceruti P, Locatelli A, et al: Accuracy of prenatal ultrasonographic diagnosis of duplex renal system. J Ultrasound Med 1999;18:463–467.

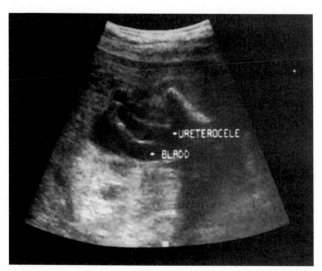

Sagittal view of the pelvic area of a prone fetus. A ureterocele can be seen impinging on the bladder (BLADD).

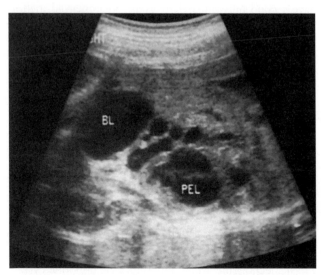

Sagittal sonographic view of the dilated renal pelvis (PEL) and the bladder (BL) in the same case. The cystic areas between the bladder and the pelvis represent portions of the tortuous dilated ureter.

5 Chest

5.1 Cystic Adenomatoid Malformation of the Lung (CCAM)

Epidemiology/Genetics

Definition Cystic adenomatoid malformations are benign hamartomatous or dysplastic lung tumors characterized by overgrowth of terminal bronchioles.

Epidemiology Unknown, but presumed rare (M1:F1).

Embryology Cystic adenomatoid malformations develop during the first 6 weeks of gestation. They are generally unilateral and classified into macrocystic (type I), mixed (type II), or microcystic (type III) forms. There is a 26% incidence of associated malformations, including pectus excavatum, hydrops, and renal agenesis.

Inheritance Patterns Sporadic.

Teratogens None.

Prognosis The majority of patients with cystic adenomatoid malformations of the lung detected antenatally have a good outcome. Many cystic adenomatoid malformations of the lung regress in utero. Others can be successfully resected and supported in modern neonatal intensive care units with normal outcomes. Early hydrops may be associated with a lethal prognosis.

Sonography

FINDINGS

1. **Fetus:**
   a. A mass is present within the lung, which is categorized by appearance into three types. In all forms, color flow Doppler sonography will show a normal blood supply from the pulmonary arteries.

   Type I (macrocystic)—Variably sized and shaped large cysts (2–10 cm) with thin intervening echogenic areas. There may be only one cyst.

   Type II (mixed)—Small to moderate-sized cysts with adjacent echogenic areas.

   Type III (microcystic)—Echogenic areas in the fetal lungs. Fetal hydrops is more common with this form.

   b. All three types may displace the fetal heart or diaphragm. With more sizable masses, fetal ascites and hydrops may be seen. The presence of hydrops makes a lethal outcome likely unless in utero surgery is performed or the lesion is cystic and can be aspirated in utero. Polyhydramnios is another sign suggesting poor outlook and is considered by some practitioners to be an indication for shunt insertion.

2. **Amniotic Fluid:** Polyhydramnios is seen often (65% of cases).

3. **Placenta:** Placentomegaly is usually present if hydrops occurs.

4. **Measurement Data:** Normal growth is expected. Umbilical artery Doppler scans may be abnormal if hydrops occurs.

5. **When Detectable:** First detectable between 12 and 18 weeks' gestation. If there is no hydrops, what appears to be a type III mass often regresses and may even disappear. Some practitioners consider that this form relates to a mucus plug in the bronchial tree, which spontaneously disappears.

Pitfalls

1. Acoustic enhancement posterior to the heart can create the impression of a microcystic mass.
2. The thymus can sometimes be seen as a subtle echopenic mass around the heart. It is a normal variant.

Differential Diagnosis

1. Diaphragmatic hernia—Can look very similar, but no diaphragm will be visible and the stomach will usually be in the chest or shifted to the right.
2. Bronchogenic and neuroenteric cysts—The single cystic form of cystic adenomatoid malformation can look similar. Neuroenteric cysts are usually central and posterior in location and are associated with vertebral anomalies.

Where Else to Look There is no association with chromosome anomalies. Renal anomalies (e.g., renal agenesis) and gastrointestinal malformations (e.g., diaphragmatic hernia and bowel atresias) should be sought.

Pregnancy Management

Investigations and Consultations Required Invasive testing is not indicated if a precise diagnosis can be made by ultrasonography. Cardiac status should be assessed by fetal echocardiography. Early consultation with a pediatric surgeon is warranted to establish a fetal management plan.

Fetal Intervention For purposes of fetal assessment, lesions are best separated into those that are predominantly macrocystic and those that are predominantly microcystic. For lesions with a single large cyst without a significant solid component, thoracoamniotic shunting may be successful in reversing fetal hydrops. Cases without hydrops, but with marked mediastinal shift, may also benefit from shunting. Multicystic lesions are generally not appropriate for shunt placement.

For cases of microcystic lesions with hydrops, open fetal surgery at specialized centers has resulted in approximately 60% survival in patients with a condition that, untreated, is uniformly fatal. Intervention must occur before the onset of placentomegaly and maternal preeclampsia, since the Mirro syndrome cannot be reversed. Conversely, surgical procedures prior to clinical evidence of fetal compromise may be unnecessary in many fetuses, as up to 20% of microcystic lesions will spontaneously regress.

Monitoring The significant incidence of pregnancy complications requires that care be coordinated at a tertiary center. Ultrasonographic examinations at least every 2 weeks are appropriate to detect early evidence of hydrops or polyhydramnios. Careful maternal assessment for the development of preeclampsia is necessary in those cases with hydrops.

Pregnancy Course Polyhydramnios may result in preterm labor. Fetal hydrops and resultant preeclampsia also may complicate obstetric management. The presence of hydrops greatly worsens the prognosis. However, many lesions regress or disappear during pregnancy.

Pregnancy Termination Issues A nondestructive procedure that provides both anatomic and microscopic evaluation is appropriate.

Delivery In the absence of fetal hydrops, delivery should be at term. After 32 weeks' gestation, any evidence of fetal compromise should prompt steroid administration to enhance fetal lung maturity and early delivery. Because immediate resuscitation may be necessary in any infant with cystic adenomatoid malformations, delivery should occur in a tertiary center with extracorporeal membrane oxygenation (ECMO) capabilities.

Neonatology

Resuscitation The two major issues affecting onset of respiration at birth are preterm delivery and the presence of fetal hydrops. Of the three histologic types, type III, microcystic, is most likely to be associated with both problems. Prompt intubation following delivery and assisted ventilation are indicated when the diagnosis is known prior to delivery, when one or both complicating factors are present, or with any evidence of early onset of respiratory distress. Care should be taken to avoid malposition of the endotracheal tube, as the malformed lung can become massively overdistended, compromising gas exchange in normal lung tissue.

Transport Immediate transfer to a tertiary center with a pediatric surgeon is essential, because the postnatal mortality rate is very high and the only successful treatment is prompt surgical excision. Maintenance of ventilatory support with avoidance of tube malposition is critical during transport. Positioning the infant with the involved side dependent may help to avoid overdistension.

Testing and Confirmation Respiratory distress is the most frequent presentation in the newborn period. Older children may present with recurrent respiratory symptoms, and some cases are detected incidentally.

If there is confusion regarding the diagnosis or the extent of the affected lung, a computed tomographic scan of the thorax is useful. Echocardiography is useful to evaluate compromise of cardiac filling and myocardial contractility.

Nursery Management Positive-pressure ventilatory support should be maintained prior to surgery. When the area of lung involvement is small, surgery in a preterm infant may be delayed until coexisting respiratory distress syndrome can be abated with surfactant replacement therapy. As discussed earlier, careful attention to tube position and to positioning the infant may reduce the overdistension of the involved segment.

If there is coexisting hydrops, restriction of fluid intake, pharmacologic diuresis, and administration of inotropic infusions may help to mobilize the fluid from the interstitial space while sustaining adequate perfusion. Rapid infusion of albumin or plasma should be avoided, as massive shifts of fluid into the intravascular space can compromise cardiac function.

Surgery

Preoperative Assessment The newborn should be evaluated in the nursery to confirm the prenatal diagnosis and exclude other associated anomalies. The infant will be at significant risk for air trapping in the congenital cystic adenomatoid malformation (CCAM), which may acutely worsen the respiratory status. In cases of unilateral CCAM, selective intubation of the contralateral bronchus may be a useful temporizing measure until resection of the CCAM can be accomplished. Pneumothorax is an additional concern in CCAM, especially in the type I or II lesions, and may require tube thoracostomy.

Operative Indications   CCAM is usually confined to a single lobe. Rare cases have been reported of multilobar involvement of one lung or bilateral lesions. Complete resection of the CCAM, usually by lobectomy, is the treatment of choice. In cases of extensive involvement of nearly the entire lung, resection of multiple lobes or pneumonectomy may be necessary. The need for immediate surgery is determined by the presence of respiratory distress requiring ventilatory support. In some patients, and particularly those with an early intrauterine diagnosis, the pulmonary symptoms are very severe and unresponsive to standard respiratory support.

The newborn with a CCAM detected antenatally that subsequently regressed needs postnatal evaluation. Often subtle abnormalities will be evident on chest radiograph, but chest computed tomography (CT) or magnetic resonance imaging (MRI) may be necessary to detect residual CCAM. Several authors have recommended that, as long as these lesions are asymptomatic, they be observed closely and managed without resection. The argument against this approach includes the reported cases of myxosarcoma, embryonal rhabdomyosarcoma, and bronchoalveolar carcinoma arising in CCAMs. Although primary lung tumors are rare in the first two decades of life, 4% of those reported were associated with congenital cystic lesions of the lung, including CCAM.

Types of Procedures   A posterolateral thoracotomy with resection of the involved lobe is the standard therapy.

Surgical Results/Prognosis   The long-term outcome of infants with CCAM following resection is excellent. If residual CCAM is left behind or the mass is not resected, the child will be at risk for complications. As noted earlier, these complications include air trapping with gradual enlargement over time, infection, and malignancy arising within the CCAM. The infants usually have remarkable compensatory growth of the residual lung following resection, with continued alveolarization for several years. These children appear to have no excessive limitations and are no more at risk for respiratory infections than other children. The children who survived open fetal surgery for CCAMs associated with hydrops are doing well 1 to 7 years after their procedure.

REFERENCES

Achiron R, Strauss S, Seidman DS, et al: Fetal lung hyperechogenicity: Prenatal ultrasonographic diagnosis, natural history and neonatal outcome. Ultrasound Obstet Gynecol 1995;6:40–42.

Adzick NS, Harrison MR, et al: Fetal cystic adenomatoid malformation: Prenatal diagnosis and natural history. J Pediatr Surg 1985;20:483–488.

Adzick NS, Harrison MR, Crombleholme TM, et al: Fetal lung lesions: Management and outcome. Am J Obstet Gynecol 1998;179:884–889.

Bagolan P, Nahom A, Giorlandino C, et al: Cystic adenomatoid malformation of the lung: Clinical evolution and management. Eur J Pediatr 1999;158:879–882.

Budorick NE, Pretorius DH, Leopold GR, Stamm ER: Spontaneous improvement of intrathoracic masses diagnosed in utero. J Ultrasound Med 1992;11:653–662.

Bunduki V, Ruano R, Silva MS, et al: Prognostic factors associated with congenital cystic adenomatoid malformation of the lung. Prenat Diagn 2000;20:459–464.

Clark SL, Vitale DJ, Minton SD, et al: Successful fetal therapy for cystic adenomatoid malformation associated with second-trimester hydrops. Am J Obstet Gynecol 1987;157:294–295.

Commergues M, Louis-Sylvestre CL, Mandelbrot L, et al: Congenital adenomatoid malformation of the lung: When is active fetal therapy indicated? Am J Obstet Gynecol 1997;177:953–958.

Graham D, Winn K, Derr W, et al: Prenatal diagnosis of cystic adenomatoid malformation of the lung. J Ultrasound Med 1982;1:9–12.

Haddon MJ, Bowen A: Bronchopulmonary and neurenteric forms of foregut anomalies: Imaging for diagnosis and management. Radiol Clin North Am 1991;29:241–254.

Johnson JA, Rumack CM, Johnson ML, et al: Cystic adenomatoid malformation: Antenatal diagnosis. Am J Roentgenol 1984;142:483–484.

Kitano Y, Flake AW, Crombleholme TM, et al: Open fetal surgery for life-threatening fetal malformations. Semin Perinat 1999;23:448–461.

Monni G, Paladinin D, Ibba RM, et al: Prenatal ultrasound diagnosis of congenital cystic adenomatoid malformation of the lung: A report of 26 cases and review of the literature. Ultrasound Obstet Gynecol 2000;16:159–162.

Neilson IR, Russo P, Laberge JM, et al: Congenital adenomatoid malformation of the lung: Current management and prognosis. J Pediatr Surg 1991;26:975–980.

Othersen B Jr: Pulmonary and bronchial malformations. In Ashcraft K, Holder T (eds): Pediatric Surgery. Philadelphia, WB Saunders, 1993.

Quinton AE, Sanoleniec JS: Congenital lobar emphysema—the disappearing chest mass: Antenatal ultrasound appearance. Ultrasound Obstet Gynecol 2001;17:169–171.

Roelofsen J, Oostendorp R, Volovics A, Hoogland H: Prenatal diagnosis and fetal outcome of cystic adenomatoid malformation of the lung: Case report and historical survey. Ultrasound Obstet Gynecol 1994;4:78–82.

Saltzman DH, Adzick NS, Benacerraf BR: Fetal cystic adenomatoid malformation of the lung: Apparent improvement in utero. Obstet Gynecol 1988;71:1000–1002.

Stocker JT, Madewell JE, Drake RM: Congenital cystic adenomatoid malformation of the lung: Classification and morphological spectrum. Hum Pathol 1977;8:155–171.

Uludag R, Medazh G, Erdogen E, et al: A case of prenatally diagnosed fetal neuroenteric cyst. Ultrasound Obstet Gynecol 2001;18:277–279.

Van Leeuwen K, Teitelbaum DH, Hirsch RB, et al: Prenatal diagnosis of congenital cystic adenomatoid malformation and its postnatal presentation, surgical indications, and natural history. J Pediatr Surg 1999;34:794–798.

Waszak P, Claris O, Lapillonne A, et al: Cystic adenomatoid malformation of the lung: Neonatal management of 21 cases. Pediatr Surg Int 1999;15:326–331.

Wesley JR, Heidelberger KP, DiPietro MA, et al: Diagnosis and management of congenital cystic disease of the lung in children. J Pediatr Surg 1986;21:202–207.

Wilson J, Maenner V: Congenital cystic adenomatoid malformation. Neonatal Netw 1993;12:15–20.

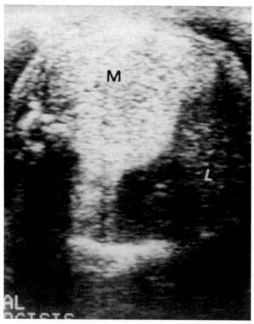

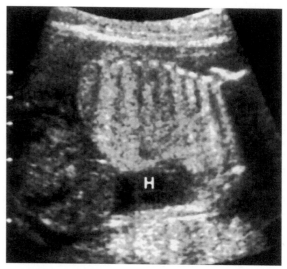

Type III cystic adenomatoid malformation of the lung (CAM). The more echogenic area of the lung (M) represents the CAM. Myriad tiny cysts are present, so no drainage procedure can be performed. This type has a worse prognosis. L, normal lung.

Another example of type III cystic adenomatoid malformation. The entire left lung is filled with small cysts, and the heart (H) is compressed.

Type I cystic adenomatoid malformation. At least two cysts are present in the lungs (M). A drainage procedure is feasible. Note the presence of a small amount of ascites around the liver (*arrow*).

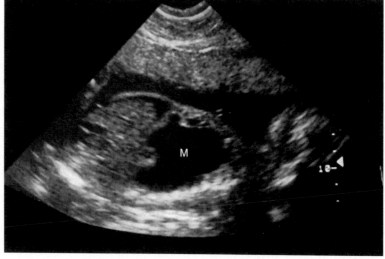

5.2 Diaphragmatic Hernia

Epidemiology/Genetics

Definition A group of diaphragmatic defects in which some portion of the abdominal contents protrude into the chest cavity. This occurs most frequently through a posterolateral (foramen of Bochdalek hernia) or retrosternal (foramen of Morgagni hernia) defect.

Epidemiology Posterolateral hernia, 15 to 20 in 100,000 births (M2:F1); retrosternal hernia, less than 1 in 1,000,000 births.

Embryology Diaphragmatic hernias probably develop between the sixth and the tenth week of gestation, when the gut is returning from the yolk sac and the diaphragm is developing. One mechanism of formation proposes an imbalance in timing of these events with thoracic migration of the gut, resulting in failure of diaphragmatic closure. Frequent associated abnormalities include cardiac malformations (20% of cases) and central nervous system malformations (30% of cases), but renal anomalies, vertebral defects, pulmonary hypoplasia, and facial clefts have also been reported. Chromosome abnormalities including trisomies 18 and 21, as well as more than 30 multiple malformation syndromes, including Fryns and Cornelia de Lange syndromes, have been described with diaphragmatic hernias.

Inheritance Patterns Generally sporadic. Less than 2% recurrence risk in siblings for isolated defects. Rare families have shown dominant, X-linked, and recessive inheritance for isolated diaphragmatic hernias. Cases with bilateral defects are more likely to be familial.

Teratogens None known.

Prognosis The two primary factors determining survival are the degree of pulmonary hypoplasia and the coexistence of other abnormalities. The severity of the pulmonary hypoplasia correlates with the volume and content of visceral herniation and is principally related to herniation of the fetal liver. The most sensitive prognostic tool is the measurement of the lung-to-head ratio (volume of contralateral lung divided by the head circumference). Fetuses with a lung-to-head ratio of greater than 1.4 have a good prognosis and those with a lung-to-head ratio of less than 0.6 are not likely to survive without in utero therapy.

In liveborn infants, survival potential has been correlated with age at presentation and severity of gas exchange problems as markers for the degree of pulmonary hypoplasia. The Liverpool group reports mortality rates of less than 5% for those who are minimally affected to asymptomatic in the first 6 hours with near normal blood gases, approximately 30% in the group who are symptomatic early but who can achieve normal blood gases with ventilatory support, and 100% in the most severe group who are symptomatic from birth and, despite maximal support, do not achieve normal blood gas values secondary to severe pulmonary hypoplasia and pulmonary hypertension. Long-term sequelae, including lower (15 IQ points) cognitive function, have been reported.

In recent years, the use of ECMO has been shown to increase survival initially in the more severely affected infants. Long-term survival may still be limited secondary to residual lung disease.

Sonography

FINDINGS

1. **Fetus:** About one third of fetuses with diaphragmatic hernia will have increased fetal nuchal translucency thickness at 11 to 14 weeks.
   a. Left-sided hernia—The heart is deviated to the right. Usually the stomach is in the chest alongside the heart, so there is no stomach or gallbladder in the abdomen. If the stomach is posteriorly located, this suggests liver herniation. The stomach may be dilated or at an odd axis. Small bowel in the chest may have a slightly mottled pattern but may look like lung. Peristalsis may be seen. The left diaphragm is not visible. The liver may be displaced into the chest, which worsens the prognosis. Findings consistent with liver herniation into the chest are color flow Doppler visualization of the lateral segment of the portal vessels pursuing a course toward or above the diaphragmatic ridge and deviation of the umbilical segment of the portal vein to the left. A soft tissue density may be seen between the lateral border of the heart and the herniated stomach.
   b. Right-sided hernia—There is liver in the chest, so the heart is deviated to the left. One may be able to see a liver-lung interface above the site of the normal diaphragm. The stomach alignment is abnormal, with the stomach moved to the right and horizontally aligned. The liver alignment is changed in the abdomen. Portal vessels can be tracked within the liver into the chest. Ascites tracking into the right chest may be seen.
   c. The ratio of the lung to head can be used to predict pulmonary hypoplasia.
   d. A CT scan with contrast in the amniotic fluid may be helpful if obesity or fetal position make detection of the diaphragmatic hernia difficult. MRI is also helpful in showing liver herniation and in measuring lung volume.

2. **Amniotic Fluid:** Normal amniotic fluid volume, unless the bowel is obstructed, in which case there is polyhydramnios. The presence of polyhydramnios is correlated with pulmonary hypoplasia and, therefore, a worse prognosis.
3. **Placenta:** Normal.
4. **Measurement Data:** Small abdomen, since much of the contents are in the chest. Overall small growth would favor a chromosomal disorder.
5. **When Detectable:** Left diaphragmatic hernia has been detected at 12 weeks with the endovaginal probe. Right-sided hernia is more subtle and can be detected at 17 to 18 weeks.

Pitfalls

1. Lung changes are easily overlooked, especially if the stomach is in the abdomen.
2. Often initially diagnosed as dextrocardia, since the lung changes are subtle.
3. The heart may be very difficult to examine in the presence of diaphragmatic hernia.

Differential Diagnosis

1. Cystic adenomatoid malformation—The diaphragm is intact and no peristalsis is seen.
2. Lung tumor, such as teratoma—Exceedingly rare, often with calcification.
3. Dextrocardia—The heart still points to the left in diaphragmatic hernia, although it is on the right side.
4. Congenital hiatal hernia—a dilated tubular structure in the thoracic cavity in the midline with a small or absent stomach may represent a hiatus hernia.

Where Else to Look   Diaphragmatic hernia is associated with chromosome disorders (trisomies 18 and 21 and tetrasomy 12p), so look at the hands, feet, heart, and face. Approximately 30% to 50% of diaphragmatic hernia cases have an anomaly elsewhere, even with normal karyotype. Look at the cardiovascular, genitourinary, musculoskeletal, and gastrointestinal systems. Diaphragmatic hernia is a component of Fryns syndrome (see Chapter 11.3).

Pregnancy Management

Investigations and Consultations Required   Fetal chromosomal evaluation by amniocentesis. Chromosomal studies on fetal blood will miss the chromosome abnormality (isochromosome 12p) seen in the Pallister-Killian syndrome, a rare but lethal cause of diaphragmatic hernia. Echocardiography is essential given the high incidence of associated cardiac abnormalities and the need for immediate surgery following birth.

Fetal Intervention   In utero repair of diaphragmatic hernia was not shown to improve survival in a controlled trial of fetal surgery and thus is no longer indicated. Currently, tracheal ligation for the most severely affected (expected to be lethal) fetuses has been successful in a few centers in avoiding immediate neonatal demise. Immediate surgical intervention is needed at delivery with pla-

cental support maintained (ex utero intrapartum treatment [EXIT] procedure) to establish a functional airway.

Monitoring   Prophylactic tocolysis, if polyhydramnios develops, may be appropriate in view of the poor results expected if prematurity complicates the surgical correction. Therefore, serial ultrasonographic examinations every 3 to 4 weeks and regular clinical assessment should be performed.

Pregnancy Course   Polyhydramnios is a common complicating factor and may result in preterm labor. The presence of polyhydramnios is correlated with pulmonary hypoplasia and, therefore, a worse prognosis.

Pregnancy Termination Issues   Diaphragmatic hernia is a component of a number of genetic syndromes. To provide appropriate counseling regarding recurrence, a complete external and internal pathologic examination of an intact fetus is required.

Delivery   Immediate resuscitation is often necessary; therefore, delivery should be in a tertiary center. There are no fetal indications for early delivery or delivery by cesarean section.

Neonatology

Resuscitation   An experienced team that is prepared to initiate full ventilatory and pharmacologic support is essential to maximize survival potential, particularly for the more severely involved neonate. Rapid, atraumatic intubation and assisted ventilation, gastric decompression, and pharmacologic paralysis are recommended initially. Hypoplastic lungs are highly prone to develop air leaks and pneumothorax with positive-pressure ventilation. The goal is to facilitate pulmonary vasodilation and promote rapid and sustained transition from the fetal to the adult circulatory pattern. Prompt correction of acidosis is essential.

Transport   Transfer to a tertiary center with pediatric surgeons is mandatory and should be done only by an experienced neonatal transport team, as these infants have very labile courses.

Testing and Confirmation   Diagnostic evaluation preoperatively should be limited to those studies that are essential to confirm the diagnosis and to exclude the presence of serious anomalies affecting long-term prognosis, such as chromosome abnormalities, cardiac, and/or CNS defects, if not done prenatally.

Nursery Management   The initial care of the infant is directed toward maintaining adequate gas exchange by mechanical ventilation and the avoidance of reflex pulmonary vasoconstriction with reversion to right-to-left shunting via fetal pathways by limiting stressful handling.

Improved early survival with ECMO treatment has been demonstrated in the group of infants previously shown to be nonsurvivors. However, overall survival remains low in this group because of late deaths secondary to severe respiratory failure. Significant CNS injury related to intracranial hemorrhage and to ischemia has been observed following ECMO treatment.

Recent reports suggest that high-frequency ventilation and surfactant replacement therapy are of benefit in improving survival rates.

Surgery

Preoperative Assessment   The acute pathophysiology of a congenital diaphragmatic hernia (CDH) postnatally results from a mechanical space-occupying lesion with accompanying lung hypoplasia, pulmonary vascular malformation, and decreased lung expansion with respiration. The hypoxemia is therefore the result of poor ventilation plus associated pulmonary hypertension. Surgery is delayed until the infant's respiratory status is stable.

Operative Indications and Techniques   The operative goals are reduction of the viscera from the thoracic cavity, closure of the diaphragmatic defect, and elimination of potential duodenal obstruction due to nonrotation of the intestine.

Surgical options include abdominal versus thoracic repair. Left posterior lateral diaphragmatic lesions occur 75% to 80% percent of the time, and most surgeons prefer an abdominal approach to accomplish the above-named goals. Some surgeons who prefer the thoracic approach do so particularly for the less frequent right posterior lateral CDH. This defect is associated with a higher incidence of hepatic herniation into the chest and may result in abnormal angulation of the suprahepatic inferior vena cava, with more difficulty in reducing the liver back into the abdomen without occluding the lower body venous return. An abdominal approach for this problem is possible, but a thoracic approach improves surgical exposure and manipulation of the vessels. Rare anterior retrosternal CDH is repaired via the abdominal approach. Posterior lateral CDH is frequently associated with insufficient remaining diaphragmatic musculature and will not allow closure of the defect. Tailored nonabsorbable woven plastic prosthetic sheets are used to cover this defect and are attached to the surrounding musculature. The ipsilateral chest is not drained by a chest tube with applied suction, since this tends to acutely shift the mobile infant mediastinum and produce hemodynamic instability.

Extracorporeal membrane oxygenation can be used as preoperative therapy either with CDH repair while the patient is on bypass therapy or after cessation of bypass therapy. It can also be used after surgical repair of CDH in infants who have had the commonly occurring postoperative "honeymoon period," with temporarily improved hypoxemia and then subsequent acute irreversible respiratory failure. ECMO is not applicable in small premature infants because of the need for anticoagulation, nor in patients who have complex, noncorrectable cardiac defects. There are significant potential acute and chronic complications of ECMO, but new access techniques, such as veno-venous circuits or heparin-bonded tubing, are improving these problems.

Surgical Results/Prognosis   The overall survival rate is 65% to 75%. This rate has improved with the use of ECMO from 50%.

A prenatal diagnosis made before 24 weeks' gestation is associated with poor long-term results. Morbidity can be related to the congenital defects but can also be iatrogenic in nature. Chronic respiratory insufficiency can occur in survivors and may be related to barotrauma induced by the need for prolonged oxygenation and ventilation. These children have an increased incidence of pathologic gastroesophageal reflux that is frequently unresponsive to standard medical therapy and increases their respiratory and nutritional complications.

Long-term problems include failure to thrive and sensorineural hearing loss due to the prolonged need for antibiotics or Lasix. Seizures and developmental delay are seen in 20 to 30% of patients. Scoliosis and pectus excavatum occur in a minority of children.

REFERENCES

Adzick NS, Harrison MR, Glick Pl, et al: Diaphragmatic hernia in the fetus: Prenatal diagnosis and outcome in 94 cases. J Pediatr Surg 1985;20:357–361.

Albanese CT, Lopoo J, Goldstein RB, et al: Fetal liver position and perinatal outcome for congenital diaphragmatic hernia. Prenat Diagn 1998;18:1138–1142.

Bahlmann F, Merz E, Hallermann C, et al: Congenital diaphragmatic hernia: Ultrasonic measurement of fetal lungs to predict pulmonary hypoplasia. Ultrasound Obstet Gynecol 1999;14:162–168.

Benacerraf BR, Greene MF: Fetal diaphragmatic hernia: Ultrasound diagnosis prior to 22 weeks' gestation. Radiology 1986;158:809–810.

Bernbaum J, Schwartz I, Gerdes M, et al: Survivors of extracorporeal membrane oxygenation at 1 year of age: The relationship of primary diagnosis with health and neurodevelopmental sequelae. Pediatrics 1994;96:907–913.

Bohn DJ, James I, Filler RM, et al: The relationship between PaCO2 and ventilation parameters in predicting survival in congenital diaphragmatic hernia. J Pediatr Surg 1984;19:666–671.

Bohn D, Tamura M, Perrin D, et al: Ventilatory predictors of pulmonary hypoplasia in congenital diaphragmatic hernia, confirmed by morphologic assessment. J Pediatr 1987;111:423–431.

Bouman NH, Koot HM, Tibboel D, et al: Children with congenital diaphragmatic hernia are at risk for lower levels of cognitive functioning and increased emotional and behavioral problems. Eur J Pediatr Surg 2000;10:3–7.

Breaux CW Jr, Rouse TM, Cain WS, et al: Congenital diaphragmatic hernia in an era of delayed repair after medical and/or extracorporeal membrane oxygenation stabilization: A prognostic and management classification. J Pediatr Surg 1992;27:1192–1196.

Crane JP: Familial congenital diaphragmatic hernia: Prenatal diagnostic approach and analysis of twelve families. Clin Genet 1979;16:244–252.

Cunniff C, Jones KL, Jones MC: Patterns of malformation in children with congenital diaphragmatic defects. J Pediatr 1990;116:258–261.

DeLorimer AA: Diaphragmatic hernia. In Aschcraft KW, Holder TM (eds): Pediatric Surgery. Philadelphia, WB Saunders, 1993, pp 204–217.

Flake AW, Cromblehome TM, Johnon MP, et al: Treatment of severe congenital diaphragmatic hernia by fetal tracheal occlusion: Clinical experience with fifteen cases. Am J Obstet Gynecol 2000;183:1059–1066.

Geary MP, Chitty LS, Morrison JJ, et al: Perinatal outcome and prognostic factors in prenatally diagnosed congenital diaphragmatic hernia. Ultrasound Obstet Gynecol 1998;12:107–111.

Harrison MR, Adzick NS, Bullard KM, et al: Correction of congenital diaphragmatic hernia in utero VII: A prospective trial. J Pediatr Surg 1997;32:1637–1642.

Harrison MR, Mychaliska GB, Albanese CR, et al: Correction of congenital diaphragmatic hernia in utero IX: Fetuses with poor prognosis (liver herniation and low lung-to-head ratio) can be saved by fetoscopic temporary tracheal occlusion. J Pediatr Surg 1998;33:1017–1022.

Haugen SE, Linker D, Eik-Nes S, et al: Congenital diaphragmatic hernia: Determination of the optimal time for operation by echocardiographic monitoring of the pulmonary arterial pressure. J Pediatr Surg 1991;26:560–562.

Hubbard AM, Adzick NS, Crombleholme TM, et al: Congenital chest lesions: Diagnosis and characterization with prenatal MR imaging. Radiology 1999;212:43–48.

Huddy CL, Boyd PA, Wilkinson AR, Chamberlain P: Congenital diaphragmatic hernia: Prenatal diagnosis, outcome and continuing morbidity in survivors. Br J Obstet Gynaecol 1999;106:1192–1196.

Irving IM, Booker PD: Congenital diaphragmatic hernia and eventration of the diaphragm. In Lister J, Irving IM (eds): Neonatal Surgery. London, Butterworths, 1990, p 199.

Kitano Y, Flake AW, Crombleholme TM, et al: Open fetal surgery for life-threatening fetal malformations. Semin Perinat 1999;23:448–461.

Lam YH, Tang MHY, Yuen ST: Ultrasound diagnosis of fetal diaphragmatic hernia and complex congenital heart disease at 12 weeks' gestation: A case report. Prenat Diagn 1998;18:1159–1162.

Langham MR, Krummel TM, Bartlett RH, et al: Mortality with extracorporeal membrane oxygenation following repair of congenital diaphragmatic hernia in 93 Infants. J Pediatr Surg 1987;22:1150.

Leung JW, Coakley FV, Hricak H, et al: Prenatal imaging of congenital diaphragmatic hernia. AJR 2000;174:1607–1612.

Lipshutz GS, Albanese CT, Feldstein VA, et al: Prospective analysis of lung-to-head ratio predicts survival for patients with prenatally diagnosed congenital diaphragmatic hernia. J Pediatr Surg 1997;32:1634–1636.

Migliazza L, Otten C, Xia H, et al: Cardiovascular malformations in congenital diaphragmatic hernia: Human and experimental studies. J Pediatr Surg 1999;34:1352–1358.

Migliazza L, Xia H, Diez-Pardo JA, Tovar JA: Skeletal malformations associated with congenital diaphragmatic hernia: Experimental and human studies. J Pediatr Surg 1999;34:1624–1629.

Mychaliska GB, Bealer JF, Graf JL, et al: Operating on placental support: The ex utero intrapartum treatment procedure. J Pediatr Surg 1997;32:227–230.

Nakayama DK, Harrison MR, Chinn DH, et al: Prenatal diagnosis and natural history of the fetus with a congenital diaphragmatic hernia: Initial clinical experience. J Pediatr Surg 1985;20:118–124.

Ogunyemi D: Serial sonographic findings in a fetus with congenital hiatus hernia. Ultrasound Obstet Gynecol 2001;17:350–353.

Paek BW, Coakley FU, Lu Y: Congenital diaphragmatic hernia: Prenatal evaluation with MR lung volumetry—preliminary experience. Radiology 2001;220:63–67.

Puri P, Gorman F: Lethal nonpulmonary anomalies associated with congenital diaphragmatic hernia: Implications for early intrauterine surgery. J Pediatr Surg 1984;19:29–32.

Reyes C, Chang LK, Waffarn F, et al: Delayed repair of congenital diaphragmatic hernia with early high-frequency oscillatory ventilation during preoperative stabilization. J Pediatr Surg 1998;33:1010–1016.

Sebire NJ, Snijders RJ, Davenport M, et al: Fetal nuchal translucency thickness at 10–14 weeks' gestation and congenital diaphragmatic hernia. Obstet Gynecol 1997;90:943–946.

Steinhorn RH, Kriesmer PJ, Green TP, et al: Congenital diaphragmatic hernia in Minnesota: Impact of antenatal diagnosis on survival. Arch Pediatr Adolesc Med 1994;148:626–631.

Suita S, Taguchi T, Yamanouchi T, et al: Fetal stabilization for antenatally diagnosed diaphragmatic hernia. J Pediatr Surg 1999;34:1652–1657.

UK Collaborative ECMO (Extracorporeal Membrane Oxygenation) Trial Group: UK collaborative randomized trial of neonatal extracorporeal membrane oxygenation. Lancet 1996;348:75–82.

UK Collaborative ECMO (Extracorporeal Membrane Oxygenation) Trial Group: UK collaborative randomized trial of neonatal extracorporeal membrane oxygenation: Follow-up to one year of age. Pediatrics 1998;101:E1.

Urban BA, Duhl AJ, Ural SH, et al: Helical CT amniography of congenital diaphragmatic hernia. Am J Roentgenol 1999;172:809–812.

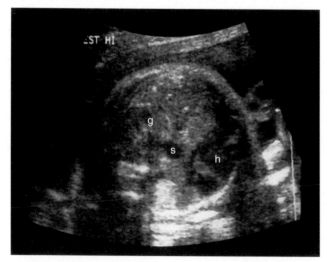

Left diaphragmatic hernia. Transverse view through the chest. The heart (h) is deviated to the right. The stomach (s) lies alongside the chest. A slight difference between the texture of the normal lung and the area that is gut-filled (g) can be seen.

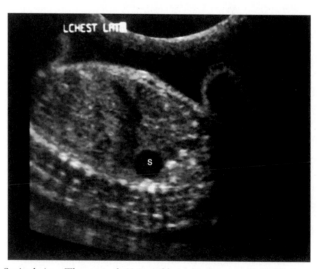

Sagittal view. The stomach (s) is visible in the chest as a fluid-filled cystic structure. An irregular texture due to small bowel can be seen superior to the stomach.

5.3 Esophageal Atresia, Tracheal Atresia, Tracheoesophageal Fistula

Epidemiology/Genetics

Definition Esophageal atresia is a congenital lack of continuity of the esophagus resulting in a blind-ending esophageal pouch. There is frequently an associated tracheoesophageal fistula.

Epidemiology One in 5000 (M1:F1); 90% of patients have esophageal atresia with a distal tracheoesophageal fistula.

Embryology Failure of the anterior foregut to divide into the anterior trachea and posterior esophagus around the fourth week of gestation results in various types of esophageal atresia and tracheoesophageal fistula. Sixty percent of patients have associated anomalies, the most common of which are cardiac (25%), genitourinary (15%), skeletal (14%), and other gut atresias (13%). The VACTERL (vertebral defects, anal atresia, tracheoesophageal fistula with esophageal atresia, radial and renal dysplasia) association occurs in approximately 10% of cases. More than 40 genetic, chromosomal, and sporadic syndromes have been described with esophageal atresia and/or tracheoesophageal fistula. Two to 3% of cases have trisomy 21.

Inheritance Patterns Sporadic.

Teratogens Retinoic acid, alcohol.

Prognosis Survival and prognosis are determined by the cause and associated malformations. Overall survival is 85 to 90%, with more than 95% of patients with isolated tracheoesophageal fistula surviving with a functional repair.

Sonography

FINDINGS

1. **Fetus:**
   a. Nonvisualization of the stomach is a finding in the type of esophageal atresia and tracheoesophageal fistula in which there is no connection between the pharynx and the stomach. A narrow connection through the lungs between the esophagus and stomach may result in a small stomach. Many other examples of tracheoesophageal fistula are not diagnosable with ultrasonography because there is a large connection between the esophagus and stomach via the lungs.
   b. A fluid-filled proximal esophagus (the pouch sign) may be seen in the neck. This sign has not been reported prior to 26 weeks' gestation.
   c. A fluid-filled distal esophageal segment and fetal regurgitation after swallowing has been reported.

2. **Amniotic Fluid:** There is massive polyhydramnios with an amniotic fluid index, which is often over 40 cm (60%) in the third trimester. Polyhydramnios may not be seen until the third trimester.
3. **Placenta:** Normal.
4. **Measurement Data:** Normal unless the fetus is chromosomally abnormal or the VACTERL syndrome is present.
5. **When Detectable:** Usually detectable only after 24 weeks, since before this point in gestation, fetal swallowing plays only a limited role in amniotic fluid dynamics.

Pitfalls

1. Nonvisualization of the stomach may be a transient normal finding.
2. Technical problems such as maternal obesity may result in an inability to visualize the stomach.
3. Brain malformations may prevent swallowing and cause nonvisualization of the stomach.
4. The stomach may be in the chest or abnormally positioned, as with diaphragmatic hernia, and therefore not seen.
5. In many examples of tracheoesophageal fistula, a connection to the stomach through the lungs exists. Consequently, the stomach will be seen and the amniotic fluid volume is normal.

Differential Diagnosis The following disorders may also cause absence of stomach visualization:

1. Facial clefts (see Chapter 7.1).
2. Central nervous system malformation that results in absent swallowing. Many of these malformations, such as the fetal akinesia sequence, or the lethal pterygium syndrome, are lethal conditions.
3. Diaphragmatic hernia.
4. Situs inversus.

Where Else to Look Associated malformations are seen in at least 50% of cases of tracheoesophageal fistula. The following abnormalities should be sought: anorectal atresia, duodenal atresia, malrotation, cardiovascular anomalies, renal obstruction, vertebral problems such as scoliosis, and hydronephrosis. Tracheoesophageal fistula is associated with the VACTERL association as well as chromosome abnormalities (trisomy 21 and 18).

Pregnancy Management

Investigations and Consultations Required Chromosome studies should be performed, as well as fetal echocardiography. Consultation with a pediatric surgeon is appropriate. A neonatology consultation also should be obtained because of the high risk of preterm delivery.

Fetal Intervention   No direct fetal intervention is indicated. Serial amniocenteses have no place in management, except for a short-term benefit in cases in which steroid therapy has been given to enhance fetal lung maturity. Decreasing amniotic fluid volume, when there is polyhydramnios, may diminish the risk of preterm labor and allow adequate time for the therapeutic effect.

Monitoring   Because of the high risk of preterm labor, care should be under the direction of a perinatologist. Tocolytic agents are often necessary. Frequent clinical and sonographic examinations are necessary to monitor the degree of polyhydramnios and for early evidence of preterm labor. Monitoring of the cervix by ultrasonography is desirable to detect early funneling of the internal os.

Pregnancy Termination Issues   In rare cases with an early diagnosis, the procedure for termination should provide an intact fetus for a complete autopsy.

Delivery   Every attempt should be made to reach term. However, significant polyhydramnios often results in preterm delivery. The site for delivery should be a tertiary center with capability of managing very premature infants.

Neonatology

Resuscitation   If the infant is born prematurely or there are associated major organ system anomalies, there may be difficulty with the onset of respiration. When the diagnosis is suspected from prenatal studies and there is delay in onset of respiration, immediate endotracheal intubation is preferable to bag and mask ventilation to avoid overdistension of the stomach. (For technique, see Nursery Management below.) Excessive oral secretions may be encountered, necessitating placement of an esophageal catheter for continuous drainage.

Transport   Transfer to a tertiary perinatal center with a pediatric surgeon is always indicated. The infant should be transported in a semi-sitting position to minimize the risk of regurgitation of gastric contents into the airway via the fistula. An esophageal catheter should be placed to drain the pooled secretions to avoid aspiration from the proximal pouch.

Testing and Confirmation   Newborns present with excessive salivation and choking with feedings. Postnatal radiologic studies will define the defect. A radiopaque catheter is carefully passed into the esophagus until resistance is met. Air is injected through the catheter and chest, and abdominal radiographs are obtained. Chromosomal analysis, if not obtained prenatally, echocardiography, and careful physical examinations for any associated anomalies are performed.

Nursery Management   The priority in the early care is to avoid aspiration of either oral or gastric secretions and

thus to decrease the likelihood of pneumonia. Continuous evacuation of esophageal secretions, positioning semi-sitting, avoiding overdistension of the stomach from crying or positive-pressure ventilation, and avoiding compression of the abdomen are useful maneuvers to prevent aspiration.

If endotracheal intubation is required, an attempt should be made to locate the tip of the tube distal to the fistula insertion. This can be accomplished either by placement under endoscopic control or with careful auscultation over the stomach as a positive-pressure breath is given, advancing the tube until air is no longer heard entering the stomach.

Surgery

Preoperative Assessment   There are several forms of tracheoesophageal anomalies, but the most common (85%) is a combination of proximal esophageal pouch with a distal tracheoesophageal fistula.

Preoperative surgical goals consist of identifying the degree of post-delivery aspiration pneumonitis and preventing further airway contamination. This includes assessment of the infant's clinical status as well as the radiographic appearance of the lungs. The latter is a late-occurring sign and more unreliable than clinical and metabolic (blood gas) determinations. A preoperative evaluation for all possible VACTERL anomalies is carried out with particular attention to cardiac lesions.

Operative Indications   The decision about whether to perform an urgent gastrostomy to relieve gastric distention and potential aspiration due to reflux or to perform an immediate thoracotomy for division of the tracheoesophageal fistula and a primary repair of the esophageal atresia is contingent on the preoperative assessment. The former approach is chosen if significant signs of pre-existing pulmonary aspiration exist, and the latter is used if no significant respiratory distress is evident, or other associated lesions contraindicate primary repair.

Types of Procedures   A right thoracotomy via a retropleural approach is used to facilitate better control of postoperative drainage in instances of an esophageal leak (5 to 20%). The tracheoesophageal fistula is divided and the tracheal opening closed carefully to prevent airway stenosis. Care must be exercised so that a double tracheal connection is not missed intraoperatively. A retropleural chest tube is left in position for any potential esophageal leakage. A separate abdominal procedure to place a gastrostomy tube may or may not be used according to surgeon's preference.

Surgical Results/Prognosis   As noted, the early complications include respiratory infection, esophageal anastomotic leak, and recurrent tracheoesophageal fistula as well as potential complications associated with the VACTERL anomalies in those patients. Late complications consist of esophageal strictures, gastroesophageal reflux, dysphagia, and various manifestations of reactive airway disease such as recurrent bronchitis or even asthmatic symptoms. The symptoms of gastroesophageal reflux can be difficult to treat.

The operative mortality rate for a full-term infant with uncomplicated esophageal atresia and tracheoesophageal fistula should approach 0% in tertiary children's centers. Premature infants with associated cardiac anomalies have a survival rate of 50 to 70%. The overall survival rate is approximately 90%.

Surviving children are frequently "slow eaters" who drink increased amounts of fluids with their meals. They also have increased susceptibility to the lodging of esophageal foreign bodies such as meat particles and especially pieces of hot dog. Both of these problems are related to a persistence of esophageal dysmotility due to the atresia.

Long-term survival is good, and further morbidity after 2 to 4 years of age is minimal; however, effects of reactive airway disease can be documented in adult post–tracheoesophageal fistula patients.

REFERENCES

Bovicelli L, Rizzo N, Orsini LF, Pilu G: Prenatal diagnosis and management of fetal gastrointestinal abnormalities. Semin Perinatol 1983;7:109–117.

Chittmittrapap S, Spitz L, Kiely EM, Brereton RJ: Oesophageal atresia and associated anomalies. Arch Dis Child 1989;64:364–368.

Choudhury SR, Ashcraft KW, Sharp RJ, et al: Survival of patients with esophageal atresia: Influence of birth weight, cardiac anomaly, and late respiratory complications. J Pediatr Surg 1999;34:70–73.

Dillon PW, Cilley RE: Newborn surgical emergencies, gastrointestinal anomalies, abdominal wall defects. Pediatr Clin North Am 1993;40:1289–1314.

Dudgeon DL, Morrison CW, Woolley MM: Congenital proximal tracheoesophageal fistula. J Pediatr Surg 1972;7:614–619.

Ein SH, Shandling B, Wesson D, Filler RM: Esophageal atresia with distal tracheoesophageal fistula: Associated anomalies and prognosis in the 1980's. J Pediatr Surg 1989;24:1055–1059.

Evans JA, Reggin J, Greenberg C: Tracheal agenesis and associated malformations: A comparison with tracheoesophageal fistula and the VACTERL association. Am J Med Genet 1985;21:21–38.

Eyheremendy E, Pfister M: Antenatal real-time diagnosis of esophageal atresia. J Clin Ultrasound 1983;11:395–397.

Greenwood RD, Rosenthal A: Cardiovascular malformations associated with tracheoesophageal fistula and esophageal atresia. Pediatrics 1976;57:87–91.

Holder TM, Ashcraft KW: Developments in the care of patients with esophageal atresia and tracheoesophageal fistula. Surg Clin North Am 1981;61:1051–1061.

Jassani MN, Gauderer MW, Faranoff AA, et al: A perinatal approach to the diagnosis and management of gastrointestinal malformations. Obstet Gynecol 1982;59:33–39.

Jolley SG, Johnson DG, Roberts CC, et al: Patterns of gastroesophageal reflux in children following repair of esophageal atresia and distal tracheoesophageal fistula. J Pediatr Surg 1980;15:857–862.

Kalache KD, Wauer R, Mau H, et al: Prognostic significance of the pouch sign in fetuses with prenatally diagnosed esophageal atresia. Am J Obstet Gynecol 2000;182:978–981.

Louhimo I, Lindahl H: Esophageal atresia: Primary results of 500 consecutively treated patients. J Pediatr Surg 1983;18:217–229.

Millener PB, Anderson NG, Chisholm RJ: Prognostic significance of nonvisualization of the fetal stomach by sonography. Am J Roentgenol 1993;160:827–830.

Nyberg DA: Intra-abdominal abnormalities. In Diagnostic Ultrasound of Fetal Anomalies: Text and Atlas. St. Louis, Mosby-Year Book, 1990, pp 358–350.

Pretorius DH, Drose JA, Dennis MA, et al: Tracheoesophageal fistula in utero: Twenty-two cases. J Ultrasound Med 1987;6:509–513.

Pretorius DH, Meier PR, Johnson ML: Diagnosis of esophageal atresia in utero. J Ultrasound Med 1983;2:475–476.

Quan L, Smith DW: The VATER association. Vertebral defects, anal atresia, T-E fistula with esophageal atresia, radial and renal dysplasia: A spectrum of associated defects. J Pediatr 1973;82:104–107.

Randolph JG, Newman KD, Anderson KD: Current results in repair of esophageal atresia with tracheoesophageal fistula using physiologic status as a guide to therapy. Ann Surg 1989;209:524–530.

Sparey C, Robson SL: Oesophageal atresia. Prenat Diagn 2000;20:251–253.

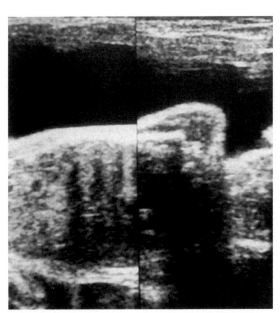

Tracheoesophageal atresia. Longitudinal view of fetus. There is severe polyhydramnios with no visible stomach.

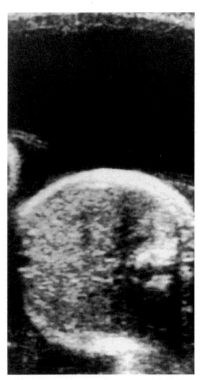

Transverse view of the abdomen. Despite prolonged observation, no stomach could be found.

5.4 Pleural Effusion (Fetal Hydrothorax)

Epidemiology/Genetics

Definition A pleural effusion is an accumulation of fluid in the pleural space. Effusions can be either chylous or clear (hydrothorax), with most primary congenital effusions being chylous and occurring on the right.

Epidemiology One in 10,000 births (M2:F1).

Embryology The cause of pleural effusions is not known, but they may result from either overproduction of lymph or impaired reabsorption. Pleural effusions are divided into primary effusions, which are usually chylous, and secondary effusions that are clear and occur as part of nonimmune hydrops. More than 50 genetic, chromosome, and sporadic syndromes have been reported that include pleural effusion.

Inheritance Patterns A number of genetic syndromes, including Caffey's cortical hyperostosis (autosomal dominant) and the Opitz-Frias hypertelorism hypospadias syndrome (autosomal dominant), have been reported with pleural effusions, hydrops, or chylothorax.

Teratogens None.

Prognosis Overall mortality for pleural effusions presenting in the neonatal period is 25%, ranging from 15% for isolated effusions to 95% for those with associated hydrops. Overall mortality for antenatally diagnosed cases is approximately 50%. Mortality is related to hydrops, pulmonary hypoplasia, and prematurity.

Sonography

FINDINGS

1. **Fetus:** Fluid surrounds the lungs on one or both sides. If the effusion is bilateral and everts the diaphragms, secondary hydrops may occur. Assess the size of the lung on the side of the pleural effusion. Lung hypoplasia or agenesis in utero is associated with pleural effusion development. The associated lung will be very small or not seen.
2. **Amniotic Fluid:** If polyhydramnios develops, the prognosis is poor.
3. **Placenta:** Usually normal. May be enlarged in the presence of fetal hydrops.
4. **Measurement Data:** Usually normal.
5. **When Detectable:** Pleural effusions have been discovered as early as 8.5 weeks. First-trimester transient pleural effusions are associated with chromosomal abnormalities.

Pitfalls Pericardial and pleural effusions may be confused. With a large pericardial effusion, the lungs are compressed posteriorly.

Differential Diagnosis Severe primary pleural effusion with secondary hydrops may be confused with primary hydrops. If the pleural effusion is the primary cause, the diaphragms are everted. A trial of pleural fluid aspiration may be necessary to make the distinction.

Where Else to Look Look for stigmata of Down syndrome (nuchal thickening, femur and humerus shortening, cardiac anomalies, duodenal atresia) and Turner syndrome (cystic hygroma). Make sure that there is no evidence of hydrops, such as skin thickening, pericardial effusions, placentomegaly, or ascites.

Pregnancy Management

Investigations and Consultations Required

1. Chromosome studies and viral cultures.
2. Maternal serum studies for TORCH (toxoplasmosis, other infections, rubella, cytomegalovirus infection, and herpes simplex) and parvovirus.
3. The significant incidence of congenital heart disease requires fetal echocardiographic evaluation of the fetus.
4. Consultation with a neonatologist or pediatric surgeon is helpful.

Fetal Intervention There is no clear evidence to support active surgical intervention. A management plan that is conservative seems to be the best approach. Following initial evaluation, a follow-up ultrasonographic scan in 2 to 3 weeks is done. If the effusion has enlarged or has increased, diagnostic/therapeutic thoracentesis should be done. If the lung expands but the effusion recurs, consideration should be given to placement of a pleuroamniotic shunt. The use of multiple thoracenteses does not appear justified. Thoracentesis just prior to delivery may be helpful, if the degree of effusion suggests that respiratory compromise may be an issue at birth.

Fetal hydrops may be secondary to either a tension hydrothorax or compression of the mediastinum. Placement of a thoracoamniotic shunt may reverse the hydrops and result in a good outcome. Before attempting any intervention, the practitioner should make every effort to determine the underlying cause of the hydrops.

Monitoring Persistent effusions require that management be coordinated at a tertiary center. Ultrasonographic examinations should be performed every 1 to 2 weeks to detect progression and/or development of fetal hydrops.

Pregnancy Course Prognosis is poor if significant effusion is diagnosed prior to 32 weeks' gestation, with a reported survival rate of 40% to 45%. However, isolated effusions treated with shunting have a much more favorable prognosis. The development of hydrops and/or polyhydramnios is associated with prematurity, pulmonary hypoplasia, and an overall survival rate of 30% or less.

Pregnancy Termination Issues In cases in which an accurate diagnosis cannot be made prior to delivery, a nondestructive method of termination should be performed to allow complete fetal evaluation.

Delivery Because immediate resuscitation may be necessary, delivery should occur at a tertiary perinatal center. Early delivery is not indicated except in cases in which hydrops occurs after 32 weeks' gestation.

Neonatology

Resuscitation Preparations should be made for intubation, assisted ventilation, and immediate post-delivery thoracentesis. Three factors are important in the decision for immediate intubation and assisted ventilation at birth: (1) gestational age, (2) bilateral collections of fluid, and (3) predelivery drainage either by thoracentesis or pleuroamniotic shunt. Term infants who have had drainage of the fluid collections within 24 hours of delivery may not require assistance with the onset of respiration. In all other cases, immediate intubation is usually required.

Transport Delivery at a tertiary perinatal center is preferable. Transfer after delivery is indicated if respiratory support is required, bilateral effusions are present, or fluid reaccumulates after initial drainage. The infant should be accompanied by a skilled neonatal transport team in transit.

Testing and Confirmation A chest radiograph will show the extent of the pleural effusion.

Nursery Management Facilitation of normal cardiorespiratory adaptation is the primary goal. Respiratory distress syndrome may complicate the course if the infant is delivered prematurely, in which case surfactant replacement therapy is indicated. Continuing pleural drainage for several days may be required.

REFERENCES

Adams H, Jones A, Hayward C: The sonographic features and implications of fetal pleural effusions. Clin Radiol 1988;39:398–401.

Bovicelli L, Rizzo N, Orsini LF, Calderoni P: Ultrasonic real-time diagnosis of fetal hydrothorax and lung hypoplasia. J Clin Ultrasound 1981;9:253–254.

Estroff JA, Parad RB, Frigoletto FD Jr, Benacerraf BR: The natural history of isolated fetal hydrothorax. Ultrasound Obstet Gynecol 1992;2:162–165.

Laberge J-M, Golbus MS, Filly RA, et al: The fetus with pleural effusions. In Harrison MR, et al (eds): The unborn patient, prenatal diagnosis and treatment. Philadelphia, W.B. Saunders, 1991, pp 314–319.

Longaker MT, Laberge JM, Dansereau J, et al: Primary fetal hydrothorax: Natural history and management. J Pediatr Surg 1989;24:573–576.

Mandelbrot L, Dommergues M, Aubry MC, et al: Reversal of fetal distress by emergency in utero decompression of hydrothorax. Am J Obstet Gynecol 1992;167:1278–1283.

Nisbet DL, Griffin DR, Chitty LS: Prenatal features of Noonan syndrome. Prenat Diagn 1999;19:642–647.

Porembski M, Laughrin TJ, Brown G, Monthei F: Ultrasonic antenatal diagnosis of pleural effusion (chylothorax). J Med Ultrasound 1981;5:51–52.

Rodeck CH, Fisk NM, Fraser DI, Nicolini U: Long-term in utero drainage of fetal hydrothorax. N Engl J Med 1988;319:1135–1138.

Shimizu T, Hashimoto K, Shimizu M, et al: Bilateral pleural efusion in the first trimester: A predictor of chromosomal abnormality and embryonic death? Am J Obstet Gynecol 1997;177:470–471.

Weber A, Phillipson EH: Fetal pleural effusion: A review and meta-analysis for prognostic indicators. Obstet Gynecol 1992;79:281–286.

Wilkins-Haug LE, Doubilet P: Successful thoracoamniotic shunting and review of the literature in unilateral pleural effusion with hydrops. J Ultrasound Med 1997;16:153–160.

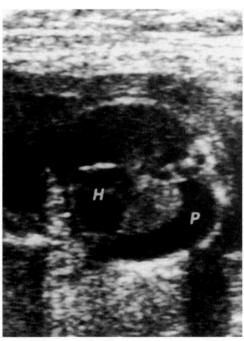

Unilateral pleural effusion (P). The heart (H) is mildly deviated to the right on this transverse view. Following neonatal aspiration of the effusion, the neonate did well.

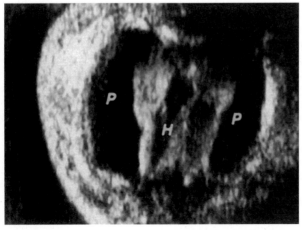

Bilateral pleural effusion (P). The heart (H) can be seen between the pleural effusions on this transverse view. This fetus was stillborn.

5.5 Pulmonary Sequestration

Epidemiology/Genetics

Definition Pulmonary sequestrations are intralobar and extralobar masses of benign pulmonary tissue lacking tracheobronchial communication and having their own vascular supply that usually arises from the thoracic or abdominal aorta.

Epidemiology One in 1000 births. Intralobar, M1:F1; extralobar, M1:F4.

Embryology Most researchers believe that sequestrations are ectopic pulmonary buds with the timing of the budding determining the type of sequestration. Early ectopic budding results in intralobar sequestration, whereas later budding results in the rarer extralobar sequestration (25%) with its own pleural covering. Ten percent of extralobar sequestrations lie below the diaphragm. Ninety percent of extralobar sequestrations are on the left side. Ten percent of intralobar and 50% of extralobar sequestrations have associated abnormalities including diaphragmatic hernias, tracheoesophageal fistulas, foregut duplications, congenital heart disease, and aneuploidy. Fetuses and newborns with significant vascular shunts can present with congestive heart failure and hydrops. Older children most commonly present with recurrent pulmonary symptoms. One half of postnatal cases are diagnosed in adults.

Inheritance Patterns Sporadic.

Teratogens None described.

Prognosis In the absence of hydrops or a severe mediastinal shift, there is an 80 to 90% survival rate. Many antenatally diagnosed cases show regression and even resolution during pregnancy, but this is currently unpredictable. Cases with residual tumor at birth have an excellent outcome with modern surgical resection.

Sonography

FINDINGS

1. **Fetus:**
   a. Intralobar form—Evenly echogenic mass involving a portion of the lung, generally at the base. It is equally frequent at left and right base and represents about 75% of sequestrations. The extralobar sequestration within the thoracic cavity occurs more frequently at the left base (80%).
   b. In most instances, the involved area is a densely echogenic mass. Since a portion of a sequestration may consist of a cystic adenomatoid malformation, a cystic component may be seen.
   c. Mediastinal shift is often present.
   d. Slow apparent disappearance of the mass over the course of the pregnancy may occur, although it may be found again after delivery.
   e. Pleural effusions can complicate either type of intrathoracic sequestration, and progression to nonimmune hydrops can occur. Nonimmune hydrops may develop as a complication of pulmonary sequestration either from a mass effect obstructing venous return or from excess protein loss if there is a cystic component to the mass.
   f. One may be able to demonstrate, with color flow Doppler sonography, a feeder artery directly arising from the descending aorta from below the diaphragm.
   g. In intralobar sequestration, venous drainage is almost always via the pulmonary veins, whereas extralobar sequestration drains via systemic veins below the diaphragm.
   h. Extrathoracic form—This rare type of sequestration (10% of cases) occurs in an infradiaphragmatic location. An echogenic mass is seen in the region of the left adrenal gland. A feeder vessel from the aorta may be visible. A CT scan will show that the mass is fluid filled, unlike many of the other similar masses in this area.
2. **Amniotic Fluid:** Normal unless there is nonimmune hydrops, in which case polyhydramnios may occur.
3. **Placenta:** Normal unless there is hydrops, in which case the placenta will be thickened.
4. **Measurement Data:** Normal unless there is hydrops, in which case abdominal measurements will be increased.
5. **When Detectable:** By about 22 weeks.

Pitfalls Type III (microcystic) cystadenomatoid malformations are indistinguishable from an intralung sequestration if a feeder vessel is not seen.

Differential Diagnosis

1. Type III cystic adenomatoid malformation—Indistinguishable from sequestration unless an aberrant feeder vessel is seen.
2. Mediastinal teratoma—Usually has a more complex pattern than sequestration and has an irregular border. Contains calcifications.
3. Diaphragmatic hernia—Typically has a more complex appearance with cystic areas. There will be stomach and liver displacement.
4. Bronchial obstruction—The lung becomes enlarged

and echogenic. May not be distinguishable from se-questration unless an aberrant feeder vessel is seen.

5. Extralobar sequestration has a wide differential diagnosis:

   • Neuroblastoma—this solid mass typically arises from the adrenal gland, which will still be visible with extralobar sequestration (see Chapter 6.9).
   • Dysplastic second collecting system—The adrenal gland should be visible superior to this cystic mass.
   • Teratoma—Has a more mixed acoustical texture with cystic and solid areas.
   • Adrenal hemorrhage—Arises from the adrenal gland and has a rapidly changing acoustical texture (see Chapter 4.1).
   • Renal tumor—Rarely echogenic and lies within the kidney (see Chapter 4.7).

Where Else to Look

1. Look for the stigmata of hydrops—Ascites, skin thickening, pleural effusion, placentomegaly, and polyhydramnios.
2. Malformations associated with sequestration include diaphragmatic hernia, cardiac defects, and gastric duplication, neuroenteric cyst, and bronchogenic cyst.

Pregnancy Management

Investigations and Consultations Required   Invasive fetal testing is not indicated because color flow Doppler sonography should provide a precise diagnosis. Cardiac status should be assessed by fetal echocardiography. Early consultation with a pediatric surgeon is warranted to establish a fetal management plan.

Fetal Intervention   The report of Lopoo et al suggests an excellent prognosis with minimal morbidity and mortality in carefully managed patients. Intervention was necessary in only 2 of 14 fetuses. Their approach consisted of placing a thoracoamniotic catheter only in those fetuses who developed hydrops (not unilateral effusions). Serial thoracentesis does not appear to have a role in management.

Fetal Monitoring   Fetuses with pleural effusion should have weekly ultrasonographic evaluations. If hydrops develops, a shunt should be considered. In those fetuses without effusions, ultrasonographic evaluation should be done every 2 to 4 weeks. A significant number of lesions will resolve over the course of the pregnancy.

Pregnancy Course   In the absence of fetal hydrops, no specific pregnancy complications are to be expected.

Pregnancy Termination Issues   If termination is chosen, a nondestructive method is necessary to establish a precise diagnosis.

Delivery   In the absence of fetal hydrops, delivery should be at term in a tertiary center. The development of hydrops after 32 weeks should prompt steroid administration to enhance fetal lung maturity, and delivery should be accom-plished. The decision to perform thoracentesis prior to delivery is controversial and should be made jointly with the neonatologist and the perinatologist.

Neonatology

Resuscitation   The prenatal presentation and course determine the immediate post-delivery management. Three distinct antenatal courses have been identified: (1) progressive enlargement with compression of thoracic viscera, pleural effusion, and/or hydrops; (2) involution of the mass prior to delivery; (3) persistent mass without associated complications. In the first instance, the presence of hydrops is the major issue for resuscitation and mortality risk is greatest. With either an involuting or static mass, intubation and ventilatory support are employed if there is respiratory distress. Only in the first group is prematurity and surfactant deficiency likely to be a complicating factor.

Transport   Transfer to a tertiary center with pediatric medical and surgical subspecialists is always indicated. An experienced neonatal transport team is essential to maintain cardiorespiratory function during the transfer.

Testing and Confirmation   The distinguishing diagnostic finding for sequestration as opposed to other chest masses is the presence of an aberrant vasculature, which may be demonstrated by Doppler color flow or by MRI. In general, on chest radiograph an opaque mass is seen. The aberrant tissues is extralobar in 75% of cases and intralobar in 25% of cases. Intra-abdominal location is found in approximately one third of cases.

Nursery Management   Initially, support of adequate pulmonary gas exchange and cardiac output is the principal focus of care. Timing of surgery is based on the clinical course and the presence of other anomalies, the degree of respiratory distress, and other complicating factors.

Surgery

Preoperative Assessment   Acute management includes evaluation of the degree of respiratory insufficiency and identification of major associated anomalies, most notably cardiac defects.

Operative Indications   The newborn with intra-abdominal bronchopulmonary sequestration (BPS) usually has no respiratory compromise and can undergo elective resection. The management of the newborn infant with an intrathoracic BPS is determined by the severity of pulmonary hypoplasia. Therapeutic needs may vary from minimal (not requiring ventilatory support) to severe (requiring ventilatory and vasopressor support, alkalinization, high-frequency oscillatory ventilation, and/or ECMO). Large pleural effusions should be treated immediately by tube thoracostomy. In the infant with pulmonary hypoplasia secondary to BPS, thoracotomy should be deferred until it is clear that the infant has stabilized. The infant's condition often deteriorates after surgery because of changes in chest wall compliance and pulmonary vascular resistance superimposed on pulmonary hypoplasia.

In the rare case of the prenatally diagnosed BPS that appears to regress, postnatal imaging studies should be performed. If the lesion is evident on plain chest radiograph, surgical resection should be planned. If the chest radiograph does not demonstrate the malformation, CT or MRI should be performed. Even though these lesions are asymptomatic, postnatal resection should be performed because of the risks of infection, hemorrhage, and malignant transformation.

Types of Procedures   A posterolateral thoracotomy with resection of the involved lobe is the standard therapy used. Intra-abdominal sequestrations are treated by resection. The surgical approach to bronchopulmonary sequestration is straightforward, with the exception of the management of anomalous blood supply. These vessels are often huge, thin-walled, and elastic, rather than muscular arteries. In 20% of cases, these vessels are subdiaphragmatic in origin; in 15%, more than one vessel is present. Subdiaphragmatic origin of anomalous vessels is more common with right-sided lesions. These vessels can retract into the mediastinum or diaphragm and continue to bleed. Intraoperative death due to hemorrhage from unrecognized anomalous vessels has been reported. Of note, one series reported that 60% of right-sided intralobar sequestrations had anomalous venous return compatible with the scimitar syndrome. The importance of preoperative assessment of venous drainage, as well as arterial supply, is underscored by the reports of postoperative fatalities due to ligation of anomalous veins that constituted the sole or major venous drainage of the entire ipsilateral lung. Occlusion of the supplying vessel by angiographic techniques is an alternative approach.

Surgical Results/Prognosis   Most children with uncomplicated cases with intrathoracic or intra-abdominal sequestration have an excellent prognosis; those with a higher incidence of associated anomalies and fetal hydrops have a much lower survival rate and poorer long-term outcome, with chronic respiratory insufficiency being the major complication. The presence of fetal hydrops is ominous, with few survivors expected if in utero therapy is not instituted.

REFERENCES

Adzick NS, Harrison MR, Crombleholme TM, et al: Fetal lung lesions: Management and outcome. Am J Obstet Gynecol 1998;179:884–889.

Anandakumar C, Biswas A, Chua TM, et al: Direct intrauterine fetal therapy in a case of bronchopulmonary sequestration associated with non-immune hydrops fetalis. Ultrasound Obstet Gynecol 1999;13: 263–265.

Barret J, Chitayat D, Sermer M, et al: The prognostic factors in the prenatal diagnosis of the echogenic fetal lung. Prenatal Diagn 1995;15: 849–853.

Becmeur F, Horta-Geraud P, Donato L, Sauvage P: Pulmonary sequestrations: Prenatal ultrasound diagnosis, treatment, and outcome. J Pediatr Surg 1998;33:492–496.

Benya EC, Bulas DI, Selby DM, Rosenbaum KN: Cystic sonographic appearance of extralobar pulmonary sequestration. Pediatr Radiol 1993;23:605–607.

Bromley B, Parad R, Estroff JA, Benacerraf BR: Fetal lung masses: Prenatal course and outcome. J Ultrasound Med 1995;14:927–936.

Curtis MR, Mooney DP, Vaccaro TJ, et al: Prenatal ultrasound characterization of the suprarenal mass: Distinction between neuroblastoma and subdiaphragmatic extralobar pulmonary sequestration. J Ultrasound Med 1997;16:75–83.

Da Silva OP, Ramanan R, Romano W, et al: Nonimmune hydrops fetalis, pulmonary sequestration, and favorable neonatal outcome. Obstet Gynecol 1996;88:681–683.

Davies RP, Ford WDA, Lequesne GW, Orell SR: Ultrasonic detection of subdiaphragmatic pulmonary sequestration in utero and postnatal diagnosis by fine-needle aspiration biopsy. J Ultrasound Med 1989;8: 47–49.

Dolkart LA, Reimers FT, Helmuth WV, et al: Antenatal diagnosis of pulmonary sequestration: A review. Obstet Gynecol Surv 1992;47:515.

Favre R, Bettahar K, Christmann D, Becmeur F: Antenatal diagnosis and treatment of fetal hydrops secondary to pulmonary extralobar sequestration. Ultrasound Obstet Gynecol 1994;4:335–338.

Gross E, Chen MK, Lobe TE, et al: Infradiaphragmatic extralobar pulmonary sequestration masquerading as an intra-abdominal, suprarenal mass. Pediatr Surg Int 1997;12:529–531.

Lopoo JB, Goldstein RB, Lipshultz GS, et al: Fetal pulmonary sequestration: A favorable congenital lung lesion. Obstet Gynecol 1999;94: 567–571.

Louie HW, Martin SM, Mulder DG: Pulmonary sequestration: 17 year experience at UCLA. Am Surgeon 1993;59:801–805.

Mariona F, McAlpin G, Zador I, et al: Sonographic detection of fetal extrathoracic pulmonary sequestration. J Ultrasound Med 1986;5: 283–285.

Morin L, Crombleholme TM, D'Alton ME, et al: Prenatal diagnosis and management of fetal thoracic lesions. Semin Perinatol 1994;18:228–253.

Plattner V, Haustein B, Llanas B, et al: Extra-lobar pulmonary sequestration with prenatal diagnosis: A report of 5 cases and review of the literature. Eur J Pediatr Surg 1995;5:235–237.

Sakala EP, Perrott WS, Grube G: Sonographic characteristics of antenatally diagnosed extralobar pulmonary sequestration and congenital cystic adenomatoid malformation. Obstet Gynecol Surv 1994;49:647.

Sauerbrei E: Lung sequestration: Duplex doppler diagnosis at 19 weeks gestation. J Ultrasound Med 1991;10:101–105.

Stocker JT, Kagan-Hallet K: Extralobar pulmonary sequestration: Analysis of 15 cases. Am J Clin Pathol 1979;72:917.

Thomas CS, Leopold GR, Hilton S, et al: Fetal hydrops associated with extralobar pulmonary sequestration. J Ultrasound Med 1986;5: 668–671.

Weiner C, Varner M, Pringle K, et al: Antenatal diagnosis and palliative treatment of nonimmune hydrops fetalis secondary to pulmonary extralobar sequestration. Obstet Gynecol 1986;68:275–280.

White J, Chan YF, Neuberger S, Wilson T: Prenatal sonographic detection of intra-abdominal extralobar pulmonary sequestration: Report of three cases and literature review. Prenat Diagn 1994;14: 653–658.

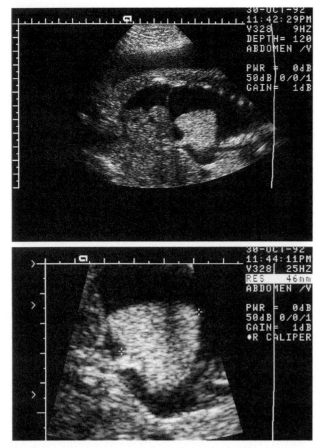

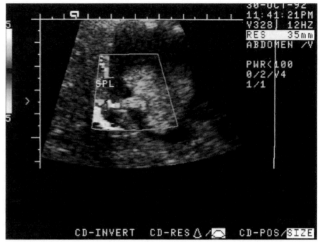

Extralobar sequestration surrounded by large pleural effusion. Note origin from diaphragm. (Courtsey of Gary Thieme, University of Colorado.)

Color flow image of the same case showing vascular supply to the sequestration from the aorta via the splenic artery below the diaphragm. (Courtesy of Gary Thieme, University of Colorado.)

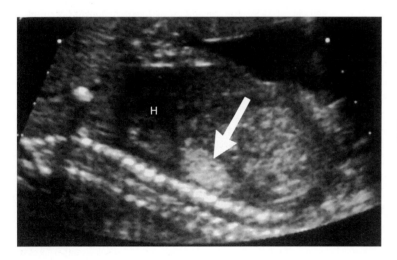

Extralobar infradiaphragmatic sequestration. The echogenic mass (*arrow*) was located superior to the left kidney. H, heart.

5.6 Tracheal/Laryngeal Atresia or CHAOS (Congenital High Airway Obstruction Syndrome)

Epidemiology/Genetics

Definition   Congenital absence of all or part of the trachea.

Epidemiology   One in 100,000 (M1.5:F1).

Embryology   Tracheal or laryngeal atresia is thought to result from aberrant pulmonary budding off the primitive foregut. Many infants with this condition are born at or near term after uncomplicated pregnancies. Oligohydramnios, intrauterine growth retardation, and congenital heart defects are associated abnormalities in some cases. Malformations seen with tracheal agenesis form patterns that overlap with the VACTERL association. Most cases have an anomalous connection with the esophagus.

Inheritance Patterns   Sporadic. No sibling recurrences have been documented.

Teratogens   None described.

Prognosis   Unrepaired complete agenesis is lethal in all cases. There is little experience with surgical intervention; so far one long-term survivor has been reported.

Sonography

FINDINGS

1. **Fetus:**
   a. Both lungs are much enlarged and densely echogenic. The diaphragms are everted.
   b. The heart is compressed by the massive lungs.
   c. Dilated bronchi filled with fluid are visible and can be traced to the level of obstruction in the trachea or larynx. Coronal views of the neck associated with color flow show no flow through the larynx with breathing movements if the obstruction is at that level.
   d. Secondary hydrops with ascites and skin thickening due to inferior vena cava compression is usual.
2. **Amniotic Fluid:** Decreased fluid is usual.
3. **Placenta:** Enlarged if hydrops is present.
4. **Measurement Data:** Enlarged abdominal circumference due to massive lungs.
5. **When Detectable:** At about 17 weeks.

Pitfalls   None reported.

Differential Diagnosis   Bilateral cystic adenomatoid malformation or sequestration has a similar appearance, but the dilated fluid-filled bronchi will not be present.

Where Else to Look

1. Make a particular effort to determine the level of obstruction, since this determines operability, by imaging the larynx with color flow sonography.
2. Look for the features of Fraser syndrome—Tracheal or laryngeal atresia, renal agenesis, microphthalmia, and poly- or syndactyly.
3. DiGeorge syndrome has been associated with tracheal atresia, so look at the heart and face.

Pregnancy Management

Investigations and Consultations Required   Most cases are isolated and sporadic. In those cases with sonographically detected abnormalities, however, chromosome studies should be done. Fetal echocardiography should be done to assess both cardiac structure and function. Consultations with a pediatric surgeon and a neonatologist are essential for planning delivery management.

Fetal Intervention   None is available at this time.

Monitoring   In the limited number of cases reported to date, there has been a high incidence of in utero deaths. There are no studies on which to base treatment recommendations, but weekly assessment of fetal status may be beneficial once the fetus has reached sufficient size that ex utero tracheotomy could be performed, should emergency delivery be deemed appropriate.

Pregnancy Termination Issues   For counseling regarding future pregnancies, an intact fetus is necessary to determine whether the airway obstruction is isolated or part of a syndrome.

Delivery   Delivery must occur in a center where a multidisciplinary team is skilled in the EXIT (ex utero intrapartum treatment) procedures. In this procedure, only the head and shoulders are delivered through the uterine incision, to maintain uterine volume. A saline infusion is used to prevent umbilical cord compression, and uterine relaxation is maintained by high concentration of inhalation anesthetics and tocolytic agents if necessary. If the fetal airway cannot be established by direct laryngoscopy or bronchoscopy, tracheostomy is performed. Only after the airway is established is the infant delivered and the umbilical cord clamped.

Mild oxygen desaturation is typical while the pulmonary vascular resistance remains elevated. As the pulmonary resistance falls, the oxygen saturation will gradually increase and symptoms of congestive heart disease may develop.

Heart failure generally develops within the first 1 to 3 weeks of life.

Neonatology

Resuscitation Few infants establish spontaneous ventilation following delivery and only rare survival of limited span is reported with palliative surgery. Satisfactory ventilation on a transient basis can be established with esophageal intubation, except in the most complex abnormalities. The occurrence of other major organ anomalies is high (85%) with cardiovascular abnormalities the most common, which further complicates the likelihood of a successful resuscitation. Given the severe prognosis, a prenatal discussion of management options with the parents is indicated. If the decision is for full effort for survival, delivery should be arranged to facilitate rapid surgical establishment of an airway if needed and with full pediatric subspecialty diagnostic and intensive care capabilities available.

Transport In most instances, the infant in distress is unlikely to survive a transport. However, if the diagnosis is made immediately at delivery, a temporary stabilization of the airway is achieved, and emergency transport with a skilled neonatal team is readily available, transport to a tertiary center with full pediatric and surgical subspecialty capabilities is indicated.

Testing and Confirmation Flexible endoscopy will confirm the blind tracheal pouch and in some cases identify the communication or communications between the esophagus and the distal airway or airways. Contrast studies may be needed to elucidate the structural anatomy of the communications in planning for surgical intervention. MRI has been useful in delineating aberrant distal airway anatomy but has the disadvantage of lack of access to an infant with an unstable airway during the examination. Multiple organ system anomalies occur in 85% of reported cases, with distal airway, pulmonary, and cardiovascular malformations being the most frequent.

Nursery Management The first priority is a stable and functional airway, which is achievable only with skilled surgical intervention. The next focus is complete evaluation, as multiple organ system anomalies occur in the preponderance of infants. The exact diagnostic and therapeutic management beyond full life support is dictated by the associated anomalies.

Surgery

Preoperative Assessment A detailed sonogram of all major organ systems should be obtained. Fraser syndrome should be excluded. In the absence of hydrops, delivery in a tertiary center familiar with the EXIT procedure is indicated. (See delivery section.)

Operative Indications CHAOS is a lethal malformation unless delivery via the EXIT procedure, followed by immediate surgery, is undertaken.

Types of Procedure Under deep general anesthesia, which allows uterine relaxation and preserves uteroplacental circulation, a bloodless hysterotomy is performed using a uterine stapling device and the fetal head and chest are delivered to secure an airway. Once the fetus is delivered, there is uterine contraction shutting down uteroplacental gas exchange. During the EXIT procedure, laryngoscopy is performed initially to evaluate the larynx. In most instances, the level of obstruction will be distal to the vocal cords and attempts to pass an endotracheal tube will be unsuccessful. Bronchoscopy should then be performed. The obstruction may be due to a simple laryngeal cyst or web, which may be amenable to bronchoscopic disruption, allowing passage into the trachea. If these efforts are unsuccessful, a formal tracheostomy should be performed. Once an airway is secured, the cord is clamped and the infant is handed over to the neonatologists. The possibility of a communication existing between trachea and esophagus must be suspected and diagnosed in all patients with CHAOS. Because of chronic tracheal obstruction, diffuse tracheobronchial malacia and diaphragmatic dysfunction are usually present.

Surgical Result/Prognosis Laryngeal webs and cysts can be easily treated, but experience with the reconstruction of an atretic trachea in a neonate with CHAOS is limited. A long-term survivor has been reported.

REFERENCES

Albanese CT, Harrison MR: Surgical treatment for fetal disease: The state of the art. Ann N Y Acad Sci 1998;847:74–85.

Crombleholme TM, Albanese CT: The fetus with airway obstruction. In Harrison MR, Evans MI, Holzgreve W, Adzick NS (eds): The Unborn Patient, 3rd ed. Philadelphia, WB Saunders, 2000.

Crombleholme TM, Sylvester K, Flake AW, et al: Salvage of a fetus with congenital high airway obstruction syndrome (CHAOS). Fetal Diagn Ther 2000;15:280–282.

DeCou JM, Jones DC, Jacobs HD, Touloukian RJ: Successful ex utero intrapartum treatment (EXIT) procedure for congenital high airway obstruction syndrome (CHAOS) owing to larygeal atresia. J Pediatr Surg 1998;33:1563–1565.

Evans JA, Greenberg CR, Erdile L: Tracheal agenesis revisited: Analysis of associated anomalies. Am J Med Genet 1999;82:415.

Evans JA, Reggin J, Greenberg C: Tracheal agenesis and associated malformations: A comparison with tracheoesophageal fistula and the VACTERL association. Am J Med Genet 1985;21:21.

Floyd J, Campbell DC, Dominy DE: Agenesis of the trachea. Am Rev Respir Dis 1962;86:557.

Hedrick MH, Martinez-Ferro, Filly RA, et al: Congenital high airway obstruction syndrome (CHAOS): A potential for perinatal intervention. J Pediatr Surg 1994;29:271–274.

Hiyama E, Yokoyama T, Ichikawa T, Matsuura Y: Surgical management of tracheal agenesis. J Thorac Cardiovasc Surg 1994;108:830.

Kalache KD, Chaoui R, Tennstedt C, Bollmann R: Prenatal diagnosis of laryngeal atresia in two cases of congenital high airway obstruction syndrome (CHAOS). Prenat Diagn 1997;17:577–581.

Kassanos D, Christodoulou CN, Agapitos E, et al: Prenatal ultrasonographic detection of the tracheal atresia sequence. Ultrasound Obstet Gynecol 1997;10:133–136.

Liechty KW, Crombleholme TM: Management of fetal airway obstruction. Semin Perinatol 1999;23:496–506.

Manschot HJ, Van Den Anker JN, Tibboel J: Tracheal agenesis. Anaesthesia 1994;49:788.

Morrison PI, Macphail S, Williams D, et al: Laryngeal atresia or stenosis presenting as second-trimester fetal ascites: Diagnosis and pathology in three independent cases. Prenat Diagn 1998;18:963–967.

Richards DS, Yancey MK, Duff P, Stieg FH: The perinatal management of severe laryngeal stenosis. Obstet Gynecol 1992;80:537–540.

Scott JN, Trevenen CL, Wiseman DA, Elliott PD: Tracheal atresia: Ultrasonographic and pathologic correlation. J Ultrasound Med 1999;18:375–377.

Skarsgard ED, Chitkara U, Krane EJ, et al: The OOPS procedure (operation on placental support): In utero airway management of the fetus with prenatally diagnosed tracheal obstruction. J Pediatr Surg 1996;31:826–828.

Watson WJ, Thorp JM Jr, Miller RC, et al: Prenatal diagnosis of laryngeal atresia. Am J Obstet Gynecol 1990;163:1456–1457.

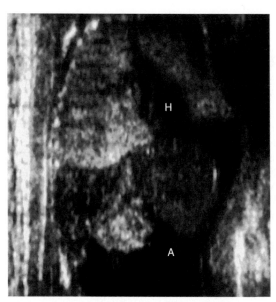

Coronal view of a fetus with CHAOS syndrome showing hyperinflated echogenic lungs depressing the diaphragm and compressing the heart (H). Fetal ascites (A) is present.

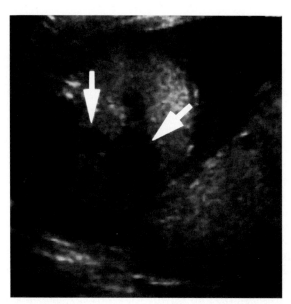

Transverse view of the fetal chest in a fetus with CHAOS syndrome showing echogenic lungs with enlarged fluid-filled bronchi (*arrows*). Note the skin thickening surrounding the chest.

6 Gastrointestinal System

6.1 Anal Atresia (Imperforate Anus, Anorectal Malformation)

Epidemiology/Genetics

Definition Anal atresia is the congenital absence of an anal opening.

Epidemiology One in 5000 births (M3:F2).

Embryology Anal atresia results from an arrest in the division of the cloaca into the urogenital sinus and rectum that occurs during the ninth week of fetal development. More than 80 genetic, chromosome, and sporadic syndromes have been reported with anal atresia. Associated abnormalities occur in 50% of cases and include spinal/skeletal abnormalities (30%), genitourinary abnormalities (38%), tracheoesophageal fistulas (10%), and cardiac malformations (5%). The VACTERL (vertebral defects, anal atresia, tracheoesophageal fistula with esophageal atresia, radial and renal dysplasia) association should be considered in these cases.

Inheritance Patterns Sporadic, with a 3 to 4% recurrence risk in first-degree relatives. Rare families show autosomal recessive inheritance.

Teratogens Alcohol, thalidomide, and maternal diabetes.

Prognosis Dependent on associated malformations. Eighty to 90% of isolated cases will have successful functional repair.

Sonography

FINDINGS

1. **Fetus:** Although rarely diagnosed prenatally, dilated colon may be noted in the pelvis or periphery of the abdomen. Echogenic foci with acoustic shadowing may be seen within the obstructed colon, representing calcified meconium.
2. **Amniotic Fluid:** Usually, the fluid volume is normal in isolated anorectal atresia but may be decreased if associated with bilateral renal dysplasia or increased if associated with tracheoesophageal fistula.
3. **Placenta:** Normal.
4. **Measurement Data:** Normal, if isolated.
5. **When Detectable:** The earliest prenatal diagnosis reported was at 29 weeks' gestation.

Pitfalls Differentiation of dilated small and large bowel may be very difficult. Location is a help if the descending colon can be traced to the rectum. Apparent haustra can be seen with large and small bowel.

Differential Diagnosis

1. Hirschsprung's disease.
2. Meconium plug syndrome.
3. Small bowel atresia, but polyhydramnios is usually present.

Where Else to Look Associated anomalies are present in 90% of cases diagnosed prenatally, and these include genitourinary (renal agenesis or dysplasia, horseshoe kidney, uterine duplications), cardiovascular, central nervous system, gastrointestinal (particularly tracheoesophageal fistula), and skeletal abnormalities. Anal atresia is associated with the VACTERL association, the syndrome of caudal regression, and trisomies 18 and 21.

Pregnancy Management

Investigations and Consultations Required

1. Fetal echocardiography should be performed to diagnose associated cardiovascular anomalies.
2. Amniocentesis can be performed for chromosomal analysis, especially if other anomalies are present.
3. Computed tomographic (CT) scan with intra-amniotic iodinated contrast injection can resolve diagnostic uncertainty.
4. Consultation with a pediatric surgeon is appropriate.

Monitoring Standard obstetric care is appropriate.

Pregnancy Course No specific obstetric complications are to be expected.

Pregnancy Termination Issues The late clinical presentation of this malformation will preclude the option of pregnancy termination.

Delivery The high association with other abnormalities makes delivery at a tertiary center with multiple pediatric and surgical subspecialists the best option. A pediatric dysmorphologist should be available to evaluate the neonate for a possible genetic syndrome.

Neonatology

Resuscitation There are no special issues for delivery room management with isolated anal atresia. If other associated anomalies exist, then management may need to be directed toward their related issues.

Transport Transfer to a tertiary center having a pediatric surgeon is always indicated. Beyond orogastric decompression, there are no special precautions during transfer.

Testing and Confirmation Obvious on newborn examination. Postnatal radiologic studies will define the defect.

Nursery Management Once the lack of patency of the anus has been established, all enteral intake is contraindicated. Maintenance intravenous fluids should be administered. Nasogastric decompression should be maintained.

Surgery

Preoperative Assessment Nasogastric decompression and intravenous access should be obtained and a physical examination and babygram radiography should be performed in the immediate postnatal period. In females, physical examination can make the diagnosis in 90% of cases. In males, examination of urine for meconium and ultrasonography are required if a perineal fistula is not found. For both sexes, the classification of types of anorectal malformations are the same. A low anorectal malformation is within 1 cm of skin, and the remainder are considered high defects. High types are classified according to where the anorectum connects with the genitourinary system (e.g., rectobulbar or prostatic urethral fistula, bladder-neck fistula, or cloaca).

Operative Indications All types of defects require operative reconstruction.

Types of Procedures Low-lying, perineal, or skin-level anomalies should be repaired in the neonatal period. High anomalies require decompressive colostomy and re-pair within 1 to 3 months. Poor postnatal weight gain and associated anomalies may alter the timing for reconstruction. However, in the presence of a colostomy, other priorities can be addressed and definitive reconstruction delayed indefinitely.

Surgical Results and Prognosis There is an excellent correlation between the degree of skeletal sacral anomaly and the functional prognosis of the newborn with an anorectal malformation. Absence of one of the five sacral vertebrae is not generally pathologic. Two or more absent sacral vertebrae is a poor prognostic sign of bowel function.

Survival is excellent unless there is a life-threatening cardiac defect or multiple associated anomalies (genitourinary, skeletal, nervous system, gastrointestinal). The majority of children who undergo reconstruction for low anorectal malformation will have some degree of postoperative constipation. This can be managed with stool softeners and cathartics. The spectrum of high anorectal malformation carries with it the postoperative problem of incontinence. In general, the higher the defect, the more likely the presence of incontinence. A Bowel Management Program, tailored to the status of colonic motility, has helped many of these children.

REFERENCES

Botto LD, Khoury MJ, Mastroiacov P, et al: The spectrum of congenital anomalies of the VATER association: An international study. Am J Med Genet 1997;71:8–15.

Grant T, Newman M, Gould R, et al: Intraluminal colonic calcifications associated with anorectal atresia: Prenatal sonographic detection. J Ultrasound Med 1990;9:411–413.

Harris RD, Nyberg DA, Mack LA, Weinberger E: Anorectal atresia: Prenatal sonographic diagnosis. Am J Roentgenol 1987;149:395–400.

Hertzberg BS, Bowie JD: Fetal gastrointestinal abnormalities. Radiol Clin North Am 1990;28:101–114.

Nyberg DA: Intra-abdominal abnormalities. In Diagnostic Ultrasound of Fetal Anomalies: Text and Atlas. St. Louis, Mosby-Year Book, 1990, pp 363–368.

Paidas CN: Fecal incontinence in children with anorectal malformations. Semin Pediatr Surg 1997;6:228–234.

Paidas CN, Pena A: Rectum and anus. In Oldham KT, Foglia RP, Colombani PM (eds): The Surgery of Infants and Children: Scientific Principles and Practice. Philadelphia, Lippincott-Raven, 1997, pp 1323–1362.

Pena A: Anorectal malformations. Semin Pediatr 1995;4:35.

Samuel N, Dicker D, Landman J, et al: Early diagnosis and intrauterine therapy of meconium plug syndrome in the fetus: Risks and benefits. J Ultrasound Med 1986;5:425–428.

Sepulveda W, Romero R, Qureshi F, et al: Prenatal diagnosis of enterolithiasis: A sign of fetal large bowel obstruction. J Ultrasound Med 1994;13:581–585.

Shalev E, Weiner E, Zuckerman H: Prenatal ultrasound diagnosis of intestinal calcifications with imperforate anus. Acta Obstet Gynecol Scand 1983;62:95–96.

Stoll C, Alembik Y, Roth MP, Dott B: Risk factors in congenital anal atresia. Ann Genet 1997;40:197–204.

Tongsong T, Wanapirak C, Piyamongkol W, Sudasan J: Prenatal sonographic diagnosis of VATER association. J Clin Ultrasound 1999;27:378–384.

Vermesh M, Mayden KL, Confino E, et al: Prenatal sonographic diagnosis of Hirschsprung's disease. J Ultrasound Med 1986;5:37–39.

Vintzeilos AM, Campbell WA, Nochimson DJ, Weinbaum PJ: Antenatal evaluation and management of ultrasonically detected fetal anomalies. Obstet Gynecol 1987;69:640–660.

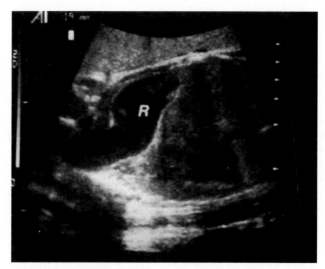

Coronal view of the fetal abdomen. A dilated loop of bowel can be seen (R). This represents a dilated rectum and sigmoid colon. Anal atresia was found at delivery.

6.2 Duodenal Atresia

Epidemiology/Genetics

Definition Duodenal atresia is characterized by complete obliteration of the lumen of the duodenum and is the most common type of congenital small bowel atresia.

Epidemiology One in 10,000 births. One third have trisomy 21.

Embryology At 5 weeks of embryonic life, the lumen of the duodenum is obliterated by proliferating epithelium. Patency is usually restored by the 11th week. Failure of this recanalization results in duodenal atresia. Associated abnormalities occur in 30 to 50% of patients and include skeletal defects (vertebral, rib, sacral agenesis, radial anomalies, and club foot), gastrointestinal abnormalities (annular pancreas, esophageal atresia, tracheoesophageal fistula, intestinal malrotation, Meckel's diverticulum, and anal atresia), cardiac malformations, and renal defects. More than 15 genetic, chromosome, and sporadic syndromes have been reported with duodenal atresia.

Inheritance Patterns Generally sporadic with rare familial reports.

Teratogens Maternal diabetes.

Prognosis Mortality is due to associated abnormalities or preterm labor and can be as high as 15%. Successful surgical repair is possible in essentially all cases of isolated duodenal atresia.

Sonography

FINDINGS

1. **Fetus:** The "double bubble" sign, an enlarged fluid-filled stomach and proximal duodenum separated by the pylorus, is seen. The stomach fails to empty. No fluid-filled bowel, distal to the duodenum, is seen.
2. **Amniotic Fluid:** Severe polyhydramnios occurs, although it may not be present until after 24 weeks.
3. **Placenta:** Normal.
4. **Measurement Data:** The abdominal circumference may be increased because of the distended stomach.
5. **When Detectable:** May be detectable as early as 18 to 20 weeks, but appearances may be normal until after 24 weeks.

Pitfalls

1. A prominent normal stomach with a visible incisura angularis may be confused with a "double bubble" sign.

The amniotic fluid will be normal and stomach dilation will not persist on repeat examinations.
2. A bile-filled gallbladder might be misinterpreted as a distended duodenum, as might other right upper quadrant cystic masses such as choledochal cyst or hepatic cyst. Appropriate angulation should show the two cystic structures of the stomach and duodenum connecting.

Where Else to Look

1. Look for the other findings of Down syndrome (there is a 30% association).
2. Skeletal problems are often found—Vertebral deformities, radial ray problems, and club feet are seen.
3. Other gastrointestinal malformations such as malrotation, other atresias, and Meckel's diverticulum should be sought.
4. Cardiovascular malformations can occur with duodenal atresia in the absence of Down syndrome.
5. Genitourinary malformations such as hydronephrosis and multicystic dysplastic kidney may be seen.
6. Examine the cervix to see if it is still long and closed in the presence of polyhydramnios.

Differential Diagnosis

1. Annular pancreas—The sonographic appearances are indistinguishable.
2. Duodenal stenosis—The obstruction site is usually at a more distal level.
3. Ladd's bands—The typical obstruction site is in the third portion of the duodenum.
4. Proximal jejunal atresia—The entire duodenum and proximal jejunum will be dilated.
5. Midgut volvulus—More dilated small bowel will be visible.
6. Proximal intestinal duplications—A normal-sized stomach should be visible as well.

Pregnancy Management

Investigations and Consultation Required Consultation with a pediatric surgeon is indicated for the family to discuss neonatal management. Chromosome studies should be done at any gestation by either amniocentesis, percutaneous umbilical blood sampling, or late chorionic villus sampling. Detailed fetal echocardiography is warranted, even in the absence of trisomy 21, because of the high association of cardiac abnormalities (20%).

Fetal Intervention No intervention is warranted. Serial amniocentesis has no benefit in prolonging pregnancy.

Monitoring   The diagnosis is usually made because of the onset of polyhydramnios. Therefore, preterm labor will occur in the majority of cases, and care should be under the direction of a perinatologist. Regularly scheduled examinations are necessary to detect evidence of preterm labor and for early institution of tocolysis.

Pregnancy Course   The major obstetric complication of this disorder is severe polyhydramnios with a high incidence of preterm labor.

Pregnancy Termination Issues   Pregnancy termination would not be indicated in a fetus with normal karyotype because of the excellent prognosis following surgical repair. Even in fetuses with Down syndrome, the options for termination are limited by the late clinical presentation of duodenal atresia.

Delivery   The site for delivery should be one capable of managing the preterm infant and one where appropriate personnel are available for surgical repair.

Neonatology

Resuscitation   With high obstruction, amniotic fluid may be green stained from regurgitated bilious secretions, giving the erroneous impression that there has been meconium passage in utero. Aspiration of bilious material into the lungs is equally damaging, as with meconium aspiration, and every effort should be made to prevent its occurrence. Fetal distress can occur, usually from reasons other than the structural anomaly. If there are other indications of distress, it is safer to assume that aspiration may have occurred and thus laryngoscopy and tracheal suction are indicated before the onset of respiration. In the absence of other markers of fetal distress and if the fluid is thin and without particulate matter, airway instrumentation is probably not indicated.

If positive-pressure ventilation is required because of respiratory depression, bag and mask ventilation should be avoided to reduce the likelihood of gaseous distension of the stomach and duodenum.

If there is known or suspected high obstruction (polyhydramnios or other ultrasonographic findings), the stomach should be emptied prior to transfer of the infant from the delivery room to reduce the risk of regurgitation and aspiration.

Transport   Transfer to a tertiary center where there is a pediatric surgeon is always indicated. Orogastric decompression and maintenance of intravenous fluid infusion in transit are essential.

Testing and Confirmation   Confirmation of the diagnosis is best established by abdominal radiographs or ultrasonograms. Air is an excellent and safe contrast media for suspected upper tract obstruction. The classic radiograph shows the double bubble of an air-filled stomach and proximal duodenum.

Additional diagnostic evaluation for associated anomalies should be obtained as indicated.

Nursery Management   If cardiorespiratory resuscitation has been required, the first priority is to facilitate cardiorespiratory adaptation with oxygen, fluids, and ventilatory support as needed.

Intravenous access should be established by the most rapid and reliable route and fluid and electrolyte support instituted. If "third spacing" or dehydration is suspected, the rate of infusion should be increased until there is urine production.

Nasogastric decompression should be maintained to minimize the risk of aspiration and respiratory complication.

Parenteral nutrition is usually required in the postoperative period, as there is usually a significant interval before adequate enteral intake is established.

Surgery

Preoperative Assessment   Acute management includes a radiographic upper gastrointestinal contrast study or radiographic enema examination to attempt to rule out an associated intestinal malrotation and potential volvulus. If this lesion can be excluded, then the surgery can be delayed long enough to rule out other significant anomalies included in the VACTERL association.

Operative Indications   If an associated intestinal malrotation can be ruled out preoperatively, then the surgical management of the duodenal atresia is semi-elective. That is, the operation can be safely delayed while possible associated anomalies are evaluated and the patient is stabilized.

Types of Procedures   Nasogastric decompression is immediately instituted as well as intravenous fluid management. The defect usually occurs at the level of the second to third portion of the duodenum and frequently is in close association with the sphincter of Oddi. The operation of choice is a duodenoduodenostomy or duodenojejunostomy. The dilated proximal duodenum can have poor peristalsis with slow emptying across the anastomotic site, making delayed enteral nutrition a possibility. Total parenteral nutrition via a central venous line can be required, or a transanastomotic feeding jejunostomy can be used for earlier enteral nutrition.

Associated VACTERL gastrointestinal deformities such as esophageal atresia with tracheoesophageal fistula or imperforate anus must be considered when establishing the order of preference for surgical repair.

Surgical Results/Prognosis   A major associated and potentially lethal problem is the presence of a cardiac defect in 20% of patients, which accounts for high mortality and chronic complication rates. Uncomplicated duodenal atresia has an excellent prognosis, with a greater than 95% survival rate.

REFERENCES

Barss VA, Benecerraf BR, Frigoletto FD Jr: Antenatal sonographic diagnosis of fetal gastrointestinal malformations. Pediatrics 1985;76:445–449.

Cragun JD, Martin ML, Moore CA, Khoury MJ: Descriptive epidemiology of small intestinal atresia, Atlanta, Georgia. Teratology 1993; 48:441–450.

Dalla Vecchia LK, Grosfeld JL, West KW, et al: Intestinal atresia and stenosis: A 25-year experience with 277 cases. Arch Surg 1998;133: 490–496.

Fonkalsrud EW, DeLorimier AA, Hays DM: Congenital atresia and stenosis of the duodenum: A review compiled from the members of the Surgical Section of the American Academy of Pediatrics. Pediatrics 1969;43:79–83.

Haller JA Jr, Tepas JJ, Pickard LR, Shermeta DW: Intestinal atresia: Current concepts of pathogenesis, pathophysiology, and operative management. Am Surg 1983;49:385–391.

Irving IM: Duodenal atresia and stenosis: Annular pancreas. In Lister J, Irving IM (eds): Neonatal Surgery, 3rd ed. London, Butterworths, 1990.

Kimura K, Tsugawa C, Ogawa K, et al: Diamond-shaped anastomosis for congenital duodenal obstruction. Arch Surg 1977;112:1262–1263.

Mooney D, Lewis JE, Connors RH, Weber TR: Newborn duodenal atresia: An improving outlook. Am J Surg 1987;153:347–349.

Nelson LH, Clark CE, Fishburne JI, et al: Value of serial sonography in the in utero detection of duodenal atresia. Obstet Gynecol 1982;59: 657–660.

Nixon HH, Tawes R: Etiology and treatment of small intestinal atresia: Analysis of a series of 127 jejunoileal atresias and comparison with 62 duodenal atresias. Surgery 1971;69:41–51.

Nyberg DA: Intra-abdominal abnormalities. In Diagnostic Ultrasound of Fetal Anomalies: Text and Atlas. St. Louis, Mosby-Year Book, 1990, pp 352–355.

Rescorla FJ, Grosfeld JL: Intestinal atresia and stenosis: Analysis of survival in 120 cases. Surgery 1985;98:668–676.

Romero R, Jeanty P, Gianluigi P, et al: The prenatal diagnosis of duodenal atresia: Does it make any difference? Obstet Gynecol 1988;71: 739.

Touloukian RJ: Intestinal atresia and stenosis. In Ashcraft KW, Holder TM (eds): Pediatric Surgery, 2nd ed. Philadelphia, WB Saunders, 1993, pp 305–319.

Wayne ER, Burrington JD: Management of 97 children with duodenal obstruction. Arch Surg 1973;107:857.

Wesley J, Mahour GH: Congenital intrinsic duodenal obstruction: A 25 year review. Surgery 1977;82:716–720.

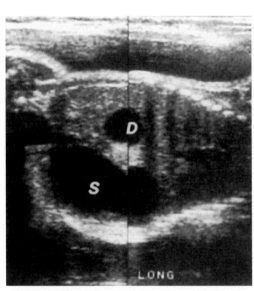

Coronal view of the fetal trunk. Two cystic structures can be seen. These represent the body of the stomach (S) and the duodenal bulb (D). Polyhydramnios was present.

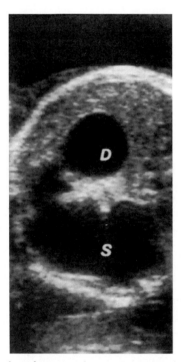

Angled view to show the two cystic structures connecting. The pylorus between the stomach (S) and the duodenum (D) is visible.

6.3 Small Bowel Atresia or Stenosis

Epidemiology/Genetics

Definition Nonduodenal bowel atresias with congenital obliteration of the lumen of segments of the large or small intestine.

Epidemiology Small intestinal atresias occur in 2 to 3 in 10,000 births (jejunal, 50%; ileal, 43%; multiple, 7%). Colonic atresia occurs in 1 in 20,000 births.

Embryology Most isolated cases of bowel atresias are thought to be due to ischemic injury from hypotension, vascular accidents, volvulus, intussusception, or vascular malformations. Forty-four percent of cases have associated findings, including small for gestational age (30%), meconium peritonitis (12%), meconium ileus (10%), cystic fibrosis (15%), omphalocele (7.5%), gastroschisis (12.5%), malrotation, imperforate anus, cardiovascular defects (7%), and chromosome abnormalities (7%). More than 15 genetic, chromosome, and sporadic syndromes have been described with intestinal atresias.

Inheritance Patterns Rare autosomal recessive genetic syndromes including multiple intestinal atresias and jejunal atresia have been described. Approximately 25% of cases of jejunal and ileal atresia have cystic fibrosis (autosomal recessive).

Teratogens Thalidomide and cocaine.

Prognosis Outcome is excellent in more than 85% of patients if the atresia occurs as an isolated abnormality, with most of the deaths due to short bowel syndrome. Prenatal diagnosis occurred in one third of cases and suggests a more proximal atresia with a poorer outcome. Otherwise, the prognosis is dependent on the associated abnormalities and/or syndrome diagnosis.

Sonography

FINDINGS

1. **Fetus:** Multiple dilated fluid-filled bowel loops are noted within the abdomen proximal to the stenotic or atretic segment. The exact site of obstruction may be difficult to determine sonographically, since large and small bowel are more or less the same size in utero. Small bowel dilation is much more common. A pattern in which there are parallel fixed bowel loops has been associated with volvulus. MRI is helpful in determining the site of obstruction.
2. **Amniotic Fluid:** Polyhydramnios is usually present and is more severe in more proximal atresias. Large bowel atresias are often not associated with polyhydramnios.
3. **Placenta:** Normal.
4. **Measurement Data:** The abdominal circumference may be large because of bowel dilation.
5. **When Detectable:** Usually detected after 24 weeks.

Pitfalls

1. Cystic abdominal masses, such as duplication, mesenteric, and ovarian cysts, may be confused with dilated bowel loops.
2. Hydronephrosis and hydroureter or very large multicystic kidneys may also be confused with fluid-filled, dilated bowel. Renal anomalies, however, are rarely associated with polyhydramnios.
3. In utero, the small and large bowel are approximately equal in size. Significantly dilated loops of bowel are much more likely to be due to small bowel atresia, especially if there is polyhydramnios. The distribution of the bowel is of limited value in determining whether it is large or small bowel.

Differential Diagnosis

1. Midgut volvulus. Dilated loops of small or large bowel encircle an echogenic area in which color flow sonography demonstrates patent mesenteric vessels. A short segment of markedly dilated bowel may form an adjacent oval cystic mass. Ascites may be present.
2. Meconium ileus.
3. Congenital chloridorrhea.

Where Else to Look

1. Meconium peritonitis (ascites, intraperitoneal calcifications, or cysts) occurs in 6% to 12% of cases due to bowel perforation. Either ascites or a meconium cyst will be visible (see Chapter 6.6).
2. Associated bowel anomalies are common and include malrotation, volvulus, intestinal duplications, gastroschisis, and other bowel atresias (anorectal, esophageal, colonic).
3. Extraintestinal anomalies are seen in less than 5% of small bowel atresias distal to the duodenum.

Pregnancy Management

Investigations and Consultations Required Chromosome studies should be performed even for more distal lesions. If sonographic findings are suggestive of meconium ileus, an evaluation for cystic fibrosis should be done. Fetal echocardiography should be performed to exclude associated cardiac malformations. A management plan should be devised in consultation with a pediatric surgeon.

Monitoring The high risk of prematurity makes it mandatory that prenatal care be under the direction of a perinatologist. Sonographic examinations should be performed every 3 to 4 weeks to detect polyhydramnios and monitor the degree of bowel dilation. Polyhydramnios is, however, rare in lesions beyond the jejunum. Careful assessment for signs of preterm labor is essential.

Pregnancy Course The risk of preterm labor is high in lesions from the proximal jejunum and higher.

Pregnancy Termination Issues Pregnancy termination is rarely entertained because of the late clinical presentation of these malformations and their potential for surgical correction.

Delivery In general, management should be delivery at term in a facility with appropriate support services. In theory, early delivery might be beneficial in cases with massive bowel dilation, but no data are available to support this approach.

Neonatology

Resuscitation With high obstruction, amniotic fluid may be green stained from regurgitated bilious secretions, giving the erroneous impression that there has been meconium passage in utero. Aspiration of bilious material into the lungs is equally damaging, as with meconium aspiration, and every effort should be made to prevent its occurrence. Fetal distress can occur, usually from reasons other than the structural anomaly. If there are other indications of distress, it is safer to assume that aspiration may have occurred and thus, laryngoscopy and tracheal suction are indicated before the onset of respiration. In the absence of other markers of fetal distress and if the fluid is thin and without particulate matter, airway instrumentation is probably not indicated.

If positive-pressure ventilation is required because of respiratory depression, bag and mask ventilation should be avoided to reduce the likelihood of gaseous distension of the stomach and proximal small bowel.

If there is known or suspected high obstruction (polyhydramnios or other ultrasonographic findings), the stomach should be emptied prior to transfer of the infant from the delivery room to reduce the risk of regurgitation and aspiration.

With known or suspected distal obstruction, there are usually no special resuscitation issues.

Transport Transfer to a tertiary center with a pediatric surgeon is always indicated. Orogastric decompression and maintenance of intravenous fluid infusion in transit are essential.

Testing and Confirmation Confirmation of the diagnosis is best established by abdominal radiographs and ultrasonograms. Air is an excellent and safe contrast medium for suspected upper tract obstruction. The typical pattern is to see multiple dilated loops and air-fluid levels proximally with no visualization of bowel distally.

Additional diagnostic evaluation for associated anomalies should be obtained as indicated.

Nursery Management If cardiorespiratory resuscitation has been required, the first priority is to facilitate cardiorespiratory adaptation with oxygen, intravenous fluids, and ventilatory support as needed.

Intravenous access should be established by the most rapid and reliable route, and fluid and electrolyte support should be instituted. If "third spacing" or dehydration is suspected, the rate of infusion should be increased until there is urine production.

Orogastric decompression should be maintained to minimize the risk of aspiration and respiratory complication.

Parenteral nutrition is usually required in the postoperative period, as there is usually a significant interval before adequate enteral intake is established.

Surgery

Operative Indications All neonates with obstructed small bowel require surgery.

Types of Procedures Intestinal decompression and intravenous access with maintenance fluids are begun immediately. Antibiotics are also started. The infant then has an exploratory laparotomy.

Surgical repair usually consists of the excision of a portion of the dilated proximal intestine and a modified end-to-end or end-to-side primary anastomosis. If the atresia involves a large portion of bowel, it can result in potential short gut syndrome. Under these circumstances, tapering of the dilated proximal bowel with primary anastomosis is utilized. This avoids increased loss of length, facilitates early gut function, and diminishes bacterial overgrowth in the proximal intestine. The use of proximal intestinal stomas is reserved only for those cases complicated by severe meconium peritonitis or perforation with bacterial contamination and secondary peritonitis.

Surgical Results/Prognosis The long-term prognosis is primarily related to the length and functional capability of the remaining small bowel and/or associated defects such as cystic fibrosis. Uncomplicated short-segment intestinal atresias have an excellent prognosis. Extensive areas of gut atresia can result in the short gut syndrome. Infants can be kept alive by intravenous alimentation but undergo progressive worsening of liver function with eventual death from portal hypertension.

REFERENCES

Benachi A, Soniogo P, Jouannic J: Determination of the antenatal intestinal occulusion by magnetic resonance imaging. Ultrasound Obstet Gynecol 2001;18:163–165.

Cragun JD, Martin ML, Moore CA, Khoury MJ: Descriptive epidemiology of small intestinal atresia, Atlanta, Georgia. Teratology 1993;48: 441–450.

Dalla Vecchia LK, Grosfeld JL, West KW, et al: Intestinal atresia and stenosis: A 25-year experience with 277 cases. Arch Surg 1998;133:490–496.

DeLorimier AA, Fonkalsrud EW, Hays DM: Congenital atresia and stenosis of the jejunum and ileum. Surgery 1969;65:819–827.

Haller JA Jr, Tepas JJ, Pickard LR, Shermeta DW: Intestinal atresia: Current concepts of pathogenesis, pathophysiology, and operative management. Am Surg 1983;49:385–391.

Howard ER, Othersen HB: Proximal jejunoplasty in the treatment of jejunal atresia. J Pediatr Surg 1973;8:685–690.

Kimble RM, Harding J, Kolbe A: Additional congenital anomalies in babies with gut atresia or stenosis: When to investigate, and which investigation. Pediatr Surg Int 1997;12:565–570.

Kjoller M, Holm-Nielsen G, Meiland H, et al: Prenatal obstruction of the ileum diagnosed by ultrasound. Prenat Diagn 1984;5:427.

Lister J: Intestinal atresis and stenosis, excluding the duodenum. In Lister J, Irving IM (eds): Neonatal Surgery. London, Butterworths, 1990.

Louw J: Resection and end to end anastomosis in the management of atresia and stenosis of the small bowel. Surgery 1967;62:940–950.

Nixon HH, Tawes R: Etiology and treatment of small intestinal atresia: Analysis of a series of 127 jejunoileal atresias and comparison with 62 duodenal atresias. Surgery 1971;69:41–51.

Nyberg DA: Intra-abdominal abnormalities. In Diagnostic Ultrasound of Fetal Anomalies: Text and Atlas. St. Louis, Mosby-Year Book, 1990, pp 355–358.

Rescorla FJ, Grosfeld JL: Intestinal atresia and stenosis: Analysis of survival in 120 cases. Surgery 1985;98:668–676.

Rickham PP, Karplus M: Familial and hereditary intestinal atresia. Helv Paediatr Acta 1971;26:561–564.

Samuel N, Dicker D, Feldberg D, Goldman JA: Ultrasound diagnosis and management of fetal intestinal obstruction and volvulus in utero. J Perinat Med 1984;12:333–337.

Schild RL, Hansmann M: Small bowel atresia: Antenatal intestinal vascular accident or parvovirus B19 infection? Ultrasound Obstet Gynecol 1998;11:227.

Tam PK, Nicholls G: Implications of antenatal diagnosis of small-intestinal atresia in the 1990s. Pediatr Surg Int 1999;15:486–487.

Touloukian RJ: Intestinal atresia and stenosis. In Ashcraft KW, Holder TM (eds): Pediatric Surgery, 2nd ed. Philadelphia, WB Saunders, 1993, pp 305–319.

Verpairjkil B, Charoenvidhya S, Tanawattanachavaoen S, et al: Fetal intestinal volvulus: Clinicosonographic findings. Ultrasound Obstet Gynecol 2001;18:186–187.

Yoo SJ, Park KW, Cho SY, et al: Definitive diagnosis of intestinal volvulus in utero. Ultrasound Obstet Gynecol 1999;13:200–203.

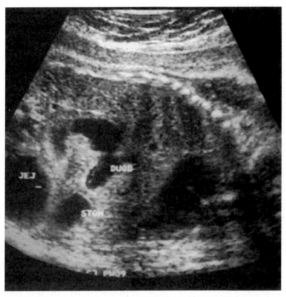

Jejeunal atresia. A few loops of distended small bowel greater than 2.5 cm wide are seen, but most of the bowel is not fluid filled. The relatively few distended loops allowed a diagnosis of a high small bowel obstruction. Polyhydramnios was present.

6.4 Gastroschisis

Epidemiology/Genetics

Definition Gastroschisis is the intrauterine evisceration of fetal intestine through a paraumbilical wall defect.

Epidemiology Occurs in 1 in 4000 births (M1:F1).

Embryology The cause is probably heterogeneous, with some cases of gastroschisis resulting from vascular accident or error in development of the right omphalomesenteric artery leading to infarction and necrosis at the base of the umbilical cord. The umbilical cord arises intact, medial to the defect. Thickening, edema, and matting together of the intestines occur in some cases. It used to be thought that these abnormalities were due to the irritating effects of amniotic fluid, but they are more likely the result of vascular compromise from kinking of the blood vessels coming through the small paraumbilical defect. Intestinal atresias and other gastrointestinal disruptions are found in approximately 5 to 10% of cases. Malrotation is almost universal. Extraintestinal abnormalities occur in less than 5% of cases.

Inheritance Patterns Rare familial recurrences suggest that a few families may have an autosomal dominant inheritance of isolated gastroschisis.

Screening Maternal serum alpha-fetoprotein measurement will detect more than 95% of gastroschisis cases. The median maternal serum alpha-fetoprotein level is 7.0 MOM for gastroschisis. Ten to 15% of affected infants have long-term developmental disabilities.

Teratogens None known.

Prognosis Liveborn infants have a greater than 90% survival rate with modern surgical treatment and neonatal intensive care.

Sonography

FINDINGS

1. **Fetus:** Small and/or large bowel herniates through the anterior abdominal wall. The bowel almost always exits through the right rather than the left lower quadrant. Cord vessels can be seen to the left of the exiting bowel. If the anterior abdominal wall defect is small, bowel loops within or outside the abdomen are dilated. Small bowel dilation to a width of greater than 1.8 cm is associated with greater long-term morbidity. Gut malrotation is very common, so the stomach may be inverted or malpositioned. The stomach and/or bladder may be included in the gastroschisis contents. Secondary hydronephrosis related to the bladder evisceration may occur.
2. **Amniotic Fluid:** Amniotic fluid volume is usually normal or slightly diminished. Polyhydramnios can occur if the gut is obstructed and carries with it a poor prognosis.
3. **Placenta:** Normal placenta.
4. **Measurement Data:** Intrauterine growth retardation often develops. Abdomen measurements are unreliable, since some of the bowel is in the gastroschisis.
5. **When Detectable:** At 13 weeks. Prior to 13 weeks, there may be confusion with physiologic gut herniation.

Pitfalls

1. The extra-abdominal bowel can be overlooked and thought to be umbilical cord coiled alongside the abdomen.
2. In large patients with oligohydramnios and in third-trimester prone fetuses, the condition can easily be missed.

Differential Diagnosis

1. Limb-body wall complex—Gastroschisis is a component of the syndrome, but, in addition, the liver will be outside of the abdomen and there will be spine and limb problems.
2. Ruptured omphalocele—In this extremely rare entity, the liver, as well as bowel, is usually outside of the abdomen.
3. Tangled cord adjacent to the fetal abdomen—Color flow Doppler sonography will show vascular flow.

Where Else to Look

1. Look for bowel dilation of greater than 18 mm in the gastroschisis or in the abdomen. This finding has a low-grade association with delay in time to oral feeding.
2. Check the stomach position for malrotation.
3. Look elsewhere for anomalies. Ruptured omphalocele containing only gut, indistinguishable by ultrasonography, is associated with chromosomal anomalies.

Pregnancy Management

Investigations and Consultations Required Although the risk of chromosomal abnormalities is low, amniocentesis should be discussed with the patient. Fetal echocardiography should be performed in all cases of gastroschisis. The family should be referred to a pediatric surgeon for a thorough discussion of the neonatal management issues.

Monitoring   Care should be coordinated in a tertiary center because of the potential need for early intervention. Serial ultrasonographic examinations should be performed every 3 to 4 weeks to detect thickening and/or dilation of the fetal bowel and to assess fetal growth. Fetal assessment, such as non-stress testing, should be initiated if there is evidence of a lag in growth. Some authors have recommended beginning biophysical testing at 30 weeks' gestation and continuing weekly until delivery.

Pregnancy Course   The increased incidence of intrauterine growth restriction in fetuses with gastroschisis may complicate the obstetric management. Preterm labor occurs in nearly one third of cases.

Pregnancy Termination Issues   There are no special concerns regarding the method or location for pregnancy termination.

Delivery   For the fetus with normal-appearing bowel on ultrasonographic examination, delivery at term is appropriate. The mode of delivery is controversial. Some studies have shown no clear benefit of cesarean section over vaginal delivery, but a recent study by Sakala et al showed an improved perinatal outcome in neonates delivered by elective cesarean section prior to labor. In the fetus in which bowel dilation and/or thickening develops, the prognosis may be improved by early delivery when fetal lung maturity is achieved.

A pediatric surgeon and a tertiary neonatal intensive care unit should be available at the delivery site.

Neonatology

Resuscitation   Assistance with the onset of respiration is usually not required, unless there is concurrent prematurity-associated respiratory distress. If assisted ventilation is required, bag and mask ventilation is contraindicated to avoid gaseous distension of the stomach and bowel.

The major concern is the protection of the extruded bowel. Extreme care must be taken to avoid torsion of the bowel loops, which would further compromise perfusion. If there is marked distension of the bowel, perfusion can be compromised by the kinking of the mesenteric vessels as they exit through the abdominal wall defect. Prompt decompression of the stomach is important. The bowel should be covered with warmed saline-soaked gauze and supported to avoid torsion, and the trunk should be encased in a sterile plastic bag with a drawstring ("bowel bag"). This not only reduces evaporative heat and water loss but also reduces the likelihood of surface contamination.

Transport   Transfer to a tertiary center that has a pediatric surgeon is always indicated. Care of the bowel, as outlined, should be provided during the transport. Reliable venous access should be established and a balanced electrolyte solution administered. Gastric decompression is essential.

Testing and Confirmation   Once the infant has recovered from the initial surgery and the exposed bowel is covered, additional diagnostic evaluation may be instituted if there is concern for associated anomalies.

Nursery Management   Protection of the bowel and intravenous fluid support as described earlier should be provided in the time prior to surgical repair.

In some instances, it may be necessary to provide ventilatory support in the early postoperative period, as there may be increased intra-abdominal pressure from the reduction of the extruded bowel back into the abdominal cavity.

Parenteral nutrition is required during the postoperative recovery period, as there is always a significant interval before adequate enteral intake is established.

Surgery

Preoperative Assessment   The immediate post-delivery goals are to preserve infant temperature, avoid excess fluid loss from the exposed bowel surface, prevent further surface contamination, and maintain circulation to the exposed bowel loops.

Nasogastric decompression is essential, and intravenous fluids calculated at 1.5 times normal maintenance rates are begun. Broad-spectrum antibiotic therapy should be started.

Operative Indications   All neonates with gastroschisis require surgery shortly after birth.

Types of Procedures   The operative repair consists of enlarging the narrowed abdominal wall opening and evaluating the exposed viscera. The abdominal wall is stretched gently and an attempt is made to reduce the extra-abdominal contents into the abdomen. If the intra-abdominal pressure is less than 20 mm Hg by intragastric or intravesical pressure measurement, a primary fascial closure can be achieved. Excessive intra-abdominal pressures necessitate delayed fascial closure utilizing temporary coverage with a silastic/Dacron intra-abdominal pouch or the use of mobilized lateral skin flaps. The former method requires a secondary closure of fascia after the bowel has been gradually reduced into the abdomen over the ensuing 5 to 7 days. The latter requires a secondary closure of fascia at several months of age. Both techniques can result in infections and a chronic incisional hernia.

Complications   The infant may have had intrauterine intestinal ischemia with necrosis of an exposed bowel loop requiring an excision and primary bowel anastomosis or possible temporary intestinal stomas. Intestinal atresias can also be a complication. Their repair as a primary or secondary procedure depends on the degree of chemical peritonitis with "matting" of the bowel that is present. Delayed intestinal function with poor enteral nutrition is expected in most patients. Central venous access and early total parenteral nutrition are therefore required. A "short bowel" syndrome can be a significant functional problem, with long-term parenteral nutrition and liver failure as potential complications.

Surgical Results/Prognosis Ultimate survival approaches 90%. A small abdominal cavity that cannot be closed with the techniques described has a poor outcome. Postoperative infection and delayed total enteral nutrition are the major acute and chronic complications. Large defects can be associated with lung hypoplasia requiring long-term ventilatory support and resulting in chronic respiratory insufficiency.

REFERENCES

Axt R, Quijano F, Boos R, et al: Omphalocele and gastroschisis: Prenatal diagnosis and peripartal management. A case analysis of the years 1989–1997 at the Department of Obstetrics and Gynecology, University of Homburg/Saar. Eur J Obstet Gynecol Reprod Biol 1999;87:47–54.

Boyd PA, Bhattacharjee A, Gould S, et al: Outcome of prenatally diagnosed anterior abdominal wall defects. Arch Dis Child Fetal Neonatal Ed 1998;78:F209–213.

Chescheir NC, Azizkhan RG, Seeds JW, et al: Counseling and care for the pregnancy complicated by gastroschisis. Am J Perinatol 1991;8:323–329.

Colombani PM, Cunningham MD: Perinatal aspects of omphalocele and gastrochisis. Am J Dis Child 1977;131:1386–1388.

Dunn JC, Fonkalsrud EW, Atkinson JB: The influence of gestational age and mode of delivery on infants with gastroschisis. J Pediatr Surg 1999;34:1393–1395.

Forrester MB, Merz RD: Epidemiology of abdominal wall defects, Hawaii, 1986–1997. Teratology 1999;60:117–123.

Fries MH, Filly RA, Callen PW, et al: Growth retardation in prenatally diagnosed cases of gastroschisis. J Ultrasound Med 1993;12:583–588.

Guzman ER: Early prenatal diagnosis of gastroschisis with transvaginal ultrasonography. Am J Obstet Gynecol 1990;162:1253–1254.

Hoyme HE, Jones MC, Jones KL: Gastroschisis: Abdominal wall disruption secondary to early gestational interruption of the omphalomesenteric artery. Semin Perinatol 1983;7:294–298.

Ikhena SE, DeChazal RC, Konje JC: Gastroschisis associated with bladder evisceration complicated by hydronephrosis presenting antenatally. Ultrasound Obstet Gynecol 1999;13:370–372.

Irving IM: Umbilical abnormalities. In Lister J, Irving IM (eds): Neonatal Surgery. London, Butterworths, 1990.

Kushnir O, Izquierdo L, Vigil D, Curet LB: Early transvaginal sonographic diagnosis of gastroschisis. J Clin Ultrasound 1990;18:194–197.

Langer JC, Khanna J, Caco C, et al: Prenatal diagnosis of gastroschisis: Development of objective sonographic criteria for predicting outcome. Obstet Gynecol 1993;81:53–56.

Luck SR, Sherman JO, Raffensperger JG, Goldstein IR: Gastroschisis in 106 consecutive newborn infants. Surgery 1985;98:677–683.

Nakayama DK, Harrison MR, Gross BH, et al: Management of the fetus with an abdominal wall defect. J Pediatr Surg 1984;19:408–413.

Paidas MJ, Crombleholme TM, Robertson FM: Prenatal diagnosis and management of the fetus with an abdominal wall defect. Semin Perinatol 1994;18:196–214.

Palomski GE, Hill LE, Knight GJ: Second-trimester maternal serum alpha-fetoprotein levels in pregnancies associated with gastroschisis and omphalocele. Obstet Gynecol 1988;71:906.

Perrella RR, Ragavendra N, Tessler FN, et al: Fetal abdominal wall mass detected on prenatal sonography: Gastroschisis vs omphalocele. Am J Roentgenol 1991;157:1065–1068.

Philippart AI, Canty TG, Filler RM: Acute fluid volume requirements in infants with anterior abdominal wall defects. J Pediatr Surg 1972;7:553–558.

Rankin J, Dillon E, Wright C: Congenital anterior abdominal wall defects in the north of England, 1986–1996: Occurrence and outcome. Prenat Diagn 1999;19:662–668.

Reiss RE, Landon MB, Jayanth VR, et al: Functional urinary tract obstruction developing in fetuses with isolated gastroschisis. Ultrasound Obstet Gynecol 2000;15:194–198.

Rubin SZ, Martin DJ, Ein SH: A critical look at delayed intestinal motility in gastroschisis. Can J Surg 1978;21:414–416.

Sakala EP, Erhard LN, White JJ: Elective caesarean section improves outcomes of neonates with gastroschisis. Am J Obstet Gynecol 1993;169:1050–1053.

Swartz KR, Harrison MW, Campbell JR, Campbell TJ: Ventral hernia in the treatment of omphalocele and gastroschisis. Ann Surg 1985;201:347–350.

Yang P, Beaty TH, Khoury MJ, et al: Genetic-epidemiologic study of omphalocele and gastroschisis: Evidence for heterogeneity. Am J Med Genet 1992;44:668–675.

Yaster M, Scherer TL, Stone MM, et al: Prediction of successful primary closure of congenital abdominal wall defects using intraoperative measurements. J Pediatr Surg 1989;24:1217–1220.

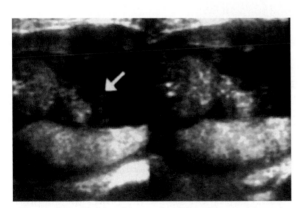

Gastroschisis. Gut is exiting to the right of the cord (*arrow*).

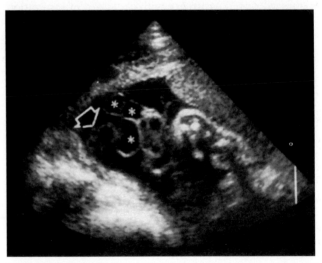

Gastroschisis. Fluid-filled bowel loops (*) are seen adjacent to the fetal abdomen. Note the different appearance of the loop of cord (*arrow*) with the two small umbilical arteries. Gastroschisis loops can be mistaken for cord loops.

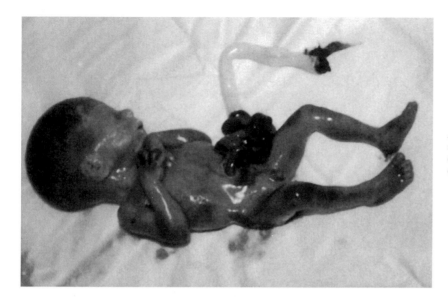

A 22-week fetus with isolated gastroschisis. Note abdominal defect is to the right of the umbilical cord with only small bowel extruding from the abdomen.

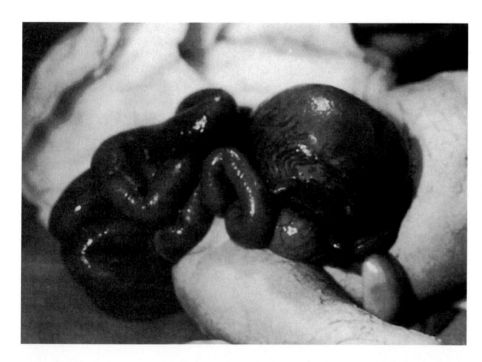

Close-up of gastroschisis in a newborn with extrusion of stomach and small bowel through a right para-umbilical defect.

6.5 Hepatic Tumors

Epidemiology/Genetics

Definition Liver tumors are the tenth most frequent pediatric tumor. Hepatic malignancy must be distinguished from benign hepatic tumors and non-neoplastic hepatomegaly. Almost 50% of primary liver tumors are benign. In older children, liver tumors more often represent metastatic disease (neuroblastoma, Wilms' tumor) than primary malignancies.

Epidemiology Occur in 1.6 in 1,000,000 births. Hepatoblastoma, M1.4:F1; vascular tumors, M:1.3:F1.

Embryology Unknown. Hepatoblastoma is associated with hemihypertrophy, the Beckwith-Wiedemann syndrome, diaphragmatic and umbilical hernias, Meckel's diverticulum, and renal anomalies. Hepatoblastomas present as an abdominal mass, with 60% detected in the first year and 90% by age 3 years. Cavernous hemangiomas occur most commonly in early childhood and may produce large masses. Diffuse congenital hemangiomatosis is a sporadic disorder that can present with heart failure and hydrops if associated with a large liver atrioventricular shunt. Isolated hepatic atrioventricular shunts with hydrops can also occur sporadically.

Inheritance Patterns Sporadic.

Teratogens None known.

Additional Investigations Postnatally, hepatoblastomas can be associated with elevated serum alpha-fetoprotein levels (66%) and intratumor calcification (30%). CT and MRI can suggest the diagnosis. Doppler flow studies can help separate benign vascular tumors from hepatoblastoma.

Prognosis Infants with vascular tumors with no evidence of heart failure or hydrops have a good prognosis. The 3-year survival rate of hepatoblastoma exceeds 90% in patients with initially resectable tumors, 65% in those with initially unresectable tumors treated first with chemotherapy, and only 10 to 20% in patients with metastatic disease.

Sonography

FINDINGS

1. **Fetus:**
   a. Hemangioma and hemangioendothelioma:
      1. Typically there is an echogenic intrahepatic mass, often containing echo-free areas. Vascularity can be much increased and the apparent cystic areas may prove to be vascular areas.
      2. Secondary hydrops due to the arteriovenous shunting through the mass may occur with skin thickening, ascites, pleural effusion, and placentomegaly. These two sonographically similar masses are benign. Hemangioma is the most common intrahepatic fetal mass.
   b. Mesenchymal hamartoma:
      1. Typically an echogenic mass honeycombed with variably sized cysts.
      2. The mass does not show increased vascularity.
      3. Other benign, not highly vascularized masses include liver adenoma and congenital peliosis hepatis.
   c. Hepatoblastoma. Highly vascular with cystic and solid areas. The fluid-filled areas are often filled with blood. Nonimmune hydrops has developed secondary to a hepatoblastoma. The tumor is very rare in utero.
   d. Liver metastases. Usually derived from neuroblastoma. These are echopenic avascular masses.
2. **Amniotic Fluid:** Polyhydramnios is common, presumably owing to gut compression.
3. **Placenta:** Normal unless there is hydrops.
4. **Measurement Data:** There may be an enlarged abdominal circumference.
5. **When Detectable:** Hemangioma has been detected at 16 weeks.

Where Else to Look

1. Look for evidence of nonimmune hydrops.
2. Hemangiomas elsewhere in the body, particularly the skin, may be present.

Pregnancy Management

Investigations and Consultations Required Because many of the hepatic tumors are associated with development of fetal hydrops, fetal echocardiography may be useful to detect early evidence of cardiac decompensation.

Fetal Intervention None is available.

Monitoring Serial ultrasonograms should be obtained to monitor growth of the mass, to detect early signs of hydrops, and to assess amniotic fluid volume. Biophysical profiles should be implemented if there is evidence of fetal compromise.

Pregnancy Course Polyhydramnios and fetal hydrops are common complications of hepatic tumors.

Pregnancy Termination Issues Pathologic confirmation of the diagnosis is essential; an intact fetus may not be necessary to obtain appropriate tissue samples.

Delivery The risk of bleeding into the tumor is unknown, but cesarean section may be the better alternative. Delivery at a tertiary center is essential for prompt evaluation and treatment of the infant.

Neonatology

Resuscitation The type, size, and systemic manifestations of a given tumor may influence the management of resuscitation. Both congestive heart failure and hydrops may occur, particularly as complications of vascular tumors and/or large, solid, infiltrative tumors. If either is present, the immediate postnatal management must address the pathophysiologic effects of each on the onset of respiration and circulatory transition. In addition, dystocia from massive abdominal enlargement may result in both traumatic injury to the viscera and asphyxial injury from obstructed delivery. Thus, volume expansion may be needed, followed by packed red cell transfusion in the former and correction of metabolic acidosis in the latter as a part of resuscitative interventions. In the absence of any of these complications, which can be anticipated from assessment of the fetus intrapartum, no special resuscitative measures are usually required.

Transport Transfer to a tertiary center with pediatric and surgical subspecialty capabilities is essential. If there is evidence of cardiorespiratory compromise, the transport should be conducted by experienced neonatal personnel.

Testing and Confirmation Vascular tumors (the most common type with presentation in the fetus) are best delineated with a combination of MRI and Doppler flow studies. Solid tumors can be recognized by either CT or MRI; histopathologic examination is necessary to determine cell type.

Nursery Management Establishing and maintaining homeostasis is the first priority, followed by expeditious diagnosis. As noted earlier, the most common neonatal hepatic tumor is a vascular hemangioma, and congestive heart failure from the shunt is the most common presentation. Management includes restriction of volume intake, diuretics, and inotropic medications. The definitive treatment is surgical. The second most common neonatal presentation is abdominal distension, which may be sufficient to embarrass both respiration and feeding. Ventilatory support and alternative modes of feeding and/or parenteral nutrition may be required. The definitive treatment of solid tumors varies with the histologic type.

Surgery

Preoperative Assessment Once an infant with a hepatic tumor is born, attention should focus on establishing a definitive diagnosis. In the cases of hepatic hemangiomas, more than 50% will have associated cutaneous hemangiomas. The infant's platelet count, fibrinogen, and fibrin split products should be checked to exclude disseminated intravascular coagulation and platelet trapping. A follow-up echocardiogram should be obtained to exclude high-output physiology. An initial bedside ultrasonogram may be helpful in establishing the diagnosis, but CT or MRI scans are usually indicated to more fully define these lesions.

The distinction between hepatic hemangioma and arteriovenous malformation is an important one. Hepatic arteriovenous malformations require embolization or surgical resection and do not respond to corticosteroids or interferon-α.

Mortality from hepatic hemangioma associated with heart failure is much decreased if corticosteroids or interferon-α is administered prior to surgery or immobilization. Currently, interferon-α is restricted to treatment of patients with serious or life-threatening hemangiomas who fail to respond to corticosteroids, develop complications of corticosteroid administration, or have a contraindication to long-term corticosteroids (gastrointestinal bleeding, vomiting, infection). An initial 2-week course of oral corticosteroids at 2 to 3 mg/kg/day is tried. If the hemangioma responds, as evidenced by shrinkage or arrest of growth, then the treatment is continued for 4 weeks before a slow taper is begun over 8 to 10 months. Interferon-α is not without potential complications, and recognized toxicities include fever, elevation of liver function test results, transient neutropenia, and anemia.

In the newborn with a hepatic mass suspected of being a hepatoblastoma, a serum alpha-fetoprotein level should be drawn. Values in normal term infants may be between 20,000 and 120,000 ng/mL, which may make interpretation difficult in the newborn, but a markedly elevated alpha-fetoprotein level is usually seen in hepatoblastoma. Color Doppler imaging is helpful in evaluating the involvement of the portal vein, hepatic veins, and inferior vena cava.

Computed tomographic scanning of the liver is helpful in defining the extent of the tumor and assessing the resectability of the tumor. MRI gives detailed information not only on segmental anatomy of a hepatic tumor but also on vascular anatomy of the liver, making angiography unnecessary.

Operative Indications Both benign and malignant tumors should be removed, since benign masses may become malignant.

Types of Procedures The combination of MRI and Doppler sonography allows the liver anatomy to be mapped. Right hepatic resections are most frequently performed. Left and extended left hepatic lobectomies may also be undertaken. The liver volume rapidly recovers to a normal size.

In cases of mesenchymal hamartoma, definitive treatment consists of a frozen section to confirm the diagnosis and exclude the possibility of malignancy and then complete resection of the mass. Surgical resection is the primary mode of treatment in hepatoblastoma. In tumors that are found to be unresectable at operative staging, however, biopsy is performed to make a diagnosis and chemotherapy is begun with reexploration for resection after several cycles of chemotherapy and evidence of tumor regression.

Surgical Results/Prognosis   A good prognosis can be anticipated for hepatic hemangiomas in the absence of complications such as congestive heart failure, platelet trapping, or rupture at the time of delivery. Most hepatic hemangiomas are asymptomatic and go unrecognized and do not develop complications. Even in the face of complications, there has been significant improvement in survival with the treatment of hepatic hemangiomas with corticosteroids and interferon-α. The natural history of hemangiomas is to progress during infancy and then to steadily regress thereafter.

There has also been steady progress in the outcome of patients treated for hepatoblastoma. The combination of surgery and chemotherapy has achieved disease-free survival rates of 100% for stage I, 75% for stage II, and 67% for stage III disease. Unfortunately, no disease-free survival has been achieved with stage IV disease.

The long-term prognosis in mesenchymal hamartoma is excellent following complete resection. These tumors are not associated with malignant transformation and do not recur following complete resection.

REFERENCES

Abuhamad AZ, Lewis D, Inati MN, et al: The use of color flow Doppler in the diagnosis of fetal hepatic hemangioma. J Ultrasound Med 1993;4:223–226.

Bracero LA, Gambon TB, Evans B, Beneck D: Ultrasonographic findings in a case of congenital peliosis hepatis. J Ultrasound Med 1995;14:483–486.

Chuileannain FN, Rowlands S, Sampson A: Ultrasonographic appearance of fetal hepatic hemangioma. J Ultrasound Med 1999;18:379–381.

Davis CF, Carachi R, Young DG: Neonatal tumors: Glasgow 1955–86. Arch Dis Child 1988;63:1075.

DeMaioribus CA, Lally KP, Sim K, et al: Mesenchymal hamartoma of the liver: A 35-year review. Arch Surg 1990;125:598.

Ehren H, Mahour G, Isaacs H Jr: Benign liver tumors in infancy and childhood: Report of 48 cases. Am J Surg 1983;145:325.

Folkman J: Towards a new understanding of vascular proliferative disease in children. Pediatrics 1984;74:850–855.

Folkman J, Mulliken JB, Ezekowitz AB: Angiogenesis and hemangiomas. In Oldham KT, Colombani PM, Foglia RP (eds): Surgery of Infants and Children: Scientific Principles and Practice. Philadelphia, Lippincott-Raven, 1997, pp 569–580.

Foucar E, Williamson RA, Yiu-Chiu V, et al: Mesenchymal hamartoma of the liver identified by fetal sonography. Am J Roentgenol 1983;140:970–972.

Gonen R, Fong K, Ciasson DA: Prenatal sonographic diagnosis of hepatic hemangioendothelioma with secondary nonimmune hydrops fetalis. Obstet Gynecol 1989;73:485–487.

Hirata GI, Matsunaga ML, Medearis AL, et al: Ultrasonographic diagnosis of a fetal abdominal mass: A case of mesenchymal hamartoma and a review of the literature. Prenat Diagn 1990;10:507.

Hubinont C, Bernard P, Khalil N, et al: Fetal liver hemangioma and chorioangioma: Two unusual cases of severe fetal anemia detected by ultrasonography and its perinatal management. Ultrasound Obstet Gynecol 1994;4:330–331.

Jones KL: Aicardi syndrome in Smith's recognizable patterns of human malformation. Philadelphia, WB Saunders, 1997, pp 534–535.

Kazzi NJ, Chang CH, Roberts EC, Shankaran S: Fetal hepatoblastoma presenting as nonimmune hydrops. Am J Perinatol 1989;6:278–280.

Keeling JW: Liver tumors in infancy and childhood. J Pathol 1971;103:69–76.

Li FP, Thurber WA, Seddon J, et al: Hepatoblastoma in families with polyposis coli. JAMA 1987;257:2475–2479.

Luks FL, Yazbeck S, Brandt ML, et al: Benign liver tumors in children: A 25-year experience. J Pediatr Surg 1991;26:1326.

Marks F, Thomas P, Lustig I, et al: In utero sonographic description of a fetal liver adenoma. J Ultrasound Med 1990;9:119–122.

Nakamoto SK, Dreilinger A, Dattel B, et al: The sonographic appearance of hepatic hemangioma in utero. J Ultrasound Med 1983;2:239–241.

Petrikovsky BM, Cohen HL, Scimeca PH, Bellucci E: Prenatal diagnosis of focal nodular hyperplasia of the liver. Prenatal Diagnosis 1994;14:406.

Platt LD, Devore GR, Benner P, et al: Antenatal diagnosis of a fetal liver mass. J Ultrasound Med 1983;2:521–522.

Raney B: Hepatoblastoma in children: A review. J Pediatr Hematol Oncol 1997;19:418–422.

Sepulveda WH, Donetch G, Giuliano A: Prenatal sonographic diagnosis of fetal hepatic hemangioma. Eur J Obstet Gynecol Reprod Biol 1993;48:73–76.

Sheu BC, Shyu MK, Lin YF, et al: Prenatal diagnosis and corticosteroid treatment of diffuse neonatal hemangiomatosis: Case report. J Ultrasound Med 1994;13:495–499.

Shih J-C, Tsao PN, Huang SF, et al: Antenatal diagnosis of congenital hepatoblastoma in utero. Ultrasound Obstet Gynecol 2000;16:94–97.

Stanley P, Geer GD, Miller JH, et al: Infantile hepatic hemangiomas: Clinical features, radiologic investigations, and treatment of 20 patients. Cancer 1989;64:936.

Stocker JT, Ishak KG: Mesenchymal hamartoma of the liver: Report of 30 cases and review of the literature. Pediatr Pathol 1983;1:245–251.

Stringer MD, Hennayake S, Howard ER, et al: Improved outcome for children with hepatoblastoma. Br J Surg 1994;82:386.

Tagge EP, Tagge DU: Hepatoblastoma and hepatocellular carcinoma. In Oldham KT, Colombani PM, Foglia RP (eds): Surgery of Infants and Children: Scientific Principles and Practice. Philadelphia, Lippincott-Raven, 1997, pp 633–643.

Tovbin J, Segal M, Tavori I, et al: Hepatic mesenchymal hamartoma: A pediatric tumor that may be diagnosed prenatally. Ultrasound Obstet Gynecol 1997;10:63–65.

Weinberg AG, Finegold MJ: Primary hepatic tumors of childhood. Hum Pathol 1983;14:512.

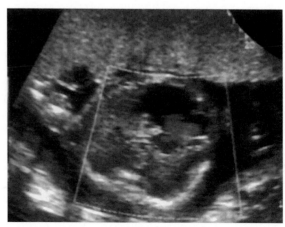

Color flow Doppler image of hemangioendothelioma in the liver. The mass is basically cystic with a large vascular component. (See color figure following p. x.)

6.6 Meconium Cyst/Meconium Peritonitis

Epidemiology/Genetics

Definition   A meconium cyst forms as the result of peritoneal inflammation from recurrent meconium spillage from an intrauterine bowel perforation.

Epidemiology   Unknown, but rare.

Embryology   Meconium peritonitis is a chemical peritonitis resulting from fetal bowel perforation of any cause. Continued leakage of meconium results in cyst formation. Sixty-five percent of cases are due to meconium ileus or small bowel atresia, with the majority of cases of meconium ileus associated with a diagnosis of cystic fibrosis. Other commonly associated conditions include volvulus and intussusception.

Inheritance Patterns   Cystic fibrosis is an autosomal recessive single gene disorder.

Teratogens   None.

Prognosis   Most meconium cysts disappear spontaneously during pregnancy. Surgery for gut torsion or other neonatal complications of meconium peritonitis is necessary in less than 25% of prenatally diagnosed cases.

Sonography

FINDINGS

1. **Fetus:**
   a. Echogenic foci, with or without shadowing, are seen anywhere in the peritoneal cavity or scrotum. Calcifications are often linear. A common site is just below the diaphragm on the right.
   b. Meconium pseudocysts—A more or less echo-free cyst with irregular echogenic borders. Calcification is often present in the wall. Cysts result from a walled-off bowel perforation. Serial sonograms will show a gradual reduction in size, often with increased calcification. They usually resolve before delivery.
   c. Generalized ascites occurs in about 50% of cases of meconium peritonitis. The ascitic fluid may appear echogenic owing to leakage of meconium through a recent bowel perforation.
   d. Dilated small bowel is seen in only about 25% of cases of prenatally diagnosed meconium peritonitis and reflects mechanical bowel obstruction leading to perforation. In prenatally diagnosed cystic fibrosis, echogenic foci are intermixed with mildly dilated small bowel loops. Calcification is rarely, if ever, seen with cystic fibrosis.
2. **Amniotic Fluid:** Polyhydramnios is present in the majority of cases (60%).
3. **Placenta:** Normal.
4. **Measurement Data:** The abdominal circumference may be large if the ascites is severe or if the bowel is markedly dilated.
5. **When Detectable:** Usually not detected until after 24 weeks.

Pitfalls

1. Very echogenic meconium may be difficult to distinguish from calcifications.
2. A few meconium cysts have smooth walls and echo-free contents.
3. Single, small intra-abdominal echogenic foci with shadowing are normal and not associated with cystic fibrosis or postpartum gut perforation.

Differential Diagnosis   Of fetal abdominal calcifications:

1. Intraluminal meconium calcification (seen in small bowel and anorectal atresia).
2. Parenchymal calcification (hepatic, splenic, adrenal, ovarian)—May be related to toxoplasmosis or cytomegalovirus.
3. Cholelithiasis. Not uncommon in utero and of no pathological consequence.
4. Echogenic small bowel—Localized echogenic small bowel of the same echogenicity as adjacent bone may be due to (a) cystic fibrosis, (b) trisomy 21, (c) cytomegalovirus infection, (d) intragut bleed, or (e) a normal variant.

Of meconium cyst:

1. Ovarian cyst (females only)—Smooth walls often echo-free.
2. Duplication cyst—Usually tubular shape, has a thick wall and may show peristalsis. Commonly alongside stomach.
3. Mesenteric cyst—Rare, may be septated.
4. Dilated gallbladder and liver cyst—Partially within, or adjacent to, the liver.
5. Abdominal lymphangioma—Multicystic, multiseptate cystic lesions usually on the left.

Where Else to Look

1. Secondary cystic fibrosis changes in pancreas, gallbladder, and lungs are not seen in utero.
2. Look for changes of cytomegalovirus (see Chapter 9.1) and Down syndrome (see Chapter 1.4).

Pregnancy Management

Investigations and Consultations Required Because the exact cause often cannot be determined by sonographic findings, amniocentesis should be performed for chromosome studies, viral cultures, and DNA studies for cystic fibrosis. Consultation with a pediatric surgeon should be arranged to plan both fetal and neonatal management.

Fetal Intervention Early delivery may be appropriate if there is marked bowel dilation. However, no guidelines exist for judging when intervention might be indicated. For cases with massive fetal ascites, fetal paracentesis just prior to delivery may prevent dystocia.

Monitoring Careful sonographic monitoring is necessary to assess fluid volume, fetal growth, degree of bowel dilation, and amount of ascites. Most cysts disappear within a few weeks.

Pregnancy Course The prognosis for obstetric complications will depend on the cause of the cyst. Significant fetal ascites may result in dystocia. Concomitant bowel obstruction may lead to polyhydramnios and preterm labor. Most meconium cysts regress and cause no problem postpartum.

Pregnancy Termination Issues Unless a precise diagnosis has been established, the technique for termination should allow for delivery of an intact fetus for a complete autopsy.

Delivery Because of the significant risk of premature delivery and the potential need for immediate surgical intervention for the neonate, the pregnancy should be managed in a tertiary center.

Neonatology

Resuscitation Severe abdominal distention may be present at birth, hindering the onset of respiration and necessitating endotracheal intubation. If ascites is known to be present from prenatal ultrasonography, then it is probably safe to perform paracentesis to relieve some of the distention.

Transport Transfer to a tertiary center that has a pediatric surgeon is always indicated. Gastric decompression during transport, to avoid aspiration, is essential. Reliable intravenous access and infusion of fluid and electrolyte solution are also indicated.

Testing and Confirmation The major diagnostic questions are the coexistence of an obstructive lesion and/or of an open perforation allowing continuing meconium spillage. Abdominal radiography without contrast media is usually sufficient to answer both concerns. If meconium ileus is determined to be the cause of the ob-

struction leading to the perforation, then iontophoresis (sweat testing) for cystic fibrosis is indicated and is known to be reliable after 1 week of age in term infants.

Nursery Management The primary issues are avoidance of aspiration by gastric decompression, maintenance of hydration and electrolyte balance, and confirmation of the diagnosis. Often, hypotension develops rapidly after birth and large volumes of plasma expanders are required to maintain perfusion.

Surgery

Preoperative Assessment Intestinal decompression and intravenous access with fluid resuscitation and antibiotics are started immediately. An evaluation for an intestinal obstruction is completed. An exploratory laparotomy is performed when and if an intestinal obstruction or peritoneal signs of infection are identified.

Operative Indications As previously noted, meconium cysts may not produce intestinal obstruction. However, a meconium cyst can maintain a fistulous connection to the bowel lumen and become secondarily infected.

Types of Procedures Such cysts require antibiotics, drainage, and eventual excision with closure of the fistula. Intestinal obstruction with meconium peritonitis presents a significant surgical challenge. Frequently, temporary enteral stomas are needed, with delayed closure after resolution of the extensive peritoneal inflammatory response.

Surgical Results/Prognosis Depending on the cause, the remaining small intestine and/or colon may be very short, resulting in chronic short gut syndrome. This may result in long-term parenteral nutrition with secondary liver failure. Long-term surgical survival for non-short gut infants is good, with the ultimate prognosis dependent on associated factors such as cystic fibrosis.

REFERENCES

Andrassy RJ, Nigiotis JG: Meconium disease of infancy: Meconium ileus, meconium plug syndrome, and meconium peritonitis in pediatric surgery. In Ashcraft K, Holder T (eds): Pediatric Surgery. Philadelphia, WB Saunders, 1993.

Boix-Ochoa J: Meconium peritonitis. J Pediatr Surg 1968;3:715.

Careskey JM, Grosfeld JL, Weber TR, Malangoni MA: Giant cystic meconium peritonitis (GCMP): Improved management based on clinical and laboratory observations. J Pediatr Surg 1982;17:482–489.

Deshpande P, Twining P, O'Neill D: Prenatal diagnosis of fetal abdominal lymphangioma by ultrasonography. Ultrasound Obstet Gynecol 2001;17:445–448.

Dirkes K, Crombleholme TM, Craigo SD, et al: The natural history of meconium peritonitis diagnosed in utero. J Pediatr Surg 1995;30:979–982.

Forouhar F: Meconium peritonitis: Pathology, evolution, and diagnosis. Am J Clin Pathol 1982;78:208–213.

Foster MA, Nyberg DA, Mahony BS, et al: Meconium peritonitis: Prenatal sonographic findings and their clinical significance. Radiology 1987;165:661–665.

Hertzberg BS, Bowie JD: Fetal gastrointestinal abnormalities. Radiol Clin North Am 1990;28:101–114.

McGahan JP, Hanson F: Meconium peritonitis with accompanying pseudo-cyst: Prenatal sonographic diagnosis. Radiology 1983;148:125–126.

Nicolaides KH, Campbell S: Ultrasound diagnosis of congenital abnormalities. In Harrison MR, Golbus MS, Filly RA (eds): The Unborn Patient: Antenatal Diagnosis and Treatment. Philadelphia, WB Saunders, 1991, pp 593–648.

Nyberg DA: Intra-abdominal abnormalities. In Diagnostic Ultrasound of Fetal Anomalies: Text and Atlas. St. Louis, Mosby-Year Book, 1990, pp 378–382.

Yankes JR, Bowie JD, Effman EL: Antenatal diagnosis of meconium peritonitis with inguinal hernias by ultrasonography. J Ultrasound Med 1988;7:211–223.

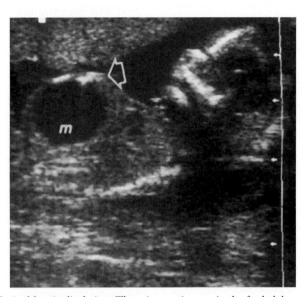

Sagittal longitudinal view. There is a cystic mass in the fetal abdomen (m). Note the echogenic areas in the wall, which represent areas of calcification (*arrow*). This meconium cyst has a relatively smooth wall. An irregular wall is not uncommon.

6.7 Meconium Ileus

Epidemiology/Genetics

Definition Meconium ileus is a cause of congenital intestinal obstruction due to inspissated meconium.

Epidemiology One in 50,000 births (M1:F1).

Embryology The cause of inspissated meconium is usually unknown, but commonly associated conditions include small bowel atresias, cystic fibrosis, volvulus, and intussusception.

Inheritance Patterns Cystic fibrosis is an autosomal recessive single gene disorder, but the other known causes are generally sporadic.

Teratogens None.

Prognosis In those cases proved to be secondary to cystic fibrosis (CF), the CF diagnosis determines the long-term outcome, although 40% of patients had neonatal complications requiring surgery. Patients with CF and meconium ileus are more likely to have chronic malnutrition than CF patients without meconium ileus. In the non–CF-related cases, the causes are mixed and the prognosis variable, although most cases resolve and patients have normal bowel function.

Sonography

FINDINGS

1. **Fetus:** Dilated bowel develops because of impacted meconium in the distal ileum. Echogenic meconium may be seen within dilated bowel or within bowel of normal caliber. Echogenic but nonshadowing masses may be seen within the abdomen and represent impacted meconium. Colonic dilation may be seen if the meconium plug obstructs the colon.
2. **Amniotic Fluid:** Polyhydramnios may be present if the bowel is dilated.
3. **Placenta:** Normal.
4. **Measurement Data:** Abdominal circumference may be increased if the bowel is significantly dilated.
5. **When Detectable:** Cases have been diagnosed prior to 24 weeks.

Pitfalls In normal fetuses, echogenic bowel may be seen prior to 20 weeks, but this is usually a transient and nonobstructive phenomenon. No small bowel dilation will be seen. Echogenic bowel is seen more often when high-frequency transducers are used.

Differential Diagnosis

1. Echogenic bowel associated with chromosomal abnormalities, particularly trisomy 21, may mimic that seen in meconium ileus.
2. Echogenic bowel may be seen in congenital infections such as cytomegalovirus.
3. Echogenic bowel may occur following ingestion of intra-amniotic blood and in association with intrauterine growth retardation.

Cases of meconium ileus with perforation will present with a sonographic picture of meconium peritonitis, and those conditions, such as cytomegalovirus infection, that have a poor prognosis must be excluded.

Where Else to Look Look for stigmata of Down syndrome or cytomegalovirus infection.

Pregnancy Management

Investigations and Consultations Required Molecular studies for cystic fibrosis should be considered. The best approach is probably amniocentesis, which also can provide information regarding chromosome status. Measurement of amniotic fluid proteins, such as alkaline phosphatase, will not be helpful, as low levels would be expected in any condition that causes intestinal obstruction. If there is a question of peritonitis, amniotic fluid culture for cytomegalovirus should be performed. Consultation with a pediatric surgeon is appropriate. If a diagnosis of cystic fibrosis is established, referral of the family to a pediatrician with special expertise in the management of cystic fibrosis should be made. In those circumstances in which the fetus is found to have only a single detectable mutation for CF, the likelihood that the fetus has CF is diminished, but the residual risk for CF ranges from 3 to 72%, depending on the ethnic background of the parents.

Fetal Intervention Theoretically, early delivery prior to bowel perforation will improve prognosis. At present, however, no criteria have been established to indicate when intervention would be appropriate.

Monitoring Serial sonograms and regular clinical assessment are essential to detect increased amniotic fluid volume and evidence of preterm labor. No other special fetal assessment is necessary. Prenatal care should be coordinated in a tertiary center.

Pregnancy Course Polyhydramnios secondary to intestinal obstructions may result in preterm labor.

Pregnancy Termination Issues There are no special concerns if a diagnosis has been established. Without a diagnosis, a complete autopsy and appropriate molecular studies on fetal tissue are essential.

Delivery   Prenatal care and delivery should be at a tertiary center. The degree of bowel distension will rarely be significant enough to cause abdominal dystocia.

Neonatology

Resuscitation   No special resuscitation measures are required.

Transport   Transfer to a tertiary perinatal center that has a pediatric surgeon is always indicated. Gastric decompression during transport is essential.

Testing and Confirmation   Reliable iontophoresis (sweat testing) is possible after 1 week in term infants.

Nursery Management   The primary issues are avoidance of aspiration by gastric decompression, maintenance of hydration and electrolyte balance, and confirmation of the diagnosis.

Relief of the obstruction by use of water-soluble, high-osmolality contrast media enemas can be obtained in the majority of cases.

Surgery

Preoperative Assessment   Initial management includes nasogastric decompression, intravenous fluid resuscitation, and a water-soluble contrast enema radiographic study. The last technique will definitely make a diagnosis and may be therapeutic by dislodging the impacted firm meconium from the distal ileum. The hypertonic intestinal contrast material can acutely dehydrate the infant. Compensation for this fluid shift must be made with increased intravenous fluids 1.5 to 2.0 times normal maintenance levels.

Operative Indications   Failure with two separate radiographic efforts or the presence of peritoneal irritation or free intraperitoneal air warrants subsequent surgical management.

Types of Procedures   Surgical management includes intraoperative irrigation of the meconium-obstructed bowel via an enterotomy. Successful evacuation is followed by primary bowel closure. Necrotic intestine, meconium peritonitis, or extensive proximal intestinal meconium blockage can necessitate the use of enteral stomas with a subsequent reanastomosis at a later time.

Surgical Results/Prognosis   The short-term prognosis is excellent (80%), and the long-term outcome is related to the cause of the meconium ileus.

REFERENCES

Benacerraf BR, Chaudhury AK: Echogenic fetal bowel in the third trimester associated with meconium ileus secondary to cystic fibrosis. J Reprod Med 1989;34:299–300.

Bosco AF, Norton ME, Lieberman E: Predicting the risk of cystic fibrosis with echogenic fetal bowel and one cystic fibrosis mutation. Obstet Gynecol 1999;94:1020–1023.

Caniano DA, Beaver BL: Meconium ileus: A fifteen-year experience with forty-two neonates. Surgery 1987;102:699–703.

Caspi B, Elchalal U, Lancet M, Chemke J: Prenatal diagnosis of cystic fibrosis: Ultrasonographic appearance of meconium ileus in the fetus. Prenat Diagn 1988;8:379–382.

Chang PY, Huang FY, Yeh ML, et al: Meconium ileus-like condition in Chinese neonates. J Pediatr Surg 1992;27:1217–1219.

Denholm TA, Crow HC, Edwards WH, et al: Prenatal sonographic appearance of meconium ileus in twins. Am J Roentgenol 1984;143:371–372.

Estroff JA, Parad RB, Benacerraf BR: Prevalence of cystic fibrosis in fetuses with dilated bowel. Radiology 1992;183:677–680.

Goldstein RB, Filly RA, Callen PW: Sonographic diagnosis of meconium ileus in utero. J Ultrasound Med 1987;6:663–666.

Hertzberg BS, Bowie JD: Fetal gastrointestinal abnormalities. Radiol Clin North Am 1990;28:101–114.

Kalayoglu M, Sieber WK, Rodnan JB, Kiesewetter WB: Meconium ileus: A critical review of treatment and eventual prognosis. J Pediatr Surg 1971;6:290–300.

Lai HC, Kosorok MR, Laxova A, et al: Nutritional status of patients with cystic fibrosis with meconium ileus: A comparison with patients without meconium ileus and diagnosed early through neonatal screening. Pediatrics 2000;105:53–61.

Muller F, Aubry MC, Gasser B, et al: Prenatal diagnosis of cystic fibrosis. II. Meconium ileus in affected fetuses. Prenat Diagn 1985;5:109–117.

Murshed R, Spitz L, Kiely E, Drake D: Meconium ileus: A ten-year review of thirty-six patients. Eur J Pediatr Surg 1997;7:275–277.

Nicolaides KH, Campbell S: Ultrasound diagnosis of congenital abnormalities. In Harrison MR, Golbus MS, Filly RA (eds): The Unborn Patient: Antenatal Diagnosis and Treatment. Philadelphia, WB Saunders, 1991, pp 593–648.

Noblett H: Treatment of uncomplicated meconium ileus by gastrografin enema: A preliminary report. J Pediatr Surg 1969;4:190–197.

Penna L, Bower S: Hyperechogenic bowel in the second trimester fetus: A review. Prenat Diagn 2000;20:909–913.

Shigemoto H, Endo S, Isomoto T, et al: Neonatal meconium obstruction in the ileum without mucoviscidosis. J Pediatr Surg 1978;13:475–479.

Vincoff NS, Callen PW, Smith-Bindman R, Goldstein RB: Effect of ultrasound transducer frequency on the appearance of the fetal bowel. J Ultrasound Med 2000;18:799–803.

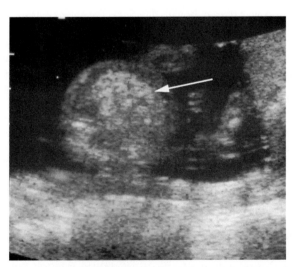

Transverse view of the abdomen of a fetus subsequently shown to have cystic fibrosis and meconium ileus. A clump of echogenic bowel is present (*arrow*).

6.8 Omphalocele

Epidemiology/Genetics

Definition An omphalocele is a transparent sac of amnion attached to the umbilical ring that contains herniated abdominal viscera.

Epidemiology Occurs in 1 in 4000 births (M1:F5).

Embryology Omphaloceles, which contain liver, are thought to result from failure of lateral body bold migration and body wall closure. Omphaloceles containing gut only are said to result from the embryonic persistence of the body stalk. Omphaloceles have associated malformations in almost two thirds of all cases, including congenital heart defects, bladder exstrophy, imperforate anus, neural tube defects, cleft lip with or without cleft palate, and diaphragmatic hernias. In addition, approximately 25% have associated chromosomal abnormalities, especially trisomies 13 and 18. The Beckwith-Wiedemann syndrome, which includes omphalocele with macrosomia, macroglossia, organomegaly, and neonatal hypoglycemia, and a number of rare skeletal dysplasias, should be considered in these patients.

Inheritance Patterns Rare autosomal dominant and X-linked recessive families have been reported with isolated omphaloceles. Some cases of the Beckwith-Wiedemann syndrome show autosomal dominant inheritance.

Teratogens None known.

Serum Screening Measurement of maternal serum alpha-fetoprotein will detect approximately 70% of omphaloceles.

Prognosis The prognosis is generally dependent on associated malformations and/or the size of the defect, and mortality may be as high as 20 to 30%. Giant lesions containing both solid and hollow viscera have limited potential for successful closure.

Sonography

FINDINGS

1. **Fetus:**
   a. Liver and/or gut bulge into a circumscribed mass at the cord insertion site can be seen. Eighty percent of omphaloceles contain liver, sometimes with small bowel. The stomach and bladder may occasionally lie in the omphalocele.
   b. A membrane consisting of amnion, peritoneum, and Wharton's jelly surrounds the mass. Ascites may be present within the omphalocele or in the abdomen.
   c. Twenty percent of omphaloceles contain gut and fluid only. Most chromosome anomalies are seen in this subgroup.
   d. Ruptured omphalocele is a rare complication—There is a similar appearance to gastroschisis, except that the liver may be present and the cord runs through the center of the mass.
2. **Amniotic Fluid:** Polyhydramnios is often present.
3. **Placenta:** Normal.
4. **Measurement Data:** The abdominal circumference cannot be accurately measured because of the omphalocele. Approximately 20% of affected fetuses have intrauterine growth restriction.
5. **When Detectable:** Can be detected at 11 weeks if liver is present within the mass.

Pitfalls

1. If the liver lies outside of the abdomen at 10 or 11 weeks, then a true omphalocele is present. In "pseudo-omphalocele" or physiologic gut herniation, only gut will be seen in the hernia.
2. A few omphaloceles are said to be only intermittently visible; presumably, they act like a hernia and return to the abdomen now and then.
3. Confusion with gastroschisis may occur. Typically, a surrounding membrane is seen with omphalocele and not with gastroschisis. It is said that omphaloceles can rupture. Liver within the ventral mass is not seen with gastroschisis, unless another anomaly, such as the limb-body wall complex, is present.
4. Undue transducer pressure on a flaccid fetal abdomen can cause an anterior bulge, which can resemble an omphalocele; however, there is no "waist" to the apparent omphalocele and it is dependant on fetal position.

Differential Diagnosis

1. Gastroschisis—A surrounding membrane is present with omphalocele. The cord exits the left side of a gastroschisis.
2. Umbilical hernia—Indistinguishable from a small omphalocele, although it is covered by skin rather than a membrane.
3. Bladder exstrophy—No bladder is visible. A mass is seen below the cord insertion site (see Chapter 4.2).
4. Cloacal exstrophy—Dilated vagina and renal systems are also seen, and the mass is inferior to the umbilicus (see Chapter 4.3).
5. Body stalk anomaly—There are usually limb problems and the placenta is attached to the fetus (see Chapter 8.11).

6. Allantoic cyst—Does not arise from the fetus. The contents are cystic and the cyst is attached to the cord. A urachal cyst may also be present so that the allantoic and urachal cysts lie adjacent.
7. Pentalogy of Cantrell—Ectopia cordis is present in addition to a large omphalocele.

Where Else to Look   At least 50% of fetuses with omphalocele have defects elsewhere.

1. Look for findings of trisomy 13 and 18, which are seen in about one third of omphalocele patients, including heart defects and facial and limb problems.
2. Look for stigmata of the Beckwith-Wiedemann syndrome, including macrosomia; renal, liver, and spleen enlargement; macroglossia; and polyhydramnios. Tumors may be seen.
3. Look for findings of body stalk anomaly and limb-body wall complex. Spinal distortion, limb absence, and ectopia cordis may be seen.
4. Omphalocele is a component of pentalogy of Cantrell (ectopia cordis and diaphragmatic and sternal defects are seen as well as omphalocele).
5. In the absence of other syndromes, cardiac defects, such as ventricular septal defect and other gastrointestinal problems, such as bowel malrotation, atresias, and stenoses, occur. Central nervous system problems such as an encephalocele and spinal dysraphism may be seen.
6. Look for cord cysts—The chances of a chromosomal anomaly increase if one or more cord cysts are present in addition to the omphalocele.

Pregnancy Management

Investigations and Consultations Required   Chromosome studies are an essential component of the initial evaluation. The high incidence of associated congenital heart defects requires that fetal echocardiography be performed in all cases. Consultation with a pediatric surgeon will prepare the family for the issues regarding neonatal management, such as primary versus secondary closure, and allow a coordinated management plan to be developed.

Monitoring   No special modifications are needed. Serial ultrasonographic examinations should be done every 4 weeks to monitor growth. Fetal evaluations, such as nonstress testing, are not necessary unless there is evidence of alteration in normal growth parameters. Preterm delivery and intrauterine growth restriction both frequently complicate cases with fetal omphalocele.

Pregnancy Course   There are no specific obstetric complications to be expected. There is a high rate of emergency caesarean sections secondary to fetal distress.

Pregnancy Termination Issues   In cases with multiple abnormalities and in which a precise cause has not been determined, consideration should be given to using a nondestructive method of termination, such as prostaglandin, followed by a careful autopsy.

Delivery   There appears to be no advantage to cesarean section except in those cases in which a large lesion might result in obstructed labor. Delivery should be performed at term, in a center with appropriate perinatal facilities for surgical management of the neonate.

Neonatology

Resuscitation   Assistance with the onset of respiration is usually not required unless there is concurrent prematurity, associated respiratory distress, or an associated anomaly that interferes with the onset of cardiorespiratory adaptation. If assisted ventilation is required, bag and mask ventilation is contraindicated to avoid gaseous distension of the stomach and bowel.

The major concern is to avoid trauma to and contamination of the omphalocele sac. Once respiration and circulation are established, the sac should be covered with warmed, saline-moistened gauze, covered by additional wrapping to avoid evaporative heat and water loss. It is always safe to enclose the trunk and legs in a sterile plastic drawstring bag ("bowel bag").

Prompt decompression of the stomach is important initially, followed by intermittent gastric suction.

Transport   Transfer to a tertiary center that has a pediatric surgeon is always indicated. Protection of the sac, as described, should be maintained during transport, as should gastric decompression.

Reliable intravenous access should be established and infusion of a balanced electrolyte solution instituted.

Testing and Confirmation   Because of the very high incidence of associated anomalies, appropriate diagnostic testing including chromosomal analysis, echocardiography, and renal sonography should be obtained expeditiously before surgical intervention.

Nursery Management   Care of the omphalocele sac, gastric decompression, and intravenous fluids, as noted earlier, should be maintained.

In some cases, it may be necessary to provide ventilatory support in the early postoperative period, as there may be increased intra-abdominal pressure from the reduction of the extruded viscera back into the abdominal cavity.

Parenteral nutrition is required during the postoperative recovery period, as there is always a significant interval before adequate enteral intake can be established.

Surgery

Preoperative Assessment   Preoperative and postdelivery goals include a thorough evaluation for associated anomalies, particularly of the cardiac system, including echocardiography. Preoperative broad-coverage antibiotics are administered.

Operative Indications   Surgical repair is required on a semi-urgent schedule, after resuscitation and evaluation for associated anomalies, to prevent further contamination of the permeable membrane covering the defect. Some surgeons prefer nonoperative management of the intact omphalocele by using frequent applications of a desiccating antiseptic solution and undertaking a delayed closure of the secondarily produced skin-covered hernia. This process is associated with acute complications of toxicity due to absorption of the antiseptic solutions and delayed complications secondary to attempted repair of the resultant hernia in the face of significant associated intraperitoneal adhesions. For these reasons, most surgeons prefer the acute reduction and total surgical repair of omphaloceles. In the case of the "giant" omphalocele, which is frequently associated with severe pulmonary insufficiency, however, the topical form of therapy may be the preferred procedure.

Types of Procedures Intraoperative management consists of removal of the amniotic sac, evaluation for associated intestinal malrotation with lysis of bands obstructing the duodenum, and evaluation of the intestine for possible associated atresias. Primary fascial and abdominal wall closure can be accomplished if intraabdominal pressure, measured by either the intragastric route using a nasogastric tube or the intravesical method using a bladder catheter, does not exceed 20 mm Hg after return of the viscera to the abdominal cavity. A temporary silastic/Dacron extra-abdominal pouch is used if the intra-abdominal pressure is too high for primary closure. Gradual reduction of the viscera can usually be accomplished over 5 to 7 days with subsequent surgical removal of the pouch and secondary abdominal wall closure.

Giant omphaloceles usually are associated with primary respiratory distress, due to lung hypoplasia, and make primary abdominal wall repair less likely. Even with the use of an initial silastic pouch, they eventually may require mobilized lateral skin flaps with prosthetic material to achieve coverage of the exposed viscera. The alternative method is the previously described acute nonoperative therapy. Secondary closure of the remaining ventral wall defect after either nonoperative or incomplete surgical closure of the fascia can be achieved following further body growth and development.

Surgical Results/Prognosis If there are no associated anomalies such as an intestinal atresia, resumption of postoperative intestinal function is prompt. Overall survival depends on the severity of the associated anomalies, most commonly cardiac defects, and can vary from 30 to 70%. Long-term morbidity is also related to the associated anomalies, most notably cardiac.

REFERENCES

Axt R, Quijano F, Boos R, et al: Omphalocele and gastroschisis: Prenatal diagnosis and peripartal management. A case analysis of the years 1989–1997 at the Department of Obstetrics and Gynecology, University of Homburg/Saar. Eur J Obstet Gynecol Reprod Biol 1999;87: 47–54.

Bowerman RA: Sonography of fetal midgut herniation: Normal size criteria and correlation with crown-rump length. J Ultrasound Med 1993;5:251–254.

Boyd PA, Bhattacharjee A, Gould S, et al: Outcome of prenatally diagnosed anterior abdominal wall defects. Arch Dis Child Fetal Neonatal Ed 1998;78:F209–213.

Colombani PM, Cunningham MD: Perinatal aspects of omphalocele and gastroschisis. Am J Dis Child 1977;131:1386–1388.

Fink IJ, Filly RA: Omphalocele associated with umbilical cord allantoic cyst: Sonographic evaluation in utero. Radiology 1983;149:473–476.

Forrester MB, Merz RD: Epidemiology of abdominal wall defects, Hawaii, 1986–1997. Teratology 1999;60:117–123.

Getachew MM, Goldstein RB, Edge V, et al: Correlation between omphalocele contents and abnormalities: Sonographic study in 37 cases. Am J Roentgenol 1992;158:133–136.

Irving IM: Umbilical abnormalities. In Lister J, Irving IM (eds): Neonatal Surgery. London, Butterworths, 1990, pp 376–402.

Kilby MD, Lander A, Usher-Somers M: Exomphalos (omphalocele). Prenat Diagn 1998;18:1283–1288.

Lodeiro JG, Byers JW III, Chuipek S, Feinstein SJ: Prenatal diagnosis and perinatal management of the Beckwith-Wiedeman syndrome: A case and review. Am J Perinatol 1989;6:446–449.

Luck SR, Sherman JO, Raffensperger JG, Goldstein IR: Gastroschisis in 106 consecutive newborn infants. Surgery 1985;98:677–683.

Nakayama DK, Harrison MR, Gross BH, et al: Management of the fetus with an abdominal wall defect. J Pediatr Surg 1984;19:408–413.

Nicolaides KH, Snijders RJM, Cheng HH, Gosden C: Fetal gastrointestinal and abdominal wall defects: Associated malformations and chromosomal abnormalities. Fetal Diagn Ther 1992;7:102–115.

Nyberg DA, Fitzsimmons J, Mack LA, et al: Chromosomal abnormalities in fetuses with omphalocele. J Ultrasound Med 1989;8:299–308.

Paidas MJ, Crombleholme TM, Robertson FM: Prenatal diagnosis and management of the fetus with an abdominal wall defect. Semin Perinatol 1994;18:196–214.

Palomski GE, Hill LE, Knight GJ: Second-trimester maternal serum alpha-fetoprotein levels in pregnancies associated with gastroschisis and omphalocele. Obstet Gynecol 1988;71:906.

Philippart AI, Canty TG, Filler RM: Acute fluid volume requirements in infants with anterior abdominal wall defects. J Pediatr Surg 1972;7: 553–558.

Rankin J, Dillon E, Wright C: Congenital anterior abdominal wall defects in the north of England, 1986–1996: Occurrence and outcome. Prenat Diagn 1999;19:662–668.

Salzman L, Kuligowska E, Semine A: Pseudoomphalocele: Pitfall in fetal sonography. AJR 1986;146:1283–1285.

Schmidt W, Yarkoni S, Crelin ES, Hobbins JC: Sonographic visualization of physiologic anterior abdominal wall hernia in the first trimester. Obstet Gynecol 1987;69:911–915.

Swartz KR, Harrison MW, Campbell JR, Campbell TJ: Ventral hernia in the treatment of omphalocele and gastroschisis. Ann Surg 1985;201: 347–350.

Van de Gijn EJ, Van Vugt JMG, Sollie JE, Van Geijn HP: Ultrasonographic diagnosis and perinatal management of fetal abdominal wall defects. Fetal Diagn Ther 1991;6:2–10.

Wakhlu A, Wakhlu AK: The management of exomphalos. J Pediatr Surg 2000;35:73–76.

Yang P, Beaty TH, Khoury MJ, et al: Genetic-epidemiologic study of omphalocele and gastroschisis: Evidence for heterogeneity. Am J Med Genet 1992;44:668–675.

Yaster M, Scherer TL, Stone MM, et al: Prediction of successful primary closure of congenital abdominal wall defects using intraoperative measurements. J Pediatr Surg 1989;24:1217–1220.

Yazbeck S, Ndoye M, Khan AD: Omphalocele: A 25 year experience. J Pediatr Surg 1986;21:761–763.

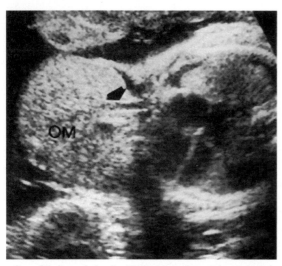

Large liver-filled omphalocele (OM). Note the cord entering the abdomen at the center of the point where the liver exits the abdomen (*arrow*). A small rim of fluid can be seen at the edge of the liver.

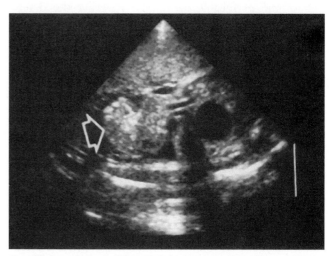

Gut-filled omphalocele. The omphalocele again exits at the cord insertion site (*arrow*), but the entire contents of the omphalocele are gut. This form of omphalocele is much more likely to occur with an abnormal karyotype.

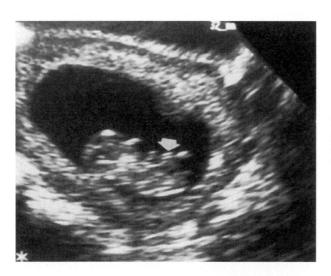

Pseudo-omphalocele. An 11-week fetus with a bulge on the anterior aspect of the abdomen (*arrow*), which represents physiologic gut herniation. A repeat sonogram a month later showed a normal anterior abdominal appearance.

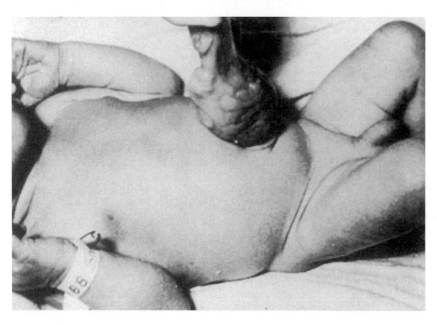

Newborn infant with isolated omphalocele containing small bowel.

Neck and Face

7.1 Cleft Lip and Palate

Epidemiology/Genetics

Definition   A facial cleft involving the upper lip and/or palate, usually occurring to the left or right of midline. Cleft lip and/or cleft palate may occur as an isolated malformation or as part of a multiple malformation syndrome. Midline facial clefts may be associated with underlying brain malformations, especially holoprosencephaly.

Epidemiology   One in 1000 births (M>F) for cleft lip and/or cleft palate; 5 in 1000 births for isolated cleft palate (M1:F2). There is marked ethnic and racial variation in incidence. Some studies suggest that maternal preconceptional folic acid supplementation decreases the incidence of nonsyndromic clefts. Medial facial clefts account for less than 1% of all facial clefts.

Embryology   The primary palate (anterior to incisive foramina) and secondary palate (posterior to the incisive foramina) are embryologically distinct. The upper lip and primary palate have usually fused by the seventh week of gestation. Formation of the secondary palate occurs by fusion of the palatal shelf by the 12th week. Cleft lip and cleft palate are due to a failure of union of the frontonasal process of the face with the lateral maxillary prominences at about 7 weeks' gestation. Almost 300 multiple malformation syndromes have been described with cleft lip or cleft palate. Midline facial clefts are the result of a deficient frontonasal development process that is normally induced by the underlying brain. Midline facial clefts with underlying brain abnormalities are seen in trisomy 13. Approximately 60% of cases are isolated. The most common associated anomalies are lumbar and cervical spine (33%) and heart (24%). Chromosomal abnormalities are seen in approximately 10% of cases.

Inheritance Patterns   Most isolated cleft lips or cleft palates show multifactorial inheritance, but up to 20% are part of dominant, recessive, and X-linked syndromes. Determining the pattern of inheritance depends on an accurate diagnosis.

Teratogens   Alcohol, maternal phenylketonuria, hyperthermia, hydantoin, trimethadione, aminopterin, and methotrexate.

Prognosis   The prognosis for a good cosmetic and functional repair with isolated cleft lip and/or cleft palate is excellent. Otherwise, the prognosis is dependent on any associated malformations or a syndrome diagnosis. Midline clefts, if they are associated with underlying brain malformations, usually carry a poor prognosis.

Sonography

FINDINGS

1. **Fetus:**
   a. Unilateral cleft lip with or without cleft palate—Obliquely aligned gap in the lip that extends up to the nose. The profile view shows a nose with a hooked appearance. A gap in the maxilla and palate is sometimes present.
   b. Bilateral cleft lip with or without palatal defect. A central mass protrudes below the nose so that there is an abnormal profile view with an infranasal premaxillary mass. Standard views of the lips are not obtainable. A bony gap in the tooth-bearing alveolar ridge of the maxilla is present if the anterior aspect of the palate is involved.
   c. Central cleft lip and palate—There is an absence of the central maxilla and upper lip with a deformed nose that may be absent and replaced by a proboscis. There may be only one nostril in a small nose. This type of cleft lip and palate is always associated with other facial findings, such as hypotelorism or cyclops, and there is usually holoprosencephaly, often with trisomy 13.
2. **Amniotic Fluid:** Amniotic fluid is generally normal but may be increased because of defective swallowing.
3. **Placenta:** Normal.
4. **Measurement Data:** Assuming this is an isolated process, growth should be normal.

5. **When Detectable:** Cleft lip is detectable by about 13 weeks' gestation, but the palatal defect may not be detectable until approximately 18 weeks. Prior to this, the maxilla is still in the process of fusion.

Pitfalls

1. Bilateral cleft lip and palate is often mistaken for a facial mass such as a teratoma or proboscis.
2. The detection of cleft lip and palate is difficult and depends on a cooperative fetus that is not always face down.
3. Isolated cleft palate is usually missed because the maxilla may be spared.
4. A central echo-free area may be seen prior to 18 weeks in the maxilla as development is completed.

Differential Diagnosis

1. Epignathus (facial teratoma)—The mass is asymmetrical and enters the mouth. Confusable with bilateral cleft lip and palate.
2. Normal variant—Delayed maxillary fusion.

Where Else to Look

1. All types of cleft lip and palate may well be associated with anomalies elsewhere, particularly congenital heart disease and intracranial malformations. Amniotic bands may be seen with unilateral clefts.
2. The central defect form is associated with midbrain fusion problems such as the various types of holoprosencephaly, septo-optic dysplasia, trisomy 13, and other facial problems such as hypotelorism and proboscis.

Pregnancy Management

Investigations and Consultations Required Chromosomal studies should be done in all cases, including apparently isolated cleft lip/palate. Fetal echocardiography is an essential component of the evaluation. The parents should be examined by a pediatric dysmorphologist for possible genetic disorders that are inherited in an autosomal dominant fashion. The need for other consultants will depend on what other structural abnormalities are present.

Monitoring Because of the significant risk of other abnormalities that may be missed by sonographic evaluations, prenatal care should be under the direction of a perinatologist. No special precautions or fetal assessment is necessary. Once a month sonography is worthwhile because additional defects may have been missed and because of the risk of polyhydramnios.

Pregnancy Course No specific obstetric complications should be expected in the fetus with cleft lip/palate. Mild polyhydramnios may be associated occasionally.

Pregnancy Termination Issues Pregnancy termination should be by a nondestructive procedure that will allow full evaluation by a fetal pathologist.

Delivery The site for delivery should be where there are appropriate facilities and support staff for the care and management of an infant with a cleft. In addition, a pediatric dysmorphologist should be available to assess the infant for possible genetic syndromes.

Neonatology

Resuscitation Fetal distress is not expected with isolated facial clefting. However, infants with multiple anomalies, including clefts, frequently develop fetal distress and require resuscitative assistance. The decision to intervene is based on the prognosis for the specific syndrome or anomaly complex.

Transport Referral to a tertiary center following birth is not indicated for isolated facial clefts unless a satisfactory feeding technique cannot be established. With multiple anomalies, referral for more extensive diagnostic evaluation is appropriate.

Testing and Confirmation Usually detected at birth during the newborn physical examination. A careful search for associated malformations is indicated.

Nursery Management Establishing a successful oral feeding technique and facilitation of parental adaptation are the initial objectives in management. There are multiple special devices available for use, and some infants are helped to feed orally by placement of a customized prosthetic device for an extensive palatal defect. Referral to a multidisciplinary orofacial team for long-term management, including surgical repair and rehabilitation, is essential.

Surgery

Preoperative Assessment Visual inspection is made to determine the type of cleft lip and palate, which can range from incomplete to complete, unilateral or bilateral, median to craniofacial. With the unilateral complete cleft lip deformity, the orbicularis muscle has an aberrant attachment to the alar wing and the columella. The premaxilla projects beyond the noncleft side and rotates outward. The nasal structures are also involved to a variable degree. The lateral alar base in invariably rotated outward and flares laterally. In craniofacial clefts, the orbital involvement may result in a dystopia, micro-ophthalmia, or anophthalmia.

Presurgical splinting or obturation of the cleft may help with feeding and nursing. Presurgical orthopedic manipulation may be necessary to reduce the size of the deformity and aid in subsequent surgical closure.

Operative Indications All patients with these types of anomalies will require surgery. The external lip and facial soft tissues are closed first within 10 weeks of life (Rule of 10's—10 weeks old, 10 g of hemoglobin, 10 lbs of weight). Closure of more extensive facial clefts involving the orbital globes with exposure of the cornea is carried out as soon as possible. The deeper structures, such as the palatal or alveolar defects, are closed at 6 months of age up to 1 year to allow good speech and language development. The alveolar bony defects or facial clefting defects are corrected at 6 to 10 years of age.

Types of Procedures The most widely used techniques for closure of the cleft lip deformities is the rotation-advancement technique for both the unilateral and bilateral deformities. The medial portion of the cleft deformity, including the skin, mucosa, and orbicularis oris muscle, is rotated from the columella into a more inferior position. Lateral lip advancement carries the flaring alar base into a better alignment with the contralateral nasal alar base and reorients the lateral component of the orbicularis muscle. In the bilateral lip deformities, the reapproximation of the orbicularis muscle will tend to realign the projection premaxilla and approximate the midfacial structures. The more extensive facial clefts are handled with layered Z-plasties that allow closure of the muscles and skin tissues of the face.

The cleft palate is closed with mucoperiosteal flaps from the hard palate to close the midline structures. The soft palate is repaired by closing the nasal lining and realigning the levator palatini muscles 90 degrees from their attachment to the hard palate. During this procedure, care is taken to elongate the palatal tissues in the midline again for purposes of improving later speech development.

Bone grafting can be carried out after the age of 5 years, but preferably at 8 to 10 years of age, to add further support or replacement to the facial skeletal foundation or contouring. This also prevents periodontal disease and allows better dental eruption and support.

Surgical Results/Prognosis Surgical results in experienced hands are good and usually restore facial aesthetics and functional speech. The rate of complications from cleft palate closure requiring late palatal lengthening or fistula closure ranges from 8 to 20%. The more extensive the deformities are, the greater the number of procedures that will be required to achieve the desired results. Surgical procedures may extend into the end of the craniofacial growth period in the teenaged years.

REFERENCES

Babcook CJ, McGahan JP: Axial ultrasonographic imaging of the fetal maxilla for accurate characterization of facial clefts. J Ultrasound Med 1997;16:619–625.

Bardach J, Morris HL: Multidisciplinary management of cleft lip and palate. Philadelphia, WB Saunders, 1990.

Bardach J, Salyer K: Surgical techniques in cleft lip and palate. Chicago, Mosby-Year Book, 1987.

Benacerraf BR, Frigoletto FD Jr, Bieber FR: The fetal face: Ultrasound examination. Radiology 1984;153:495–497.

Benacerraf BR, Mulliken JB: Fetal cleft lip and palate: Sonographic diagnosis and postnatal outcome. Plast Reconstr Surg 1993;92:1045–1051.

Berge SJ, Plath H, Vondel PT: Fetal cleft lip and palate: Sonographic diagnosis, chromosomal abnormalities, associated anomalies and postnatal outcome in 70 fetuses. Ultrasound Obstet Gynecol 2001;18:422–431.

Bronshtein M, Mashiah N, Blumenfeld I, et al: Pseudoprognathism: An auxiliary ultrasonographic sign for transvaginal ultrasonographic diagnosis of cleft lip and palate in the early second trimester. Am J Obstet Gynecol 1991;165:1314–1316.

Chervenak FA, Tortora M, Mayden K, et al: Antenatal diagnosis of median cleft face syndrome: Sonographic demonstration of cleft lip and hypertelorism. Am J Obstet Gynecol 1984;149:94–97.

Cockell A, Lees M: Prenatal diagnosis and management of orofacial clefts. Prenat Diagn 2000;20:149–151.

Dufresne C, Jelks G: Classification of craniofacial anomalies. In Smith B (ed): Ophthalmic Plastic and Reconstructive Surgery. Philadelphia, Mosby-Year Book, 1987, p 1185.

Dufresne C, So I: Facial clefting malformations. In Dufresne C, Carson B, Zinreich SJ (eds): Complex Craniofacial Problems. New York, Churchill Livingstone, 1992, p 195.

Hartridge T, Illing HM, Sandy JR: The role of folic acid in oral clefting. Br J Orthod 1999;26:115–120.

Jones MC: Etiology of facial clefts: Prospective evaluation of 428 patients. Cleft Palate 1988;25:16–20.

Kaufman FL: Managing the cleft lip and palate patient. Pediatr Clin North Am 1991;38:1127–1147.

Nyberg DA, Hegge FN, Kramer D, et al: Premaxillary protrusion: A sonographic clue to bilateral cleft lip and palate. J Ultrasound Med 1993;12:331–335.

Pilu G, Reece A, Romero R, et al: Prenatal diagnosis of craniofacial malformations with ultrasonography. Am J Obstet Gynecol 1986;155:45–50.

Saltzman DH, Benacerraf BR, Frigoletto FD Jr: Diagnosis and management of fetal facial clefts. Am J Obstet Gynecol 1986;155:377–379.

Shields ED: Cleft palate: A genetic and epidemiologic investigation. Clin Genet 1981;20:13–24.

Tolarova MM, Cervenka J: Classification and birth prevalence of orofacial clefts. Am J Med Genet 1998;75:126–137.

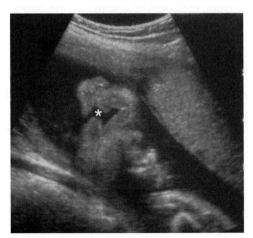

Unilateral cleft lip. Note that the defect (*) extends to the base of the nose.

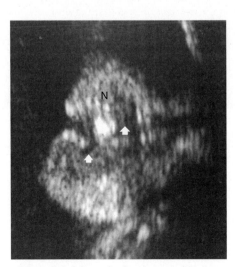

Bilateral cleft lip and palate (*arrows*). N, nose.

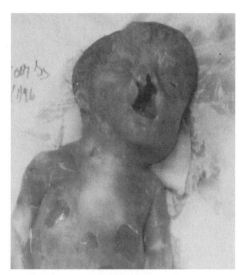

Autopsy view of the same fetus showing an extensive central defect.

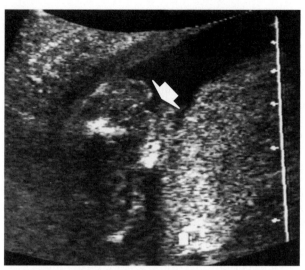

Central cleft lip and palate (*arrow*). This form of cleft lip is associated with gross facial malformations, such as cyclops and absent nose, and intracranial malformation, such as holoprosencephaly.

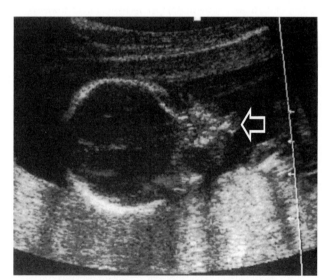

This coronal view of the face shows the apparent central mass that develops when the cleft is bilateral (*arrow*).

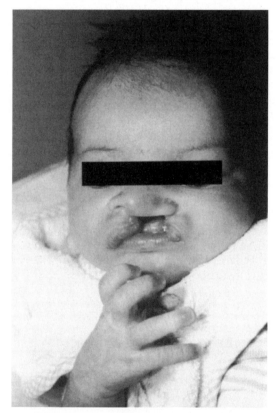

A 2-week-old infant with unilateral cleft lip and palate deformity with the typical flaring of the nasal alar cartilage and aberrant muscular insertions of the orbicularis oris onto the base of the columella and lateral alar nasal base. Bunching of the orbicularis muscle is noted both medial and lateral to the cleft. The greater segment of the cleft alveolus and palate is rotated outward, accentuating the size of the cleft.

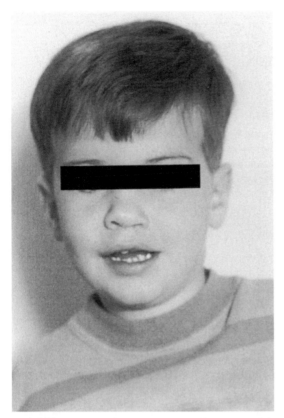

The same child approximately 2½ years later after repair of the cleft lip, palate, and nasal components. Facial esthetics and palatal function are also restored.

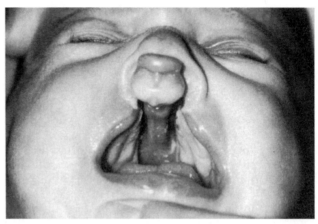

A 3-week-old female infant with a typical bilateral cleft lip and palate deformity. The premaxilla is projecting forward from the lateral palatal segments, exaggerating the deformity. The lateral palatal shelves are more upright than normal and the vomer is readily noted. The lower lip has two paramedian lip pits, which establishes the diagnosis of Van der Wouds syndrome. The lip pits will be removed at the time of the bilateral lip repairs at 10 weeks of age.

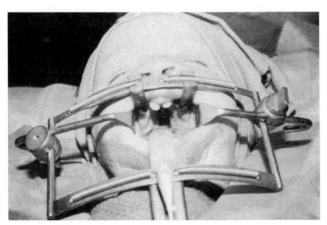

At 6 months of age, the palate is repaired as shown intraoperatively. Following the lip repair, the premaxilla and palatal shelves are in better approximation.

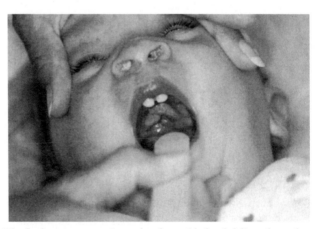

The final appearance at 8 months of age with the cleft lip and nose having been repaired and the palate also repaired.

7.2 Cystic Hygroma

Epidemiology/Genetics

Definition Nuchal cystic hygromas are characterized by single or multiple congenital cysts of the lymphatic system most commonly found within the soft tissues of the neck.

Epidemiology One in 875 spontaneous abortions (M<1:F1).

Embryology Nuchal cystic hygromas are the clinical consequence of a delay in development or absence of the communications that normally develop between the jugular lymph sacs and the internal jugular veins at approximately 40 days' gestation. The obstructed jugular lymph sacs dilate along the paths of least resistance into the posterior and lateral cervical areas. Late communication of the sacs with the internal jugular vein may be manifest by redundancy of the posterior nuchal skin, neck webbing, and elevation and anterior rotation of the ears. Complete lymphatic obstruction may be associated with nonimmune fetal hydrops, which is frequently fatal.

Inheritance Patterns Multiple malformation syndromes with cystic hygromas include the Turner syndrome, multiple pterygium syndrome (autosomal recessive, X-linked), Noonan syndrome (autosomal dominant), and the Robert's syndrome (autosomal recessive).

Teratogens Alcohol.

Prognosis Almost all fetuses with cystic hygroma and hydrops die antenatally. Survivors with lymphatic recanalization may present with a webbed neck or redundant nuchal skin.

Sonography

FINDINGS

1. **Fetus:**
   a. Large bilateral cystic areas termed *cystic hygromas* develop within the skin in the posterolateral aspect of the neck. They may grow so large that they lie adjacent to each other. It then appears that there is a cystic mass arising from the back of the neck with one to three septa in the center.
   b. Skin thickening—Skin thickening, most pronounced in the upper torso and cranium, soon develops. Septa can be seen within the thickened skin and, as the thickening becomes more severe, lakes of fluid can be seen within the skin.
   c. Hydrops—In more severe examples, hydrops develops with large pleural effusions, pericardial effusions, and ascites. The fetus adopts a Buddha-like position.

2. **Amniotic Fluid:** The amniotic fluid is often reduced.
3. **Placenta:** Normal or thickened with hydrops.
4. **Measurement Data:** Normal, if hydrops does not develop.
5. **When Detectable:** This entity can be first detected at 10 weeks, preferably using the endovaginal probe.

Pitfalls

1. Since small cystic hygromas can spontaneously disappear, patients who had cystic hygromas early on may later appear normal and yet have syndromes such as Turner syndrome at birth.
2. A separate entity, also called cystic hygroma, is a unilateral mass in the lateral aspect of the neck or upper torso seen close to term or in neonates. This mass is not associated with karyotypic abnormalities. There is a complex internal structure with multiple septa. Surgical removal is required.
3. If the cystic hygroma is incompletely seen, the amniotic band syndrome may be suggested. Skin thickening is not seen with the amniotic band syndrome.

Differential Diagnosis

1. Nuchal translucency is a similar, although not identical, process in which there is fluid within the skin along the fetal back without the bilateral cystic areas in the neck (see Chapter 1.4).
2. Encephalocele or meningocele—The mass is posterior and is a single mass. Septum and solid contents may be seen within. It is associated with a cranial defect (see Chapter 2.10).
3. Unfused amniotic membrane—Before 13 weeks, an unfused amniotic membrane may lie adjacent to the fetus and be confused with a cystic hygroma.

Where Else to Look Several syndromes are associated with cystic hygromas:

1. Turner syndrome—see Chapter 1.5 for details. Look for other stigmata of Turner syndrome: congenital heart disease and renal anomalies (see chromosomal section).
2. Noonan syndrome—Fetuses with a syndrome similar to Turner syndrome, but with normal chromosomes. Cardiac disease with pulmonary stenosis is typical. Micropenis and cryptorchidism are present in males. Hemivertebrae may occur.
3. Pena-Shokeir syndrome—A chromosomally normal syndrome with features similar to trisomy 18 but without chromosome abnormality (see Chapter 11.5).
4. Down syndrome (see Chapter 1.4).
5. Robert's syndrome.
6. Multiple pterygium syndrome. Pterygia—bands of tough skin—prevent the arms from extending. The fe-

tal limbs are acutely flexed and do not move (see Chapter 8.12).

Pregnancy Management

Investigations and Consultations Required About 60% of patients with cystic hygromas are chromosomally abnormal, with most having Turner syndrome but a minority having Down syndrome and a few trisomy 18. Chromosomal analysis and fetal echocardiography are essential components of the evaluation of isolated cystic hygroma. The consultants used will depend very much on the cause that is established for the cystic hygroma.

Fetal Intervention In utero drainage procedures have no role in management. Spontaneous resolution is common. Progression to fetal hydrops suggests a generalized severe condition that will not respond to drainage of one body cavity.

Monitoring Serial sonographic examinations every 3 to 4 weeks should be performed for those conditions likely to progress to fetal hydrops. Assessment for signs of polyhydramnios and preeclampsia should be done in cases with hydrops.

Pregnancy Course Both polyhydramnios and preeclampsia may complicate conditions that are associated with fetal hydrops. Cystic hygroma with hydrops is almost always a lethal combination, with death within a short time period. Cystic hygromas without hydrops usually regress completely.

Pregnancy Termination Issues Unless a precise diagnosis has been established prenatally, the method of termination should be nondestructive and examinations by both a fetal pathologist and a dysmorphologist should be performed.

Delivery Except in the case of markedly excessive size, the presence of a cystic hygroma should not necessitate a cesarean section. Delivery should occur in a tertiary center with capabilities for managing any complications that may arise.

Neonatology

Resuscitation Airway compromise at birth occurs infrequently because the form of cystic hygroma that presents as a mass, cervical cystic hygroma, is not usually located midline. However, extensive invasion of the tongue and pharyngeal structures can occur, and airway compromise may then be seen. If a large mass is suspected from prenatal sonography, delivery should be planned at a tertiary center with an appropriate team available to establish a reliable airway.

Transport Time of transfer is dictated by the presence of airway compromise. If the airway is functional, then transfer to a tertiary center that has a pediatric surgeon can be delayed until cardiorespiratory adaptation is established.

Testing and Confirmation Cystic hygromas are usually obvious on physical examination in the newborn unless the hygromas are small. A webbed neck and excessive nuchal skin, suggesting a resolved antenatal cystic hygroma, are also noted on the newborn examination. Diagnostic evaluation should be directed toward excluding other coexisting abnormalities, as indicated by prenatal findings and physical examination. Computed tomographic (CT) scan or magnetic resonance imaging (MRI) of the neck and upper thorax are the better imaging studies to delineate the extent and anatomic location of neck masses.

REFERENCES

Azar GB, Snijders RJM, Gosden C, Nicolaides KH: Fetal nuchal cystic hygromata: Associated malformations and chromosomal defects. Fetal Diagn Ther 1991;6:46–57.

Bronshtein M, Bar-Hava I, Blumenfeld I, et al: The difference between septated and nonseptated nuchal cystic hygroma in the early second trimester. Obstet Gynecol 1993;81:683–687.

Byrne J: The significance of cystic hygroma in fetuses. Hum Pathol 1984;15:61–67.

Chervenak FA, Isaacson G, Blakemore KJ, et al: Fetal cystic hygroma: Cause and natural history. N Engl J Med 1983;309:822–825.

Gallagher PG, Mahoney MJ, Gosche JR: Cystic hygroma in the fetus and newborn. Semin Perinatal 1999;23:341–356.

Johnson MP, Johnson A, Holzgreve W, et al: First-trimester simple hygroma: Cause and outcome. Am J Obstet Gynecol 1993;168:156–161.

Langer JC, Fitzgerald PG, Desa D, et al: Cervical cystic hygroma in the fetus: Clinical spectrum and outcome. J Pediatr Surg 1990;25:58–61.

Ninh TN, Ninh TX: Cystic hygroma in children: A report of 126 cases. J Pediatr Surg 1974;9:191.

Van Zalen-Sprock MM, Van Vugt JMG, Van der Harten HJ, Van Geijn HP: Cephalocele and cystic hygroma: Diagnosis and differentiation in the first trimester of pregnancy with transvaginal sonography: Report of two cases. Ultrasound Obstet Gynecol 1992;2:289–292.

Zimmer EZ, Drugan A, Ofir C, et al: Ultrasound imaging of fetal neck anomalies: Implications for the risk of aneuploidy and structural anomalies. Prenat Diagn 1997;17:1055–1058.

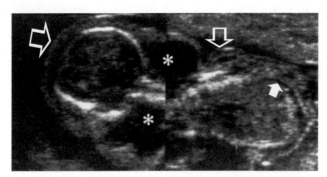

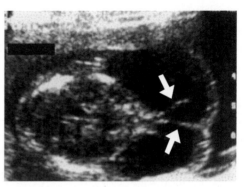

Bilateral cystic hygromata with hydrops. The bilateral cystic masses (*) by the neck are the cystic hygroma. There is skin thickening around the body (*open arrow*). A small amount of ascites is present (*closed arrow*).

Transverse view through the neck and base of the head showing a large cystic hygroma. The two sacs (*arrows*) have enlarged so much that they lie alongside each other. The two central septa lie close to each other.

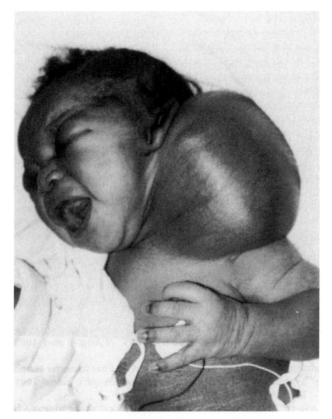

Newborn with large lateral neck lymphangioma. Surgical removal resulted in normal function with an excellent cosmetic repair.

7.3
Facial Asymmetry (Goldenhar's Syndrome) (Hemifacial Microsomia; Oculoauriculovertebral Dysplasia)

Epidemiology/Genetics

Definition Significant facial asymmetry involving the maxilla and mandible, often with associated ipsilateral ocular and auricular abnormalities. The malformation involves the embryologic structures of the first and second branchial arches.

Epidemiology Facial asymmetry secondary to intrauterine constraint is relatively prevalent but occurs late in gestation. Significant degrees of facial asymmetry (detectable on second-trimester antenatal ultrasonogram) are much less common. Most studies suggest a 1 in 5600 birth frequency, with a male-to-female ratio at least 3:2 and a 3:2 predilection for right-sided involvement.

Embryology Minor degrees of facial asymmetry, arising late in pregnancy due to intrauterine constraint, are frequently seen in infants. Common primary causes of serious facial asymmetry include Goldenhar's syndrome (oculoauriculovertebral dysplasia, hemifacial microsomia), amniotic band disruptions, craniosynostosis syndromes, and CHARGE association. Goldenhar's syndrome features a wide range of manifestations, including facial asymmetry, ipsilateral abnormalities of the external ear (anotia, microtia, preauricular abnormalities), ocular defects (epibulbar lipodermoid, lid colomba), cardiac abnormalities (30%), renal malformations (30%), and vertebral anomalies, often with torticollis (50%). Approximately 15% of children have some bilateral involvement.

Inheritance Patterns Dependent on underlying cause. Goldenhar's syndrome is generally sporadic, with an estimated 2% recurrence risk.

Teratogens Retinoic acid (Accutane) embryopathy can have mild facial asymmetry with bilateral microtia/anotia.

Differential Diagnosis Treacher-Collins syndrome, craniosynostosis syndromes, acrofacial dysostoses, and chromosome 4p- syndrome may have facial asymmetry with auricular abnormalities.

Additional Investigations Fetal karyotype and aneuploid fluorescent in situ hybridization should be considered, especially if additional malformations are detected.

Prognosis Minor degrees of facial asymmetry may improve over time. More severe forms of facial asymmetry require major reconstructive surgery. Intelligence in most patients with Goldenhar's syndrome is normal unless the central nervous system is involved. In the presence of microphthalmia, the syndrome is likely to include mental retardation. There is an increased frequency of conductive hearing loss on the affected side.

Sonography

FINDINGS

1. **Fetus:** The findings are variable, but there is generally unilateral hypoplasia of the mandible involving the temporomandibular joint with marked asymmetry of the soft tissues of the jaw. A unilateral cleft lip and palate may be present. One eye is usually small (microphthalmia) or absent (anophthalmia), and there is zygomatic and maxillary asymmetry. A small, absent, or deformed ear on the affected side may be seen. Hemivertebrae are usually present in the cervical and occasionally the thoracic vertebrae. Cardiac and renal anomalies are common.
2. **Amniotic Fluid:** Polyhydramnios is common.
3. **Placenta:** Normal.
4. **Measurement Data:** Normal apart from cranial measurements.
5. **When Detectable:** The entity has been detected at 14 weeks, but milder facial deformities are generally picked up at 18 weeks.

Pitfalls

1. If the fetus is persistently prone, the findings cannot be seen.
2. Isolated palatal defects are common and will not be detected if they do not involve the maxilla and lip.
3. Mild bilateral defects are most unlikely to be detected.

Differential Diagnosis

1. Fraser syndrome—Cryptophthalmos with depressed nasal bridge and ear abnormalities. Other features are urinary tract abnormalities, syndactyly, and laryngeal atresia or stenosis.
2. Nager syndrome—Mandibular hypoplasia, malformed low-set ears, and an abnormal radial aspect of the hand and forearm.
3. Treacher-Collins syndrome—Micrognathia, abnormal orbits with ocular fissures slanted downward, hypoplastic zygomas, and malformed ears. Cleft palate and choanal atresia are other features (see Chapter 7.6).
4. Trisomies 13 and 18 (see Chapters 1.2 and 1.3).

Where Else to Look

1. Look at the heart for cardiac anomalies such as ventricular septal defect.
2. Look for kidney abnormalities.
3. Look in the brain for ventriculomegaly.

Pregnancy Management

Investigations and Consultations Required   Precise prenatal diagnosis is unlikely; therefore, chromosomal studies and fetal echocardiography should be performed to exclude other genetic conditions. Consultation with a pediatric dysmorphologist may provide the family with important information about the natural history of the disorder.

Fetal Intervention   None is indicated or necessary.

Monitoring   Normal obstetric management is appropriate in most cases. Should there be significant fetal micrognathia, monthly sonographic assessment of amniotic volume may be beneficial to detect polyhydramnios. An early third-trimester scan to assess fetal growth should be performed in all cases.

Pregnancy Course   Usually uncomplicated. Occasionally there will be prenatal growth deficiency.

Pregnancy Termination Issues   If termination is chosen, an intact fetus is essential to establish this diagnosis.

Delivery   Site of delivery will depend on the presence of cardiac malformations, the degree of micrognathia, and the presence of other associated cardiac malformations. In most cases, delivery at a tertiary center is the most prudent option.

Neonatology

Resuscitation   Several components of spectrums of anomalies may necessitate special consideration for resuscitation. Mandibular hypoplasia is the most common of the group, although difficulties with maintaining an adequate airway have not been reported in neonates. Much less frequent are cardiac anomalies and anomalies of the foregut derivatives; tracheoesophageal fistula and developmental defects of the bronchopulmonary system are very uncommon. If such are diagnosed prenatally, then delivery room management of the onset of respiration should follow the directions for the individual anomalies.

Transfer   Transport to a tertiary center with pediatric and surgical subspecialty capabilities is indicated in the neonatal period to confirm the diagnosis, identify all the component abnormalities, and initiate a multidisciplinary long-term care plan.

Testing and Confirmation   The specific diagnostic imaging to be performed will be dictated by the associated abnormalities suspected from the clinical course and physical examination. All infants should undergo imaging of the cervical spine as an initial assessment.

Nursery Management   Again, the specifics of management will be dictated by the spectrum of anomalies present in an individual infant. Priority should be given

to establishing a long-term plan for reconstructive surgery and sensorineural habilitation after the more functionally disabling issues have been addressed, such as corrective cardiac and/or genitourinary surgery.

Surgery

Preoperative Assessment   The goal of treatment in patients with mandibular deformities as seen in hemifacial microsomia and Treacher-Collins syndrome is improvement of function and optimization of aesthetic facial appearance and symmetry when craniofacial growth is completed. Treatment includes correction of the secondary deformities of the maxilla and orbit and improvement of the deficiencies of the facial soft tissues. Treatment varies according to the age of the patient, the degree of malformation, and the anticipated distortion of future growth potential. The thrust of treatment is the creation of an environment that both potentiates normal facial growth and minimizes secondary distortion of the neighboring structures. Often the mandibular configuration not only indicates the severity of the defect but also predicts the rate of progression into secondary and tertiary deformities.

Craniofacial microsomia is a progressive skeletal and soft tissue deformity; the earliest skeletal manifestation is found in the mandible. The mandibular asymmetry progresses with time. As growth proceeds, deformation results in progressive asymmetry of the neighboring maxilla, orbit, and nose. Psychological problems in patients also increase with progression of the facial deformity.

A good treatment plan is essential for management of these complex deformities. Surgical management is based on analysis of facial skeletal radiographs in the frontal, sagittal, and transverse planes. With today's technological advances, a three-dimensional CT scan provides the best evaluation of the frontal plane, demonstrating the asymmetry of the mandible, maxilla, piriform apertures, and orbits. The obliquity and rotation of the maxillary and mandibular midlines can also be evaluated by this method. In affected patients, the dental midline is deviated toward the abnormal side. A lateral cephalogram offers a demonstration of the sagittal plane. In this view or in the three-dimensional scan, the discrepancies in the ramus height and the shape of the temporomandibular joint can be studied. A lateral cephalogram also demonstrates the relationship between the maxilla and the mandible and between the maxillomandibular complex and the base of the skull. The submental vertex radiograph helps to evaluate the transverse plane, revealing the shape, width, and asymmetry of the mandibular body and zygomatic arches, and the medial and anterior displacement of the temporomandibular joint.

Operative Indications   The main objectives of surgical management are (1) improvement of symmetry of the mandible (by performing bilateral vertical osteotomies of the rami during the period of mixed dentition, allowing the affected mandibular body to move forward, laterally, and downward into a more normal position); (2) provision for downgrowth of the maxilla by lengthening of the anteromedial displacement; (3) restoration of functional dental occlusion by proper positioning of the mandibular symphyseal midlines; and (4) expansion of the facial skeleton at an early age to fill out the soft tissue on the affected side of the face.

Types of Procedures   In the surgical phase of treatment, the mandible is reconstructed by either elongation or extension of the mandible. Elongation is performed on patients who have a functioning temporomandibular joint. This can be accomplished by osteotomies or bone distraction. The pseudojoint or functioning condyle is maintained, and bone grafting (with rib) is used at the level of the ramus. Vertical osteotomies of the ramus can be performed with interpositional bone grafts if there is a need to increase the anteroposterior dimension of the ramus. If the ramus is minimally hypoplastic, a sagittal split technique can be used. The mandible is extended if there is a congenitally missing condyle or if the condyle must be removed. Concomitant maxillary osteotomies, either segmental or Le Fort, are performed in older patients depending on the severity of the deformity. Elongation or impaction of the maxillary occlusal plane must be determined so that the rotation of the maxilla is freed from the muscle and ligamentous attachments on the affected side and is repositioned as the splint is wired between the jaws. The mandible is then placed in intermaxillary fixation for 8 to 10 weeks for immobilization.

When a Le Fort I osteotomy is planned, the fulcrum of rotation is determined by the desired postoperative length of the midface. If maximal midface lengthening is required, the fulcrum of rotation should be located at the piriform aperture of the nasal septum, with impaction of the maxilla superiorly on the normal side. If exposure of the maxillary incisor teeth below the upper lip is excessive, the rotational fulcrum should be the molar region of the abnormal side to produce the maximal impaction of the normal side.

If asymmetry is very severe, two surgical lengthening procedures may be necessary, with the first procedure completed when the patient is 8 to 10 years of age and the second completed when the patient is 16 to 18 years of age. When mandibular lengthening is performed early, the existing maxillary deficiency is treated orthodontically by active extrusion of individual teeth on the affected side, resulting in closure of the open bite by the repositioning of the mandible.

Surgical Results/Prognosis   The key to success in this type of craniofacial surgery is the realization that the osteotomies and grafts are part of a complex engineering project. The long-term stability is ensured by detailed preoperative planning, precision during surgery, and rigid fixation of the skeletal framework. Decisions for early surgery must be based on the character of the anatomic deformity, taking into account the spatial relationship of the condylar process of the mandible to the temporal bone and the pterygoid process of the sphenoid bone and the functional activity of the muscles attached to these bones. Because soft tissue has little resistance to mandibular advancement, the lack of sufficient cutaneous tissues to resist the mandibular advancement constitutes an indication for early surgery. Repair of the soft tissue constitutes a

secondary surgery after the facial skeleton has been restored. This leads to an overall favorable prognosis, but one that requires multiple surgeries over an extended period of time to replace the orbital and zygomatic deficiencies.

REFERENCES

Aleksic S, Budzilovich G, Choy P, et al: Congenital ophthalmoplegia in auriculovertebral dysplasia: A clinicopathologic study and review of the literature. Neurology 1976;26:638.

Benacerraf BR, Frigoletto FD: Prenatal ultrasound recognition of Goldenhar's syndrome. Am J Obstet Gynecol 1988;159:950–952.

Berman MD, Feingold M: Oculo-auriculo-vertebral dysplasia. Br J Ophthalmol 1971;55:145.

Boles DJ, Bodurtha J, Nance WE: Goldenhar complex in discordant monozygotic twins: A case report and review of the literature. Am J Med Genet 1987;28:103.

Bowen P, Harley F: Mandibulofacial dysostosis with limb malformations (Nager's acrofacial dysostosis). Birth Defects 1974;10:109.

Bromley B, Benacerraf B: Fetal micrognathia: Associated anomalies and outcomes. J Ultrasound Med 1994;13:529–533.

Caldarelli DD, Hutchinson J, Pruzansky S, Valvassori G: A comparison of microtic and temporal bone anomalies in hemifacial microsomia and mandibulofacial dyostosis. Cleft Palate J 1980;17:103.

Coccaro PJ, Becker MH, Conoverse JM: Clinical and radiographic variations in hemifacial microsoma. Birth Defects 1975;11:314.

Cohen MM: Oculoauriculovertebral spectrum: An updated critique. Cleft Palate J 1989;26:276.

Cohen MM Jr, Rollnick BR, Kaye CI: Oculoauriculovertebral spectrum: An updated critique. Cleft Palate J 1989;26:276.

Converse JM, Coccaro PJ, Becker H, et al: On hemifacial microsomia: The first and second branchial arch syndrome. Plast Reconstr Surg 1973;51:268.

Converse JM, Horowitz SL, Coccaro PJ, et al: Corrective treatment of craniofacial microsomia. In Converse JM (ed): Reconstructive Plastic Surgery. Philadelphia, WB Saunders, 1977, p 2359.

Converse JM, McCarthy JG, Coccaro PJ, et al: Clinical aspects of craniofacial microsomia. In Converse JM, McCarthy JG, Wood-Smith D (eds): Symposium on Diagnosis and Treatment or Craniofacial Anomalies. St. Louis, CV Mosby, 1979.

Converse JM, Wood-Smith D, McCarthy JG, et al: Bilateral facial microsomia: Diagnosis, classification, treatment. Plast Reconstr Surg 1974;54:413.

DeCatte L, Laubach M, Legein J, Goossens A: Early prenatal diagnosis of oculoauriculovertebral dysplasia or the Goldenhar syndrome. Ultrasound Obstet Gynecol 1996;8:422–424.

Dufresne C: Treacher Collins syndrome. In Dufresne C, Carason B, Zinreich S (eds): Complex Craniofacial Problems. New York, Churchill Livingstone, 1992, p 281.

Elmore SG: Antenatal sonographic demonstration of Goldenhar-Gorlin syndrome. J Diagn Med Sonogr 1995;11:324–326.

Franceschetti A, Klein D: Mandibulofacial dysostosis: New hereditary syndrome. Acta Ophthalmol 1949;27:143.

Godin RJ, Cohen MM, Levin LS: Syndromes of the Head and Neck, 3rd ed. New York, Oxford University Press, 1990.

Hsieh YY, Chang CC, Tsai HD, et al: The prenatal diagnosis of Pierre-Robin sequence. Prenat Diagn 1999;19:567–569.

Lin HJ, Owens TR, Sinow RM, et al: Anomalous inferior and superior venae cavae with oculoauriculovertebral defect: Review of Goldenhar complex and malformations of left-right asymmetry. Am J Med Genet 1998;75:88–94.

Ritchey ML, Norbeck J, Huang C, et al: Urologic manifestations of Goldenhar syndrome. Urology 1994;43:88–91.

Rollnick BR, Kaye CI, Nagatoshi K, et al: Oculoauriculovertebral dysplasia and variants: Phenotypic characteristics of 294 patients. Am J Med Genet 1987;28:103.

Stoll C, Viville B, Treisser A, Gasser B: A family with dominant oculoauriculovertebral spectrum. Am J Med Genet 1998;78:345–349.

Tamas DE, Mahony BS, Bowie JD, et al: Prenatal sonographic diagnosis of hemifacial microsomia (Goldenhar-Gorlin syndrome). J Ultrasound Med 1986;5:461–463.

Wilson GN: Cranial defects in the Goldenhar syndrome. Am J Med Genet 1983;14:435.

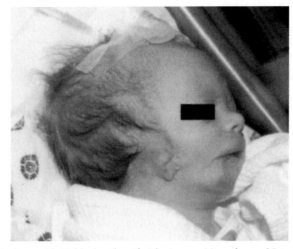

Newborn with Goldenhar (hemifacial microsomia) syndrome. Note absent right ear with right mandibular hypoplasia and lateral macrostomia.

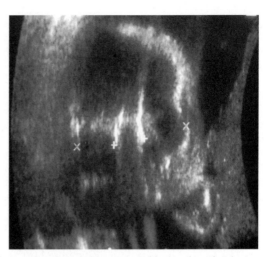

Facial view of a 20-week fetus with Goldenhar (hemifacial microsomia) syndrome showing asymmetrical orbits.

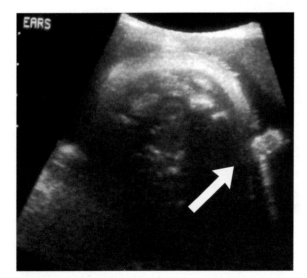

Same fetus. View of the cranium showing a markedly distorted ear on one side (*arrow*). The contralateral ear was normal.

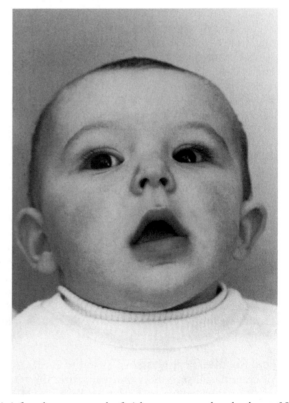

This infant demonstrates the facial asymmetry and occlusal cant. Note the skeletal hypoplasia as well as the soft tissue hypoplasia.

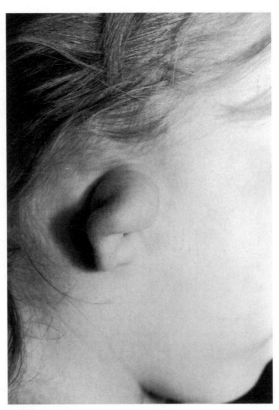

Various degrees of microtia are also involved with this syndrome on the affected side.

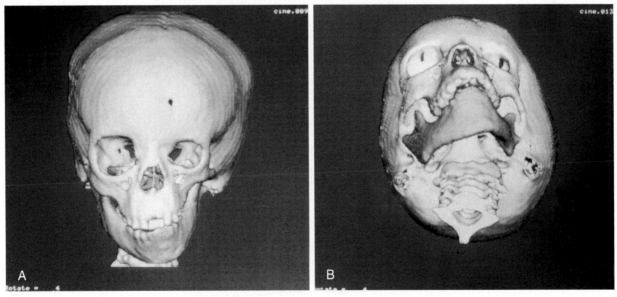

Three-dimensional computed tomographic scans will often clearly show the skeletal asymmetry as demonstrated here. The patient also has congenital anophthalmia on the affected side.

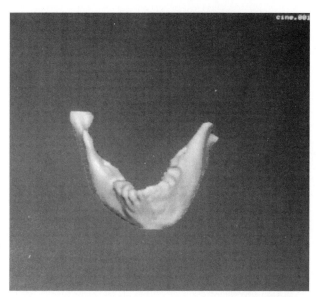

Scan shows that the mandible is twisted and the ramus and condyle fore-shortened and hypoplastic.

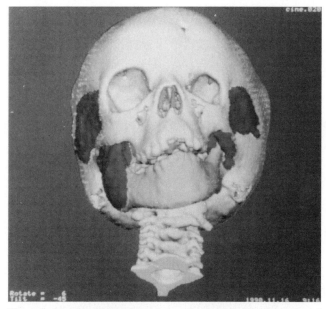

The soft tissues including the muscles of mastication (temporalis and masseter muscles) are hypoplastic on the affected side, noted here as the dark gray structures.

7.4 Pierre Robin Sequence

Epidemiology/Genetics

Definition The Pierre Robin sequence consists of the triad of micrognathia, cleft palate, and glossoptosis (posteriorly displaced tongue). It has a heterogeneous cause and can be part of a number of genetic syndromes including the Stickler syndrome.

Epidemiology One in 5000 to 1 in 10,000 births (M1:F1).

Embryology It is hypothesized that severe micrognathia is the initiating event in this sequence, displacing the developing tongue upward and posteriorly to prevent normal palatal closure. Approximately 14% of patients have associated congenital heart disease and/or other abnormalities. Although the cause is heterogeneous, approximately 20 to 30% of cases are associated with the Stickler syndrome, which is a connective tissue disorder caused by mutations in various collagen genes. It is also seen with many severe or lethal skeletal dysplasias and numerous other genetic and chromosomal syndromes.

Inheritance Patterns Dependent on the cause. Autosomal dominant for the Stickler syndrome.

Teratogens Retinoic acid.

Prognosis Dependent on the cause and syndrome association. Patients with isolated, nonsyndromic cases often have a good outcome with normal cognitive function. Patients with severe cases may need temporary tracheostomies and feeding gastrostomies because of the micrognathia.

Sonography

FINDINGS

1. **Fetus:**
   a. Micrognathia is characterized by a small mandible and receding chin. It can be assessed only on a profile view that does not show the orbit and is truly at right angles.
   b. Usually the assessment is subjective, but the mandibular length can be measured between the temporomandibular joint and the junction of the mandibular rami, the symphysis mentis. A table of normal lengths has been produced.
   c. A cleft palate is present but is usually not detected sonographically because it does not involve the maxilla or lips.
2. **Amniotic Fluid:** Mild or severe polyhydramnios is common (70%), presumably due to poor swallowing ability.
3. **Placenta:** Normal.
4. **Measurement Data:** Intrauterine growth restriction associated with the underlying cause is common.
5. **When detectable:** At about 15 weeks' gestation.

Pitfalls It is very easy to create false micrognathia if an oblique profile view is obtained.

Differential Diagnosis

1. Trisomy 13 and 18 (about 60% of fetuses with micrognathia have a chromosomal anomaly).
2. Treacher-Collins syndrome—The features are severe micrognathia, malar hypoplasia, and malformation of the external ears. Cleft palate may be present (see Chapter 7.6).
3. Goldenhar-Gorlin syndrome—The facial structures are asymmetrical (see Chapter 7.3).
4. Harlequin syndrome.
5. Pena-Shokeir syndrome (see Chapter 11.5).
6. Multiple pterygium syndrome (see Chapter 8.12).
7. Nager acrodysostosis.

Where Else to Look Most fetuses with micrognathia have abnormalities elsewhere, so a thorough study should be performed, including the cardiac and skeletal systems.

Pregnancy Management

Investigations and Consultations Required Chromosomal studies and deletion 22q11.2 fluorescent in situ hybridization should be offered. Fetal echocardiography and a generalized fetal anomalies survey are recommended.

Fetal Intervention No fetal intervention is indicated.

Monitoring In some cases, polyhydramnios may develop. Monthly sonographic evaluations should be performed to detect changes in amniotic fluid index.

Pregnancy Course No significant changes are expected unless polyhydramnios develops. Polyhydramnios may be associated with preterm labor.

Pregnancy Termination Issues Should a couple choose pregnancy termination, labor induction and delivery of an intact fetus are essential to establish a precise diagnosis.

Delivery Delivery should occur in a tertiary center because severe respiratory complications and difficult intubation may result from the more severe cases of mandibular hypoplasia.

Neonatology

Resuscitation   Airway obstruction from mandibular hypoplasia and glossoptosis may be present from birth, necessitating airway support for the onset of respiration. Use of a nasal trumpet or an appropriately sized oral airway with bag and mask ventilation may be sufficient initially. When the diagnosis is known prior to delivery, arrangements should be made for a physician skilled in neonatal airway management to be present at delivery. Emergency tracheostomy is rarely required.

Transport   Immediate transport by an experienced neonatal transport team to a tertiary center with pediatric otolaryngology expertise may be indicated.

Testing and Confirmation   The diagnostic triad of mandibular hypoplasia, glossoptosis, and a large, usually U-shaped palatal defect form the basis of the diagnosis. Careful physical examination will confirm the presence or absence of other abnormalities. The triad of findings occurs in isolation in approximately one third of cases, as a component of Stickler syndrome in another third, and as part of other multiple malformation syndromes in the remaining third. The concomitant occurrence of airway obstruction and feeding difficulties is more frequent and more severe in infants from the latter two thirds. The presence of other malformations or organ malfunction will dictate the other diagnostic studies needed to complete the assessment. Flexible endoscopy is recommended to determine the most appropriate management approach if airway obstruction is a significant issue.

Nursery Management   The major objectives of care are to establish a definitive diagnosis, a stable airway, and an adequate feeding mode as expeditiously as possible. Concurrent abnormalities in other systems should raise the concern for a syndromic diagnosis. Frequently, prone positioning with the head forward will ameliorate the airway obstruction. If not, evaluation by flexible endoscopy may be indicated to elucidate the exact mechanics of the airway malfunction and thus indicate the most appropriate approach to management. Progression in the severity of airway obstruction in the first several weeks has been observed. Thus, a period of several weeks' observation in the nursery is recommended, followed by a prolonged period of home cardiorespiratory monitoring. Oral feeding is often a difficult problem because of the combination of a large palatal defect and an abnormal tongue position. Use of specialized feeding systems and, in extreme circumstances, gastrostomy may be required. Binaural hearing deficiency occurs more frequently than with isolated cleft palate; thus, long-term care should include careful audiologic assessment to allow early intervention.

Surgery

Preoperative Assessment   The goal of treatment in patients with Pierre Robin sequence is improvement of function and optimization of aesthetic facial appearance. Treatment includes correction of the secondary deformities of the maxilla and orbit and improvement of the deficiencies of the facial soft tissues. Treatment varies according to the age of the patient, the degree of malformation, and the anticipated distortion of future growth potential.

A good treatment plan is essential for management of these complex deformities. Surgical management is based on analysis of facial skeletal radiographs and often a three-dimensional CT scan.

Types of Procedures   In patients with the Pierre Robin sequence, the deformities are approached early, starting at 3 years of age with calvarial grafts, either free or vascularized, to replace the orbital and zygomatic deficiencies. An extended Le Fort II maxillary osteotomy, rotating the midface and advancing the mandible, will help the airways and improve aesthetics. Additional soft tissue surgery may be required when skeletal stability is achieved.

Surgical Results/Prognosis   The key to success in this type of craniofacial surgery is the realization that the osteotomies and grafts are part of a complex engineering project. Repair of the soft tissue constitutes a secondary surgery after the facial skeleton has been restored. This leads to an overall favorable prognosis, but one that requires multiple surgeries over an extended period of time.

REFERENCES

Bromley B, Benacerref B: Fetal micrognathia: Associated anomalies and outcomes. J Ultrasound Med 1994;13:529–533.

Bull MJ, Givan DC, Sadove AM, et al: Improved outcome in Pierre Robin Sequence: Effect of multidisciplinary evaluation and management. Pediatrics 1990;86:294.

Marques IL, Barbieri MA, Bettol H: Etiopathogenesis of isolated Robin sequence. Cleft Palate Craniofac J 1998;35:517.

Myers CM III, Reed MJ, Cotton RT, et al: Airway management in Pierre Robin sequence. Otolaryngol Head Neck Surg 1998;118:630.

Otto C, Platt LD: The fetal mandible measurement: An objective determination of fetal jaw size. Ultrasound Obstet Gynecol 1991;1:12–17.

Paladini D, Morra T, Teodoro A, et al: Objective diagnosis of micrognathia in the fetus: The jaw index. Obstet Gynecol 1999;93:382–386.

Perkins JA, Sie KCY, Milczuk H, et al: Airway management in children with craniofacial anomalies. Cleft Palate Craniofac J 1997;34:135.

Sadewitz VL: Robin sequence: Changes in thinking leading to changes in patient care. Cleft Palate Craniofac J 1992;29:246.

Sher AE: Mechanisms of airway obstruction in Robin sequence: Implications for treatment. Cleft Palate Craniofac J 1992;29:224.

Shprintzen RJ: The implications of the diagnosis of Robin sequence. Cleft Palate Craniofac J 1992;29:205.

Tomaske SM, Zalzal GH, Saal HM: Airway obstruction in the Pierre Robin sequence. Laryngoscopy 1995;105:111.

Turner GM, Twining P: The facial profile in the diagnosis of fetal abnormalities. Clin Radiol 1993;47:389–395.

Williams AJ, Williams MA, Walker CA, et al: The Robin anomalad (Pierre Robin syndrome): A follow up study. Arch Dis Child 1981;56:663.

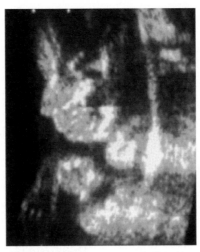

Sonogram profile view showing marked micrognathia.

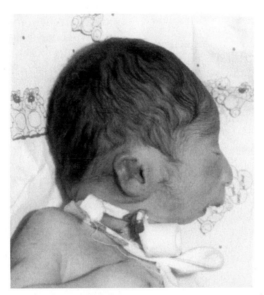

A 32-week neonate with tracheal atresia and severe retrognathia.

7.5 Thyroid Enlargement/Goiter

Epidemiology/Genetics

Definition   A goiter is an enlarged thyroid gland.

Epidemiology   Rare.

Embryology   Goiters can be associated with hypothyroidism (most common), hyperthyroidism, or a euthyroid state. Goiters associated with hypothyroidism are due to iodine deficiency, iodine intoxication, maternal antithyroid medications, or inborn errors in thyroid hormone synthesis. Goiters associated with hyperthyroidism are the result of transplacental passage of maternal thyroid-stimulating antibodies, whether or not the mother has active Graves' disease. One in 70 women with Graves' disease will have a fetus with a goiter.

Inheritance Patterns   Generally sporadic. The Pendred syndrome, however, is an autosomal recessive disorder with sensorineural deafness and goiter caused by an inborn error in thyroid hormone synthesis.

Teratogens   Propylthiouracil, iodine preparations, lithium.

Prognosis   The prognosis depends on the cause of the goiter. Polyhydramnios may induce prematurity.

Sonography

FINDINGS

1. **Fetus:** The fetal thyroid is visibly enlarged. There will be a symmetrical anterior echogenic mass in the neck, which is considered abnormal if it is 2 SD above normal. This goiter may result in posterior extension of the neck. Normal thyroid size measurements exist. Skeletal maturation may be delayed with failure to see more than two sternal ossification centers after 22 weeks' gestation or absence of the femoral epiphyseal ossification center after 33 weeks. The fetal heart rate may be increased above 160 bpm.
2. **Amniotic Fluid:** Severe polyhydramnios may occur if the esophagus is compressed.
3. **Placenta:** Normal.
4. **Measurement Data:** Intrauterine growth restriction is common.
5. **When Detectable:** This entity has not been reported as detected before 23 weeks' gestation.

Pitfalls   The extended head position may make it difficult to examine the anterior aspect of the neck if the fetus is prone.

Differential Diagnosis   Cervical teratoma—The mass will have a much more coarse and varied internal texture and will extend above or below the thyroid region. The mass may well be asymmetric.

Where Else to Look   Look for cardiomegaly and cardiac rhythm problems: tachycardia and heart block.

Pregnancy Management

Investigations and Consultations Required   Amniocentesis should be performed for chromosomal studies, measurement of alpha-fetoprotein level, and determination of thyroid-stimulating hormone concentration. Fetal MRI may be of value in delivery planning when airway compromise is a concern.

Fetal Intervention   Cases of fetal goiter secondary to hypothyroidism may be successfully treated by intra-amniotic injection of thyroid hormone.

Monitoring   No specific changes in obstetric management are indicated. Serial sonograms about every 3 weeks, to check for polyhydramnios, are helpful.

Pregnancy Course   Goiter may cause dystocia by preventing the normal flexion of the fetal head during labor.

Pregnancy Termination Issues   In the absence of a precise diagnosis, termination should be done by a non-destructive approach.

Delivery   Because of the high potential for respiratory complications, delivery should be in a tertiary center. Cesarean section may be required as a result of the excessive extension of the fetal head.

Neonatology

Resuscitation   In the delivery room, the establishment of an adequate airway is the major concern. Rarely does this require emergency tracheostomy, but if the mass is very large, endotracheal intubation can be difficult. Once an airway is secured, other specific resuscitative measures usually are not required.

Transport   Referral to a tertiary perinatal center is always indicated for diagnostic evaluation and treatment. If airway compromise is present, emergency transfer by an experienced neonatal transport team is important.

Testing and Confirmation   Thyroid enlargement will be visible on clinical examination. Radionuclide scanning, thyroid function studies, and cervical sonography are useful to define both the anatomy and the functional status of the gland.

Nursery Management   Once adequate ventilation is ensured, the focus of care is the diagnosis of the functional abnormality in thyroid production causing the goiter. Prompt relief of a congenital hypothyroid state or control of neonatal thyrotoxicosis is necessary to suppress the stimulus for hyperplasia and cause resolution of the goiter.

REFERENCES

Achiron R, Rotstein Z, Lipitz S, et al: The development of the foetal thyroid: In utero ultrasonographic measurements. Clin Endocrinol 1998;48:259–264.

Asteria C, Rajanayagam O, Collingwood TN, et al: Prenatal diagnosis of thyroid hormone resistance. J Clin Endocrinol Metab 1999;84:405–410.

Avni EF, Rodesch F, Vandemerckt C, Vermeylen D: Detection and evaluation of fetal goiter by ultrasound. Br J Radiol 1992;65:302–305.

Belfar HL, Foley TP Jr, Hill LM, Kislak S: Sonographic findings in maternal hyperthyroidism. J Ultrasound Med 1991;10:281–284.

Bromley B, Frigoletto FD Jr, Cramer D: The fetal thyroid: Normal and abnormal sonographic measurements. J Ultrasound Med 1992;11:25–28.

Bruner JP, Dellinger EH: Antenatal diagnosis and treatment of fetal hypothyroidism: A report of two cases. Fetal Diagn Ther 1997;12:200–204.

Fraser GR: Association of congenital deafness with goiter (Pendred's syndrome): A study of 207 families. Ann Hum Genet 1965;28:201–249.

Hubbard AM, Crombleholme TM, Adzick NS: Prenatal MRI evaluation of giant neck masses in preparation for the fetal exit procedure. Am J Perinatol 1998;15:253–257.

Muir A, Daneman D, Daneman A, Ehrlich R: Thyroid scanning, ultrasound, and serum thyroglobulin in determining the origin of congenital hypothyroidism. Am J Dis Child 1988;142:214–216.

VanLoon AJ, Derksen JT, Bos AF, Rouwe CW: In utero diagnosis and treatment of fetal goitrous hypothyroidism, caused by maternal use of propylthiouracil. Prenat Diagn 1995;15:599–604.

Volumenie JL, Polak M, Guibourdenche J, et al: Management of fetal thyroid goiters: A report of 11 cases in a single perinatal unit. Prenat Diagn 2000;20:799–806.

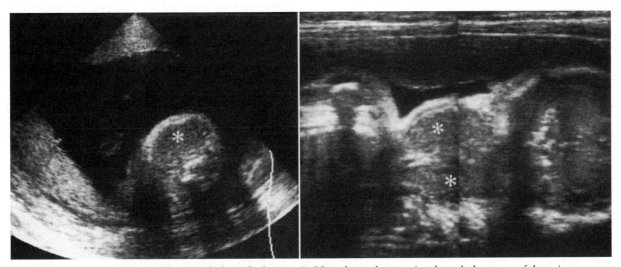

Transverse and longitudinal views of a large fetal goiter (*). Note the trachea running through the center of the goiter.

7.6   Treacher-Collins Syndrome (Mandibulofacial Dysostosis)

Epidemiology/Genetics

Definition Treacher-Collins syndrome is an autosomal dominant craniofacial disorder characterized by symmetrical malar hypoplasia, down-slanting palpebral fissures, lower lid coloboma (70%), mandibular hypoplasia, external ear abnormalities, and hearing loss.

Epidemiology One in 10,000 to 1 in 25,000 (M1:F1).

Embryology This syndrome results from dominant mutations in the *TREACLE* gene located at 5q32-q33.1. While it is assumed that the *TREACLE* gene is a developmental gene important for early craniofacial development, its exact function is not yet understood.

Inheritance Patterns Autosomal dominant, with approximately 50% of cases resulting from new mutations. DNA mutation analysis is becoming available and will aid in antenatal confirmation of suspected cases.

Teratogens None.

Prognosis In severe cases, extensive craniofacial reconstruction with staged operations is required. Temporary tracheostomies and gastrostomies may be required. Although intelligence is usually normal (90–95% of cases), conductive deafness occurs in approximately 40% of cases.

Additional Investigations Extracranial abnormalities are rare. Genetic testing for the Treacher-Collins syndrome is becoming available.

Sonography

FINDINGS

1. **Fetus:**
   a. Micrognathia is characterized by a small mandible and receding chin. It can be assessed only on a profile view that does not show the orbit and is truly at right angles.
   b. Usually the assessment is subjective, but the mandibular length can be measured between the temporomandibular joint and the junction of the mandibular rami, the symphysis mentis. A table of normal lengths has been produced.
   c. Malformed ears that are low-set.
   d. The nose may be absent or very small.
2. **Amniotic Fluid:** Mild or severe polyhydramnios is common (70%), presumably due to poor swallowing ability.
3. **Placenta:** Normal.

4. **Measurement Data:** Intrauterine growth restriction associated with the underlying cause is common.
5. **When Detectable:** The syndrome has been detected at 15 weeks.

Pitfalls It is very easy to create false micrognathia if an oblique profile view is obtained.

Differential Diagnosis

1. Trisomy 13 and 18 (about 60% of fetuses with micrognathia have a chromosomal anomaly).
2. Goldenhar-Gorlin syndrome—The facial structures are asymmetrical (see Chapter 7.3).
3. Robin anomalad—The features are micrognathia and glossoptosis. Cleft palate is present in about 50% of cases. Congenital heart disease is common (see Chapter 7.6).
4. Harlequin syndrome.
5. Pena-Shokeir syndrome (see Chapter 11.5).
6. Multiple pterygium syndrome (see Chapter 8.12).
7. Nager acrodysostosis.

Where Else to Look Most fetuses with micrognathia have abnormalities elsewhere, so a thorough study should be performed, including the cardiac and skeletal systems.

Pregnancy Management

Investigations and Consultations Required Extracranial abnormalities are rare, although fetal echocardiography and a generalized fetal anomalies survey are recommended. DNA mutation analysis for the Treacher-Collins syndrome is becoming available. In unconfirmed cases, chromosomal studies and deletion 22q11.2 fluorescent in situ hybridization should be offered.

Fetal Intervention No fetal intervention is indicated.

Monitoring In some cases, polyhydramnios may develop. Monthly sonographic evaluations should be performed to detect changes in amniotic fluid index.

Pregnancy Course No significant changes are expected unless polyhydramnios develops. Polyhydramnios may be associated with preterm labor.

Pregnancy Termination Issues Should a couple choose pregnancy termination, labor induction and delivery of an intact fetus are essential to establish a precise diagnosis.

Delivery Delivery should occur in a tertiary center because severe respiratory complications and difficult intubation may result from the more severe cases of mandibular hypoplasia.

Neonatology

Resuscitation   Airway obstruction may be present from birth secondary to mandibular hypoplasia and glossoptosis obstructing the oropharyngeal airway. Neonatal deaths have been reported from an inability to establish and/or maintain an adequate airway. In cases of severe mandibular hypoplasia, emergency tracheostomy may be required.

Transport   Transport by an experienced neonatal transport team to a tertiary center with multiple pediatric medical and surgical subspecialty capabilities, diagnostic imaging, and neonatal intensive care may be indicated.

Testing and Confirmation   Consultation with a clinical geneticist to confirm the characteristic physical findings is recommended. Diagnostic imaging and flexible endoscopy of the upper airway may be necessary to determine the need for early surgical intervention. DNA mutation analysis is becoming available for confirmation of the diagnosis.

Nursery Management   The major objectives of care are to establish a definitive diagnosis, a stable airway, and an adequate feeding mode as expeditiously as possible. Significant risks for acute airway obstruction may persist for several months, necessitating home cardiorespiratory monitoring. Extensive parental education in specialized care and monitor use is essential, particularly if alternative feeding modes and/or tracheostomy are required. Long-term management should be arranged with a multidisciplinary team because extensive reconstructive surgery, audiologic evaluation, and speech therapy are often required for satisfactory habilitation.

Surgery

Preoperative Assessment   The goal of treatment in patients with Treacher-Collins syndrome is improvement of function and optimization of aesthetic facial appearance. Treatment includes correction of the secondary deformities of the maxilla and orbit and improvement of the deficiencies of the facial soft tissues. Treatment varies according to the age of the patient, the degree of malformation, and the anticipated distortion of future growth potential.

A good treatment plan is essential for management of these complex deformities. Surgical management is based on analysis of facial skeletal radiographs and often a three-dimensional CT scan.

Types of Procedures   In patients with the Treacher-Collins syndrome, the deformities are approached early, starting at 3 years of age with calvarial grafts, either free or vascularized, to replace the orbital and zygomatic deficiencies. An extended Le Fort II maxillary osteotomy, rotating the midface and advancing the mandible, will help the airways and improve aesthetics. Additional soft tissue surgery may be required when the skeletal stability is achieved.

Surgical Results/Prognosis   The key to success in this type of craniofacial surgery is the realization that the osteotomies and grafts are part of a complex engineering project. Repair of the soft tissue constitutes a secondary surgery after the facial skeleton has been restored. This leads to an overall favorable prognosis but one that requires multiple surgeries over an extended period of time.

REFERENCES

Behrents RA, McNamara JA, Avewry JK: Prenatal mandibulofacial dysostosis (Treacher Collins syndrome). Cleft Palate J 1977;14:13.

Campbell W: The Treacher Collins syndrome. Br J Radiol 1954;27:639.

McKenzie J, Craig J: Mandibulofacial dysostosis (Treacher Collins syndrome). Arch Dis Child 1955;30:391.

Munro IR, Kay PB: Mandibulofacial dysostosis (Treacher Collins syndrome). In McCarthy JG (ed): Plastic Surgery. Philadelphia, WB Saunders, 1990.

Nicolaides DK, Johansson D, Donnai D, Rodeck CH: Prenatal diagnosis of mandibulofacial dysostosis. Prenatal Diagn 1984;4:201.

Poswillo D: The pathogenesis of the Treacher Collins syndrome (mandibulofacial dysostosis). Br J Oral Surg 1975;13:1.

Raulo Y: Treacher Collins syndrome: Analysis and principles of surgery. In Caronni EP (ed): Craniofacial Surgery. Boston, Little, Brown & Co, 1985, p 371.

Rogers BO: Berry-Treacher Collins syndrome: A review of 200 cases (mandibulofacial dysostosis: Franceschetti-Zwahlen-Klein syndrome). Br J Plast Surg 1964;17:109.

Rogers BO: The surgical treatment of mandibulofacial dysostosis (Berry syndrome; Treacher Collins syndrome; Franceschetti-Zwahlen-Klein syndrome). Clin Plast Surg 1976;3:653.

Rogers BO: Mandibulofacial dysostosis. In Converse JM (ed): Plastic and Reconstructive Surgery. Philadelphia, WB Saunders, 1977.

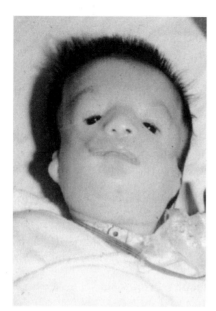

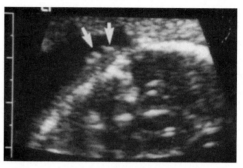

A 3-month-old child with Treacher-Collins (mandibulofacial dysostosis) syndrome. Note the bilateral microtia, downslanting palpebral fissures, and macrostomia.

Semiaxial ultrasonographic scan through the fetal head shows rudimentary, abnormal auricular components (*arrows*) in a 19-week fetus with Treacher-Collins syndrome. (From Wagner RC, Koenigsberg M, Goldberg RB: US case of the day. Radiographics 1996;16:1517–1520.)

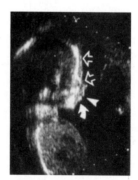

Midsagittal profile ultrasonographic scan of the fetal face shows the forehead (*top open arrow*), nose (*bottom open arrow*), mouth (*arrowhead*), and chin (*curved arrow*). There is marked micrognathia with an obvious receding chin, as well as flattening of the nasofrontal angle. (From Wagner RC, Koenigsberg M, Goldberg RB: US case of the day. Radiographics 1996;16:1517–1520.)

This infant demonstrates the appearance of Treacher-Collins syndrome with mandibular hypoplasia requiring emergency tracheostomy, absent zygomas and lateral orbital walls, and bilateral microtia. A three-dimensional computed tomographic scan of this child reveals the characteristic skeletal malformations of the mandible, condyles, maxilla, and missing orbital walls and zygomatic arch.

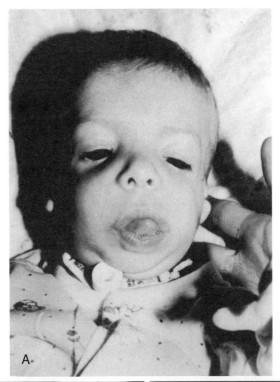

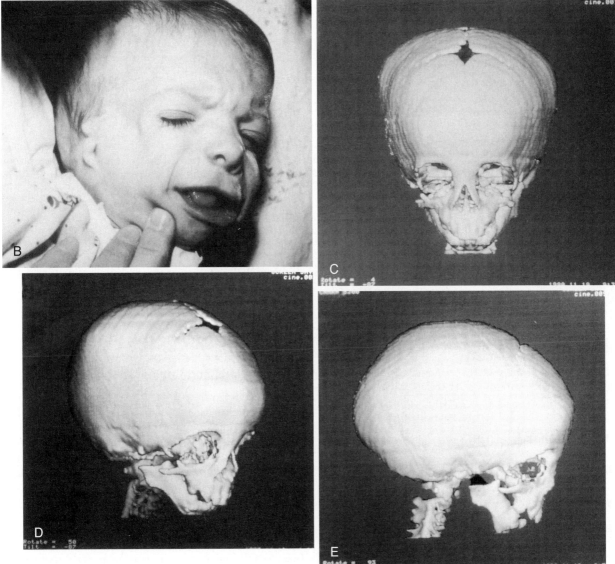

8 Skeletal Abnormalities

8.1 Achondrogenesis

Epidemiology/Genetics

Definition   Achondrogenesis is a group of lethal skeletal dysplasias characterized by severe limb and trunk shortening with a disproportionately large head.

Epidemiology   Rare. Presumably M1:F1, but reported cases show an excess of males.

Embryology   These fetuses have severe micromelia, trunk shortening, edema of the soft tissues, and a disproportionately large head. Ossification of the lumbar vertebrae is minimal (type I) or absent (type II), and the sacral, pubic, and ischial bones show little ossification. The ribs are thin and often fracture. Characteristic craniofacial features include micrognathia, flat face, and frontal bossing. Molecular defects, in type II collagen, have been found in cases of type II achondrogenesis with dominant inheritance. Mutations in the diastrophic dysplasia sulfate transporter (*DTDST*) gene on chromosome 5q have been found in achondrogenesis type I, which has autosomal recessive inheritance. Consultation with a geneticist or genetic counselor is recommended when this group of disorders is suspected.

Inheritance Patterns   Type I is inherited as an autosomal recessive disorder. Type II achondrogenesis is a new dominant mutation.

Teratogens   None.

Screening   DNA analysis for recurrence in a family with a previously identified type II collagen defect is possible. Genetic heterogeneity is a major concern, so linkage studies are not useful for prenatal diagnosis.

Prognosis   Lethal antenatally or in the newborn period.

Sonography

FINDINGS

1. **Fetus:** There are two main subtypes:
   a. Type 1—There is gross shortening of the limbs (micromelia) with flaring of the ribs or fractures and
lack of ossification of the calvarium and spine. Micrognathia is seen. Hydrops may occur.
   b. Type 2 (Langer-Saldino)—There is no flaring of the ribs or rib fractures and there is a relatively normal skull, but otherwise the features are similar.
   c. Increased nuchal translucency may occur between 11 and 14 weeks' gestation.
2. **Amniotic Fluid:** Severe polyhydramnios is invariable.
3. **Placenta:** Normal.
4. **Measurement Data:** The abdomen and head are relatively large. The limbs and chest are extremely small.
5. **When Detectable:** At 13 or 14 weeks.

Pitfalls   Easily confused with osteogenesis imperfecta because both have deossified spine and skull, but in achondrogenesis, the cranium is not compressible and limb fractures are not seen.

Differential Diagnosis

1. Thanatophoric dwarfism—The bones are more ossified (see Chapter 8.16).
2. Osteogenesis imperfecta (see Pitfalls, Chapter 8.13).

Where Else to Look   An entire fetal survey is required.

Pregnancy Management

Investigations and Consultations Required:

1. Fetal echocardiography should be performed, looking for congenital heart disease, a feature of a number of skeletal dysplasias but not of achondrogenesis.
2. Fetal radiographs should be reviewed by an individual experienced in the diagnosis of skeletal dysplasias.
3. Once a diagnosis of a lethal condition is established, and if the pregnancy is beyond the legal limits for termination, the family should meet with a neonatologist to discuss neonatal management.

Monitoring   Once a diagnosis of a lethal condition has been established, routine maternal care and supportive psychological service should be provided. No attempts to treat preterm labor or to monitor fetal status are appropriate.

Pregnancy Course   Polyhydramnios is a common complicating factor and may result in preterm labor.

Pregnancy Termination Issues   An intact fetus must be delivered and the postmortem examination, including radiologic, morphologic, biochemical, and molecular studies, must be performed by individuals with extensive experience in skeletal dysplasias. Cultured cell lines and frozen chondro-osseous tissue should be obtained.

Delivery   Vaginal delivery without electronic monitoring is appropriate. Delivery should occur in a center with expertise in the diagnostic evaluation of skeletal dysplasias, or one with an interest and expertise in fetal pathology.

Neonatology

Neonatal Resuscitation   When the diagnosis is known prior to delivery, a prenatal decision for nonintervention, made after discussion with the family, is appropriate. If the diagnosis is uncertain, resuscitation and ventilatory support are appropriate to allow time for diagnostic evaluation and parental adaptation.

Neonatal Transport   Referral to a tertiary perinatal center is appropriate for confirmation of a diagnosis. Mechanical ventilatory support is often required during the transport.

Testing and Confirmation   Postnatal radiographs can help determine the specific type of achondrogenesis.

Nursery Management   Confirmation of the diagnosis, comfort care for the infant, and counseling and support of the family are the primary goals. Provision of mechanical life support in the interim is appropriate. Liveborn infants that were not given life support survived less than 24 hours.

REFERENCES

Borochowitz Z, Lachman R, Adomian GE, et al: Achondrogenesis type I: Delineation of further heterogeneity and identification of two distinct subgroups. J Pediatr 1988;112:23–31.

Borochowitz Z, Ornoy A, Lachman R, Rimoin DL: Achondrogenesis II—Hypochondrogenesis: Variability versus heterogeneity. Am J Med Genet 1986;24:273–288.

Cai G, Nakayama M, Hiraki Y, Ozono K: Mutational analysis of the DTDST gene in a fetus with achondrogenesis type 1B. Am J Med Genet 1998;78:58–60.

Dreyer SD, Zhou G, Lee B: The long and short of it: Developmental genetics of the skeletal dysplasias. Clin Genet 1998;54:464–473.

Godfrey M, Hollister DW: Type II achondrogenesis—Hypochondrogenesis: Identification of abnormal type I collagen. Am J Hum Genet 1988;43:904–913.

Graham D, Tracey J, Winn K, et al: Early second trimester sonographic diagnosis of achondrogenesis. J Clin Ultrasound 1983;11:336–338.

Mahony BS, Filly RA, Cooperberg PL: Antenatal sonographic diagnosis of achondrogenesis. J Ultrasound Med 1984;3:333–335.

Tretter AE, Sanders RC, Meyers CM, et al: Antenatal diagnosis of lethal skeletal dysplasias. Am J Med Genet 1998;75:518–522.

Whitley CB, Gorlin RJ: Achondrogenesis: Nosology with evidence of genetic heterogeneity. Radiology 1983;148:693–698.

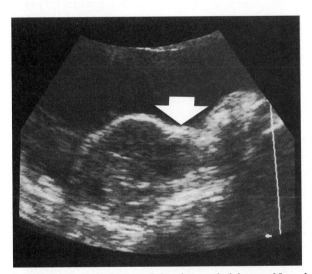

Achondrogenesis, sagittal view of the chest and abdomen. Note the poorly ossified spine and tiny chest (*arrow*) with a bell-shaped, relatively large abdomen. There is polyhydramnios.

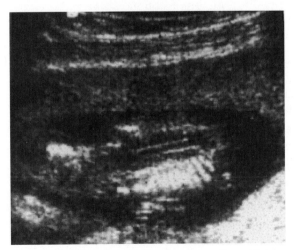

Coronal view of the spine showing the poor-quality ossification.

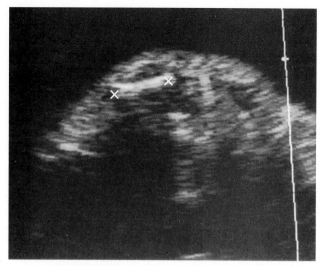

View of the femur (between the x's). It is much shorter than normal and fairly well ossified. Redundant soft tissue is present.

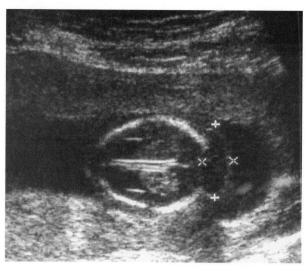

View of cranium with nuchal thickening (between x's) posterior to the skull, a common finding in achondrogenesis.

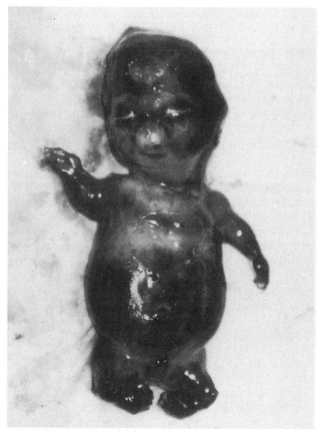

A 19-week fetus with achondrogenesis. Note the very short limbs and normal proportion of head in relation to trunk.

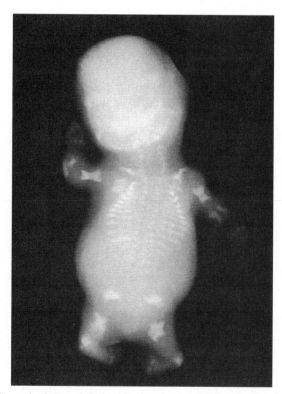

Radiograph of 19-week fetus with achondrogenesis. Note the short limbs and deficient ossification of spine.

8.2 Achondroplasia

Epidemiology/Genetics

Definition Achondroplasia is the most common non-lethal skeletal dysplasia and is characterized by rhizomelic limb shortening with macrocephaly.

Epidemiology Five to 15 in 10,000 live births (M1:F1).

Embryology The phenotype is due to decreased endochondral ossification and is characterized by rhizomelic micromelia, macroencephaly with frontal bossing, and midface hypoplasia. Achondroplasia is due to mutations in the fibroblast growth factor receptor-3 (*FGFR3*) gene that maps to the distal end of chromosome 4p. Antenatal diagnosis using DNA mutation analysis is widely available.

Inheritance Patterns Autosomal dominant with 80% of cases representing new gene mutations.

Teratogens None.

Prognosis Intelligence and life span are usually normal. Affected individuals are at risk for neurologic complications, including spinal cord compression at the foramen magnum and the thoracolumbar region. Other complications include obstructive sleep apnea and obesity. Homozygosity for achondroplasia, which occurs when both parents are affected, is lethal, with either stillbirth or early neonatal death from respiratory failure.

Sonography

FINDINGS

1. **Fetus:** Very short limbs (below the fifth percentile) developing in third trimester. There is a similar limb configuration to thanatophoric dwarfism, with a relatively small chest and a bell-shaped abdomen. A small spine width is seen with accentuated lumbar lordosis. The head is large, with low, flat nasal bridge and frontal bossing. There is brachycephaly. Short, trident-like hands with fingers of similar lengths are seen.
2. **Amniotic Fluid:** Polyhydramnios, developing in the third trimester.
3. **Placenta:** Normal.
4. **Measurement Data:** Large abdomen and head; short limbs.
5. **When Detectable:** After 24 weeks.

Pitfalls Cannot be diagnosed before 22 weeks' gestation in most instances.

Differential Diagnosis

1. Severe intrauterine growth restriction—The limbs will not be as short and there will be markedly decreased fluid.
2. Thanatophoric dwarfism—Similar appearance, but it develops earlier and is much more severe (see Chapter 8.16).
3. Homozygous achondroplasia has a similar appearance to thanatophoric dwarfism and presents at 13 weeks.
4. Hypochondroplasia—This syndrome also presents in the third trimester and has similar features to achondroplasia. Features not seen with achondroplasia are cataracts and postaxial polydactyly of the feet.

Pregnancy Management

Investigations and Consultations Required

1. Fetal echocardiography and chromosomal studies should be performed to exclude other conditions, with mild shortening of the long bones. DNA testing is available for confirmation of a suspected diagnosis.
2. *FGFR3* DNA mutation analysis is available to confirm the diagnosis on amniocentesis or other blood or tissue samples.
3. Consultation with a pediatric geneticist should be done to assist the family with an understanding of the disorder and the implications for further care.
4. To date, all cases of achondroplasia have been on the basis of two mutations in the *FGFR3* gene. Therefore, if a precise diagnosis is deemed necessary, amniocentesis would allow a precise molecular confirmation of the presumptive sonographic diagnosis. However, because the diagnosis of heterozygous achondroplasia is rarely made prior to 24 weeks' gestation, the risk of preterm rupture of the membranes from amniocentesis must be weighed against the potential benefit of a precise diagnosis.

Monitoring No change in standard obstetric practice is necessary.

Pregnancy Course Mild polyhydramnios may develop, but preterm labor or other obstetric complications are unusual.

Pregnancy Termination Issues The shortening of long bones is not evident until after 24 weeks' gestation, the legal limit for termination in most states. A diagnosis of achondroplasia prior to 24 weeks should raise suspicion of other diagnoses (usually thanatophoric dwarfism).

Delivery   Delivery should occur in a tertiary center with full capabilities for neonatal resuscitation, in the event of an incorrect diagnosis. Because of the narrow foramen magnum and upper cervical spine, spinal cord compression is a significant risk with neck manipulation. Therefore, consideration should be given to delivery by elective cesarean section.

Neonatology

Resuscitation   In the absence of known homozygosity, there are no contraindications to full resuscitative efforts following delivery, if there is delay in spontaneous onset of respiration.

Transport   The primary indication for referral in the immediate neonatal period is for confirmation of diagnosis.

Testing and Confirmation   Postnatal skeletal radiographs are pathognomonic and can confirm the clinical phenotype.

Nursery Management   Hydrocephalus may develop, although not usually in the neonatal period, except in infants with the homozygous form.

Surgery

Preoperative Assessment   During the first 3 years of life, attention is directed toward spinal development, to detect and prevent thoracolumbar kyphosis and foramen magnum stenosis. After walking age, more attention is placed on the problems of angular deformities (usually varus knees). By the age of 8 to 10 years, discussions about lengthening begin, to determine the child's and family interest. Plain radiographs help to plan lengthening and angular corrections. During the adult years, spinal stenosis is the major problem to be addressed.

Operative Indications   Thoracolumbar kyphosis in the infant to toddler age usually responds well to nonoperative treatment (bracing). Genu varum (bow legs) requires surgery in the form of either osteotomy or occasionally fibulectomy. If desired, the short stature and disproportion can be treated surgically by limb lengthening of the femurs, tibias, and humeri. Spinal stenosis in adults can be treated with surgical decompression to relieve pain and neurologic deficits.

Types of Procedures   Genu varum with fibular overgrowth leads to lateral collateral ligament laxity. Treatment consists of proximal tibial osteotomy with distraction to pull down the fibular head and tighten the lateral collateral ligament with the Ilizarov technique. This can be coordinated with lengthening.

Lengthening for stature is a complex program to achieve minimum normal height for sex for the patient at skeletal maturity. This requires 10 to 12 inches (25–30 cm) of lengthening in most patients with achondroplasia and 6 to 8 inches (15–20 cm) in most patients with hypochondroplasia. The first lengthening can be done between the ages of 8 and 10 years for 10 cm in both femurs and both tibias (5 cm each). A repeat lengthening can then be undertaken in the tibia for 10 cm of lengthening at age 12. At age 12, a 10 to 12 cm bilateral humeral lengthening is done. Near skeletal maturity, bilateral femoral lengthenings are done. The newest method of femoral lengthening combines external fixation with intramedullary nails in the femurs. This shortens the external fixation treatment time. An even newer iteration involves the use of an implanted telescopic self-lengthening nail, which eliminates the need for external fixation.

If patients develop neurologic compromise, which can range from apnea related to foramen magnum stenosis to more common lumbar spinal stenosis and kyphosis with bladder symptomatology, then decompression of the spinal cord and frequently stabilization of the spine are required.

Surgical Results/Prognosis   Realignment of the tibia by the Ilizarov method has a very low complication rate, with the exception of pin tract infection, which is managed by oral antibiotics. The main risk is that of recurrence, since the growth rate of the fibula continues to be faster than that of the tibia. Care must be taken to avoid injury to the peroneal nerve. An alternative procedure is resection of the fibula, which leaves a nonunion of the fibular bone. However, this does not tighten the loose lateral collateral ligament.

There are many potential risks of lengthening for stature, including neurovascular injury, stiffness of the ankle or knee joint with a femoral lengthening, joint contractures, premature consolidation requiring re-osteotomy, and delayed consolidation. The most common complication is pin tract infection, which can be treated with oral antibiotics, usually without any sequela. The risk of late arthritis is a possibility. Extended limb lengthening should be performed only in centers with significant experience with limb lengthening. The goals of 10 to 12 inches of lengthening over three or four lengthening procedures is achievable in many cases. Deformity correction can be combined with the lengthening.

Spinal surgery for achondroplasia is fraught with complications and should be carried out only by experienced individuals. There is a risk of paraplegia with lumbar spinal level surgery and quadriplegia with cervical level surgery. These procedures should be done only when the risk of not proceeding significantly outweighs the risk of surgery.

REFERENCES

Andersen PE Jr, Hauge M: Congenital generalized bone dysplasias: A clinical, radiological, and epidemiological survey. J Med Genet 1989;26:37–44.

Bellus GA, Hefferon TW, Ortiz de Luna RI, et al: Achondroplasia is defined by recurrent G380R mutations of FGFR3. Am J Hum Genet 1995;56:368–373.

Clark RN: Congenital dysplasias and dwarfism. Pediatr Rev 1990;12:149–159.

Cohen MM Jr: Achondroplasia, hypochondroplasia and thanatophoric dysplasia: Clinically related skeletal dysplasias that are also related at the molecular level. Int J Oral Maxillofac Surg 1998;27:451–455.

Elejalde BR, de Elejalde MM, Hamilton PR, Lombardi JM: Prenatal diagnosis in two pregnancies of an achondroplastic woman. Am J Med Genet 1983;15:437–439.

Herzenberg JE, Paley D: Methods and strategies in limb lengthening and realignment for skeletal dysplasia. In Laron Z (ed): Limb Lengthening—For Whom, When and How? Tel Aviv, Freund Publishing, 1995.

Kurtz AB, Filly RA, Wapner RJ, et al: In utero analysis of heterozygous achondroplasia: Variable time of onset as detected by femur length measurements. J Ultrasound Med 1986;5:137–140.

Lemyre E, Azouz EM, Teebi AS, et al: Bone dysplasia series. Achondroplasia, hypochondroplasia and thanatophoric dysplasia: Review and update. Can Assoc Radiol J 1999;50:185–197.

Leonard CO, Sanders RC, Lau HL: Prenatal diagnosis of the Turner syndrome, a familial chromosomal rearrangement and achondroplasia by amniocentesis and ultrasonography. Johns Hopkins Med J 1979;145:25–30.

Margolin D, Benoit B: Three dimensional sonographic aspects in the antenatal diagnosis of achondroplasia. Ultrasound Obstet Gynecol 2001;18:81–84.

Modaff P, Horton K, Pauli RM: Errors in the prenatal diagnosis of children with achondroplasia. Prenat Diag 1996;16:525–530.

Nelson FW, Hecht JT, Horton WA, et al: Neurological basis of respiratory complications in achondroplasia. Ann Neurol 1988;24:89–93.

Patel MD, Filly RA: Homozygous achondroplasia: US distinction between homozygous, heterozygous and unaffected fetuses in the second trimester. Radiology 1995;196:541–545.

Ozeren S, Yuksel A, Tukel T: Prenatal sonographic diagnosis of type I achondrogenesis with a large cystic hygroma. Ultrasound Obstet Gynecol 1999;13:75–76.

Won HS, Yoo HK, Lee PR, et al: A case of achondrogenesis type II associated with huge cystic hygroma: Prenatal diagnosis by ultrasonography. Ultrasound Obstet Gynecol 1999;14:288–291.

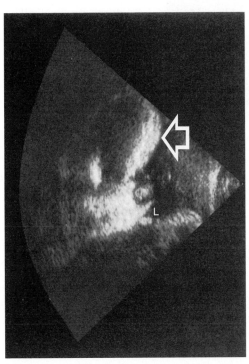

Achondroplasia. Face and forehead view. There is frontal bossing (*arrow*). L, lips.

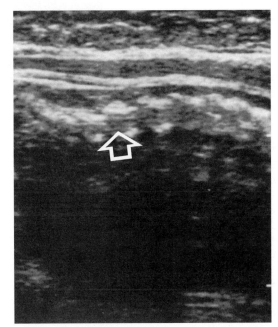

Fetal spine in achondroplasia. The intervertebral distance is decreased and the spinal canal is narrowed (*arrow*).

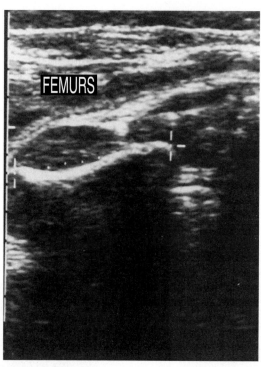

Femur view. The femur (between x's) is short and bowed, so there is a resemblance to a telephone receiver.

8.3 Amniotic Band Syndrome

Epidemiology/Genetics

Definition *Amniotic band syndrome* refers to a spectrum of asymmetric disruptive abnormalities and limb amputations thought to result from antenatal rupture of the amnion.

Epidemiology One in 1300 live births (M1:F1).

Embryology The disruptions and deformities seen in the amniotic band syndrome are asymmetric and highly variable, depending on the gestational timing of amnion rupture and the regions of the fetus involved. Early amnion rupture severely disrupts intrauterine development and may lead to anencephaly, encephaloceles, facial clefting, abdominal wall defects, and ectopia cordis. Later amnion rupture is characteristically associated with ring constrictions, limb amputations, and distal digital fusion, simulating syndactyly.

Inheritance Patterns Most often sporadic. Very rare cases may be associated with heritable disorders of connective tissue, including Ehlers-Danlos syndromes and epidermolysis bullosa.

Teratogens None.

Prognosis In the absence of central nervous system involvement, intelligence is normal. The degree of developmental disruption by the bands will determine the clinical outcome. Digital function is often excellent, despite major amputations.

Sonography

FINDINGS

1. **Fetus:** There are numerous forms of amniotic band syndrome, which may occur as isolated problems or as combinations:
   a. Absent digits or portions of limbs; for example, absent hand or end of digit.
   b. Swollen distal arm—A constriction ring related to an amniotic band causes the hand or foot and adjacent area to swell. This has been observed to progress to limb amputation but may regress spontaneously.
   c. Facial problems—Cleft lip and occasionally palate, asymmetrical microphthalmia, and severe nasal deformity.
   d. Cranial problems—Encephalocele and anencephaly may be due to bands (the encephalocele, unlike the type associated with neural crest anomalies, is usu-

ally eccentrically placed in, for example, a parietal location).
   e. Club feet or club hands.
   f. Gastroschisis may be due to amniotic bands, especially when both gut and liver lie outside the body. Omphalocele is also occasionally due to amniotic bands.
   g. Amniotic bands are also seen in the limb-body wall complex syndrome, which is considered separately (see Chapter 8.11).
2. **Amniotic Fluid:** Amniotic bands are occasionally seen in the amniotic fluid, although they are subtle and difficult to see (indeed, they are easy to miss at pathologic assessment). In the first trimester, a cobweb-like appearance to amniotic bands may be seen.
3. **Placenta:** Normal.
4. **Measurement Data:** Providing that a structure is not affected by amniotic bands, measurements should be normal.
5. **When Detectable:** At 12 to 13 weeks with the vaginal probe.

Pitfalls The combination of findings with amniotic band syndrome may suggest a neural crest problem, such as club feet and encephalocele.

Differential Diagnosis

1. Neural crest problems.
2. Radial ray problems such as Fanconi's syndrome or VACTERL (vertebral defects, anal atresia, tracheoesophageal fistula with esophageal atresia, radial and renal dysplasia) association, if the arms are affected.
3. Limb swelling may suggest Klippel-Trenaunay-Weber syndrome, but there is no increased vascularity (see Chapter 8.10).
4. Membranes within the amniotic fluid, unless associated with the sonographic findings described earlier, are probably due to (a) amniotic sheets—infolding of the amnion related to prior synechiae; (b) a remnant of a blighted twin sac; (c) displaced amnion from chorion due to previous amniocentesis, chorionic villus sampling, or prior subamniotic bleed; or (d) marginal bleed in a subamniotic location with echopenic blood.

Where Else to Look Look everywhere—virtually any anatomical structure can be affected.

Pregnancy Management

Investigations and Consultations Required

1. Depending on the pattern of malformations, chromosomal evaluation should be performed. Major limb

malformations and large non-membrane-covered ventral wall malformations are not likely to be caused by aneuploidy.
2. Fetal echocardiography, however, should be performed in all cases, for both diagnostic and prognostic purposes.

Monitoring   Because oligohydramnios may be associated with amniotic band syndrome, a decision must be made regarding the overall prognosis for the fetus before an obstetric management plan can be formulated. Fetal assessment, such as non-stress testing, is inappropriate in cases with major structural malformations or early onset of oligohydramnios in which survival is unlikely, even in a full-term infant. Encephaloceles need monitoring for developing hydrocephalus.

Pregnancy Course   No obstetric complications should be expected as a result of the amniotic band sequence, except in those cases complicated by oligohydramnios.

Pregnancy Termination Issues   A precise diagnosis is dependent on the demonstration of amniotic bands. Therefore, the method of termination must ensure an intact fetus and placenta.

Delivery   In cases with uncorrectable structural malformations or prolonged oligohydramnios, strong consideration should be given to labor without fetal monitoring and vaginal delivery.

Neonatology

Resuscitation   The decision to begin resuscitative measures is contingent on the extent of the body structure disruption known to be present prior to the onset of labor. With only extremity involvement, full resuscitation is always indicated.

Transport   Referral to a tertiary perinatal center after birth is indicated only if the degree of body structure disruption does not appear to be lethal and appears to be amenable to reconstructive surgery. Exposed viscera and denuded surfaces should be covered with sterile, moist dressings to prevent excess heat and water loss and to protect from contamination.

Nursery Management   With severe disruption of an uncorrectable nature, comfort care for the infant and counseling and supportive care for the family are the most appropriate measures. Provision of mechanical life support is appropriate when the prognosis is uncertain, to allow time for delineation of the defects and for parental adaptation.

With extremity involvement only, referral to a multidisciplinary clinic or team for children with limb deficiencies should be made prior to hospital discharge.

Surgery

Preoperative Assessment   Classification is according to degree of involvement:
1. Simple ring constriction
2. Ring constriction with distal bone fusions
3. Ring constriction with distal soft tissue fusions
4. Intrauterine amputation

A search for associated problems such as syndactyly, club foot, and cleft lip or palate should be made. Mild leg length discrepancy can develop during childhood in certain cases.

Operative Indications   In most cases, surgery is largely cosmetic, to eliminate the deep grooves caused by the constriction bands. Urgent surgery is occasionally indicated for unusual cases of impending lymphatic or venous gangrene.

Types of Procedures   Z-plasty skin releases eliminate the cosmetic groove deformity. Although successful single-stage releases (360 degrees) have been reported, many surgeons prefer to stage the release, correcting one half at a time to prevent the possibility of vascular compromise.

Surgical Results/Prognosis   Recurrence is unlikely after the bands are released. Parents should be warned, however, that they are trading a groove for a scar.

REFERENCES

Higginbottom MC, Jones KL, Hall BD, Smith DW: The amniotic band disruption complex: Timing of amniotic rupture and variable spectra of consequent defects. J Pediatr 1979;95:544–549.
Hill LM, Kislak S, Jones N: Prenatal ultrasound diagnosis of a forearm constriction band. J Ultrasound Med 1988;7:293–295.
Jones MC: The spectrum of structural defects produced as a result of amnion rupture. Semin Perinatol 1983;7:281–284.
Lockwood C, Ghidini A, Romero R: Amniotic band syndrome in monozygotic twins: Prenatal diagnosis and pathogenesis. Obstet Gynecol 1988;71:1012–1016.
Lubinsky M, Sujansky E, Sanger W, et al: Familial amniotic bands. Am J Med Genet 1983;14:81–87.
Mahony BS, Filly RA, Callen PW, Golbus MS. The amniotic band syndrome: Antenatal sonographic diagnosis and potential pitfalls. Am J Obstet Gynecol 1985;152:63–68.
Schwarzler P, Moscoso G, Senat MV, et al: The cobweb syndrome: First trimester diagnosis of multiple amniotic bands confirmed by fetoscopy and pathological examination. Hum Reprod 1998;13:2966–2969.
Seeds JW, Cefalo RC, Herbert WNP: Clinical opinion: Amniotic band syndrome. Am J Obstet Gynecol 1982;144:243–248.
Tadmor OP, Kreisberg GA, Achiron R, et al: Limb amputation in amniotic band syndrome: Serial ultrasonographic and Doppler observations. Ultrasound Obstet Gynecol 1997;10:312–315.

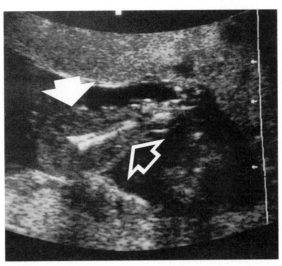

Amniotic band syndrome. Localized swelling of the proximal arm (*closed arrow*) due to a constriction band above the wrist (*open arrow*).

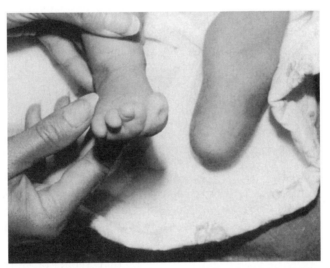

A 3-month-old infant with amniotic band amputations of the left leg and toes of the right foot.

8.4 Arthrogryposis

Epidemiology/Genetics

Definition *Arthrogryposis* is a term for a group of disorders characterized by congenital, usually nonprogressive, joint contractures at multiple sites.

Epidemiology One to 3 in 10,000 births (M1:F1).

Embryology Arthrogryposis is a physical finding that results from a heterogeneous group of disorders. These include more than 120 genetic, chromosomal, and sporadic multiple malformation syndromes. The arthrogryposes are divided into three groups: (1) those with only limb involvement; (2) those with generalized neuromuscular involvement; and (3) those with central nervous system as well as neuromuscular involvement. Only one half of children with arthrogryposis receive a specific diagnosis. Trisomy 18 is the most common chromosomal diagnosis. Myotonic dystrophy is an autosomal dominant disorder with a severe arthrogrypotic congenital form. It occurs only in offspring of mothers with myotonic dystrophy and can be diagnosed by DNA analysis in amniocytes or chorionic villi.

Inheritance Patterns Autosomal dominant, recessive, and X-linked syndromes have been described.

Teratogens Maternal hyperthermia and congenital infections.

Prognosis Prognosis is dependent on an accurate diagnosis and may range from perinatal lethal disorders to those with only mild to moderate orthopedic limitations.

Sonography

FINDINGS

1. **Fetus:** Nuchal edema is present at 10 to 14 weeks' gestation, regressing by the end of the second trimester. The legs are held in one position, either in extension and crossed or persistently flexed. The arms are flexed. The fetus, in the most severe form, is immobile. If the condition affects only the feet, the remainder of the body may have normal movement. The hands are clenched with overlapping of the fingers. The feet are extended, so they are almost in the same axis as the legs, although clubbing is also present. Muscle tissue, particularly in the lower limbs, is markedly diminished; however, limb edema is sometimes seen.
2. **Amniotic Fluid:** Some examples of arthrogryposis are due to constriction of the cavity by fibroids, uterine anomalies, membranes, or oligohydramnios. In other cases, there is polyhydramnios.
3. **Placenta:** Normal.
4. **Measurement Data:** Normal measurement data or intrauterine growth restriction.
5. **When Detectable:** The presence of nuchal thickening allows diagnosis at 10 to 14 weeks' gestation, although the limb manifestations may not be evident until about 17 weeks.

Differential Diagnosis

1. Multiple pterygium syndrome—Cystic hygroma is present and feet are flexed, rather than extended as in arthrogryposis. All limbs are involved. The webs causing the contractures may be visible at joints (see Chapter 8.12).
2. Pena-Shokeir syndrome—Contractures are less extreme. Rocker-bottom feet with severe growth deficiency are present (see Chapter 11.5).

Where Else to Look The entire fetus should be surveyed to ensure that the limb abnormalities are not part of a generalized syndrome, such as trisomy 18. Additional findings often seen with arthrogryposis are micrognathia, cataracts, microcephaly, and facial defect.

Pregnancy Management

Investigations and Consultations Required

1. Fetal karyotype and studies to rule out congenital infections should be considered, especially if additional malformations are detected.
2. Fetal echocardiography may be helpful in establishing a diagnosis and determining prognosis.

Monitoring Standard obstetric care is appropriate. Serial ultrasonograms to assess fluid volume are helpful for prognostic purposes.

Pregnancy Course Breech presentation is common in fetuses with arthrogryposis syndromes. Polyhydramnios is rare except in lethal disorders.

Pregnancy Termination Issues The heterogeneous group of disorders that has arthrogryposis as a feature require that a complete autopsy on an intact fetus be performed. Accurate recurrence risk counseling requires a precise diagnosis.

Delivery The mode of delivery should be based on obstetric indications only. Because an exact diagnosis will rarely be established prenatally, delivery at a tertiary center is appropriate.

Neonatology

Resuscitation   The decision not to offer resuscitation is easiest when there is a definite diagnosis of a concomitant lethal condition. In all other circumstances, resuscitation should be initiated and support continued, if needed, while a diagnostic evaluation is completed.

Transport   Referral to a tertiary perinatal center for diagnostic evaluation is appropriate. With an otherwise asymptomatic infant, referral for outpatient evaluation and treatment planning is also acceptable.

Testing and Confirmation   Because long-term prognosis is heavily influenced by associated or coexisting disorders, complete diagnostic evaluation and etiologic determination are the top priorities. Muscle biopsy and nerve conduction studies are important in determining the potential for habilitation.

Nursery Management   Treatment is directed toward achieving stable functional weight-bearing and manual dexterity. Initially, positioning, physical therapy, and bracing are used, followed by surgery in later infancy and childhood.

Surgery

Preoperative Assessment   The diagnosis is made by physical examination alone. The affected joints are stiff and contracted and have diminished or absent joint skin creases. Involvement usually includes both hands, both feet, and often both hips, elbows, shoulders, and knees. The joints are typically flexed, with webbing seen on the flexion side in severe cases. Some children have isolated single limb involvement. Scoliosis develops in about 10% of cases.

Operative Indications   The need for surgery depends on the location and extent of involvement. The most common surgery required for arthrogrypotic children in the first year of life is for correction of club foot and reduction of dislocated hips. As these children grow, they often require release of knee flexion contractures in order to stand upright. Upper extremity surgery is occasionally indicated to treat elbow and wrist flexion contractures.

Types of Procedures   Soft tissue releases (cutting tight muscles and ligaments) are the mainstay of treatment. Instead of tight tendons being lengthened, they are simply cut, to diminish the chance of recurrence. In nearly every case, the joint capsular ligaments must also be sectioned. For dislocated hips, the tight structures are cut and the hip is placed into the acetabulum. Scoliosis is treated by distraction instrumentation and fusion in older children.

Recurrence of foot deformities often requires talectomy or triple arthrodesis. More recently, the Ilizarov distraction external fixator has been sized to treat recurrent club foot deformities in arthrogryptics. In older children and teenagers with recurrent contractures, external fixators have been used to gradually correct contracted knees and elbows. Gradual correction with distraction devices (Ilizarov apparatus) is safer for the contracted neurovascular structures than acute correction.

Surgical Results/Prognosis   Prognosis is largely dependent on the initial degree of involvement and cause. Total body involvement may render a child wheelchair-bound. More commonly, involvement of all four extremities responds to surgery, but the child often requires braces and crutches to walk. Isolated single limb involvement has the best prognosis. Hand deformities preclude many activities, but most children do remarkably well. Mentation is normal in most cases.

REFERENCES

Bui TH, Lindholm H, Demir N, Thomassen P: Prenatal diagnosis of distal arthrogryposis type I by ultrasonography. Prenat Diagn 1992;12:1047–1053.

Degani S, Shapiro I, Lewinsky R, Sharf M: Prenatal ultrasound diagnosis of isolated arthrogryposis. Acta Obstet Gynecol Scand 1989;68:461–462.

Fahy MJ, Hall JG: A retrospective study of pregnancy complications among 828 cases of arthrogryposis. Genet Couns 1990;1:3–11.

Geifman-Holtzman O, Fay K: Prenatal diagnosis of congenital myotonic dystrophy and counseling of the pregnant mother: Case report and literature review. Am J Med Genet 1998;78:250–253.

Goldberg JD, Chervenak FA, Lipman RA, Berkowitz RL: Antenatal sonographic diagnosis of arthrogryposis multiplex congenita. Prenat Diagn 1986;6:45–49.

Gorczyca DP, McGahan JP, Lindfors KK, et al: Arthrogryposis multiplex congenita: Prenatal ultrasonographic diagnosis. J Clin Ultrasound 1989;17:40–44.

Hageman G, Willemse J: Arthrogryposis multiplex congenita: Review with comment. Neuropediatrics 1983;14:6–11.

Hall JG: Arthrogryposis (congenital contractures). In Emery AA, Rimoin DL (eds): Principles and Practice of Medical Genetics. Edinburgh, Churchill Livingstone, 1983, pp 781–811.

Herzenberg JE, Paley D: Ilizarov management of clubfoot deformity in young children. Foot Clinics/Foot and Ankle Clinics 1998; 3:649–661.

Hyett J, Noble P, Sebire NJ, et al: Lethal congenital arthrogryposis presents with increased nuchal translucency at 10–14 weeks of gestation. Ultrasound Obstet Gynecol 1997;9:310–313.

Miskin M, Rothberg R, Rudd NL, et al: Arthrogryposis multiplex congenita-prenatal assessment with diagnostic ultrasound and fetoscopy. J Pediatr 1979;95:463–464.

Robinson YJ, Rouse GA, De Lange M: Sonographic evaluation of arthrogrypotic conditions. J Dent Maxillofac Surg 1994;10:18–22.

Scott H, Hunger A, Bedard B: Non-lethal arthrogryposis multiplex congenita presenting with cystic hygroma at 13 weeks gestational age. Prenat Diagn 1999;19:966–971.

Silberstein EP, Kakulas BA: Arthrogryposis multiplex congenita in western Australia. J Paediatr Child Health 1998;34:518–523.

Wynne-Davies R, Lloyd-Roberts GC: Arthrogryposis multiplex congenita: Search for prenatal factors in 66 sporadic cases. Arch Dis Child 1976;51:618–623.

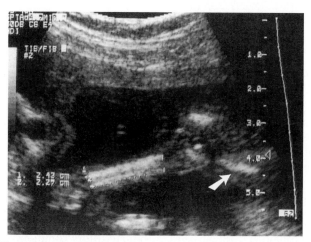

View of the tibia and fibula in a patient with arthrogryposis. Note the almost complete absence of soft tissue due to severe muscle wasting. The femur can be seen to the right (*arrow*). No change in the alignment of the upper and lower leg was seen over a prolonged period.

8.5 Campomelic Dysplasia

Epidemiology/Genetics

Definition Campomelic dysplasia is a heterogeneous group of lethal skeletal dysplasias with characteristic bowing deformities of the femur and tibia.

Epidemiology Rare. Phenotypic sex ratio, M1:F2.3; karyotypic sex ratio, M2:F1.

Embryology The campomelic dysplasias comprise both short-boned and long-boned types, and affected infants have a flat facial profile, cleft palate, and tracheal abnormalities. An apparent preponderance of females is due to 46,XY males with sex-reversal. The gene associated with the disorder is located on chromosome 17 and is designated *SOX*-9 (*SRY*-related *HMG*-box 9) gene. Mutations in the gene and proximal to the gene have been reported in cases of campomelic dysplasia.

Inheritance Patterns Autosomal dominant. Campomelic dysplasia is due to mutations in the *SOX*9 gene on chromosome 17q. Consultation with a geneticist or genetic counselor concerning antenatal testing should be done in suspected cases.

Teratogens None.

Prognosis Usually lethal in the neonatal period. Survival duration is related to the degree of respiratory compromise at birth. Infants with less severe manifestations may occasionally survive into early infancy but with significant respiratory and feeding difficulties. All have delayed development and are mentally retarded.

Sonography

FINDINGS

1. **Fetus:**
   a. Bowed and shortened lower limbs, particularly the tibia and femur. There may be acute angulation of the femur suggesting fracture with a "chevron" configuration. The fibulae are hypoplastic or absent.
   b. A bell-shaped chest and abdomen is seen, owing to the narrow chest.
   c. Severe micrognathia with elongated philtrum and flattened nose. Hypotelorism may occur. Cleft palate may be present.
   d. Club feet with brachydactyly.
   e. Lateral ventriculomegaly may develop.
   f. Hypoplastic scapulae with normally ossified unfractured ribs.
   g. Poorly formed or ambiguous genitalia may be seen.
   h. Renal pelvic dilation is sometimes seen.

2. **Amniotic Fluid:** Increased fluid is usual, since the thorax is small.
3. **Placenta:** Normal.
4. **Measurement Data:** Small chest circumference and markedly shortened lower limbs.
5. **When Detectable:** At about 17 weeks.

Differential Diagnosis Osteogenesis imperfecta—the lower limbs are also most affected by osteogenesis imperfecta and bowing is often seen. The facial and cranial findings and club feet seen with campomelic dwarfism do not occur with osteogenesis imperfecta. Bony structures are deossified in osteogenesis imperfecta but normally ossified in campomelic dysplasia (see Chapter 8.13).

Where Else to Look Other occasional abnormalities are heart defects and club feet.

Pregnancy Management

Investigations and Consultations Required

1. Fetal echocardiography should be performed to exclude congenital heart defects, which are not usually a feature of campomelic dysplasia. The status of DNA mutation analysis should be checked.
2. Neonatology specialists should be consulted to plan the perinatal management approach that will be taken.

Monitoring Tocolytic agents are contraindicated. There are no benefits to prolonging pregnancy.

Pregnancy Course Polyhydramnios and preterm labor frequently complicate the fetal malformation.

Pregnancy Termination Issues An intact fetus must be delivered, and the postmortem examination, including radiologic, morphologic, biochemical, and molecular studies, must be performed by individuals with extensive experience in skeletal dysplasias. Culture cell lines and frozen chondro-osseous tissue should be obtained.

Delivery The site for delivery should be one where all personnel are comfortable with a nonaggressive approach to labor, delivery, and neonatal care.

Neonatology

Resuscitation When the diagnosis is known prior to delivery, a prenatal decision for nonintervention, made after discussion with the family, is appropriate. If the diagnosis is uncertain, resuscitation and ventilatory support are instituted to allow time for diagnostic evaluation and parental adaptation.

Transport   Referral to a tertiary perinatal center is appropriate for confirmation of a diagnosis. Mechanical ventilatory support is often required during the transport.

Testing and Confirmation   Skeletal radiographs postnatally will establish the diagnosis.

Nursery Management   Confirmation of the diagnosis and counseling and support of the family are the primary goals. Provision of mechanical life support initially is appropriate with concurrence of the family. Withdrawal of support may become a problem subsequently if respiratory insufficiency persists.

REFERENCES

Balcari I, Bieber FR: Sonographic and radiologic findings in camptomelic dysplasia. Am J Roentgenol 1983;141:481–482.

Carlan SJ, Parsons MT, Flasher J: Camptomelic skeletal dysplasia with a narrow thorax. J Dent Maxillofac Surg 1990;1:40–42.

Cordone M, Lituania M, Zampatti C, et al: In utero ultrasonographic features of camptomelic dysplasia. Prenat Diagn 1989;9:745–750.

Dreyer SD, Zhou G, Lee B: The long and short of it: Developmental genetics of the skeletal dysplasias. Clin Genet 1998;54:464–473.

Gillerot Y, Vanheck CA, Foulon M, et al: Camptomelic syndrome: Manifestations in a 20 week fetus and case history of a 5-year-old child. Am J Med Genet 1989;34:589–592.

Hall BD, Spranger JW: Camptomelic dysplasia: Further elucidation of a distinct entity. Am J Dis Child 1980;134:285–289.

Houston CS, Opitz JM, Spranger JW, et al: The camptomelic syndrome: Review, report of 17 cases, and follow-up on the currently 17-year-old boy first reported by Maroteaux et al in 1971. Am J Med Genet 1983;15:3–28.

Kozlowski K, Butzler HO, Galatius-Jensen F, Tulloch A: Syndromes of congenital bowing of the long bones. Pediatr Radiol 1978;7:40–48.

McDowall S, Argentaro A, Ranganathan S, et al: Functional and structural studies of wild type SOX9 and mutations causing camptomelic dysplasia. J Biol Chem 1999;274:24023–24030.

Tongson T, Wanapirak C, Pongsatha S: Prenatal diagnosis of camptomelic dysplasia. Ultrasound Obstet Gynecol 2000;15:428–430.

Tretter AE, Sanders RC, Meyers CM, et al: Antenatal diagnosis of lethal skeletal dysplasias. Am J Med Genet 1998;75:518–522.

Winter R, Rosenkranz W, Hofmann H, et al: Prenatal diagnosis of camptomelic dysplasia by ultrasonography. Prenat Diagn 1985;5:1–8.

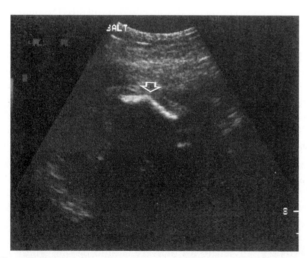

Campomelic dwarfism. Shortened angulated femur initially thought to be due to osteogenesis imperfecta. Note the apparent fracture (*arrow*) and "chevron" shape of the femur.

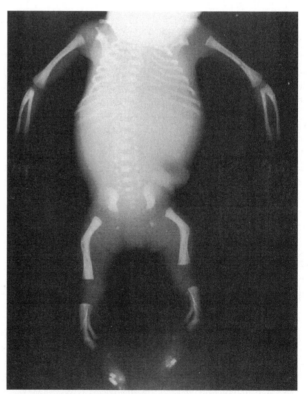

Radiograph showing angulated shortened femurs and shortened bowed tibia and fibula. (From Sanders RC, Greyson-Flag RT, Hogge WA, et al: Osteogenesis imperfecta and camptomelic dysplasia: Difficulties in prenatal diagnosis. J Ultrasound Med 1994;13:691–700.)

8.6 Club and Rocker-Bottom Feet (Vertical Talus)

Epidemiology/Genetics

Definition   A club foot is a foot malformation characterized by equinus and inversion of the foot with associated abnormalities in the musculature of the lower leg. A rocker-bottom foot is the phenotypic description of a foot characterized by dorsiflexion of the forefoot, equinus of the heel, and a convex sole.

Epidemiology   Club foot occurs with a frequency of 1 to 3 in 1000 live births. The frequency of rocker-bottom feet is unknown but is much less common.

Embryology   Club foot can occur as an isolated abnormality or as part of more than 200 chromosomal, genetic, or sporadic multiple malformation syndromes. It is frequently secondary to lower extremity paralysis from a neural tube defect. Rocker-bottom feet have been described in association with more than 30 chromosomal, genetic, or sporadic multiple malformation syndromes, especially trisomy 18.

Inheritance Patterns   Dependent on the cause of the foot abnormalities.

Teratogens   None specific.

Prognosis   Dependent on the cause of the foot abnormalities.

Sonography

FINDINGS

1. **Fetus:**
   a. Club feet—The two long bones of the leg can be seen at the same time as the lateral aspect of the feet because the foot is inverted or, more likely, extraverted. The foot is either flexed or extended (see diagram for the various different types). It is fixed in position. With talipes equinovarus, there is adduction of the forefoot, inversion of the heel, and plantar flexion of the forefoot and ankle. With talipes calcaneovalgus, there is dorsal flexion of the forefoot and the plantar surfaces face laterally. With metatarsus adductus, there is inversion and adduction of the forefoot alone.
   b. Rocker-bottom foot—The heel of the foot extends posterior to the leg. The mid-portion of the foot may be inferior to the proximal and distal portions of the foot.
2. **Amniotic Fluid:** If the condition is isolated, the amniotic fluid is normal.

3. **Placenta:** If the condition is isolated, the placenta is normal.
4. **Measurement Data:** Normal, if the condition is isolated.
5. **When Detectable:** At about 13 weeks' gestation using the vaginal probe.

Pitfalls   The foot may be held in a deviated flexed position, as a normal variant, if there is little fluid and the foot is pushing against the uterine wall. Because of the difficulty in aligning the leg and feet at the same time by in utero visualization, there may be overdiagnosis of club feet. The diagnosis of rocker-bottom foot by ultrasound is subtle without well-defined criteria.

Differential Diagnosis   Arthrogryposis—The foot is very extended but not necessarily deviated to right or left, and there is soft tissue loss.

Where Else to Look   Many club and rocker-bottom feet are associated with syndromes that involve every structure. Look particularly for chromosomal malformations, neural tube defects and caudal regression, amniotic band syndrome, and dwarfing syndromes such as diastrophic dysplasia and camptomelic dysplasia.

Pregnancy Management

Investigations and Consultations Required   Chromosomal studies and fetal echocardiography are essential components of the work-up, except for an isolated club foot. Consultation with a pediatric geneticist or dysmorphologist with evaluation of the parents may be helpful in establishing a diagnosis. Because club feet may be a manifestation of primary central nervous system disorders, myelomeningocele, fetal akinesia syndromes, and a host of genetic syndromes, the diagnosis of isolated club foot must be made with caution.

Monitoring   No change in standard obstetric management is necessary.

Pregnancy Course   No obstetric complications should be expected, if these conditions are isolated.

Pregnancy Termination Issues   Should termination be chosen, the method used should provide an intact fetus for complete morphologic and pathologic examination.

Delivery   The high likelihood that these conditions are not isolated makes delivery in a tertiary center, with full diagnostic and treatment capabilities, the preferable approach.

Surgery

Preoperative Assessment   The diagnosis of neonatal club foot is made on clinical examination, with uncorrectable hindfoot equinus and rigid forefoot adductus. The entire foot is internally rotated, relative to the tibia. Radiographs of club feet in the neonatal period are less helpful, since the bones are largely nonossified.

The physical findings in rocker-bottom feet are more subtle. The arch of the foot is "flat." In a true vertical talus, the foot is rigid, not flexible. Radiographic confirmation of the vertical talus is required to confirm the diagnosis. In a true vertical talus, stress plantar flexion lateral views of the foot show that the first metatarsal never lies in line with the long axis of the talus. Other causes of flatfoot should be considered in the preoperative assessment, including tarsal coalition, flexible flatfoot, and benign calcaneovalgus flatfoot (from intrauterine molding).

Operative Indications   Nearly every foot with vertical talus will require surgery to obtain a plantigrade, shoeable foot. Treatment for club foot always begins with serial casting. Idiopathic cases may require only tenotomy of the Achilles tendon, but syndromic cases require extensive posteromedial surgical release.

Types of Procedures   The initial treatment for club foot or vertical talus is serial casting. This helps to stretch the contracted soft tissues in preparation for surgery. The optimal age for surgery is 6 to 12 months. For both disorders, surgery consists of tendon lengthenings combined with ligament releases. This allows the bones to be repositioned into normal alignment. Usually, small temporary steel pins are inserted to hold the alignment for the first 6 weeks after surgery. Casts are worn for 6 to 12 weeks after surgery. In more severe cases, follow-up bracing is used to prevent recurrence, particularly in neurogenic and severe cases associated with syndromes. For idiopathic club foot, the Ponseti method is gaining popularity. This method uses serial casting, percutaneous Achilles tenotomy, and prolonged splinting with a foot abduction orthosis.

Surgical Results/Prognosis   For most idiopathic cases, the results of surgery are a nearly normal foot. Most children can walk without a limp. The corrected club foot is always stiffer than a normal foot, and thus may be prone to develop arthritis in middle age. The calf is noticeably thinner in diameter on the affected side, and this may be of cosmetic concern in girls who wear skirts or dresses. Recurrence after surgery is not unusual, especially in teratologic and neurogenic cases. Recurrence requires further surgery, such as triple arthrodesis (fusion of the hindfoot joints). More recently, external fixators (Ilizarov) have been used to stretch out recurrent contracted foot deformities.

REFERENCES

Bronshtein M, Zimmer EZ: Transvaginal ultrasound diagnosis of fetal club feet at 13 weeks, menstrual age. J Clin Ultrasound 1989;17:518–520.

Carroll SCM, Lockyer H, Andrews H: Outcome of fetal talipes following in utero sonographic diagnosis. Ultrasound Obstet Gynecol 2001;18:437–441.

Malone FD, Marino T, Bianchi DW, et al: Isolated clubfoot diagnosed prenatally: Is karyotyping indicated? Obstet Gynecol 2000;95:437–440.

Paley D, Herzenberg JE: Applications of external fixation to foot and ankle reconstruction. In Myerson MS: Foot and Ankle Disorders. Philadelphia, WB Saunders, 1999, pp 1135–1188.

Ponseti IV: Clubfoot management. J Pediatr Orthop 2000;20(6):699–700.

Rijhsinghani A, Yankowitz J, Kanis AB, et al: Antenatal sonographic diagnosis of club foot with particular attention to the implications and outcomes of isolated club foot. Ultrasound Obstet Gynecol 1998;11:103–106.

Tillett RL, Fisk NM, Murphy D, Hunt DM: Clinical outcome of congenital talipes equinovarus diagnosed antenatally by ultrasound. J Bone Joint Surg Br 2000;82:976–980.

Woodrow N, Tran T, Umstad M, et al: Mid-trimester ultrasound diagnosis of isolated talipes equinovarus: Accuracy and outcome for infants. Aust N Z J Obstet Gynaecol 1998;38:301–305.

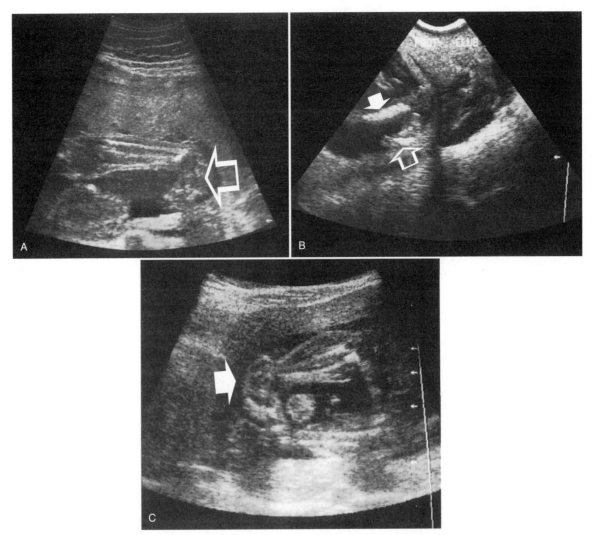

Different forms of club foot with either extension or flexion and abduction or inversion deformities (*arrows*).

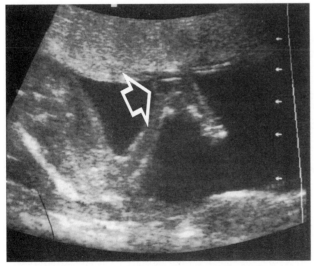

Rocker-bottom foot. Note the prominent heel (*arrow*).

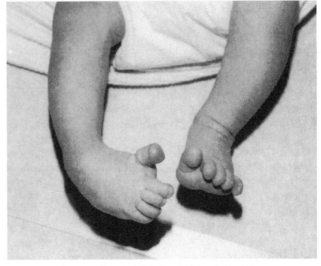

Term newborn with isolated right clubbed foot.

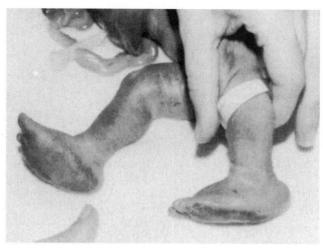

A 28-week stillborn with trisomy 13. Note typical rocker-bottom feet with prominent calcaneus.

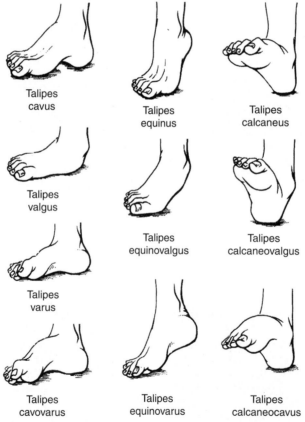

Talipes
cavus

Talipes
equinus

Talipes
calcaneus

Talipes
valgus

Talipes
equinovalgus

Talipes
calcaneovalgus

Talipes
varus

Talipes
cavovarus

Talipes
equinovarus

Talipes
calcaneocavus

Diagram showing the different types of club feet. (From Dorland's Illustrated Medical Dictionary, 29th ed. Philadelphia, WB Saunders, 2000.)

8.7 Diastrophic Dysplasia

Epidemiology/Genetics

Definition Diastrophic dysplasia is a short-limbed skeletal dysplasia characterized by club feet, ear swelling, and progressive joint and spine deformity.

Epidemiology Very rare (M1:F1).

Embryology Diastrophic dysplasia is characterized by club feet, an abducted "hitchhiker" thumb, inflammatory cystic swelling of the ear pinna, and cleft palate. The gene for diastrophic dysplasia has been cloned and is called the diastrophic dysplasia sulfate transporter (*DTDST*) gene and is located on chromosome 5q31–34. Consultation with a geneticist or genetic counselor should be sought to determine the status of antenatal DNA mutation analysis.

Inheritance Patterns Autosomal recessive.

Teratogens None.

Prognosis Rare neonatal death has been described, but most patients have a normal life span and intellectual development. Adult height is generally less than 4 feet, with severe orthopedic abnormalities. A lethal variant has been reported with associated cardiac defects and a high incidence of intrauterine growth retardation. All affected infants succumbed shortly after birth or in early infancy.

Sonography

FINDINGS

1. **Fetus:** The sonographic features involve much of the body:
   a. Micromelia—All limbs are very short throughout their extent.
   b. Ulnar deviation of the hands with short phalanges—The thumbs are abducted and proximally inserted (hitchhiker thumbs). The big toes have a similar deformity. The feet are severely extended and clubbed.
   c. Micrognathia.
   d. Cleft lip and palate.
   e. Cervical kyphoscoliosis, a major finding later in life, is subtle in utero.
   f. Flexion deformity of the elbows and knees.
   g. The chest is relatively normal-sized, considering the small limb size.
   h. Congenital heart defects.
2. **Amniotic Fluid:** Polyhydramnios may be seen.
3. **Placenta:** Normal.
4. **Measurement Data:** All limb measurements are well below the fifth percentile.
5. **When Detectable:** At about 13 weeks.

Differential Diagnosis Other lethal dwarfing syndromes. In diastrophic dwarfism, unlike most other lethal syndromes, the long bones are not bowed. The hitchhiker thumb and kyphoscoliosis make for a relatively distinct picture.

Where Else to Look The entire body needs to be surveyed in detail.

Pregnancy Management

Investigations and Consultations Required

1. The gene for diastrophic dysplasia has been cloned (*DTDST*), and prenatal diagnosis is available for at-risk families.
2. Fetal echocardiography should be performed; the presence of a congenital heart defect would suggest another type of skeletal dysplasia other than diastrophic dysplasia.
3. A neonatology consultation should be obtained to assist in planning perinatal management.

Monitoring Preterm labor secondary to polyhydramnios may occur. Therefore, obstetric care should be coordinated by a perinatologist. Despite the severity of the disorder, it is not usually lethal, and severe prematurity will only further complicate management.

Pregnancy Course Polyhydramnios is an occasional complication of this skeletal dysplasia and may result in preterm labor. As is the case for all skeletal dysplasias, the lethal forms should be excluded before an obstetric management plan is established.

Pregnancy Termination Issues An intact fetus must be delivered and the postmortem examination, including radiologic, morphologic, biochemical, and molecular studies, must be performed by individuals with extensive experience in skeletal dysplasias. Cultured cell lines and frozen chondro-osseous tissue should be obtained.

Delivery Respiratory complications are common, and intubation may be complicated because of micrognathia. Delivery should occur in a tertiary center with the capabilities to manage these complications.

Neonatology

Resuscitation Initiation of resuscitation in liveborn infants is appropriate when the prognosis is in doubt.

Testing and Confirmation Confirmation of the diagnosis and prognosis are the first priorities. Careful physical examination, skeletal radiographs, echocardiography, and genetic testing are useful in the evaluation.

Nursery Management   Respiratory insufficiency secondary to laryngeal obstruction appears to be the mode of death in the lethal variant. Response to ventilatory support and a mechanical airway is unknown.

The long-term treatment plan is directed toward orthopedic correction of the club feet and kyphoscoliosis, should the latter develop.

Surgery

Preoperative Assessment   Initial problems may include severe club feet and dislocated hips. Flexion contractures develop in upper and lower extremities. Scoliosis or kyphoscoliosis occurs in early childhood. Growth is retarded, with a mean adult height less than 4 feet tall. In addition to the orthopedic problems, assess for cleft palate, which is seen in two thirds of cases.

Operative Indications   Orthopedic surgical efforts are directed primarily toward the club feet and hip dysplasia problems. Knee flexion deformity and patellar subluxation can also benefit from surgery. Scoliosis is initially treated with bracing but ultimately may require surgery to stabilize deformities.

Types of Procedures   These club feet are some of the most difficult club feet to treat. They are very stiff and frequently recur after surgical treatment. Conventional releases frequently cannot achieve full correction, and recurrence of deformity is common. Newer alternatives for treatment include application of a distraction apparatus such as the Ilizarov device. Conventional treatment re-

sorts to talectomy in the most severe cases. Talectomy, unfortunately, has not had good long-term results and frequently presents with recurrent deformities that are almost impossible to treat.

Surgical Results/Prognosis   Cervical spinal kyphosis in diastrophic dysplasia can lead to neurologic complications if untreated. Flexion contractures frequently lead to severe joint deformities, which can preclude walking ability. This is one of the more difficult orthopedic conditions to treat. Occasionally, involvement is mild, and prognosis is much better.

REFERENCES

Clark RN: Congenital dysplasias and dwarfism. Pediatr Rev 1990;12: 149–159.

Dreyer SD, Zhou G, Lee B: The long and short of it: Developmental genetics of the skeletal dysplasias. Clin Genet 1998;54:464–473.

Gembruch U, Niesen M, Kehrberg H, Hansmann M: Diastrophic dysplasia: A specific prenatal diagnosis by ultrasound. Prenat Diagn 1988;8:539–545.

Gollop TR, Eigier A: Prenatal ultrasound diagnosis of diastrophic dysplasia at sixteen weeks. Am J Med Genet 1987;27:321–324.

Gustavson KH, Holmgren G, Jagell S, Jorulf H: Lethal and non-lethal diastrophic dysplasia: A study of 14 Swedish cases. Clin Genet 1985;28:321–334.

Hastbacka J, Salonen R, Laurilap, et al: Prenatal diagnosis of diastrophic dysplasia with polymorphic DNA markers. J Med Genet 1993;30: 265–268.

Jung C, Sohn C, Sergi C: Case report: Prenatal diagnosis of diastrophic dysplasia by ultrasound at 21 weeks of gestation in a mother with massive obesity. Prenat Diagn 1998;18:378–383.

Kaitila I, Ammala P, Karjalainen O, et al: Early prenatal detection of diastrophic dysplasia. Prenat Diagn 1983;3:237–244.

Mantagos S, Weiss RR, Mahoney M, Hobbins JC: Prenatal diagnosis of diastrophic dwarfism. Am J Obstet Gynecol 1981;139:111–113.

Rossi A, Van Der Harten HJ, Beemer FA, et al: Phenotypic and genotypic overlap between atelosteogenesis type 2 and diastrophic dysplasia. Hum Genet 1996;98:657–661.

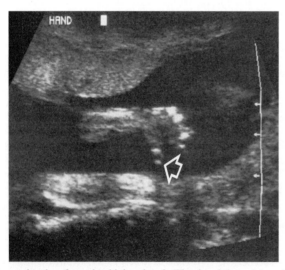

Diastrophic dwarfism—hitchhiker thumb. The thumb (*arrow*) is at right angles to the remaining digits. All are short and stubby.

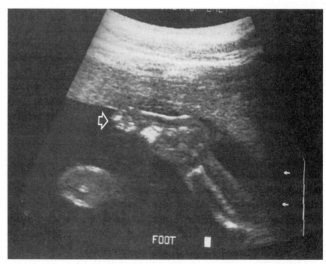

Severely extended foot (*arrow*) in diastrophic dysplasia. Note the short tibia.

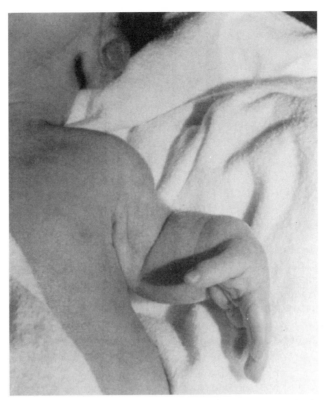

A 2-month-old infant with diastrophic dysplasia. Note angulated (hitch-hiker) thumb and ear cartilage hematomas (cauliflower ear).

8.8 Focal Femoral Hypoplasia (FFH)

Epidemiology/Genetics

Definition Focal femoral hypoplasia (FFH) is characterized by shortening and/or deformity of the femur.

Epidemiology Rare (M2:F3).

Embryology Focal femoral hypoplasia is a physical finding that may be seen in more than 25 genetic and sporadic multiple malformation syndromes, including a number of skeletal dysplasias. It is often associated with abnormalities of the ipsilateral tibia and fibula.

Inheritance Patterns Dependent on diagnosis, but includes dominant and recessive genetic syndromes.

Teratogens Maternal diabetes and fetal vitamin A exposure.

Prognosis Prognosis depends on cause and can range from lethal skeletal dysplasias (rare) to disorders with only mild orthopedic abnormalities.

Sonography

FINDINGS

1. **Fetus:**
   a. The proximal portion of one femur, including the femoral head, is usually absent. The femur is often angulated or bowed.
   b. Absence, or partial absence, of other long bones or digits may occur. Bowing of the tibia may occur if the fibula is absent.
   c. The femur-fibula-ulna complex consists of bilateral femoral hypoplasia and partial or complete absence of the fibula and ulna. There may be partial or complete absence of the arm.
   d. The femoral hypoplasia/unusual facies syndrome consists of cleft palate, micrognathia, short or absent femora, and vertebral and genitourinary malformations such as ambiguous genitalia.
2. **Amniotic Fluid:** Normal.
3. **Placenta:** Normal.
4. **Measurement Data:** Normal, except in the affected limb or limbs.
5. **When Detectable:** As early as 14 weeks. The abnormality becomes progressively more obvious.

Pitfalls The deformity with angulation of the femur can create an impression of osteogenesis imperfecta with a fracture. However, no additional fractures are seen.

Differential Diagnosis Osteogenesis imperfecta—see Pitfalls. The severe forms of this disorder must be differentiated from sirenomelia, which is generally associated with lethal renal abnormalities.

Where Else to Look

1. Look elsewhere for findings associated with osteogenesis imperfecta. Acute angulation of the hypoplastic femur may occur.
2. Cleft palate and micrognathia are a rare association.
3. If the condition is bilateral, look for the features of the femur-fibula-ulna syndrome and femoral hypoplasia/unusual facies syndrome.

Pregnancy Management

Investigations and Consultations Required

1. To exclude other syndromes, fetal echocardiography should be performed. The presence of a congenital heart defect should prompt a reassessment of the diagnosis of FFH, unless it occurs in association with maternal diabetes.
2. An orthopedic surgeon should meet with the family to discuss the prognosis for the child.
3. Karyotype should be considered if other anomalies are detected.

Monitoring The severity of the degree of shortening can be predicted by the rate of growth of the femur, so serial ultrasonographic studies are worthwhile for surgical preparation.

Pregnancy Course No specific obstetric complications are associated with FFH.

Pregnancy Termination Issues An intact fetus should be delivered so that the diagnosis can be confirmed. There would be no increased risk for recurrence if FFH is the only finding.

Delivery There should be no perinatal complications associated with FFH that would require delivery in a tertiary center.

Neonatology

Resuscitation No specific resuscitation measures are required.

Transport Referral in the immediate neonatal period is not necessary unless there are associated malformations requiring evaluation and management.

Testing and Confirmation   The diagnostic evaluation should include careful physical examination, skeletal radiographs, and pediatric orthopedic consultation. These may be obtained through an outpatient referral.

Surgery

Preoperative Assessment   The predicted leg length discrepancy is estimated by measuring the length of the long and short legs following birth and expressing the difference as a percentage of the longer. The percentage of shortening tends to remain constant, whereas the absolute discrepancy increases with age. Radiographs define both length and angular deformities. Next, determine the stability of the hip and knee and look for contractures.

Operative Indications   All children with this diagnosis will require some form of surgery. Problems to be addressed may include the following: femoral shortening, tibial shortening, unstable knee, varus hip, acetabular insufficiency, and external rotation deformity. Usually the necessary corrective surgeries are staged over a series of years. The most important decision to make is whether to lengthen or to amputate. Traditional thinking recommends amputation and prosthetic rehabilitation. The indications for leg lengthening are evolving, but the tendency is to recommend lengthening for predicted discrepancies of up to 20 cm and even more. For mild cases, epiphysiodesis (growth arrest) of the normal side can easily equalize length.

Types of Procedures   The management controversy for this diagnosis has been reconstruction with lengthening and deformity correction versus Symes amputation with above-knee prosthetic fitting. A modification of amputation has been described in which the joint is removed, and the foot and ankle rotated 180 degrees, thus becoming a "knee" and allowing below-knee prosthetic fitting. Amputations reduce the number of surgeries required. Lengthening requires greater commitment of time and effort.

Surgical lengthening involves application of an external fixator, cutting the short bone, and then gradually distracting the gap, which fills in with regenerated bone. Simultaneous correction of angular and rotational deformities is possible. Since the knee cruciate ligaments are deficient, the external fixator must cross the knee with hinges to prevent joint subluxation. If the hip joint is shallow, a prelengthening pelvic osteotomy is done to stabilize the hip joint. Usually no more than 8 cm of lengthening should be carried out in the femur at any one time. This can be combined with 4 to 6 cm of tibial lengthening. Recently, it has been demonstrated that femoral lengthening can be carried out as early as toddler age.

Surgical Results/Prognosis   The main risk of lengthening is loss of knee motion. An intensive rehabilitation program is necessary. Knee and hip subluxation are additional risks and may be prevented by adhering to certain technical points.

When a hip and knee are present, the results of lengthening are potentially excellent. It is possible, in most children, to equalize the leg length and maintain the function of the knee and hip and restore the patient to a normal gait pattern. Many children receive amputation instead of reconstruction because of the surgeon's lack of experience in lengthening. Both options (amputation and lengthening) should be offered, along with referral to major centers if needed. The cost of lengthenings is initially higher than that of amputation, but when considering lifetime costs for changing prostheses, lengthening is cost-effective. Amputation surgery is quite reliable and has withstood the test of time. Long-term outcome studies are needed to determine the relative place of amputation versus lengthening.

REFERENCES

Burn J, Winter RM, Baraitser M, et al: The femoral hypoplasia—Unusual facies syndrome. J Med Genet 1984;21:331–340.

Camera G, Dodero D, Parodi M, et al: Antenatal ultrasonographic diagnosis of a proximal femoral focal deficiency. J Clin Ultrasound 1993;21:475–479.

Florio I, Wisser J, Huch R, Huch A: Prenatal ultrasound diagnosis of a femur-fibula-ulna complex during the first half of pregnancy. Fetal Diagn Ther 1999;14:310–312.

Goncalves LF, De Luca GR, Vitorello DA, et al: Prenatal diagnosis of bilateral proximal femoral hypoplasia. Ultrasound Obstet Gynecol 1996;8:127–130.

Jeanty P, Kleinman G: Proximal femoral focal deficiency. J Ultrasound Med 1989;8:639–642.

Sabharwal S, Paley D, Bhave A, Herzenberg JE: Growth patterns after lengthening of congenitally short lower limbs in young children. J Pediatr Orthop 2000;20(2):137–145.

Urban JE, Ramus RM, Stannard MW, Rogers BB: Autopsy, radiographic and prenatal ultrasonographic examination of a stillborn fetus with femoral facial syndrome. Am J Med Genet 1997;71:76–79.

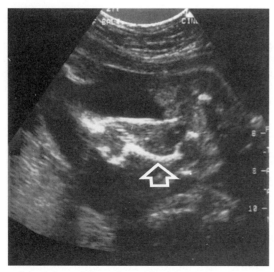

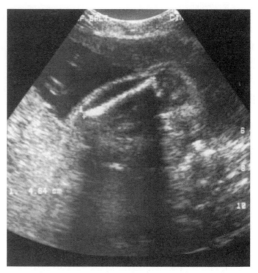

Proximal focal femoral hypoplasia. The left femur is markedly short-ened and bowed. In this example, the femoral head (*arrow*) is present. All other bones were of normal length and appearance.

Normal right femur in the same patient.

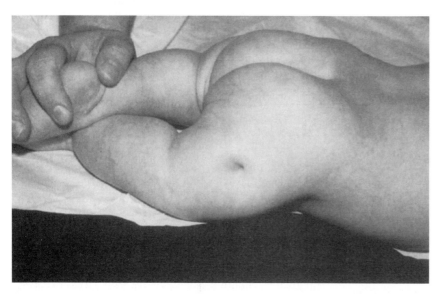

Newborn with focal femoral hypoplasia associated with maternal diabetes. Note skin dimple that overlies bent right femur.

8.9 Jeune's Thoracic Dystropy (Asphyxiating Thoracic Dystrophy)

Epidemiology/Genetics

Definition Autosomal recessive skeletal dysplasia with very narrow thorax, pulmonary hypoplasia, short limbs, renal dysplasia, and high lethality.

Epidemiology The genetic abnormality is unknown and there is phenotypic overlap with the short-rib polydactyly syndromes and the Ellis-van Creveld syndrome. Ribs are short and horizontal with irregular costochondral junctions, and the iliac wings are hypoplastic and appear square. Renal dysplasia with proteinuria and renal insufficiency may occur in survivors. Polydactyly may be present in some cases, and antenatal sonographic differentiation from other lethal skeletal dysplasias is difficult.

Inheritance Patterns Autosomal recessive with a 25% recurrence risk for future pregnancies. The gene has not yet been localized.

Teratogens None known.

Differential Diagnosis Other skeletal dysplasias such as the short-rib polydactyly, thanatophoric dysplasia, and Ellis-van Creveld syndromes.

Prognosis Most infants do not survive the neonatal period because of pulmonary hypoplasia and pneumonia. Neonatal survivors usually have improved growth of the thorax with only moderate short stature. Renal insufficiency and failure is a serious complication in survivors, with hepatic failure also possible but less likely. Retinal degeneration has been described in some surviving patients.

Sonography

FINDINGS

1. **Fetus:**
   a. Increased nuchal translucency at 14 weeks.
   b. The chest is very small with an abnormal thoracic/abdominal ratio and very short ribs. The heart occupies most of the chest and may show decreased contractility, pericardial fluid, and leftward axis deviation.
   c. Limbs are of normal length or, more often, mildly shortened with mild bowing. The femur and humerus are more likely to be shortened than other long bones.
   d. Small cysts may be seen in the kidneys.
2. **Measurement Data:** The limbs are often mildly shortened.

3. **Amniotic Fluid:** Polyhydramnios is usual due to esophageal compression.
4. **Placenta:** Normal
5. **When Detectable:** The syndrome has been detected at 14 weeks' gestation by the nuchal thickening. By 17 weeks the small chest size is obvious and the long bone length is usally below the 10th percentile.

Pitfalls The syndrome may be overlooked because the limb lengths are only mildly shortened and the important findings are in the chest, which is not measured in the standard obstetric ultrasonographic series.

Differential Diagnosis

1. Ellis-van Creveld syndrome—Polydactyly will be present and all limbs will be very short.
2. Majewski syndrome—There will be polydactyly with syndactyly and very short limbs.

Where Else to Look Renal dysplasia with cysts and pancreatic cysts have been reported at pathologic examination on autopsy cases.

Pregnancy Management

Investigations and Consultations Required Consultation with a pediatric dysmorphologist may be beneficial to the family, to discuss the natural history of those infants who survive.

Fetal Intervention Not applicable in this disorder.

Monitoring For those couples choosing to continue a pregnancy, monthly assessment is appropriate to detect the onset of polyhydramnios.

Pregnancy Course No changes are expected unless there is development of polyhydramnios, which may result in preterm labor. Polyhydramnios likely represents cases with significantly small chest size and therefore a higher likelihood of severe pulmonary hypoplasia.

Pregnancy Termination Issues In the first case in a family, it may be difficult to make a precise diagnosis by ultrasonography. Therefore, delivery of an intact fetus and skeletal radiographs may be necessary to establish a precise diagnosis.

Delivery In the absence of polyhydramnios, standard obstetric practice should be followed. Cases in which a significantly small chest is found by ultrasonography and those associated with polyhydramnios likely represent the lethal form of the disorder. Consultation with the family and the neonatologist is appropriate to develop a plan for intrapartum and immediate neonatal management.

Neonatology

Resuscitation A full discussion with the parents regarding the potential for an early death from respiratory failure, severe renal dysfunction with progressive renal failure, and multiple surgical procedures to alleviate the restriction of lung volume is essential. Although the prognosis for early demise is substantial in the neonatal period, successful surgical reconstruction has been reported. The initiation of ventilatory support is indicated to allow confirmation of the diagnosis and evaluation for surgical correction. A decision for limited or non-support of the infant following birth is also an option.

Transport Transfer by experienced neonatal transport personnel to a tertiary center with multiple pediatric medical and surgical subspecialists and a neonatal intensive care unit should be arranged if delivery at such a center is not feasible.

Testing and Confirmation Diagnostic imaging with conventional radiography, ultrasonogaphy, and magnetic resonance imaging will confirm the typical skeletal abnormalities and the coexistence of renal and liver (biliary) dysplasias.

Nursery Management Maintenance of adequate ventilatory gas exchange and nutritional support are essential from birth, while the delineation of the skeletal and other organ system abnormalities is completed. The timing of the initial surgical procedure to relieve the chest wall constriction is not well established. It would seem prudent to avoid prolonged ventilatory support and thus to decrease the potential of lung injury prior to surgery, if such is planned.

REFERENCES

Barnes ND, Hull D, Milner AD: Chest reconstruction in thoracic dystrophy. Arch Dis Child 1971;46:833.

Denhollander NS, Robben SGF, Hoggeboom AJM, et al: Early prenatal sonographic diagnosis and follow-up of Jeune syndrome. Ultrasound Obstet Gynecol 2001;18:378–383.

Elejalde BR, de Elejalde MM, Pansch D: Prenatal diagnosis of Jeune syndrome. Am J Med Genet 1985;21:433.

Herdman RC, Langer LO: Thoracic asphyxiant dystrophy and renal disease. Am J Dis Child 1968;116:192.

Hudgins L, Rosengren S, Treem W, Hyams J: Early cirrhosis in survivors with Jeune thoracic dystrophy.

Jeune M, Beraud C, Carron R: Dystrophie thoracique asphyxiante de caractere familial. Arch Francais de Pediatr 1955;12:886.

Jeune M, Carron R, Beraud C: Polycondrodystrophy avec biocage thoracic d'evolution fatal. Pediatrie 1954;9:390.

Sharoni EE, Chorev G, Dagan O, Vidne BA: Chest reconstruction in asphyxiating thoracic dystrophy. J Pediatr Surg 1998;33:1578.

Sharony R, Browne C, Lachman RS, Rimoin DL: Prenatal diagnosis of the skeletal dysplasias. Am J Gynecol 1993;169:668.

Todd DW, Tinguely SJ, Norberg WJ: Thoracic expansion technique for Jeune's asphyxiating thoracic dystrophy. J Pediatr Surg 1986;21:161.

Tongsong T, Chanprapaph P, Thongpadungroj T: Prenatal sonographic findings associated with asphyxiating thoracic dystrophy (Jeune syndrome). J Ultrasound Med 1999;18:573.

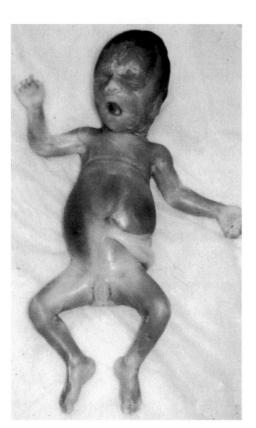

A 22-week fetus with Jeune syndrome. Note narrow chest.

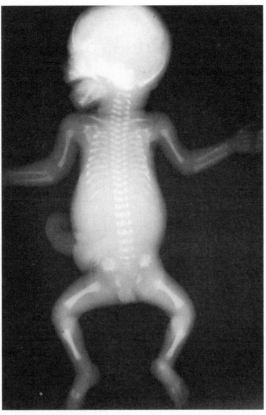

Radiograph of 22-week fetus with Jeune syndrome. Note short horizontal ribs.

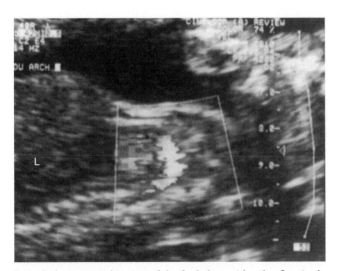

Sagittal ultrasonographic view of the fetal chest with color flow in the aortic arch. Note small chest size and bell-shaped abdomen.

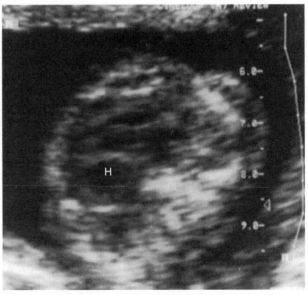

Transverse sonographic view of fetal chest. The heart (H) appears unduly large because the chest is so small.

8.10 Klippel-Trenaunay-Weber (KTW) Syndrome

Epidemiology/Genetics

Definition Klippel-Trenaunay-Weber syndrome is the association of various cutaneous hemangiomas, vascular abnormalities, and hemihypertrophy and/or segmental overgrowth.

Epidemiology Rare (M1:F1).

Embryology The pathogenesis of this disorder is unknown but may be due to abnormalities in the regulation of local vascular and other growth factors. The location of the cutaneous hemangiomas, vascular abnormalities, and overgrowth may not correspond and makes simple vascular explanations for the overgrowth unlikely.

Inheritance Patterns Sporadic.

Teratogens None known.

Prognosis Prognosis depends on the type and extent of involvement.

Sonography

FINDINGS

1. **Fetus:** One or more areas of localized enlargement of one or more limbs. There may be focal enlargement of a portion of the torso. Color flow Doppler sonography will demonstrate greatly increased arterial flow in the involved area. It is important to determine whether the vascular malformation extends from a limb to the trunk. This makes the prognosis much worse, since an amputation will not remove the complete malformation. When there is a large arteriovenous shunt, there may be cardiomegaly and other findings of hydrops.
2. **Amniotic Fluid:** Normal.
3. **Placenta:** Normal unless there is hydrops.
4. **Measurement Data:** Measurement data will be enlarged locally by the abnormal trunk and limb masses.
5. **When Detectable:** At about 16 weeks.

Pitfalls A high-quality ultrasonographic system is required to see the abnormal blood flow.

Differential Diagnosis

1. Amniotic band syndrome—Although there may be localized limb enlargement, no increased blood flow will be seen.
2. Localized vascular malformation such as hemangio-lymphangioma—The lesion will show arterial flow but will be limited to one area. There is no limb hypertrophy.
3. Hemangioma—A single localized mass will be present, which will not show vascular flow with color flow Doppler sonography.
4. Proteus syndrome—Hemihypertrophy with subcutaneous hemangioma.
5. Tumor such as rhabdomyosarcoma—A solid mass with echogenic areas will be present.

Where Else to Look Look for evidence of hydrops.

Pregnancy Management

Investigations and Consultations Required

1. Although the yield will be low, chromosomal analysis should be considered, especially if other abnormalities are noted.
2. Fetal echocardiography should be performed to establish baseline parameters.
3. Magnetic resonance imaging may be considered if it is uncertain whether there is increased vascularity.
4. Consultations should be obtained with neonatology and pediatric surgery practitioners to discuss neonatal management with the family.

Fetal Intervention Theoretically, the administration of digoxin or similar medication to the mother and subsequent placental transfer may have some benefit in cases with high output cardiac failure. At 32 weeks' gestation or greater, early delivery and ex utero management are preferable.

Monitoring The pregnancy should be monitored by serial sonographic examinations to detect signs of fetal hydrops. Fetal echocardiography may be helpful in the early detection of cardiac decompensation. The high risk of pregnancy complications requires that prenatal care be under the direction of a perinatologist.

Pregnancy Course Nonimmune fetal hydrops and/or polyhydramnios may complicate pregnancy management.

Pregnancy Termination Issues Pregnancy termination should be by a nondestructive procedure, and an autopsy should be performed in a center with expertise in fetal pathology.

Delivery Delivery should be in a tertiary center because of the significant risk of obstetric and neonatal complications. The size and location of the mass may require cesarean section.

Neonatology

Resuscitation   No specific resuscitation measures are required, unless there is evidence of fetal cardiac decompensation and/or hydrops fetalis. See Chapter 13.2 for details of management.

Transport   Referral in the immediate neonatal period for diagnostic evaluation, to exclude other causes, is indicated only for marked asymmetry of the extremities or for hydrops.

Testing and Confirmation   Findings on physical examination after birth easily confirm the diagnosis.

Nursery Management   In the absence of congestive heart failure and/or hydrops fetalis, routine newborn care is appropriate. Lymphatic obstruction has also been described. Surgical intervention has been delayed, usually to early childhood or later in adulthood.

Surgery

Preoperative Assessment   Diagnostic evaluation of the vascularity of the involved extremity with noninvasive imaging techniques such as ultrasonography and magnetic resonance imaging may demonstrate either venous obstruction or an arteriovenous malformation. Extremity bone radiographs of the involved and contralateral limbs are important for future consideration in therapy for bony hypertrophy.

Operative Indications   Therapy depends on the degree of vascular involvement and bony hypertrophy. The vascular component is frequently associated with lymphatic obstruction and edema. Angiomatosis with rapidly proliferating skin and subcutaneous lesions may also be present.

Types of Procedures   Compression treatment is effective if it is started early and strict patient compliance is achieved. Intermittent pneumatic compression can be applied, particularly at night. The technique is improved with associated use of static compression (Jobst) garments. This therapy is particularly difficult in infants and growing children because the garments are warm, require frequent changes in size, and, if not used properly, can pro-

duce local irritation over the damaged skin. Local vascular procedures to correct atrioventricular fistulae and varicose veins result in marginal success. Intermittent bouts of cellulitis require antibiotic therapy, but prophylactic antibiotics are not routinely used. Severe limb hypertrophy can require epiphysiodesis, and functional impairment may require major limb procedures and/or amputations.

Surgical Results/Prognosis   These children may be severely handicapped both functionally and cosmetically. This lesion is not usually associated with malignant degeneration or secondary tumors.

REFERENCES

Baskerville PA, Ackroyd JS, Lea Thomas M, Browse NL: The Klippel-Trenaunay syndrome: Clinical, radiological and haemodynamic features and management. Br J Surg 1985;72:232–236.

Drose JA, Thickman D, Wiggins J, Haverkamp AB: Fetal echocardiographic findings in the Klippel-Trenaunay-Weber syndrome. J Ultrasound Med 1991;10:525–527.

Edgerton MT: The treatment of hemangiomas with special reference to the role of steroid therapy. Ann Surg 1976;183:517–532.

Martin WL, Ismail KMK, Brace V: Klippel-Trenaunay-Weber (KTW) syndrome: The use of in utero magnetic resonance imaging (MRI). Prenat Diagn 2001;21:311–313.

McCullough CJ, Kenwright S: The prognosis in congenital lower limb hypertrophy. Acta Orthop Scand 1979;50:307–313.

Meholic AJ, Freimanis AK, Stucka J, LoPiccolo ML: Sonographic in utero diagnosis of Klippel-Trenaunay-Weber syndrome. J Ultrasound Med 1991;10:111–114.

Meiner A, Faber R, Horn LC, et al: Prenatal detection of a giant bilateral thoracic vascular lesion: Prognostic evaluation and genetic aspects. Prenat Diagn 1999;19:583–586.

Mor Z, Schreyer P, Wainraub Z, et al: Nonimmune hydrops fetalis associated with angioosteohypertrophy (Klippel-Trenaunay) syndrome. Am J Obstet Gynecol 1988;159:1185–1186.

Paladini D, Lamberti A, Teodoro A, et al: Prenatal diagnosis and hemodynamic evaluation of Klippel-Trenaunay-Weber syndrome. Ultrasound Obstet Gynecol 1998;12:215–217.

Senoh D, Hanaoka U, Tanaka Y: Antenatal ultrasonographic features of fetal giant hemangiolymphangioma. Ultrasound Obstet Gynecol 2001;17:252–254.

Servelle M: Klippel and Trenaunay's syndrome: 768 operated cases. Ann Surg 1985;201:365–373.

Stringel G, Dastous J: Klippel-Trenaunay syndrome and other cases of lower limb hypertrophy: Pediatric surgical implications. J Pediatr Surg 1987;22:645–650.

Viljoen D, Saxe N, Pearn J, Beighton P: The cutaneous manifestations of the Klippel-Trenaunay-Weber syndrome. Clin Exp Dermatol 1987;12:12–17.

Warhit JM, Goldman MA, Sachs L, et al: Klippel-Trenaunay-Weber syndrome: Appearance in utero. J Ultrasound Med 1983;2:515–518.

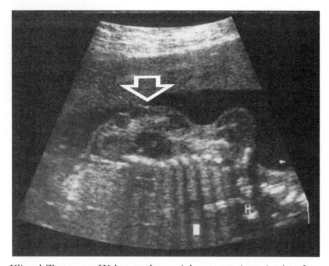

Klippel-Trenaunay-Weber syndrome A large mass (*arrow*) arises from the chest wall. The mass was pulsatile and involved the shoulder joint.

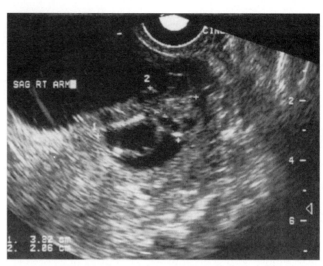

There was a second mass involving the right hand (between x's). The arm and hand were swollen and a large soft tissue mass was present.

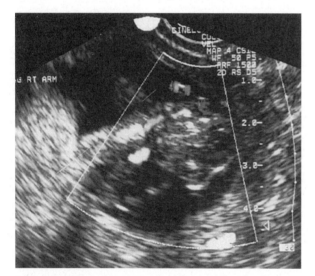

Color flow Doppler image of the same hand. The highly echogenic areas (within box) represent blood flow related to the enlarged, abnormal vasculature of this a-v malformation.

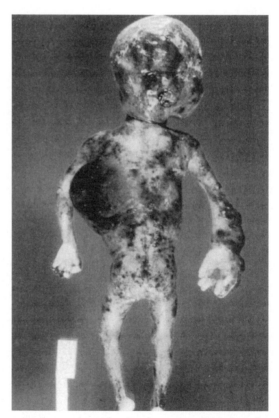

Post-termination specimen showing the masses arising from the trunk and right hand.

8.11 Limb-Body Wall Complex (Body Stalk Complex, Cyllosoma)

Epidemiology/Genetics

Definition   Limb-body wall complex is generally defined as consisting of two of the three following abnormalities: (1) myelomeningocele and/or caudal regression; (2) thoraco- and/or abdominoschisis; and (3) limb defects.

Epidemiology   Rare.

Embryology   At least two mechanisms exist. Limb-body wall complex is most frequently thought to arise as a result of early amnion disruptions and usually shows other features of amniotic band disruptions. In other cases, the amniotic band disruption is thought to be due to early embryonic maldevelopment.

Inheritance Patterns   Sporadic.

Teratogens   None known.

Prognosis   If all components of the syndrome are present, the condition is lethal. Milder forms of amniotic band syndrome, with gastroschisis and absent limb, for example, may be grouped with limb-body wall complex but have a better prognosis.

Sonography

FINDINGS

1. **Fetus:** A complex array of sonographic findings is seen:
   a. One or more limbs, or segments of limbs, are missing. Club feet may be present.
   b. Intestines, liver, and even the bladder extend outside of the abdominal wall and may be attached to the placenta. Diaphragmatic absence and bowel atresia usually occur.
   c. A short, curved spine with sacral regression is common.
   d. Myelomeningocele is frequent, with secondary Arnold-Chiari malformation and hydrocephalus. Encephalocele may occur.
   e. Ectopia cordis or other cardiac anomalies may be present.
   f. Facial clefts may be present.
   g. Hydronephrosis due to bladder positional changes may be seen.
2. **Amniotic Fluid:** There is often oligohydramnios.
3. **Placenta:** The placenta may be attached to the fetus. A single umbilical artery is common. The umbilical cord is usually short and is adherent to placental membranes. Occasionally, amniotic membrane remnants are visible.
4. **Measurement Data:** Normal where measurable, but most structures are affected by the process.

5. **When Detectable:** 13 to 14 weeks.

Pitfalls   Limited fluid may make limb visualization difficult.

Differential Diagnosis

1. The body stalk anomaly is a variant of the same condition in which the placenta is attached to the trunk of the fetus, and similar deformities occur.
2. Cloacal exstrophy—A large omphalocele, distorted spine, club feet, and meningomyelocele are features of cloacal exstrophy, however, without partial or complete loss of an extremity. An absent bladder is a feature of cloacal exstrophy not seen with limb-body wall complex (see Chapter 4.3).

Where Else to Look   The entire fetus needs to be scanned in detail, since anomalies can affect any organ.

Pregnancy Management

Investigations and Consultations Required   The pattern and severity of the malformations are inconsistent with the usual chromosomal abnormalities, but chromosomal studies should be considered to exclude unbalanced chromosome rearrangements that may have implications for subsequent pregnancies. If the condition does not appear lethal, consultation with a pediatric surgeon may be helpful for discussion with the parents regarding the complications of the malformations.

Monitoring   The classic form of limb-body wall complex is lethal, and prenatal care should focus on maternal issues. Fetal assessment is not appropriate.

Pregnancy Course   No specific obstetric complications should be expected.

Pregnancy Termination Issues   To establish a precise diagnosis, a termination technique should be used that allows an intact fetus to be delivered.

Delivery   A diagnosis of limb-body wall complex should be an indication for vaginal delivery only, without fetal monitoring.

Neonatology

Resuscitation   Resuscitation is not indicated, because this anomaly, as reported in the literature, is lethal.

Transport   Not indicated unless the fetus survives delivery and the diagnosis is uncertain.

Testing and Confirmation   Careful physical examination and sonography are usually all that are required to determine the extent of organ involvement.

Nursery Management   Supportive care is appropriate until the diagnosis is confirmed and time has been allowed for parental adaptation to the lethal prognosis.

REFERENCES

Lockwood CJ, Scioscia AL, Hobbins JC: Congenital absence of the umbilical cord resulting from maldevelopment of embryonic body folding. Am J Obstet Gynecol 1986;155:1049–1051.

Martinez-Frias ML, Bermejo E, Rodriguez-Pinilla E: Body stalk defects, body wall defects, amniotic bands with and without body wall defects and gastroschisis. Comp Epidemiol Am J Med Genet 2000;92:13–18.

Moerman P, Fryns J-P, Vanderberghe K, Lauweryns JM: Constrictive amniotic bands, amniotic adhesions, and limb-body wall complex: Discrete disruption sequences with pathogenetic overlap. Am J Med Genet 1992;42:470–479.

Negishi H, Yaegishi M, Kato EH, et al: Prenatal diagnosis of limb-body wall complex. J Reprod Med 1998;43:659–664.

Patten RM, Van Allen M, Mack LA, et al: Limb-body wall complex: In utero sonographic diagnosis of a complicated fetal malformation. Am J Roentgenol 1986;146:1019–1024.

Russo R, D'Armiento M, Angrisani P, Vecchione R: Limb body wall complex: A critical review and a nosological proposal. Am J Med Genet 1993;47:893–900.

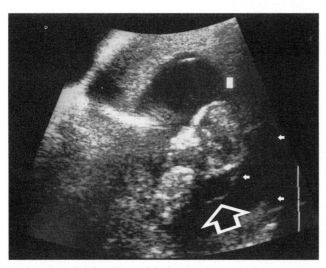

Limb-body wall defect. View of the head and upper body. An amniotic band is visible attached to the head (*arrow*).

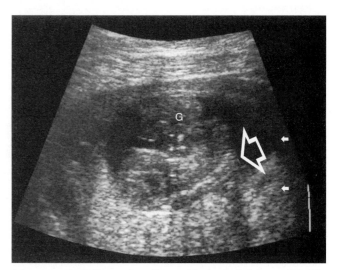

A large mass with liver and gut lies outside the fetal abdomen (G). The spine (*arrow*) is short owing to caudal regression.

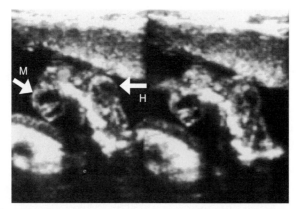

View of scoliotic shortened spine with abnormal vertebra in a fetus with limb-body wall syndrome. There is a myelomeningocele (M) and ectopia cordis (H).

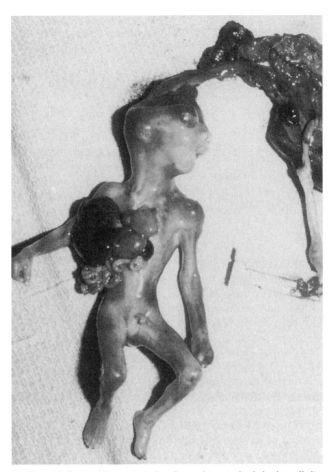

An 18-week fetus with amniotic bands resulting in limb-body wall disruption. Extruded visceral contents included heart, liver, and gastrointestinal tract components.

A 24-week fetus with limb-body wall disruption showing right clubbed foot and massive evisceration.

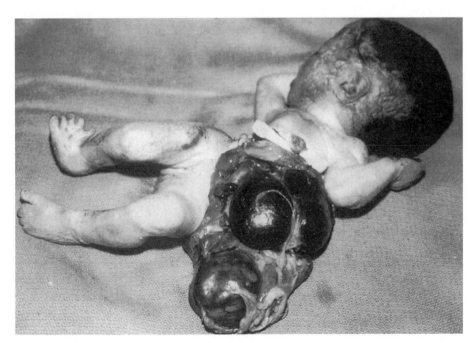

8.12 Multiple Pterygium Syndrome

Epidemiology/Genetics

Definition The multiple pterygium syndromes are a heterogeneous group of disorders characterized by pterygia or webbing across the neck and other joints.

Epidemiology Rare (M1:F1).

Embryology Pterygia, or webs that occur across joint spaces, are thought to be the result of limited in utero movement. More than 25 multiple malformation syndromes have been described with pterygia and have been divided into lethal and nonlethal forms. The lethal forms generally have growth retardation, cystic hygroma, and/or fetal hydrops.

Inheritance Patterns Most nonlethal cases are sporadic, whereas lethal cases usually show autosomal recessive inheritance. Rare X-linked recessive families have been reported. Because of the rapid progress in mapping of genes and subsequent development of genetic testing, consultation with a medical geneticist or genetic counselor to determine the availability of clinical genetic testing for this disorder (or disorders) is advised.

Teratogens None.

Prognosis Life span and intellectual development in nonlethal cases is generally normal. Ambulation and function are dependent on the severity of the pterygia and success of orthopedic correction.

Sonography

FINDINGS

1. **Fetus:**
   a. Persistent, severely flexed arms and flexed hips with extended, crossed legs. Cutaneous webs, known as pterygia, may be visible at the elbow and knee joints. Fetal movement is almost absent.
   b. Nuchal thickening is present at 10 to 14 weeks' gestation. Hydrops may occur.
   c. Club feet may be present and the hands are also in a clubbed position. Syndactyly of the second to fourth fingers gives the hands an odd shape.
   d. Micrognathia and cleft palate may be present.
   e. Hypertelorism with corneal opacities may be seen.
   f. The stomach may not be seen because of defective swallowing.
   g. The long bones are bowed.
   h. Hydronephrosis, microcephaly, cardiac defects, and ventriculomegaly are occasional findings.

2. **Amniotic Fluid:** Polyhydramnios is often present.
3. **Placenta:** Normal unless there is hydrops.
4. **Measurement Data:** Intrauterine growth retardation may be present.
5. **When Detectable:** At 11 to 14 weeks by the presence of nuchal edema and from abnormal fixed limb position at about 16 weeks.

Pitfalls The condition can be confused with a normal fetus that holds its limbs in a flexed position owing to a confined space, as with oligohydramnios.

Differential Diagnosis

1. Arthrogryposis—A similar limb position is assumed, along with absent fetal movement, but pterygia are absent (see Chapter 8.4).
2. Caudal regression syndrome—Although the limbs are flexed and contracted, the arms are unaffected (see Chapter 2.5).
3. Other syndromes with nuchal translucency and fixed position such as trisomy 18 and Pena-Shokeir syndrome.

Where Else to Look This is a generalized syndrome, so look throughout the body.

Pregnancy Management

Investigations and Consultations Required Chromosomal studies should be done, as trisomy 18 may present with a similar clinical picture on rare occasions. Fetal echocardiography should be performed, as cardiac hypoplasia (generalized) is a frequent feature.

Monitoring Standard obstetric care without fetal assessment is appropriate. No attempt to stop preterm labor should be made.

Pregnancy Course Polyhydramnios is a common complication and may be severe, resulting in preterm labor.

Pregnancy Termination Issues Delivery of an intact fetus for careful assessment of external features and neuropathologic evaluation is essential to establish a precise diagnosis.

Delivery The site of delivery should be one where the staff is comfortable with a noninterventional approach to labor management and newborn resuscitation. Fetal monitoring during labor is not appropriate.

Neonatology

Resuscitation If a lethal variant is suspected from prenatal diagnosis, a decision for nonintervention at delivery is appropriate with concurrence of the family. There may be difficulty in establishing a reliable airway if jaw mobility is affected.

Transport Referral to a tertiary perinatal center in the immediate neonatal period is appropriate for diagnostic evaluation and confirmation of the prognosis. Mechanical respiratory support during transport may be needed for infants with the lethal variant.

Testing and Confirmation The diagnostic evaluation should include careful physical examination, genetic consultation, and skeletal radiographs.

Nursery Management Mechanical life support, to allow time for diagnostic evaluation and parental adaptation, is appropriate. Deaths in the lethal variant are from respiratory failure secondary to pulmonary hypoplasia, which implies that long-term mechanical ventilation is unlikely to be beneficial.

The long-term treatment goal for an infant without respiratory failure is to establish joint mobility with physical therapy and soft tissue release surgery.

Surgery

Preoperative Assessment Determine the degree of contracture. Splinting and serial casting are indicated in young infants.

Operative Indications Knee flexion contracture greater than 25 degrees, elbow flexion contracture greater than 45 degrees, and equinus contracture of the foot are all indications for surgery.

Types of Procedures Osteotomies to extend the bones give only temporary correction, as the flexion recurs with bone remodeling.

Open resection of contracted fascia, Z-plasty of the skin, and joint releases are all required to straighten a limb affected by pterygium. Gradual distraction with an Ilizarov device is useful, but recurrence is common.

REFERENCES

Anthony J, Mascarenhas L, O'Brien J, et al: Lethal multiple pterygium syndrome—The importance of fetal posture in mid-trimester diagnosis by ultrasound: Discussion and case report. Ultrasound Obstet Gynecol 1993;3:212–216.

Baty B, Cubberley D, Morris C, Carey J: Prenatal diagnosis of distal arthrogryposis. Am J Med Genet 1988;29:501–510.

de Die-Smulders CEM, Vonsee HJ, Zandvoort JA, Fryns JP: The lethal multiple pterygium syndrome: Prenatal ultrasonographic and postmortem findings: A case report. Eur J Obstet Gynecol Reprod Biol 1990;35:283–289.

Froster UG, Stallmach T, Wisser J, et al: Lethal multiple pterygium syndrome: Suggestion for a consistent pathological workup and review of reported cases. Am J Med Genet 1997;68:82–85.

Hall JG, Reed SD, Rosenbaum KN, et al: Limb pterygium syndromes: A review and report of eleven patients. Am J Med Genet 1982;12:377–409.

Lockwood CL, Irons M, Troiani J, et al: The prenatal sonographic diagnosis of lethal multiple pterygium syndrome: A heritable cause of recurrent abortions. Am J Obstet Gynecol 1988;159:474–476.

Meizner I, Hershkovit R, Carmi R, Katz M: Prenatal ultrasound diagnosis of a rare occurrence of lethal multiple pterygium syndrome in two siblings. Ultrasound Obstet Gynecol 1993;3:432–436.

Meyer-Cohen J, Dillon A, Pai GS, Conradi S: Lethal multiple pterygium syndrome in four male fetuses in a family: Evidence for an X-linked recessive subtype? Am J Med Genet 1999;82:97–99.

Moerman P, Fryns JP, Cornelis A, et al: Pathogenesis of the lethal multiple pterygium syndrome. Am J Med Genet 1990;35:415–421.

Sciarrone A, Verdiglione P, Botta G, et al: Prenatal diagnosis of lethal multiple pterygium syndrome in mid-pregnancy. Ultrasound Obstet Gynecol 1998;12:218–219.

Shenker L, Reed K, Anderson C, et al: Syndrome of camptodactyly, ankyloses, facial anomalies, and pulmonary hypoplasia (Pena-Shokeir syndrome): Obstetric and ultrasound aspects. Am J Obstet Gynecol 1985;152:303–307.

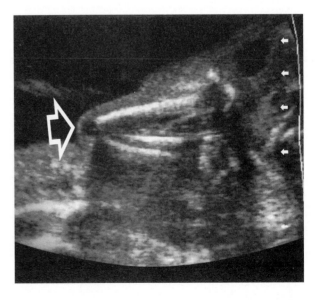

An 18-week fetus with multiple pterygian syndrome. View of the arm. The *arrow* shows the elbow. The proximal and distal portions of the arm are close together because the arm was in a constantly severely flexed position. Note the pterygium between the two limbs.

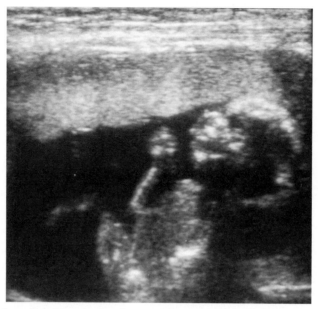

Same fetus. Note the flexed arm and unusual profile. There was a cleft lip present.

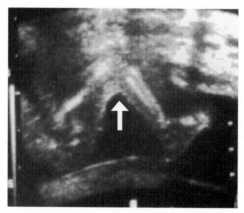

Flexed leg of the same fetus with multiple pterygian syndrome. The pterygium is visible behind the knee (*arrow*).

8.13 Osteogenesis Imperfecta

Epidemiology/Genetics

Definition Osteogenesis imperfecta is a heterogeneous group of brittle bone diseases characterized by an excessive tendency to antenatal and/or postnatal fractures.

Epidemiology An Australian study found an incidence of 1.6 to 3.5 in 100,000 live births (M1:F1).

Embryology Most types of osteogenesis imperfecta are due to type I collagen abnormalities and exhibit a highly variable phenotype. The Sillence classification is frequently used to divide these disorders into phenotypic groups. Type I is the classic form of osteogenesis imperfecta, with moderate fractures, blue sclera, variable degrees of hearing loss, and dentinogenesis imperfecta; type II is a severe neonatal lethal form with multiple antenatal fractures; type III is a progressively deforming disorder with severe disability by middle age; and type IV is a variable phenotype with normal sclerae.

Inheritance Patterns Most families demonstrate autosomal dominant inheritance. In the lethal forms, the mutations are new dominant mutations, but the presence of germ-line mosaicism results in recurrence risks for the family that range from approximately 2% if there is one affected child to 28% if there are two previously affected children.

Teratogens None.

Screening If the precise abnormality in a particular family is known, biochemical analysis of type I collagen or another biochemical or DNA marker may be studied on chorionic villus samples or amniocytes. Because some families do not have type I collagen defects, linkage studies cannot be routinely done. Collagen testing can take up to 30 days and may be most useful for post-delivery diagnosis. Gonadal mosaicism for type I collagen mutations have been found in phenotypically normal parents, complicating genetic counseling.

Prognosis Highly variable, depending on clinical type. Infants with type II disease are born with multiple fractures and most often die in the neonatal period from respiratory compromise. In the milder types I and IV, fractures may not occur until later in life.

Sonography

FINDINGS

1. **Fetus:**
   a. Types I and IV—There are one or two fractures with normal or mildly shortened bones. Bone length of limbs, on each side, is not equal. Callus formation is visible, the bone is angulated, there is bowing, or the bone has an irregular contour. There may be no findings until after birth.
   b. Type II—Most in utero cases fall in this group. There is generalized bony deossification with many rib deformities. The head is compressible with too easily seen intracranial structures and absence of skull reverberations. The bones are variably shortened with callus and bone angulation.
   c. Lethal form of type II—Intracranial structures are too well seen with little or no skull ossification. All bones are extremely short, with marked fragmentation. There is a very small chest. The long bones are "transparent," so the back wall of the long bone is visible. The ribs have a concave appearance.
   d. Type III—Multiple fractures are detected in the second trimester. The findings are less severe than with type II.
2. **Amniotic Fluid:** Normal or increased fluid.
3. **Placenta:** Normal placenta.
4. **Measurement Data:** Variably shortened long bones. Normal head and abdomen size.
5. **When Detectable:** Can be detected at 13 or 14 weeks.

Pitfalls Variable short limb length may be the only clue to the more mild form.

Differential Diagnosis

1. Achondrogenesis—Leg shortening and a small chest may be the predominant findings, so the process may be mistaken for achondrogenesis, since bones are echopenic in achondrogenesis (see Chapter 8.1).
2. Campomelic dwarfism—Tibial and femoral bowing may be the predominant features (the legs are usually more affected than the arms in osteogenesis imperfecta), so campomelic dwarfism may be diagnosed (see Chapter 8.5).
3. Hypophosphatasia—Although the long bones are hypoechoic, no fractures are seen. Long bones tend to be thin or absent and considerably shortened. The vertebrae and cranium are deossified.
4. Cleidocranial dysostosis—The skull is deossified, but long bones are normal. The clavicles are absent or hypoplastic.

Where Else to Look Look at the eyes for cataract.

Pregnancy Management

Investigations and Consultations Required

1. Many of the skeletal dysplasias, but not osteogenesis imperfecta, are associated with congenital heart dis-

ease. Therefore, a fetal echocardiogram should be done.

2. Fetal radiographs may be helpful in establishing a more precise diagnosis.
3. A neonatologist should be consulted to plan perinatal management, if a lethal dwarfism is expected.

Monitoring   No obstetric intervention should be performed for the fetus with osteogenesis imperfecta type II. Other types are not lethal; they are associated with a less severe deformity, and standard obstetric management should be employed.

Pregnancy Course   Polyhydramnios may occur but, if present, is usually mild.

Pregnancy Termination Issues   An intact fetus must be delivered for a complete postmortem evaluation, including radiologic, morphologic, biochemical, and molecular studies. There is a special need for establishing cultured cell lines to determine the exact molecular or biochemical defect so that early diagnosis will be possible in future pregnancies.

Delivery   For the nonlethal forms of osteogenesis imperfecta, cesarean delivery is theoretically of benefit to decrease the risk of fractures and intracranial hemorrhage. Delivery should occur in a tertiary center.

Neonatology

Resuscitation   Given that the prenatal differentiation between the various types may be difficult, it is appropriate to initiate resuscitative efforts. However, if the prenatal diagnosis of osteogenesis imperfecta type II is definite, a prenatal decision for nonintervention, after discussion with the parents, is appropriate.

Transport   Referral to a tertiary perinatal center for confirmation of the diagnosis is always indicated for a live-born infant with osteogenesis imperfecta. Mechanical ventilatory support may be required during transport. Caution in handling is required to reduce the risk of inadvertent fractures.

Testing and Confirmation   Careful physical examination and skeletal radiographs are helpful in determining classification. Multiple prenatal fractures and blue sclerae at birth strongly suggest osteogenesis imperfecta type II, the ultimately lethal form.

Nursery Management   Assistive devices (plastic shells) may be needed to facilitate handling while protecting the infant from additional fractures.

Long-term ventilatory support is possible but controversial for some infants with osteogenesis imperfecta type II. Survival beyond early childhood has not been reported.

Surgery

Preoperative Assessment   Type II osteogenesis imperfecta patients generally die in early infancy, although we are aware of one child who survived and is ventilator-dependent and wheelchair-bound at the age of 9 years. In general, the severity of the phenotype will determine the level of treatment needed. Radiographs show osteoporosis and healed or healing fractures. Mild cases may be confused with child abuse.

Operative Indications   When children have an osteogenesis imperfecta fracture, they generally heal at a normal rate. The important issue is to prevent progressive bowing deformities from developing in the long bones. The usual treatment for childhood fractures is cast immobilization. More aggressive treatment with internal or external fixation is occasionally indicated to prevent deformity. In severe cases, such as type III, this is often a losing battle, with the patient eventually becoming wheelchair-bound. For more functional patients, bowing deformities represent a mechanical and cosmetic problem.

Corrective osteotomies can help, although the technical nature of these procedures can be difficult in thin, gracile, bowed bones. Scoliosis frequently develops in severe cases and requires operative stabilization with special techniques to accommodate the frail bone. Bracing is not helpful in controlling spinal deformities in osteogenesis imperfecta. However, leg braces can help improve walking ability in selected cases.

Types of Procedures   Acute fractures are usually treated with casts or splints, occasionally with surgery and internal fixation. Established bowing and angular deformities may be treated by corrective osteotomies and internal fixation. Severely bowed bones require the so-called "shish-ka-bob" procedure, in which the bowed bone is cut at multiple levels into small sections and then "skewered" onto a straight intramedullary rod to heal in the corrected alignment. Special telescopic intramedullary nails that elongate during growth are used in young children.

Surgical Results/Prognosis   Ultimate prognosis depends on the severity of the specific phenotype. In general, if fractures appear before walking age, there is a 30% chance that the child will eventually be wheelchair-bound. Nonunion of fractures, while rare in normal children, can be seen in up to 20% of children with osteogenesis imperfecta.

REFERENCES

Andersen PE Jr, Hauge M: Osteogenesis imperfecta: A genetic, radiological, and epidemiological study. Clin Genet 1989;36:250–255.

Chervenak FA, Romero R, Berkowitz RL, et al: Antenatal sonographic findings of osteogenesis imperfecta. Am J Obstet Gynecol 1982;143: 228–230.

Palmer TM, Rouse GA, Song A, DeLange M: Transparent bone and concave ribs: Additional sonographic features of lethal osteogenesis imperfecta. J Diagn Med Sonogr 1998;14:246–250.

Pepin M, Atkinson M, Starman BJ, Byers PH: Strategies and outcomes of prenatal diagnosis for osteogenesis imperfecta: A review of biochemical and molecular studies completed in 129 pregnancies. Prenat Diagn 1997;17:559–570.

Sillence DO: Osteogenesis imperfecta nosology and genetics. Ann N Y Acad Sci 1988;543:1–15.

Sillence DO, Barlow KK, Garber AP, et al: Osteogenesis imperfecta type II: Delineation of the phenotype with reference to genetic heterogeneity. Am J Med Genet 1984;17:407–423.

Stewart PA, Wallerstein R, Moran E, Lee MJ: Early prenatal diagnosis of cleidocranial dysplasia. Ultrasound Obstet Gynecol 2000;15:154–156.

Tongsong T, Pongthsa S: Early prenatal diagnosis of congenital hypophosphatasia. Ultrasound Obstet Gynecol 2000;15:252–255.

Tretter AE, Sanders RC, Meyers CM, et al: Antenatal diagnosis of lethal skeletal dysplasias. Am J Med Genet 1998;75:518–522.

Willing MC, Pruchno CJ, Byers PH: Molecular heterogeneity in osteogenesis imperfecta. Am J Med Genet 1993;45:223–227.

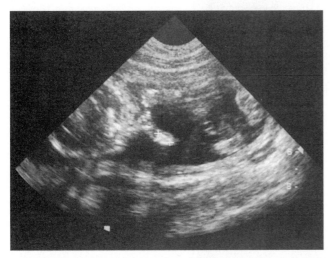

Lethal form of osteogenesis imperfecta. The humerus (between +'s) is extremely short and fractured into several fragments.

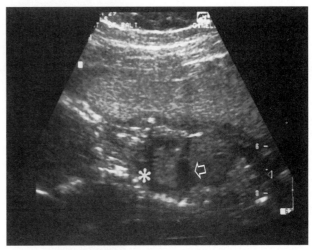

Type III osteogenesis imperfecta. There is a fracture of the midpoint of the tibia (+).

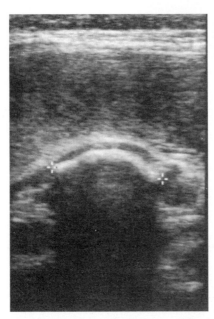

Type II osteogenesis imperfecta. The femur is mildly shortened and bowed (between +'s). Note the irregular texture indicating previous fractures.

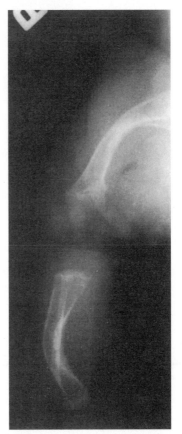

Radiograph of the same bone after birth. There has been remodeling with repair of the fracture. The bones are deossified.

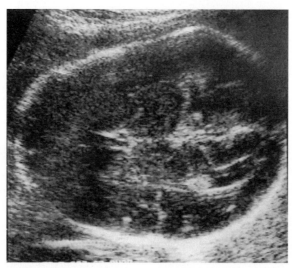

View of the head. Note the unduly well-seen intracranial structures and the poorly ossified cranium. The area closest to the transducer is flattened by the transducer pressure because the skull is so weak.

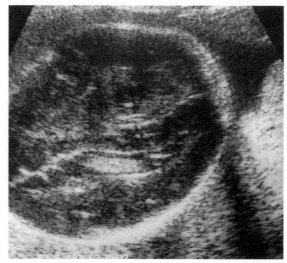

The same skull reexamined with a light touch. The skull deformity is no longer present.

8.14 Polydactyly

Epidemiology/Genetics

Definition Polydactyly is a phenotypic abnormality of the limbs characterized by excessive partitioning of the digital rays of the hands and feet. This is clinically manifested as extra digits, broad digits, or bifid digits.

Epidemiology Postaxial (ulnar or fibular side of the limb) polydactyly occurs in 1 in 3000 live births of white infants, but it is 10 times more common in blacks than whites (M1.5:F1). Preaxial (radial or tibial side of limb) polydactyly is much less common, with a frequency in whites of 0.15 in 1000.

Embryology More than 100 multiple malformation syndromes have been described with polydactyly, including many short-limbed skeletal dysplasias, and chromosome abnormalities, including trisomies 13, 18, and 21. The combination of low maternal estriol, postaxial polydactyly, and congenital heart disease should raise the suspicion of the Smith-Lemli-Opitz syndrome. Antenatal testing for this autosomal recessive defect in cholesterol metabolism is available.

Inheritance Patterns Isolated postaxial polydactyly is most often inherited as an autosomal dominant trait. Isolated preaxial polydactyly is most often unilateral and not familial.

Teratogens Alcohol, valproate, maternal diabetes.

Prognosis Excellent for isolated polydactylies; otherwise, it is dependent on the associated abnormalities and syndrome diagnosis.

Sonography

FINDINGS

1. **Fetus:** Hands and/or feet have one or more extra digits, which may be normally sited and sized as a sixth finger or small, abnormally located, and angled. The extra digit can be located proximal to the rest of the digits on the radial or tibial side (preaxial) or alongside the remaining digits on the ulnar or fibular side (postaxial).
2. **Amniotic Fluid:** Normal, if the only finding is polydactyly.
3. **Placenta:** Normal, if the only finding is polydactyly.
4. **Measurement Data:** Normal, if isolated.
5. **When Detectable:** About 13 weeks.

Pitfalls Inappropriate oblique angulation can create an appearance of polydactyly when none exists.

Differential Diagnosis Abnormally located fifth digit.

Where Else to Look

1. Meckel-Gruber syndrome, see Chapter 11.4.
2. Ellis van Creveld syndrome—Short extremities, narrow chest with short ribs, and cardiac defects.
3. Short rib polydactyly—Short ribs and limbs and narrow chest.
4. Smith-Lemli-Opitz syndrome, see Chapter 11.6.
5. Trisomy 13—Look for stigmata; commonly has polydactyly (see Chapter 1.2).

Pregnancy Management

Investigations and Consultations Required

1. Chromosomal analysis to exclude trisomy 13 is essential.
2. Fetal echocardiography is necessary because a number of the syndromes with polydactyly also have congenital heart defects.
3. Additional consultations will depend on the presumptive diagnosis and the types of malformations seen in association with the polydactyly.

Monitoring Unless the condition can clearly be established as lethal (e.g., Meckel-Gruber syndrome, short-rib polydactyly syndrome), obstetric management should not be modified.

Pregnancy Course Obstetric complications will vary, depending on the associated abnormalities. Those conditions with skeletal dysplasias may be associated with polyhydramnios.

Pregnancy Termination Issues Except for cases with trisomy 13, all other situations require a nondestructive termination procedure and a complete postmortem evaluation by a fetal pathologist and a dysmorphologist.

Delivery Because an exact diagnosis may be difficult to establish prenatally, delivery should occur in a tertiary center where a full array of diagnostic and management options exist.

Surgery

Referral to a hand surgery specialist is recommended for evaluation and treatment. Surgical procedures range from simple amputation to complex reconstruction, depending on the severity and specific nature of the problem.

REFERENCES

Bromley B, Shipp TD, Benacerraf B: Isolated polydactyly: Prenatal diagnosis and perinatal outcome. Prenat Diagn 2000;20:905–908.

Guschmann M, Horn D, Gasiorek-Wiens A, et al: Ellis-van Creveld syndrome: Examination at 15 weeks' gestation. Prenat Diagn 1999;19:879–883.

Kratz LE, Kelley RI: Prenatal diagnosis of the RSH/Smith-Lemli-Opitz syndrome. Am J Med Genet 1999;82:376–381.

Temtany SA, McKusick VA: The Genetics of Hand Malformations. New York, Alan R. Liss, for the National Foundation-March of Dimes, 1987.

Zimmer EZ, Bronshtein M: Fetal polydactyly diagnosis during early pregnancy: Clinical applications. Obstet Gynecol 2000;183:755–758.

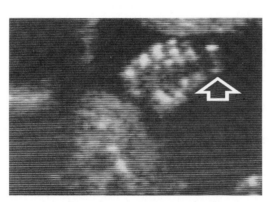

Polydactyly. An extra digit (*arrow*) is present, of about the same size and location as the others in a postaxial location.

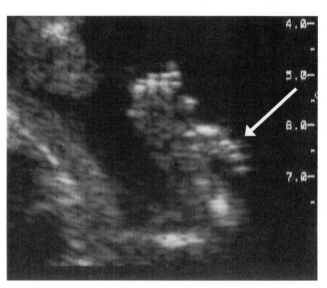

Large extra digit in a preaxial location (*arrow*).

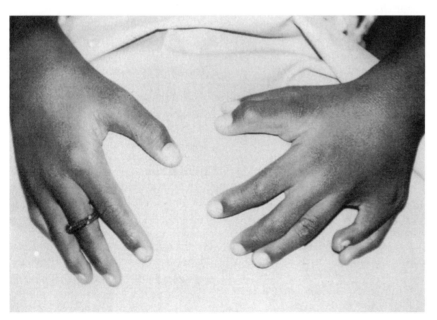

Pre- and postaxial polydactyly in a child with orofaciodigital syndrome type IV.

8.15   Radial Ray Problems
Radial Ray Aplasia/Hypoplasia

Epidemiology/Genetics

Definition   Radial aplasia/hypoplasia is a physical and radiographic abnormality characterized by partial or complete absence of the radius and/or radial ray structures (thumb and radial carpal bones). The etiology is heterogeneous, with most defects being unilateral and sporadic.

Epidemiology   Occurs in 0.3 to 0.8 in 10,000 births.

Embryology   The distal upper limbs are composed of two major developmental fields, a radial (preaxial) field and an ulnar (postaxial) field. Most major limb defects result from abnormalities in one of these fields, causing pre- and/or postaxial limb defects. Defects occurring at the junction of these fields result in split hand (ectrodactyly) malformations.

Inheritance Patterns   Most radial defects are unilateral and sporadic, with bilateral defects being much more likely to be part of a multiple malformation syndrome. Syndromes with radial aplasia/hypoplasia (see index) include hematologic syndromes such as Fanconi anemia, Aase syndrome, and thrombocytopenia-absent radius (TAR) syndrome; sporadic associations such as the VACTERL (vertebral defects, anal atresia, tracheoesophageal fistula with esophageal atresia, radial and renal dysplasia) association and the Goldenhar syndrome (see Chapter 7.3); chromosome syndromes including trisomy 13, 18, and triploidy; and some miscellaneous syndromes such as acrofacial dysostoses, Baller-Gerold syndrome, Cornelia de Lange syndrome, Townes-Brock syndrome, and Holt-Oram syndrome. Because of the rapid progress in mapping of genes and subsequent development of genetic testing, consultation with a medical geneticist or genetic counselor to determine the availability of clinical genetic testing for this disorder (or disorders) is advised.

Teratogens   Thalidomide, cocaine, valproate, and vitamin A.

Prognosis   Dependent on associated abnormalities and syndrome diagnosis. Good function is possible in most cases with aggressive orthopedic treatment.

Sonography

FINDINGS

1. **Fetus:** Arm bones—The radius can be short or absent. The ulna can be short, bowed, or sometimes also absent. The hand is usually "clubbed" and the thumb may be absent, along with some of the carpal bones.

   a. In TAR syndrome, the lower limbs may also be short or absent. The thumbs and metacarpals are always present. The condition is symmetrical.
   b. In Holt-Oram syndrome, the bony deformity may be asymmetrical and lower limb involvement does not occur. There may be absence of the entire arm long bones with phocomelia. The scaphoid and the trapezium may be absent.
2. **Amniotic Fluid:** Generally normal, but may be decreased with some etiologic origins.
3. **Placenta:** Normal.
4. **Measurement Data:** Abdomen and head measurements are normal.
5. **When Detectable:** Early second trimester.

Pitfalls   One arm may lie behind the trunk, so it cannot be seen.

Differential Diagnosis   Osteogenesis imperfecta—Usually affects lower limbs more than arms (see Chapter 8.13).

Where Else to Look

1. With Holt-Oram syndrome, perform fetal echocardiography looking for cardiac malformations such as common atrium ventricular septal defect, transposition, or tetralogy of Fallot.
2. Additional findings in the TAR complex include cardiac abnormalities (25%) and micrognathia (15%).
3. Radial ray problems can be a feature of the VACTERL complex, so look for heart anomalies, kidney deformities, spina bifida, hemivertebrae, and gut atresia (see Chapter 11.8).
4. Trisomy 18 can present with radial ray problems, so look for intrauterine growth retardation, cardiac anomalies, and choroid plexus cysts.
5. Valproic acid can result in radial ray defects—Look at the face for cleft palate and the spine for myelomeningocele if there is an appropriate history.

Pregnancy Management

Investigations and Consultations Required   Fetal karyotype should be considered, especially if other malformations are detected. A careful history is essential to assess for presence of limb or cardiac abnormalities in the parents or previous children. The history also should include information regarding consanguinity, since many of the disorders are autosomal recessive. Any potential teratogen exposure, specifically valproic acid, should be ascertained.

Both amniocentesis and cordocentesis should be performed. Fetal hematologic status must be assessed to exclude TAR syndrome, Fanconi anemia, and Aase syndrome. Amniotic fluid cultures should be established to look for chromosome breakage (Fanconi anemia) or premature centromere splitting (Robert's syndrome). Fetal echocardiography should be performed, as cardiac defects are associated with a number of the possible etiologic conditions.

Other consultations should be based on the presumptive diagnosis and the need for neonatal medical or surgical therapy.

Fetal Intervention   None is indicated.

Monitoring   Ultrasonographic examinations every 3 to 4 weeks should be performed to assess amniotic fluid status.

Pregnancy Termination Issues   Unless a precise diagnosis has been established prenatally, the method of termination should provide an intact fetus for a complete morphologic and radiologic examination.

Delivery   The complex nature of these multiple malformation conditions requires that delivery and neonatal management occur in a tertiary center. In cases of TAR syndrome and Fanconi anemia with platelet counts less than 50,000/mm³, consideration must be given to elective cesarean section or platelet transfusion just prior to elective induction of labor.

Neonatology

Resuscitation   In general, any special issues for resuscitation are determined by the associated or underlying cause of the skeletal defect.

Transport   Referral to a tertiary perinatal center following birth is indicated for definitive diagnosis, particularly if cardiac or chromosomal abnormalities are suspected.

Testing and Confirmation   In general, careful physical examination, blood cell morphology, extremity radiographs, an echocardiogram, and chromosomal analysis if there are other dysmorphic features complete the basic evaluation.

Nursery Management   The primary issue is a definitive etiologic diagnosis. Long-term prognosis is determined by the associated or underlying cause. Palliative procedures are possible to create a prehensile grasp.

REFERENCES

Auerbach AD, Sagi M, Adler B: Fanconi anemia: Prenatal diagnosis in 30 fetuses at risk. Pediatrics 1985;76:794–800.

Brons JTJ, Van Geijn HP, Wladimiroff JW, et al: Prenatal ultrasound diagnosis of the Holt-Oram syndrome. Prenat Diagn 1988;8:175–181.

Brons JTJ, Van Der Harten HJ, Van Geijn HP, et al: Prenatal ultrasonographic diagnosis of radial-ray reduction malformations. Prenat Diagn 1990;10:279–288.

Donnenfeld AE, Wiseman B, Lavi E, Weiner S: Prenatal diagnosis of thrombocytopenia absent radius syndrome by ultrasound and cordocentesis. Prenat Diagn 1990;10:29–35.

Luthy DA, Mack L, Hirsch J, Cheng E: Prenatal ultrasound diagnosis of thrombocytopenia with absent radii. Am J Obstet Gynecol 1981; 141:350–352.

Meizner I, Bar-Ziv J, Barki Y, Abeliovich D: Prenatal ultrasonic diagnosis of radial-ray aplasia and renal anomalies (acro-renal syndrome). Prenat Diagn 1986;6:223–225.

Shelton SD, Paulyson K, Kay HH: Prenatal diagnosis of thrombocytopenia absent radius (TAR) syndrome and vaginal delivery. Prenat Diagn 1999;19:54–57.

Tongsong T, Chanprapaph P: Prenatal sonographic diagnosis of Holt-Oram syndrome. J Clin Ultrasound 2000;28:98–100.

Tongsong T, Sirichotiyakul S, Chanprapaph P: Prenatal diagnosis of thrombocytopenia-absent-radius (TAR) syndrome. Ultrasound Obstet Gynecol 2000;15:256–258.

Varaiter M, Winter RM: Oxford Dysmorphology Database. Oxford, England, Oxford University Press, 1993.

Wood VE: Congenital thumb deformities. Clin Orthop 1985;195:7–25.

Ylagan LR, Budorick NE: Radial ray aplasia in utero: A prenatal finding associated with valproic acid exposure. J Ultrasound Med 1994;13: 408–411.

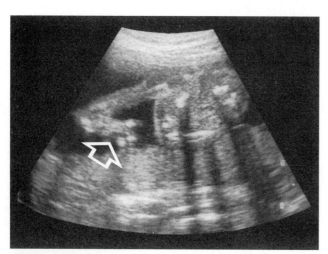

Radial ray anomaly. View of the humerus, forearm, and hand. Note that the forearm (*arrow*) is very short and that the hand is deformed.

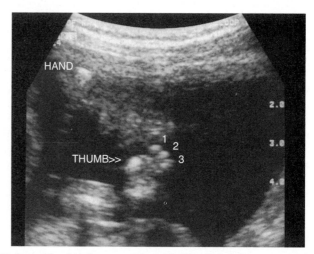

Deformed hand in the same patient. The thumb is rudimentary and the first finger is missing.

8.16 Thanatophoric Dysplasia (Dwarfism)

Epidemiology/Genetics

Definition Thanatophoric dysplasia is the most common lethal short-limbed skeletal dysplasia and is characterized by micromelia, narrow thorax, and a relatively large head.

Epidemiology One in 40,000 live births.

Embryology Thanatophoric dysplasia has characteristic radiographic findings, including telephone receiver–shaped femurs and short ribs. Cloverleaf skull is an uncommon feature.

Inheritance Patterns Most cases are sporadic and represent new dominant mutations in the fibroblast growth factor receptor-3 (*FGFR*-3) gene on chromosome 4p. Antenatal diagnosis using DNA mutation analysis is widely available.

Prognosis Thanatophoric dysplasia is invariably fatal, usually shortly after birth.

Sonography

FINDINGS

1. **Fetus:**
   a. Type I (most common):
      1. Very short limbs with telephone receiver–shaped femurs are seen. There is a rhizomelic pattern to the limb shortening.
      2. A very small chest expands into a bell-shaped abdomen.
      3. The hands have a trident shape, with short stubby fingers that are widely separated. Redundant soft tissue surrounds the limb bones.
      4. The intravertebral distance is shortened and the spine is short.
      5. There is a depressed nasal bridge with a bossed forehead.
   b. Type II:
      1. Short long bones, which are straight and longer than in type I.
      2. A cloverleaf deformity of the skull (Kleeblattschadel) in which there is a bulge arising from the superior aspect of the head.
2. **Amniotic Fluid:** Very severe polyhydramnios is always seen.
3. **Placenta:** Normal.
4. **Measurement Data:** Large abdomen and head. Very small chest and bones.
5. **When Detectable:** About 14 weeks' gestation.

Pitfalls None reported.

Differential Diagnosis

1. Achondrogenesis—Some varieties are indistinguishable from thanatophoric dwarfism. In the most typical form, the spine is echopenic and there is nuchal translucency at 11 to 14 weeks' gestation (see Chapter 8.1).
2. Achondroplasia—In the heterozygous form, the sonographic features are similar but less severe and all of the findings are seen at a later date. Before 20 to 24 weeks, the sonographic appearances are within normal limits. The homozygous form has similar features to thanatophoric dwarfism. Both parents will have heterozygous achondroplasia (see Chapter 8.2).
3. Asphyxiating thoracic dystrophy (Jeune's syndrome). Very small chest but relatively long, straight long bones (see Chapter 8.9).

Where Else to Look This is a generalized process, involving most structures.

Pregnancy Management

Investigations and Consultations Required Fetal echocardiography, to detect congenital heart defects, may assist in establishing a precise diagnosis. A neonatologist should be consulted to plan perinatal management.

Monitoring Supportive psychological care for the family is necessary in localities where late termination is not an option. No obstetric intervention should be undertaken for fetal indications.

Pregnancy Course Nearly 75% of cases of thanatophoric dwarfism will be complicated by severe polyhydramnios.

Pregnancy Termination Issues An intact fetus must be delivered for confirmation of the prenatal diagnosis. As with other skeletal dysplasias, a complete postmortem evaluation of the fetus, including radiologic, morphologic, biochemical, and molecular studies, should be performed by individuals with extensive experience in skeletal dysplasias.

Delivery Cesarean section is contraindicated, except for dystocia. Cephalocentesis is appropriate to facilitate delivery in those cases with severe hydrocephalus.

Neonatology

Resuscitation   When the diagnosis is known prior to delivery, a prenatal decision for nonintervention, made after discussion with the family, is appropriate. If the diagnosis is uncertain, resuscitation and ventilatory support are appropriate to allow time for diagnostic evaluation and parental adaptation.

Transport   Referral to a tertiary perinatal center is appropriate for confirmation of a diagnosis. Mechanical ventilatory support is often required during the transport.

Testing and Confirmation   Postnatal skeletal radiographs and careful physical examination will establish the diagnosis.

Nursery Management   Confirmation of the diagnosis, comfort care for the infant, and counseling and support of the family are the primary goals. Provision of mechanical life support in the interim is appropriate, although withdrawal of support may subsequently become a problem.

REFERENCES

Chen C, Schu-Revn C, Shih J: Prenatal diagnosis and genetic analysis of type 1 and type 2 thanatophoric dysplasia. Prenat Diagn 2001;21: 89–95.

Chervenak FA, Blakemore KJ, Isaacson G, et al: Antenatal sonographic findings of thanatophoric dysplasia with cloverleaf skull. Am J Obstet Gynecol 1983;146:984–985.

Cremin BJ, Shaff MI: Ultrasonic diagnosis of thanatophoric dwarfism in utero. Radiology 1977;124:479–480.

Elejalde BR, de Elejalde MM: Thanatophoric dwarfism: Fetal manifestations and prenatal diagnosis. Am J Med Genet 1985;22:669–683.

Martinez-Frias ML, Ramos-Arroyo MA, Salvador J: Thanatophoric dysplasia: An autosomal dominant condition? Am J Med Genet 1988;31: 815–820.

Schild RL, Hunt GH, Moore J, et al: Antenatal sonographic diagnosis of thanatophoric dysplasia: A report of three cases and a review of the literature with special emphasis on differential diagnosis. Ultrasound Obstet Gynecol 1996;8:62–67.

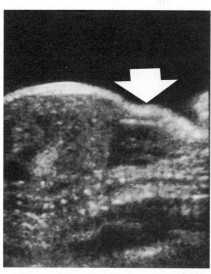

Thanatophoric dwarfism. Sagittal view of the chest and abdomen. Note the small size of the chest and relatively large abdomen. There is severe polyhydramnios.

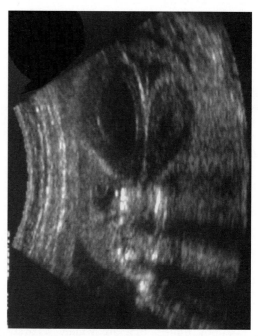

Kleeblattschadel (cloverleaf) skull deformity with huge forehead in fetus with type II thanatophoric dwarfism.

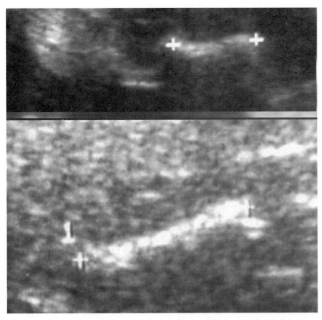

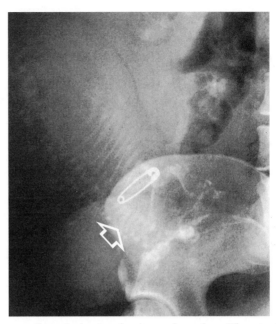

Thanatophoric dwarfism type I femur shown *above* with telephone receiver shape compared with the straight longer thanatophoric dwarfism type II femur shown *below* (at same scale).

In utero radiograph showing the abnormal vertebrae. There is platyspondyly (*arrow*).

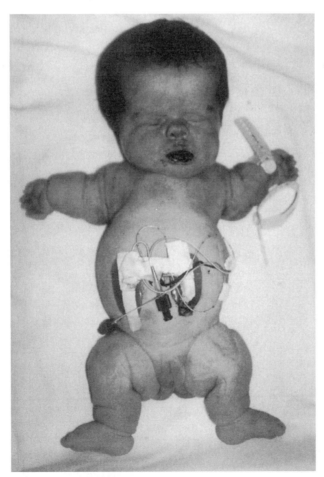

Newborn with thanatophoric dysplasia. Note rhizomelic shortening of limbs and relative macrocephaly.

9 Infections

9.1 Cytomegalic Inclusion Disease

Epidemiology/Genetics

Definition Cytomegalovirus is a large, enveloped DNA herpes virus. Adult infection is frequently asymptomatic, but fetal infection may cause severe damage. Cytomegalovirus is transmitted via secretions, by sexual contact, and transplacentally.

Epidemiology Approximately 0.5 to 1% of pregnant women are infected with cytomegalovirus. Twenty percent of their infants will show severe sequelae during pregnancy or at birth, with an additional 17% having audiologic deficits at 1 year. Primary maternal infection, in pregnancy, poses the greatest risk to the fetus: 30% of fetuses become infected. Transmission of virus in the first half of pregnancy is associated with more severe disease.

Embryology Cytomegalovirus kills infected cells. Symptoms of severe congenital infection include intrauterine growth restriction (IUGR), hemolytic anemia, pneumonitis, hepatitis, thrombocytopenia, and intracranial calcifications. Microcephaly is frequent and hydrocephaly is uncommon.

Inheritance Patterns Not genetic.

Screening Primary maternal infection can be documented by IgM seroconversion and IgG avidity testing. For women with a positive IgG test during pregnancy, a presumptive diagnosis of primary infection can be made on the basis of a positive IgM titer, which may persist for up to 4 months after infection. Polymerase chain reaction (PCR) for cytomegalovirus DNA can determine viral load. Rapid changes in testing technology are occurring and should prompt appropriate consultation.

Prognosis Approximately 95% of infants who secrete cytomegalovirus at birth are asymptomatic, but of those who show symptoms, 80% will have central nervous system sequelae and 30% will die. Asymptomatic survivors may still manifest visual defects, neurologic problems, and deafness later in life. Early pregnancy infection usually results in a more severe outcome:

- Sensorineural hearing loss, 50%
- Microcephaly, 70%
- Mental retardation, 61%
- Cerebral palsy, 35%
- Chorioretinitis or optic atrophy, 22%
- Dental enamel defects, 40%

Late-occurring sequelae in clinically inapparent infection are as follows:

- Sensorineural hearing loss, 10–25%
- Chorioretinitis, 1%
- Microcephaly, usually with mental retardation, 2%
- Dental enamel defects, 5%

Sonography

FINDINGS

1. **Fetus:**
   a. Calcification occurs in a number of sites:
      1. Clumps of "echogenic bowel" may be seen. Suspect areas should be as echogenic as neighboring bone.
      2. Echogenic foci may be seen in the liver or spleen.
      3. Calcification in the lateral borders of lateral ventricles is diagnostic of cytomegalovirus. The calcification occurs in the subependymal area, related to cell necrosis.
      4. Branching linear calcifications in the basal ganglia.
   b. Nonimmune hydrops due to anemia—Pleural and pericardial effusions and ascites.
   c. Hepatosplenomegaly.
   d. Microcephaly and ventriculomegaly individually or together. The ventriculomegaly may be unilateral.
   e. Cardiomegaly, tachyarrhythmia, and bradyarrhythmia.

f. Hydronephrosis (usually unilateral).
2. **Amniotic Fluid:** Polyhydramnios is seen with nonimmune hydrops and oligohydramnios with IUGR. Oligohydramnios is more common (25%).
3. **Placenta:** Placentomegaly will occur in association with hydrops or as an isolated finding.
4. **Measurement Data:** IUGR may occur at an early gestational age.
5. **When Detectable:** Cytomegalovirus has been detected as early as 20 weeks' gestation.

Pitfalls

1. The fetus may appear normal yet be infected.
2. It is easy to overdiagnose echogenic bowel if a high-frequency transducer is used. Make sure the suspect area is as echogenic as neighboring bowel.

Differential Diagnosis

1. Echogenic gut areas are also seen as a normal variant, in trisomy 21, with cystic fibrosis, and following ingestion of intra-amniotic blood.
2. All of the other causes of nonimmune hydrops.
3. Microcephaly may also be familial or related to vascular causes.

Where Else to Look   A detailed survey of the entire fetus, except for the limbs, is required.

Pregnancy Management

Investigations and Consultations Required

1. Maternal viral titers should be performed with appropriate confirmatory studies, when a positive IgM titer is found. Amniotic fluid culture is the most reliable diagnostic test. PCR molecular testing may increase the reliability of amniotic fluid evaluations for cytomegalovirus infections.
2. Consultations with a neonatologist may be appropriate to plan delivery management, depending on the severity of the structural malformations.

3. Computed tomographic scanning is helpful in confirming intracranial or liver calcification.

Fetal Intervention   Fetal blood sampling can detect thrombocytopenia, anemia, and cytomegalovirus-specific IgM in fetal serum (see the table below).

Monitoring   The severity of the central nervous system effects of cytomegalovirus cannot be assessed, except in the case of severe hydrocephalus or microcephaly. To prevent further damage from hypoxic causes, fetal evaluation and monitoring may be appropriate in selected cases. Sonograms should be performed every 2 to 3 weeks, since nonimmune hydrops may develop.

Pregnancy Course   The presence of IUGR or severe hydrocephalus may require that decisions be made with the family regarding the desirability and type of obstetric intervention to be instituted.

Pregnancy Termination Issues   If a precise diagnosis has been established, there are no special recommendations regarding pregnancy termination.

Delivery   In the presence of severe hydrocephalus resulting in dystocia, consideration should be given to cephalocentesis. Cases diagnosed on the basis of IUGR or mild ventriculomegaly should be managed in similar fashion to normal pregnancies to prevent any further central nervous system damage.

Neonatology

Resuscitation   Respiratory depression or distress is likely if hydrops or severe anemia is present. In those circumstances, assistance with the initiation of respiration is usually required. See Chapter 13.2 for management of hydrops.

Transport   Referral to a tertiary perinatal center is indicated for treatment of respiratory distress, severe ane-

Outcomes of Cytomegalovirus (CMV) Infection in Pregnancy*

At Onset of Pregnancy	During Pregnancy	Infection	At Birth	Final Outcome
CMV seronegative at conception	1–4% pregnant women develop primary CMV	40% of babies born to mothers with primary CMV are congenitally infected	5–15% congenitally infected babies are symptomatic (4)	10% normal 60% die with sequelae (2.4)* 30% die within 2 years (1.2)
(10,000)*	(100)*	(40)*	85–95% congenitally infected babies are asymptomatic (36)*	5–15% survive with sequelae (2.5)* 85–95% normal
CMV seropositive at conception	Recurrent CMV	0.5–1.5% of all babies born to seropositive mothers are congenitally infected	Almost all babies are asymptomatic at birth	1–15% survive with sequelae (1–15)* 85–99% normal
(10,000)*	(7)*	(50–150)*	(50–150)*	

*If 10,000 pregnant women (seropositive and seronegative) are followed, the estimated number of babies affected is shown in parentheses.

mia, and/or hydrops. The infant may require ventilatory assistance in transit.

Testing and Confirmation   Cytomegalovirus can be isolated from urine or saliva within the first 3 weeks of life. Rapid diagnosis using monoclonal antibodies for cytomegalovirus or PCR is available. After that, positive serum titers may suggest antenatal infection.

Diagnosis is best confirmed by virus recovery from urine or secretions. Specific antibodies can be identified.

Nursery Management   Supportive and symptomatic care only once the diagnosis has been confirmed.

Blood and body fluid precautions need to be observed during the hospital stay, and direct contact by pregnant women should be avoided.

No specific treatment is available for congenitally acquired infection, as organ damage has already occurred. Ganciclovir may be of use in postnatally acquired infection.

REFERENCES

Bale J, Murph J: Congenital infections and the nervous system. Pediatr Neurol 1992;39:669–690.

Casteels A, Naessens A, Gordts F, et al: Neonatal screening for congenital cytomegalovirus infections. J Perinat Med 1999;27:116–121.

Drose JA, Dennis MA, Thickman D: Infection in utero: US findings in 19 cases. Radiology 1991;178:369–374.

Estroff JA, Parad RB, Teele RL, Benacerraf BR: Echogenic vessels in the fetal thalami and basal ganglia associated with cytomegalovirus infection. J Ultrasound Med 1992;11:686–688.

Fakhry J, Khoury A: Fetal intracranial calcifications: The importance of periventricular hyperechoic foci without shadowing. J Ultrasound Med 1991;10:51–54.

Forouzan I: Fetal abdominal echogenic mass: An early sign of in-trauterine cytomegalovirus infection. Obstet Gynecol 1992;80:535–537.

Freij BJ, Sever JL: Herpesvirus infections in pregnancy: Risks to embryo, fetus, and neonate. Clin Perinatol 1988;15:203–231.

Grose C, Itani O, Weiner C: Prenatal diagnosis of fetal infection: Advances from amniocentesis to cordocentesis—congenital toxoplasmosis, rubella, cytomegalovirus, varicella virus, parvovirus, and human immunodeficiency virus. Pediatr Infect Dis J 1989;8:459–468.

Grose C, Weiner CP: Prenatal diagnosis of congenital cytomegalovirus infection: Two decades later. Am J Obstet Gynecol 1990;163:447–450.

Guerra B, Lazzarotto T, Quarta S, et al: Prenatal diagnosis of symptomatic congenital cytomegalovirus infection. Am J Obstet Gynecol 2000;183:476–482.

Hohlfeld P, Vial Y, Maillard-Brignon C, et al: Cytomegalovirus fetal infection: Prenatal diagnosis. Obstet Gynecol 1991;78:615–618.

Kumar ML, Nankervis GA, Jacobs IB, et al: Congenital and postnatally acquired cytomegalovirus infections: Long-term follow-up. J Pediatr 1984;104:674–679.

Lazzarotto T, Varani S, Guerra B, et al: Prenatal indicators of congenital cytomegalovirus infection. J Pediatr 2000;137:90–95.

Liesnard C, Donner C, Brancart F, et al: Prenatal diagnosis of congenital cytomegalovirus infection: Prospective study of 237 pregnancies at risk. Obstet Gynecol 2000;95:881–888.

Lynch L, Daffos F, Emanuel D, et al: Prenatal diagnosis of fetal cytomegalovirus infection. Am J Obstet Gynecol 1991;165:714–718.

Pass RF, Stagno S, Myers GJ, Alford CA: Outcome of symptomatic congenital cytomegalovirus infection: Results of long-term longitudinal follow-up. Pediatrics 1980;66:758–762.

Stagno S, Whitley RK: Herpesvirus infections of pregnancy. Part I: Cytomegalovirus and Epstein-Barr virus infections. N Engl J Med 1985;313:1270–1274.

Stagno S, Pass RF, Could G, et al: Primary cytomegalovirus infection in pregnancy. Incidence, transmission to fetus, and clinical outcome. JAMA 1986;256:1904–1908.

Twickler DM, Perlman J, Maberry MC: Congenital cytomegalovirus infection presenting as cerebral ventriculomegaly on antenatal sonography. Am J Perinatol 1993;10:404–406.

Ville Y: The megalovirus. Ultrasound Obstet Gynecol 1998;12:151–153.

Weiner CP, Grose C: Prenatal diagnosis of congenital cytomegalovirus infection by virus isolation from amniotic fluid. Am J Obstet Gynecol 1990;163:1253–1255.

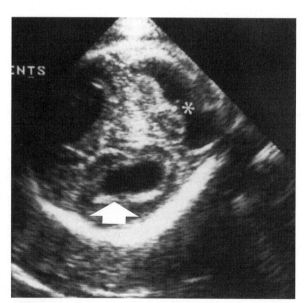

Microcephaly with ventriculomegaly due to cytomegalovirus (CMV). Note the large cisterna magna suggesting atrophy (*). The border of the lateral ventricle (*arrow*) is densely echogenic because it is calcified. Calcification in this area is typical of CMV.

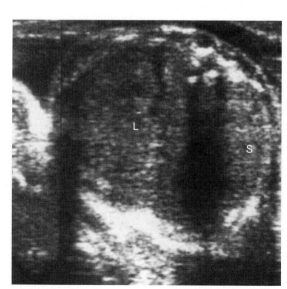

The liver (L) and spleen (S) are enlarged due to cytomegalovirus.

9.2 Parvovirus (Fifth Disease)

Epidemiology/Genetics

Definition Parvovirus is a single-stranded DNA virus that causes erythema infectiosum (fifth disease) in children and adults. Infected individuals may be asymptomatic. In the fetus, parvovirus may result in anemia with nonimmune hydrops.

Epidemiology Congenital infection rates vary depending on the prevalence in the community. Approximately 50 to 75% of adult women are immune. The risk of congenital infection from an infected mother is between 10 and 20% and is highest in the first and second trimesters.

Embryology Parvovirus destroys host cells, particularly red blood cell precursors, and has an affinity for rapidly dividing cells. Congenital infection can cause hydrops fetalis, with resultant stillbirth, or neonatal death. Associated findings include hepatosplenomegaly, polyhydramnios, and liver disease. Transplacental transmission can occur any time during pregnancy.

Inheritance Patterns Not genetic.

Screening Maternal serum alpha-fetoprotein may be elevated because of hydrops.

Prognosis There is a 10% risk of fetal death due to hydrops from severe fetal anemia. The risk of fetal death in utero is 17% before 20 weeks' gestation and 6% after 20 weeks, if the fetus is infected. Most infected women, however, give birth to apparently normal babies.

Sonography

FINDINGS

1. **Fetus:**
   a. Ascites is usually the presenting finding.
   b. Other findings of hydrops—pleural effusion, pericardial effusion, and skin thickening—develop later.
   c. There is cardiomegaly and decreased movement in severe cases. The cardiac biventricular diameter is increased.
   d. Hepatosplenomegaly may be seen.
   e. Hydrocephalus, microcephaly, with intracranial and hepatic calcification, may occur in severely affected cases.
   f. There is increased peak velocity in the middle cerebral artery in fetuses with moderate or severe anemia.
2. **Amniotic Fluid:** Normal amniotic fluid is usual.
3. **Placenta:** Placentomegaly may develop.
4. **Measurement Data:** Growth is reported as normal.

When Detectable Hydrops develops between 3 and 13 weeks after maternal infection. Most cases occur between 16 and 32 weeks. If a mother has had a documented parvovirus infection, weekly sonograms for the next 6 weeks to detect the onset of fetal hydrops are recommended.

Pitfalls Pseudopericardial effusion and pseudoascites due to fat deposits may mimic hydrops.

Differential Diagnosis Numerous other causes of hydrops exist. Ask for a history of maculopapular rash and arthralgia.

Where Else to Look

1. Look for hydrocephalus, which has been seen occasionally in fetuses with parvovirus.
2. A case of vasculitis causing myocarditis and dystrophic calcification in spleen and liver has been reported in a fetus with parvovirus.
3. Look for other causes of hydrops, such as heart problems, chromosomal abnormalities, cytomegalovirus, or syphilis.

Pregnancy Management

Investigations and Consultations Required

1. Maternal serum titers for infectious agents should be performed.
2. Evaluation should be done to exclude other causes of both immune and nonimmune hydrops, including assessment of fetal hematologic status by percutaneous umbilical blood sampling. Fetal blood sampling can detect anemia and IgM-specific antibody to human parvovirus. PCR testing of amniotic fluid or fetal blood allows precise detection of fetal infection.

Fetal Intervention Because the major fetal manifestation of parvovirus infection is anemia, treatment by in utero transfusions is appropriate when a presumptive diagnosis of parvovirus infection is made in the fetus with hydrops. Although spontaneous resolution has been reported, the presence of a severe anemia (hematocrit of less than 25%) in a hydropic fetus warrants transfusion.

Monitoring Hydrops has been reported as developing between 3 and, in one instance, 13 weeks following exposure. Weekly sonograms up to 13 weeks after well-documented exposure are desirable. Following transfusion, weekly sonographic evaluation is appropriate to monitor resolution of the hydrops. Because of the self-limited nature of the disease, repeat transfusions may not be necessary.

Pregnancy Course   No specific obstetric complications are to be expected if the hydrops resolves.

Pregnancy Termination Issues   There should be no indication for termination, but if this option is chosen, careful pathologic examinations must be performed to confirm the diagnosis.

Delivery   The site for delivery will depend on the clinical condition of the fetus. The presence of hydrops or a recent transfusion should be an indication for delivery in a tertiary center. Those fetuses in which resolution of hydrops has occurred require no special delivery precautions.

Neonatology

Resuscitation   Respiratory depression and distress are likely if hydrops or severe anemia is present. The neonatologist must be prepared to remove serous fluid collections (pleural, pericardial, peritoneal).

Transport   Neonatal transport is indicated for treatment of respiratory distress, severe anemia, and/or hydrops. The infant may require ventilatory assistance in transit.

Nursery Management

1. Transfusion—Approach the management as if the neonate had nonimmune hydrops. Indications for replacement transfusion are a hematocrit of less than 36% with symptoms and of less than 32% irrespective of symptoms. Use packed red blood cells with high hematocrit (75% or greater).
2. Treatment of hydrops—Mobilize the anasarca, interstitial, and serosal fluid collections by direct removal or forced diuresis in accompaniment with infusion of plasma proteins. Peritoneal dialysis is rarely needed.

Respiratory support may be required with severe hydrops.

REFERENCES

Anderson LJ, Hurwitz ES: Human parvovirus B19 and pregnancy. Clin Perinatol 1988;15:273–286.

Bale J, Murphy J: Congenital infections and the nervous system. Pediatr Neurol 1992;39:669–690.

Dieck D, Schild RL, Hansmann M, Eis-Hubinger AM: Prenatal diagnosis of congenital parvovirus B19 infection: Value of serological and PCR techniques in maternal and fetal serum. Prenatal Diagn 1999;19:1119–1123.

Grose C, Itani O, Weiner C: Prenatal diagnosis of fetal infection: Advances from amniocentesis to cordocentesis—congenital toxoplasmosis, rubella, cytomegalovirus, varicella virus, parvovirus, and human immunodeficiency virus. Pediatr Infect Dis J 1989;8:459–468.

Humphrey W, Magoon M, O'Shaughnessy R: Severe nonimmune hydrops secondary to parvovirus B-19 infection: Spontaneous reversal in utero and survival of a term infant. Obstet Gynecol 1991;78:900–902.

Katz VL, McCoy C, Kuller JA, Hansen WF: Association between fetal parvovirus B19 infection and fetal anomalies: A report of two cases. Am J Perinatol 1996;13:43–45.

Kumar ML: Human parvovirus B19 and its associated diseases. Clin Perinatol 1991;18:209–225.

Pryde PG, Nugent CE, Pridjian G, et al: Spontaneous resolution of nonimmune hydrops fetalis secondary to human parvovirus B19 infection. Obstet Gynecol 1992;79:859–861.

Rodis JF, Borgida AF, Wilson M, et al: Management of parvovirus infection in pregnancy and outcomes of hydrops: A survey of members of the Society of Perinatal Obstetricians. Am J Obstet Gynecol 1998;179:985–988.

Rodis JF, Quinn DL, Gary GW Jr, et al: Management and outcomes of pregnancies complicated by human B19 parvovirus infection: A prospective study. Am J Obstet Gynecol 1990;163:1168–1171.

Sahakian V, Weiner CP, Naides SJ, et al: Intrauterine transfusion treatment of nonimmune hydrops fetalis secondary to human parvovirus B19 infection. Am J Obstet Gynecol 1991;164:1090–1091.

Sheikh AU, Ernest JM, O'Shea M: Long-term outcome in fetal hydrops from parvovirus B19 infection. Am J Obstet Gynecol 1992;167:337–341.

Swain S, Cameron AD, MacNay MB, Howatson AG: Prenatal diagnosis and management of nonimmune hydrops fetalis. Aust N Z Obstet Gynecol 1999;39:285–290.

Von Daiserburg CS, Jonat W: Fetal parvovirus infection. Ultrasound Obstet Gynecol 2001;18:280–288.

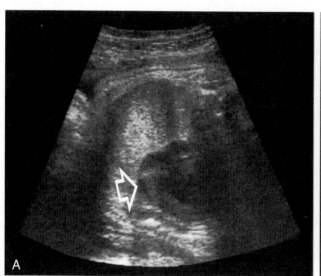 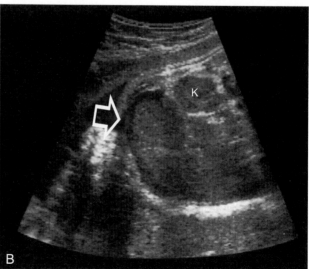

Early hydrops due to parvovirus. In *A*, a small pericardial effusion can be seen around the heart (*arrow*). In *B*, a small amount of ascites is present around the liver (*arrow*). K, kidney.

9.3 Congenital Syphilis

Epidemiology/Genetics

Definition Syphilis is a sexually transmitted infection caused by the spirochete *Treponema pallidum*, which can damage the developing fetus.

Epidemiology Common. The prevalence of infection is dependent on the population being studied. The infection rate is on the rise in the United States. The incidence of syphilis peaked in 1990 and has recently declined. In 1993 the incidence of congenital syphilis was 80.9 per 100,000 live births in the United States, whereas in 1997 the incidence had fallen to 26.9 per 100,000 live births. The rate of congenital infection correlates to the duration of maternal infection and degree of spirochetemia. The greatest risk occurs with recent onset or current secondary syphilis, as both are associated with the greatest load of organisms.

Embryology *T. pallidum* can cross the placenta and infect the developing fetus at any time during pregnancy. Clinical manifestations include characteristic skin and osseous lesions (seen in 90% of infants with untreated congenital syphilis), meningeal inflammation, nephritis, and hepatosplenomegaly. Features become apparent after 18 to 20 weeks' gestation, when immunocompetence of the fetus is established. More than 50% of pregnancies with untreated syphilis spontaneously abort or result in stillbirth.

Inheritance Patterns Not genetic.

Prognosis Varies with the amount of fetal damage and the timing of treatment. Infants can appear normal at birth and develop signs of infection later in life. Mental retardation, blindness, and sensorineural deafness all occur as the result of fetal infection.

Sonography

FINDINGS

1. **Fetus:** Hepatosplenomegaly (above the 90th percentile for size in longitudinal view) is the first, and often the only, finding. In severe cases, there is fetal hydrops (pleural effusion, ascites, pericardial effusion, and skin thickening).
2. **Amniotic Fluid:** Polyhydramnios is a late and uncommon finding.
3. **Placenta:** Placentomegaly occurs but is uncommon in the early stages of the disease.
4. **Measurement Data:** Growth is normal.
5. **When Detectable:** First detected at about 24 weeks.

Differential Diagnosis

1. Look for other causes of hydrops.
2. Isolated hepatosplenomegaly may be due to other infectious causes, such as cytomegalovirus.

Where Else to Look Look at the maternal liver for stigmata of syphilis.

Pregnancy Management

Investigations and Consultations Required Maternal serologic testing should include not only nonspecific tests such as Venereal Disease Research Laboratories test (VDRL) or the rapid plasma reagin test (RPR), but also a specific treponemal test such as fluorescent treponemal antibody absorption test (FTA-ABS). If hydrops is present, a complete evaluation, as outlined in Chapter 13.2, should be performed.

Fetal Intervention Fetal intervention is contraindicated if a diagnosis of congenital syphilis is established.

Monitoring Antibiotic therapy should be instituted at once for maternal treatment. The effects of fetal infection are not reversible; however, the severity of the infection may be modified. Fetal assessment modalities are not appropriate once a diagnosis has been established.

Pregnancy Course As in other cases of hydrops, polyhydramnios is a commonly associated finding. The incidence of stillbirth is high.

Pregnancy Termination Issues If a precise diagnosis has been established, no special precautions are necessary. If a diagnosis has not been made in the case of a fetal demise, amniotic fluid should be obtained prior to termination for dark-field evaluation looking for spirochetes. Complete gross and microscopic examinations of the fetus and placenta are necessary to confirm the diagnosis.

Delivery The dismal prognosis for these infants will not be altered by aggressive management. The site of delivery should be one chosen by the patient in consultation with her physician.

Neonatology

Resuscitation There are usually no specific resuscitation issues for the majority of congenital syphilis cases. If there is prenatal evidence of congenital syphilis, however, there is a high likelihood that the infant will experience difficulty with the onset of cardiorespiratory adaptation. Infrequently, aspiration of serous fluid accumulation—pleural or peritoneal—may be necessary to facilitate breathing, and anemia may be of such severity as to cause difficulty.

Blood and body fluid precautions are important, as both substances may be highly contagious in severe cases of congenital syphilis.

Transport   Transfer to a tertiary perinatal center is indicated for extreme prematurity, uncertain diagnosis, or severe organ involvement such as peritonitis, nephrotic syndrome, or hydrops.

Testing and Confirmation   Clinical features may be present at birth. Radiographic studies will demonstrate the osseous lesions. Testing for treponemal specific IgM antibodies confirms the diagnosis. Diagnosis should be confirmed by serologic testing, including serum and cerebrospinal fluid VDRL, serum IgM FTA-ABS, dark-field examination of skin lesions, body fluids and nasal secretions, and long-bone radiographs. Other evaluations should be directed toward determining the extent and severity of organ involvement.

Nursery Management   Neonatal manifestations presenting in the first several days in overt cases include hepatosplenomegaly, 91%; anemia, 64%; jaundice, 49%; periostitis, 37%; skin rash, 31%; cerebrospinal fluid abnormalities, 44%. Hydrops, peritonitis, and nephrotic syndrome are infrequent to rare clinical findings. Most neonatal cases have serologic evidence only.

The recommended antibiotic therapy is aqueous penicillin G 50,000 U/kg daily for 10 days. In addition, other therapy such as transfusion, cardiorespiratory support, and phototherapy for hyperbilirubinemia should be determined by type and severity of organ involvement.

REFERENCES

Barton JR, Thorpe EM Jr, Shaver DC, et al: Nonimmune hydrops fetalis associated with maternal infection with syphilis. Am J Obstet Gynecol 1992;167:56–58.

Centers for Disease Control: Congenital syphilis. Morbid Mortal Week Rep 1989;38:825.

Hira SH, Ganapati JB: Early congenital syphilis: Clinico-radiologic features in 202 patients. Sex Trans Dis 1985;12:177.

Hollier LM, Harstad TW, Sanchez PJ: Fetal syphilis: Clinical laboratory characteristics. Obstet Gynecol 2001;97:447–453.

Minkoff HL: Preventing fetal damage from sexually transmitted diseases. Clin Obstet Gynecol 1991;34:336–344.

Nathan L, Bohman VR, Sanchez PJ, et al: In utero infection with Treponema pallidum in early pregnancy. Prenat Diagn 1997;17:119–123.

Nathan L, Twickler DM, Peters MT, et al: Fetal syphilis: Correlation of sonographic findings and rabbit infectivity testing of amniotic fluid. J Ultrasound Med 1993;12:97–101.

Raafat NA, Birch AA, Altieri LA, et al: Sonographic osseous manifestations of fetal syphilis: A case report. J Ultrasound Med 1993;12:783–785.

Rawstron SA, Jenkins S, Blanchard S, et al: Maternal and congenital syphilis in Brooklyn, NY. Epidemiology, transmission, and diagnosis. Am J Dis Child 1993;147:727–731.

Wendel GD: Gestational and congenital syphilis. Clin Perinatol 1989;15:287.

9.4 Toxoplasmosis

Epidemiology/Genetics

Definition An infection by the parasite *Toxoplasma gondii*. There are three forms: the tachyzoite or obligate intracellular form, the tissue cyst, and the oocyst found only in cats. Infection in adults occurs from ingestion of raw meats or contact with cat feces, and fetal transmission is transplacental.

Epidemiology Occurrence differs widely with different populations and climates. An estimated 3000 congenitally infected births occur each year in the United States. Exact infection rates for exposed fetuses are unknown but may be as high as 40%. It is estimated that over 75% of infected fetuses are unaffected and 10% have severe disease. The risk for severe disease is greatest in first- and second-trimester infection; congenital infection is more likely to be acquired in the third trimester. Fetal infection occurs only with primary maternal infection.

Embryology Tachyzoites proliferate and destroy fetal cells. Severe congenital infection results in chorioretinitis, microcephaly, hydrocephaly, intracranial calcifications, thrombocytopenia, anemia, and hydrops fetalis. More severe disease is generally associated with early pregnancy transmission.

Inheritance Patterns Not genetic.

Screening A precise diagnosis is established if there is the appearance of IgG antibodies in a woman who had previously been seronegative. An initial low level of IgG antibodies should be repeated in 3 weeks and the paired samples tested in parallel. A fourfold rise in titer is indicative of recent infection. In the patient with an initial high titer (>1024), assessment of specific IgM antibodies should be performed to differentiate recent from old infection.

Prognosis Most congenital infections are asymptomatic. The mortality rate, including stillbirth, is 12% for those with severe disease. Ocular and central nervous system abnormalities are seen in about 80% of infants who show severe infection. Apparently asymptomatic infants are at risk for the later development of mental retardation, deafness, and ocular problems.

Sonography

FINDINGS

1. **Fetus:**
   a. Random calcification in the brain is seen usually as echogenic areas rather than high-level echoes with shadowing. Cataracts may be visible as hyperechogenicity of the lens borders. Microcephaly may develop.
   b. Hepatosplenomegaly with intrahepatic echogenic densities occurs.
   c. Cranial ventriculomegaly may be seen starting in the occipital horns.
   d. Ascites—Pleural and pericardial effusions are seen either separately or together. Full-blown hydrops may develop.
2. **Amniotic Fluid:** Polyhydramnios may occur with hydrops.
3. **Placenta:** Placentomegaly with variation in placental texture may occur.
4. **Measurement Data:** Hepatosplenomegaly may cause abdominal circumference increase. Normal tables for liver and spleen size exist. IUGR may be present.
5. **When Detectable:** Reported as being first detected in the second trimester.

Differential Diagnosis Cytomegalic inclusion disease (cytomegalovirus)—Calcification in cytomegalovirus is periventricular rather than random throughout the brain. Cardiac abnormalities favor cytomegalovirus.

Where Else to Look A generalized disease, so all organs need to be examined.

Pregnancy Management

Investigations and Consultations Required The work-up should include maternal serum analysis for viral specific IgG and IgM for common viral infections. Previous studies have documented the reliability of percutaneous umbilical blood sampling at 20 to 22 weeks' gestation for the prenatal diagnosis of toxoplasmosis. Detection of toxoplasma specific IgM and isolation of the parasite by mouse inoculation are the primary diagnostic tests. Nonspecific signs of fetal infection, such as elevated liver enzymes, low platelet counts, and high eosinophil counts provide additional diagnostic information. More recently, a PCR test has been developed that may allow reliable detection of infection from an amniotic fluid sample.

Fetal Intervention No specific interventions are indicated. Aggressive maternal treatment with pyrimethamine and sulfadiazine has been shown to be beneficial in the fetus with asymptomatic infection. There is no benefit to therapy in the fetus with sonographically detected abnormalities.

Monitoring Sonographic monitoring for the development of severe hydrocephalus is appropriate, but most cases of ventriculomegaly caused by toxoplasmosis will not be associated with an increase in biparietal diameter.

Pregnancy Course   Usually uncomplicated except in cases in which hydrops develops.

Pregnancy Termination Issues   If a precise microbiologic diagnosis has been established, no special precautions are necessary. If not, an intact fetus is necessary for full evaluation by an individual with special expertise in fetal neuropathology.

Delivery   The presence of severe hydrocephalus requires an informed decision by the parents regarding either cephalocentesis or caesarian section. In cases without hydrocephalus, delivery management should not be altered, as the degree of central nervous system damage cannot be ascertained by ultrasonographic examination. In all circumstances, delivery should take place in a tertiary center.

Neonatology

Resuscitation   No specific measures are called for other than infection precautions for the resuscitation team (maternal and fetal blood and body fluids).

Hydrocephalus and/or hydrops fetalis may predispose to perinatal asphyxia, resulting in the need for resuscitation. Removal of pleural and/or peritoneal fluid may be necessary to facilitate lung expansion.

Transport   Referral to a tertiary perinatal center is indicated for treatment of respiratory distress, central nervous system disorders, and/or hydrops. The infant may require ventilatory assistance in transit.

Testing and Confirmation   Infection can be confirmed by detection of anti-toxoplasma IgM, the persistence of anti-toxoplasma IgG in the infant's serum, or the detection of parasites in tissues, blood, or cerebrospinal fluid. Confirm diagnosis with serologic testing and central nervous system diagnostic imaging.

Nursery Management   Cerebrospinal fluid findings of lymphocytosis and elevated protein may be found in otherwise asymptomatic infants.

Neonatal manifestations:

- Low birth weight (<2500 g), 28%
- Hepatomegaly, 37%
- Splenomegaly, 40%
- Jaundice, 42%
- Petechiae/purpura, 10%
- Pneumonia, 12%
- Cataracts, 2%

- Chorioretinitis, 90%
- Microcephaly, 10%
- Hydrocephaly, 20%
- Intracranial calcifications, 38%

Two clinical syndromes:

1. Generalized disease—Jaundice, anemia, visceral involvement, birth to 1 month.
2. Neurologic disease—Seizures, meningoencephalitis after 1 month.

Treatment is both nonspecific, directed at symptoms of jaundice, anemia, and respiratory distress, and specifically antimicrobial, with pyrimethamine and sulfadiazine.

Ninety percent of survivors of neonatal clinical disease have serious neurologic sequelae: mental retardation, seizures, cerebral palsy, visual impairment, hydrocephalus, microcephaly, and sensorineural deafness.

Asymptomatic disease in the neonatal period progresses to clinical disease as late as 9 to 10 years of age with chorioretinitis and neurologic manifestations.

REFERENCES

Bale J, Murph J: Congenital infections and the nervous system. Ped Neurol 1992;39:669–690.

Carter AO, Frank JW: Congenital toxoplasmosis: Epidemiologic features and control. Can Med Assoc J 1986;135:618–623.

Daffos F, Forestier F, Capella-Pavlovksy M, et al: Prenatal management of 746 pregnancies at risk for congenital toxoplasmosis. N Engl J Med 1988;318:271–275.

Desmonts G, Convreur J: Congenital toxoplasmosis: A prospective study of 378 pregnancies. N Engl J Med 1974;290:1110–1116.

Desmonts G, Convreur J: Toxoplasmosis: Epidemiologic and serologic aspects of perinatal infection. In Drugman S, Gershon AA (eds): Infections of the Fetus and Newborn Infant. New York, Alan R. Liss, 1975.

Foulon W, Pinon JM, Stray-Pedersen B, et al: Prenatal diagnosis of congenital toxoplasmosis: A multicenter evaluation of different diagnostic parameters. Am J Obstet Gynecol 1999;181:843–847.

Friedman S, Ford-Jones LE, Toi A, et al: Congenital toxoplasmosis: Prenatal diagnosis, treatment and postnatal outcome. Prenat Diagn 1999;19:330–333.

Grose C, Itani O, Weiner C: Prenatal diagnosis of fetal infection: Advances from amniocentesis to cordocentesis—congenital toxoplasmosis, rubella, cytomegalovirus, varicella virus, parvovirus, and human immunodeficiency virus. Pediatr Infect Dis J 1989;8:459–468.

Hohlfeld P, MacAleese J, Capella-Pavlovski M, et al: Fetal toxoplasmosis: Ultrasonographic signs. Ultrasound Obstet Gynecol 1991;1:241–244.

Lee RV: Parasites and pregnancy: The problems of malaria and toxoplasmosis. Clin Perinatol 1988;15:351–363.

Naessens A, Jenum PA, Pollak A, et al: Diagnosis of congenital toxoplasmosis in the neonatal period: A multicenter evaluation. J Pediatr 1999;135:714–719.

Pedreira DAL, Camargo ME, Leser PG: Toxoplasmosis: Will the time ever come? Ultrasound Obstet Gynecol 2001;17:459–463.

Pedreira DAL, Diniz EMA, Schultz R, et al: Fetal cataract in congenital toxoplasmosis. Ultrasound Obstet Gynecol 1999;13:266–267.

Robert-Gangneux F, Gavinet MF, Ancelle T, et al: Value of prenatal diagnosis and early postnatal diagnosis of congenital toxoplasmosis: Retrospective study of 110 cases. J Clin Microbiol 1999;37:2893–2898.

Sever JL, Ellenberg JH, Ley AC, et al: Toxoplasmosis: Maternal and pediatric findings in 23,000 pregnancies. Pediatrics 1988;82:181–192.

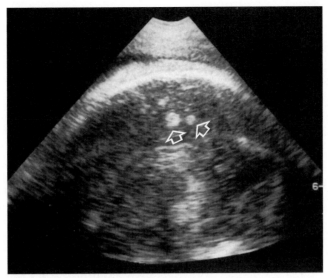

Intracranial calcifications due to toxoplasmosis (*arrows*). They are randomly located throughout the brain.

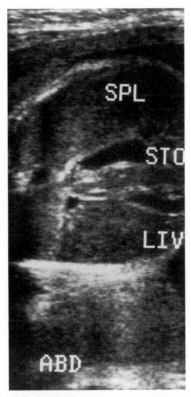

Massive spleen (SPL) and less marked liver (LIV) enlargement due to toxoplasmosis. The stomach (STO) is squashed between the two enlarged organs. ABD, abdomen.

9.5 Varicella Infection (Varicella-Zoster Virus)

Epidemiology/Genetics

Definition Varicella-zoster is a DNA herpes virus. Primary infection causes chicken pox and may lead to latency of the virus in sensory dorsal root ganglia. Reactivation of the virus later in life causes shingles.

Epidemiology The incidence of varicella-zoster infection during pregnancy is 1 to 5 per 10,000 births (as of 1989). The risk to the fetus of congenital infection differs during the course of pregnancy but is low. Of the fetuses infected, less than 5% will have congenital abnormalities. Observed male-to-female ratio is 1:4 for severe disease.

Embryology The virus is transmitted transplacentally. It is neurotropic and denervates fetal structures. The most severe features are associated with first-trimester infection and include focal cutaneous ulcerations with scarring, reduction deformity of limbs, microphthalmia, microcephaly, and other central nervous system abnormalities.

Inheritance Patterns Not genetic.

Prognosis Prognosis is dependent on the timing and severity of infection, with most infected infants being asymptomatic. As many as one third of severely infected infants die in the newborn period, however. When only skin scarring is present, the prognosis is good.

Sonography

FINDINGS

1. **Fetus:**
   a. Ascites—Pleural effusion and other features of hydrops may occur.
   b. There may be echogenic foci related to calcification in the liver, heart, or kidneys. These have been found at autopsy in other organs.
   c. Club feet, limb contractures, or shortened limbs may occur.
   d. Decreased fetal motion with a limb fixed in position adjacent to the fetal trunk may be present.
   e. Ventriculomegaly may develop. Echogenic thickening of the lens due to cataract may be seen.
2. **Amniotic Fluid:** Polyhydramnios is common.
3. **Placenta:** Normal.
4. **Measurement Data:** IUGR may occur.
5. **When Detectable:** Three to 12 weeks after maternal exposure. Detection has been reported at 15 weeks' gestation.

Pitfalls Overdiagnosis of calcification or echogenic bowel due to a sonographic system, which enhances echogenicity.

Differential Diagnosis Cytomegalovirus and toxoplasmosis also give intraorgan calcification.

Where Else to Look Look for calcification in all organs. See if all limbs move, since limb adherence to the trunk is a known complication.

Pregnancy Management

Investigations and Consultations Required Maternal viral titers for common viral infections should be performed. Invasive testing should await the results of this testing. Because the sensitivity and specificity of fetal IgM, amniotic fluid culture, and PCR assay of chorionic villi are all unknown, the presence of suggestive sonographic features and evidence of recent maternal infection (clinical and serologic) may be sufficient for a presumptive diagnosis of the congenital varicella syndrome.

Monitoring Sonographic monitoring for the detection of ventriculomegaly is appropriate. Sonographic evidence of central nervous system damage suggests a dismal prognosis, and a nonaggressive approach to pregnancy management and delivery should be discussed with the family.

Pregnancy Course The development of severe hydrocephalus and polyhydramnios has been reported and may complicate delivery management.

Pregnancy Termination Issues The difficulty in establishing a precise diagnosis prenatally may warrant a nondestructive approach to pregnancy termination in those cases without classic sonographic features of the congenital varicella syndrome.

Delivery Those cases without evidence of central nervous system involvement should be managed in standard fashion for uninfected pregnancies. Those fetuses with severe ventriculomegaly are candidates for cephalocentesis and/or no electronic monitoring during pregnancy.

Neonatology

Resuscitation No specific issues.

Transport Referral to a tertiary perinatal center is indicated if the infant is symptomatic or the diagnosis is uncertain.

Testing and Confirmation Anti-varicella-zoster antibodies may persist after birth. Evaluation for central nervous system and ophthalmic involvement is required.

Nursery Management Delineation of extent of organ involvement and supportive care are the principal components of management. Isolation of infants with structural defects secondary to varicella is not necessary, as the virus is not shed. However, such infants may have episodic skin lesions and become infectious while the lesions are acute. Treatment with acyclovir may be considered during such episodes.

REFERENCES

Bale J, Murph J: Congenital infections and the nervous system. Pediatr Neurol 1992;39:669–690.

Chapman SJ: Varicella in pregnancy. Semin Perinatol 1998;22:339–346.

Grose C, Itani O, Weiner C: Prenatal diagnosis of fetal infection: Advances from amniocentesis to cordocentesis—congenital toxoplasmosis, rubella, cytomegalovirus, varicella virus, parvovirus, and human immunodeficiency virus. Pediatr Infect Dis J 1989;8:459–468.

Hartung J, Enders G, Chaoui R, et al: Prenatal diagnosis of congenital varicella syndrome and detection of varicella-zoster virus in the fetus: A case report. Prenat Diagn 1999;19:163–166.

Mouly F, Mirlesse V, Meritet JF, et al: Prenatal diagnosis of fetal varicella-zoster virus infection with polymerase chain reaction of amniotic fluid in 107 cases. Am J Obstet Gynecol 1997;177:894–898.

Paryani SJ, Arvin AM: Intrauterine infection with varicella-zoster virus after maternal varicella. N Engl J Med 1986;314:1542–1546.

Petignat P, Vial Y, Lavrini R, et al: Fetal varicella-herpes zoster syndrome in early pregnancy: Ultrasonographic and morphological correlations. Prenat Diagn 2001;21:121–124.

Pretorius DH, Hayward I, Jones KL, Stamm E: Sonographic evaluation of pregnancies with maternal varicella infection. J Ultrasound Med 1992;11:459–463.

Stagno S, Whitney RJ: Herpesvirus infections of pregnancy. Part II. Herpes simplex virus and varicella-zoster virus infections. N Engl J Med 1985;313:1327–1330.

Williamson AP: The varicella-zoster virus in the etiology of severe congenital defects: A survey of eleven reported instances. Clin Pediatr 1975;14:553–555.

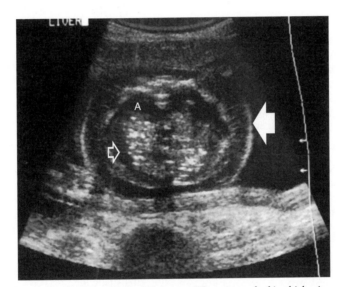

Transverse view of the fetal abdomen. There is much skin thickening (*arrow*). Fetal ascites (A) surrounds the liver (*open arrow*). The liver contains numerous calcific foci.

10 Drugs

10.1 Fetal Alcohol Syndrome

Epidemiology/Genetics

Definition Fetal alcohol syndrome is a characteristic pattern of physical malformations, including growth and mental retardation, seen in the offspring of chronically alcoholic women.

Epidemiology The incidence of fetal alcohol syndrome varies with the population being studied, with estimates ranging from 1 in 1000 to as high as 1 in 100 in some American Indian populations. The risk of a chronically alcoholic mother having a child with fetal alcohol syndrome is between 20 and 40%, but effects on fetal mental development have been reported with exposures of greater than two drinks per day (M1:F1).

Embryology Alcohol and its metabolites easily cross the placenta. Alcohol causes cell death and inhibits cell growth. The diagnostic criteria for fetal alcohol syndrome include prenatal and/or postnatal growth retardation, a characteristic face (midface hypoplasia, epicanthal folds, smooth philtrum with thin upper lip, and ear malformations), and central nervous system involvement. Associated abnormalities include cardiovascular defects (70%), microcephaly (80%), microphthalmia, genitourinary tract malformations (10%), and skeletal abnormalities. Spina bifida and cleft lip/palate have also been reported.

Inheritance Patterns Not genetic.

Prognosis Dependent on the timing and amount of alcohol exposure. The average IQ of children with fetal alcohol syndrome is about 65. In addition to mental retardation, many children have serious behavioral disturbances.

Sonography

FINDINGS

1. **Fetus:** Most fetuses with fetal alcohol syndrome appear sonographically normal. Sonographically visible congenital anomalies include the following:

   a. Cardiac malformations such as ventricular septal defect, atrial septal defect, double-outlet right ventricle, pulmonary atresia, dextrocardia, and tetralogy of Fallot.
   b. Central nervous system anomalies including microcephaly, agenesis of the corpus callosum, and neural tube defects. There is a reduction in frontal cortex size.
   c. Facial abnormalities such as micrognathia, cleft palate and lip, and hypoplastic maxilla.
   d. Truncal and skeletal anomalies including diaphragmatic hernia, pectus excavatum, and cervical vertebral malformations.
   e. Genitourinary malformations such as hypoplastic external genitalia.
2. **Amniotic Fluid:** Oligohydramnios may be seen accompanying intrauterine growth retardation (IUGR).
3. **Placenta:** Normal
4. **Measurement Data:** IUGR is a common feature of this disorder.
5. **When Detectable:** Most features are not detectable until late second trimester, when the findings may be subtle.

Pitfalls This is a syndrome affecting multiple organ systems, and any one anomaly may have alternate causes.

Differential Diagnosis The two features of the fetal alcohol syndrome most likely to cause confusion with other entities are congenital heart defects and intrauterine growth retardation.

Pregnancy Management

Investigations and Consultations Required

1. Chromosomal studies and TORCH (toxoplasmosis, other infections, rubella, cytomegalovirus infection, and herpes simplex) titers should be done.
2. An evaluation for maternal medical disorders, including phenylketonuria, should be done.

3. A history of maternal drug exposure should be obtained.
4. A fetal echocardiogram should be performed.
5. Consultation with a neonatologist is necessary to plan perinatal management.

Monitoring With IUGR, serial sonographic examinations, to monitor growth and appropriate fetal assessment modalities, are the major additions to standard obstetric care.

Pregnancy Course The presence of prenatal growth deficiency in these infants is likely to present as intrauterine growth restriction in the third trimester.

Pregnancy Termination Issues The lack of a precise risk figure for fetal alcohol syndrome makes pregnancy termination a controversial issue. The subtle features of fetal alcohol syndrome are not likely to be seen in a fetus except by a very experienced dysmorphologist.

Delivery Except in circumstances when neonatal withdrawal is likely to be a complication, there is no specific need for delivery in a tertiary center.

Neonatology

Resuscitation There may be a slight increased risk for fetal distress and a low 1-minute Apgar score in fetal alcohol syndrome infants. No special resuscitation measures are required.

Transport Referral to a tertiary center in the neonatal period is indicated only if a major central nervous system or cardiac malformation is present.

Testing and Confirmation Careful assessment for cardiac and or central nervous system malformations is important when fetal alcohol syndrome is suspected and prenatal evaluation has not been done.

Nursery Management An alcohol withdrawal syndrome with tremors, agitation, metabolic acidosis, hypoglycemia, and seizures has been described in newborns who are born to severely alcoholic mothers who are intoxicated at the time of delivery.

REFERENCES

Abel EL: Fetal alcohol effects: Advice to the advisors. Alcohol 1985;20:189–193.
Abel EL, Sokol RJ: Incidence of fetal alcohol syndrome and economic impact of FAS-related anomalies. Drug Alcohol Depend 1987;19:51–70.
Eliason MJ, Williams JK: Fetal alcohol syndrome and the neonate. Perinat Neonatal Nurs 1990;3:64–72.
Ernhart CB, Sokol RJ, Martier S, et al: Alcohol teratogenicity in the human: A detailed assessment of specificity, critical period, and threshold. Am J Obstet Gynecol 1987;156:33–39.
Hannigan JH, Armant DR: Alcohol in pregnancy and neonatal outcome. Semin Neonatol 2000;5:243–254.
Hill RM, Hegemier S, Tennyson LM: The fetal alcohol syndrome: A multihandicapped child. Neurotoxicology 1989;10:585–595.
Johnson VP, Swayze VW, Sato Y, Andreason NC: Fetal alcohol syndrome: Craniofacial and central nervous system manifestations. Am J Med Genet 1996;61:329–339.
Jones KL: Fetal alcohol syndrome. Pediatr Rev 1986;8:122–126.
Koren G, Edwards MB, Miskin M: Antenatal sonography of fetal malformations associated with drugs and chemicals: A guide. Am J Obstet Gynecol 1987;156:79–85.
Little BB, Snell LM, Rosenfeld CR, et al: Failure to recognize fetal alcohol syndrome in newborn infants. Am J Dis Child 1990;144:1142–1146.
Russell M: The impact of alcohol-related birth defects (ARBD) on New York State. Neurobeh Toxicol 1980;2:277.
Streissguth AP, Aase JM, Clarren SK, et al: Fetal alcohol syndrome in adolescents and adults. JAMA 1991;265:1961–1967.
Sulaiman ND, Florey CD, Taylor DJ, Ogston SA: Alcohol consumption in Dundee primigravidas and its effects on outcome of pregnancy. Br Med J 1988;296:1500–1503.
Walpole I, Zubrick S, Pontre J: Confounding variables in studying the effects of maternal alcohol consumption before and during pregnancy. J Epidemiol Community Health 1989;43:153–161.
Wass TS, Persutte WH, Hobbins JC: The impact of prenatal alcohol exposure on the frontal cortex. Am J Obstet Gynecol 2001;185:731–742.
Werler MM, Lammer EJ, Rosenberg L, Mitchell AA: Maternal alcohol use in relation to selected birth defects. Am J Epidemiol 1991;134:691–698.

10.2
Anti-Seizure Drugs (Phenytoin, Carbamazepine, Valproic Acid, and Phenobarbital)

Epidemiology/Genetics

Definition   A variety of medications are used to control seizures, with the four most common being phenytoin (Dilantin), phenobarbital, carbamazepine (Tegretol), and valproic acid (Depakote). These drugs are used either alone or in combination with each other, and each has been implicated as a potential teratogen.

Epidemiology   All epileptic women have an overall two- to threefold increase in the risk for congenital anomalies in their offspring with cleft lip, with or without cleft palate, and cardiovascular abnormalities being most common. A specific syndrome is associated with phenytoin use, consisting of a characteristic facies, microcephaly, digital and nail hypoplasia, and growth and mental delay. A similar phenotype is seen in infants exposed to carbamazepine during pregnancy. In addition, valproic acid and carbamazepine have been associated with a 1% risk for spina bifida. An overall risk for a "fetal anticonvulsant syndrome" may be about 10%.

Embryology   Teratogenicity of several anticonvulsants has been associated with the activity of the enzyme epoxide hydrolase. This enzyme activity is inherited in an autosomal recessive pattern, with homozygotes for decreased activity being at the greatest risk for congenital abnormalities.

Inheritance Patterns   Not genetic.

Prognosis   Over 90% of all women with epilepsy have normal babies. Prognosis is dependent on the type of involvement and the severity of the developmental delays.

Sonography

FINDINGS

1. **Fetus:** Ultrasonographically visible side effects of anticonvulsants include the following:
   a. Central nervous system abnormalities—Microcephaly and, rarely, holoprosencephaly. Myelomeningocele and Arnold-Chiari malformation are seen with valproic acid.
   b. Facial anomalies—Ocular hypertelorism, cleft lip and/or palate, short nose, and broad nasal bridge.
   c. Skeletal malformations—Absence of the radial ray (valproic acid), hypoplasia of the distal phalanges, digitalized thumb, hip dislocation, short webbed neck, and rib or sternal anomalies may occur.
   d. Cardiac anomalies—Ventricular septal defects and pulmonary and aortic valvular stenoses.
   e. Genitourinary abnormalities—Ambiguous genitalia and rare renal malformations.
2. **Amniotic Fluid:** Oligohydramnios may be associated with IUGR.
3. **Placenta:** Normal.
4. **Measurement Data:** Mild to moderate IUGR is a common feature with or without associated antenatally detectable anomalies.
5. **When Detectable:** Most associated anomalies are subtle and not detectable until well into the second trimester.

Pitfalls   Myelomeningocele associated with valproic acid may be small and at a sacral level.

Differential Diagnosis   The two categories of malformation most commonly associated with these medications that will cause a management dilemma are congenital heart defects and neural tube defects. Because of the relatively low incidence of the findings in patients exposed to antiepileptic medications, a careful search for other causes must be made.

Pregnancy Management

Investigations and Consultations Required   Other causes such as chromosome abnormalities should be excluded.

Monitoring   The obstetric management should be based on the specific type of malformation seen. In the absence of structural malformations, standard obstetric care should be performed.

Pregnancy Course   No specific obstetric complications are to be expected, although mild prenatal growth deficiency may be a feature in some cases.

Pregnancy Termination Issues   Pregnancy termination, if chosen, must be done in such a way as to provide an intact fetus. The subtle features that are seen with exposure to these drugs require that a trained dysmorphologist and fetal pathologist evaluate the fetus.

Delivery   In the absence of structural malformations, delivery does not need to occur in a tertiary center. Delivery management of the fetus with a malformation will be as outlined for that specific abnormality.

A small risk of intracranial hemorrhage with fetal hydantoin exposure in the fetus has been reported, thus the recommendation that vitamin K be given early in labor to the mother. Hydantoin is known to depress liver production of vitamin K–dependent coagulation factors.

Neonatology

Resuscitation   No anti-epileptic agent has been reported to produce fetal depression or delay in onset of respirations. As all are teratogenic, the management at birth will be dictated by the specific defect manifested by the infant (see Chapters 2.17, 3.1 through 3.18, and 7.1).

Transport   Referral to a tertiary center is not indicated for antenatal exposure only but is indicated for diagnosis and management of major organ anomalies. Referral to a multidisciplinary program for orofacial abnormalities is indicated for infants having a cleft lip and/or palate.

Nursery Management   If cleft lip and/or palate is present, care is directed toward establishing an appropriate feeding technique and initiating a plan for repair and rehabilitation.

In the case of hydantoin exposure and if intrapartum vitamin K was not given to the mother, it is important that the infant receive it immediately after birth and that close monitoring for intracranial hemorrhage be done.

Once a specific organ defect is identified, care requirements are based on the diagnosis.

Carbamazepine has been associated with postnatal growth failure and developmental delay; therefore, careful monitoring for both should continue through infancy and early childhood.

REFERENCES

Bradai R, Robert E: Prenatal ultrasonographic diagnosis in the epileptic mother on valproic acid: Retrospective study of 161 cases in the central eastern France register of congenital malformations. J Gynecol Obstet Biol Reprod 1998;27:413–419.

Buehler BA, Delimont D, Van Waes M, Finnell RH: Prenatal prediction of risk of the fetal hydantoin syndrome. N Engl J Med 1990; 332:1567–1572.

Hanson JW, Buehler BA: Fetal hydantoin syndrome: Current status. J Pediatr 1982;101:816–818.

Hanson JW, Myrianthopoulos NC, Harvey MA, Smith DW: Risks to the offspring of women treated with hydantoin anticonvulsants, with emphasis on the fetal hydantoin syndrome. J Pediatr 1976;89:662–668.

Jones KL, Lacro RV, Johnson KA, Adams J: Pattern of malformations in the children of women treated with carbamazepine during pregnancy. N Engl J Med 1989;320:1661–1666.

Koren G, Edwards MB, Miskin M: Antenatal sonography of fetal malformations associated with drugs and chemicals: A guide. Am J Obstet Gynecol 1987;156:79–85.

Morrell MJ: Guidelines for the care of women with epilepsy. Neurology 1998;51:S21–27.

Rosa FW: Spina bifida in infants of women treated with carbamazepine during pregnancy. N Engl J Med 1991;324:674–677.

Weinbaum PJ, Cassidy SB, Vintzileos AM, et al: Prenatal detection of a neural tube defect after fetal exposure to valproic acid. Obstet Gynecol 1986;67:31S–37S.

10.3 Illegal Drugs (Cocaine, Heroin)

Epidemiology/Genetics

Definition Cocaine and heroin are commonly abused drugs that are both central nervous system stimulants and local anesthetics. As drugs of abuse, they can be sniffed, injected intravenously, or smoked.

Epidemiology Drug use is dependent on population. Teratogenic effects in exposed fetuses are probably uncommon. Methadone maintenance treatment does not seem to improve pregnancy outcome, as individuals continue with other drug abuse.

Embryology Cocaine and heroin cause a transient rise in maternal blood pressure, placental vasoconstriction, and interruptions of blood flow to the fetus. Vascular hypotension, vascular constriction, and disruption of blood flow has been proposed as a possible mechanism for the teratogenic effects of cocaine and heroin. A small increase in urogenital anomalies, craniofacial defects, cardiovascular abnormalities, and central nervous system disruptions has been reported with exposure. Additional abnormalities have included limb reduction defects, ocular defects, and IUGR. Heroin decreases cell multiplication and is associated with IUGR.

Inheritance Patterns Not genetic.

Prognosis The most significant effects associated with cocaine and heroin use appear to be for adverse pregnancy outcomes and include placental abruption, stillbirth, and premature birth. The exact risk for congenital malformations in a cocaine- or heroin-exposed pregnancy is unknown but is probably low.

Sonography

FINDINGS

1. **Fetus:** Most fetuses are normal. Antenatal sonographic findings in the fetus involve multiple organ systems. The following findings have been reported as associated with illegal drug use. The quality of documentation for these associations is variable:
   a. Central nervous system acquired anomalies include cerebral infarctions or hemorrhage, porencephaly, hydrocephalus, and hydranencephaly. Congenital malformations include microcephaly, midline abnormalities such as agenesis of the corpus callosum, septo-optic dysplasia, schizencephaly, encephalocele, and teratoma.
   b. Genitourinary and cardiac malformations.
   c. Limb reduction abnormalities with limb shortening or amputation.
   d. Intestinal atresia and perforation with meconium peritonitis.
   e. Spontaneous abortion.
   f. Occasional facial anomalies such as cleft palate and lip.
2. **Amniotic Fluid:** IUGR and premature rupture of membranes are often seen in cocaine and heroin abusers, so oligohydramnios may be found.
3. **Placenta:** Placental abruption is more common in cocaine abusers. A hematoma may be seen in a (1) marginal location, (2) retroplacental location, (3) preplacental location, (4) intra-amniotic location, or (5) intraplacental location.
4. **Measurement Data:** Symmetric growth restriction is a common finding.
5. **When Detectable:** Depends on the severity of the anomaly and the frequency of substance abuse.

Pitfalls Multisubstance abuse is common, and the simultaneous use of other drugs such as heroin and cocaine, cigarettes, and alcohol or the presence of congenital infections must always be considered as alternate causes for congenital anomalies.

Pregnancy Management

Investigations and Consultations Required The presence of a structural malformation should prompt chromosomal studies and fetal echocardiography to exclude associated cardiac malformations. Other consultations should be based on the specific malformations detected. The neonatology staff should be made aware of the potential for neonatal withdrawal.

Monitoring No specific change in standard obstetric care is required, unless IUGR complicates the pregnancy. Pregnancy management should be coordinated by a perinatologist.

Pregnancy Course The increased risk of placental abruption in patients using cocaine may be the major risk to fetal well-being. Intrauterine growth restriction also occurs more commonly in these patients.

Pregnancy Termination Issues Should pregnancy termination be chosen because of a fetal malformation, delivery of an intact fetus is essential to establish a precise diagnosis.

Delivery The significant risk associated with maternal and neonatal withdrawal requires that delivery occur in a tertiary center.

Neonatology

Resuscitation An increased incidence of fetal distress is associated with maternal cocaine use precipitating preterm labor and placental abruption. No special resuscitative measures are required, although acute volume expansion may be needed if there is an abruption.

Transport Referral to a tertiary center is required for management of problems associated with prematurity or structural defects resulting from vascular disruptions.

Nursery Management The gestational age at delivery and the presence of anomalies resulting from vascular disruptions determine the neonatal management problems and care needed.

There appears to be an increased risk for early-onset necrotizing enterocolitis in larger infants with maternal cocaine exposure.

REFERENCES

Brown HL, Britton KA, Mahaffey D, et al: Methadone maintenance in pregnancy: A reappraisal. Am J Obstet Gynecol 1998;179:459–463.

Chasnoff IJ, Burns WJ, Schnoll SH, Burns KA: Cocaine use in pregnancy. N Engl J Med 1985;313:666–669.

Chavez GF, Mulinare J, Cordero JF: Maternal cocaine use during early pregnancy as a risk factor for congenital urogenital anomalies. JAMA 1989;262:795–798.

Cohen HL, Sloves JH, Laungani S, et al: Neurosonographic findings in full-term infants born to maternal cocaine abusers: Visualization of subependymal and periventricular cysts. J Clin Ultrasound 1994;22:327–333.

Dominguez R, Aguirre Vila-Coro A, Slopis JM, Bohan TP: Brain and ocular abnormalities in infants with in utero exposure to cocaine and other street drugs. Am J Dis Child 1991;145:688–695.

Frank DA, McCarten KM, Robson CD, et al: Levels of in utero cocaine exposure and neonatal ultrasound findings. Pediatrics 1999;104:1101–1105.

Hall TR, Zaninovic A, Lewin D, et al: Neonatal intestinal ischemia with bowel perforation: An in utero complication of maternal cocaine abuse. Am J Roentgenol 1992;158:1303–1304.

Heier LA, Carpanzano CR, Mast J, et al: Maternal cocaine abuse: The spectrum of radiologic abnormalities in the neonatal CNS. Am J Neuroradiol 1991;12:951–956.

Hollingsworth DR: Drugs and reproduction: Maternal and fetal risks. In Hollingsworth DR, Resnik R (eds): Medical Counseling Before Pregnancy. New York, Churchill Livingston, 1988, pp 59–63.

Hoyme HE, Jones KL, Dixon SD, et al: Prenatal cocaine exposure and fetal vascular disruption. Pediatrics 1990;85:743–747.

Malanga CJ, Kosofsky BE: Mechanisms of drugs of abuse on the developing fetal brain. Clin Perinatol 1999;26:17–37.

Viscarello RR, Ferguson DD, Nores J, Hobbins JC: Limb-body wall complex associated with cocaine abuse: Further evidence of cocaine's teratogenicity. Obstet Gynecol 1992;80:523–526.

Volpe JJ: Effect of cocaine use on the fetus. N Engl J Med 1992;327:399–407.

Wagner CL, Katikaneni LD, Cox TH, Ryan RM: The impact of prenatal drug exposure on the neonate. Obstet Gynecol Clin North Am 1998;25:169–194.

11

Syndromes

11.1 Beckwith-Wiedemann Syndrome

Epidemiology/Genetics

Definition Beckwith-Wiedemann syndrome is a somatic overgrowth syndrome characterized by macrosomia, macroglossia, and visceromegaly.

Epidemiology One in 15,000 births (M1:F1).

Embryology Rare cases showing small chromosome duplications have localized the critical region for this disorder to chromosome 11p15. Insulin-like growth factor II is a candidate gene in the genesis of this condition. Ventral wall defects including omphalocele, diastasis recti, and umbilical hernia (80%) and congenital heart defects (6.5%) are the most common major malformations. Additional clinical findings include neonatal hypoglycemia, ear pits or creases, hemihypertrophy, Wilms tumor (6%), neuroblastoma, and hepatoblastoma.

Inheritance Patterns Complex. Most cases are sporadic, but some families have shown autosomal dominant inheritance with variable expressivity and decreased penetrance. A preponderance of females identified as transmitting parents suggests that genomic imprinting is occurring. Careful examination of parents and genetic counseling are recommended to provide accurate recurrence risk.

Teratogens None.

Prognosis Good, with successful surgical repair of omphaloceles and control of neonatal hypoglycemia. Some children require tracheostomy because of macroglossia until surgical tongue reduction can be achieved. Intelligence is generally within the normal range, but learning disabilities are increased. Presence of hemihypertrophy is a risk factor for tumor development.

Sonography

FINDINGS

1. **Fetus:**
   a. Omphalocele or ventral hernia is a common but not universal finding.
   b. Macroglossia is present in almost all cases. The tongue is constantly protruded beyond the lips on profile views.
   c. There is enlargement and increased echogenicity of the kidneys. The kidneys measure over the 90th percentile for length.
   d. A markedly enlarged liver and spleen may occupy most of the abdomen.
   e. Cardiomegaly may be present.
2. **Amniotic Fluid:** Severe polyhydramnios is usual.
3. **Placenta:** Placental enlargement with cysts within the placenta is often present.
4. **Measurement Data:** Macrosomia occurring in the second or third trimester is usual.
5. **When Detectable:** If an omphalocele is present, detection is possible from 12 weeks' gestation on. In the absence of an omphalocele, the syndrome may not be detectable until the late second trimester.

Pitfalls Do not mistake a mass such as a hemangioma for a persistently protruded tongue.

Differential Diagnosis

1. Macrosomia with maternal diabetes, but macroglossia is not present.
2. Down syndrome—Some cases present with macroglossia, but there are usually other features such as short humerus and femur and echogenic focus in the heart. Most fetuses with Down syndrome are of normal size or large.
3. With congenital hypothyroidism, there may also be an omphalocele; however, the thyroid will most likely be enlarged.
4. Facial masses may be mistaken for the tongue, such as neurofibroma, hemangioma, and lymphangioma.
5. Simpson-Golabi-Behnel syndrome.
6. Sotos syndrome.
7. Weaver syndrome.

Where Else to Look Measure the size of internal organs, which will be enlarged. Tumors of the liver and kidneys detected in utero have not been reported but should be sought.

Pregnancy Management

Investigations and Consultations Required The most likely feature to be detected by ultrasonography is omphalocele. Therefore, chromosomal studies and fetal echocardiography should be performed to exclude other causes for the omphalocele. A pediatric surgeon and neonatologist should be consulted to discuss the immediate neonatal management of the infant.

Fetal Intervention None is available.

Monitoring Third trimester sonographic evaluations should be performed to assess fetal weight. To prevent the complications of extreme macrosomia, assessment of lung maturity and induction of labor may be appropriate in some situations.

Pregnancy Course The third trimester may be complicated by polyhydramnios and preterm labor. Aggressive therapy for preterm labor is appropriate to allow time for fetal lung maturity.

Pregnancy Termination Issues The subtle features of the Beckwith-Wiedemann syndrome would require an intact fetus to establish a precise diagnosis.

Delivery The significant neonatal complications in this disorder require delivery in a tertiary center. The obstetrician should be prepared for the possible complications of macrosomia, especially shoulder dystocia.

Neonatology

Resuscitation Most newborns with this disorder do not require intervention for the onset of breathing, although respiratory distress may be noted in association with preterm delivery as a consequence of polyhydramnios, which occurs frequently. On occasion, the macroglossia can be severe enough to compromise the airway. Oral intubation may be difficult. Use of a nasal trumpet airway is an alternative. The co-occurrence of major cardiothoracic anomalies may also complicate early adaptation. Management of an omphalocele, if present, consists of avoiding gastric distension and encasing the lower body in a sterile plastic bag. A bowel bag helps to prevent evaporative heat and water loss and to protect the omphalocele sac and its contents.

Transport Transfer to a tertiary center with pediatric surgery capability is necessary if there is an omphalocele and/or airway compromise. It is recommended to confirm diagnosis, manage the almost universal hypoglycemia, and establish the multidisciplinary follow-up usually required.

Testing and Confirmation Careful physical examination combined with diagnostic imaging form the primary methods of diagnosis. Chromosomal karyotyping is indicated, if not done prenatally, as is careful assessment of the parents to facilitate further genetic counseling.

Nursery Management In addition to the unique management requirements for surgical repair of an omphalocele, management of hyperinsulinemic hypoglycemia, which can be severe and prolonged, and stabilization of the airway are the two major issues. Suckle feeding can be compromised by the macroglossia, necessitating alternative feeding methods in some cases. Because there is a significant association of embryonally derived neoplasia, a thorough search for such is essential. The most frequently reported site is renal, but hepatic and adrenal tumors have also been seen.

REFERENCES

DeBaun MR, Tucker MA: Risk of cancer during the first four years of life in children from the Beckwith-Wiedemann syndrome registry. J Pediatr 1998;132:398–400.

Elliott M, Bayly R, Cole T, et al: Clinical features and natural history of Beckwith-Wiedemann syndrome: Presentation of 74 new cases. Clin Genet 1994;46:168–174.

Harker CP, Winter T III, Mack L: Prenatal diagnosis of Beckwith-Wiedemann syndrome. Am J Roentgenol 1997;168:520–522.

Hewitt B, Bankier A: Prenatal ultrasound diagnosis of Beckwith-Wiedemann syndrome. Aust N Z J Obstet Gynaecol 1994;34:488–490.

Lenke RR, Schmidt EK: Diagnosis of Beckwith-Wiedemann syndrome in the second trimester of pregnancy. J Reprod Med 1986;31:514.

Lodeiro JG, Byers JW III, Chuipek S, Feinstein SJ: Prenatal diagnosis and perinatal management of the Beckwith-Wiedemann syndrome: A case and review. Am J Perinatol 1989;6:446–449.

McCowan LME, Becroft DMO: Beckwith-Wiedemann syndrome, placental abnormalities, and gestational proteinuric hypertension. Obstet Gynecol 1994;83:813–817.

Nowotny T, Bollmann R, Pfeifer L, Windt E: Beckwith-Wiedemann syndrome: Difficulties with prenatal diagnosis. Fetal Diagn Ther 1994;9:256–260.

Orozco-Florian R, McBride JA, Favara BE, et al: Congenital hepatoblastoma and Beckwith-Wiedemann Syndrome: A case study including DNA ploidy profiles of tumor and adrenal cytomegaly. Pediatr Pathol 1991;11:131.

Pettenati MJ, Haines JL, Higgins RR, et al: Wiedemann-Beckwith syndrome: Presentation of clinical and cytogenetic data on 22 new cases and review of the literature. Hum Genet 1986;74:143.

Ranzini AC, Day-Salvatore D, Turner T, et al: Intrauterine growth and ultrasound findings in fetuses with Beckwith-Wiedemann syndrome. Obstet Gynecol 1997;89:538–542.

Sotelo-Avila C, Gonzalez-Crussi F, Fowler JW: Complete and incomplete forms of Beckwith-Wiedemann syndrome: Their oncogenic potential. J Pediatr 1980;96:47.

Sotelo-Avila C, Singer DB: Syndrome of hyperplastic fetal visceromegaly and neonatal hypoglycemia (Beckwith's syndrome): A report of seven cases. Pediatrics 1970;46:240.

Weissman A, Mashiach S, Achiron R: Macroglossia: Prenatal ultrasonographic diagnosis and proposed management. Prenat Diagn 1995;15:66–69.

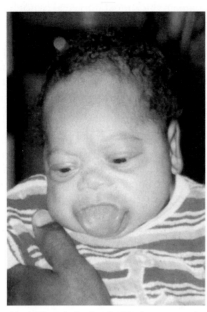

A 9-month-old child with Beckwith-Wiedemann syndrome showing macroglossia.

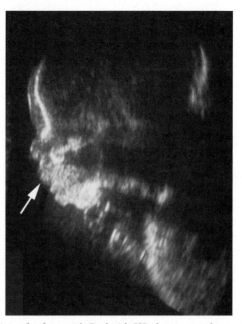

Profile view of a fetus with Beckwith-Wiedemann syndrome showing tongue (*arrow*) protruding beyond the lips. (Courtesy of Sheila Sheth, MD, Johns Hopkins Medical Institutions.)

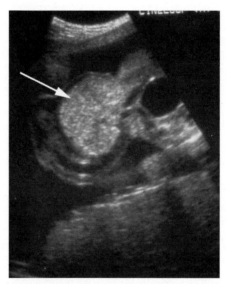

Liver-containing omphalocele (*arrow*) associated with Beckwith-Wiedemann syndrome, surrounded by umbilical cord. (Courtesy of Sheila Sheth, MD, Johns Hopkins Medical Institutions.)

11.2 Deletion 22q11.2 Syndrome (DiGeorge Syndrome, Velocardiofacial Syndrome, Shprintzen Syndrome)

Epidemiology/Genetics

Definition Deletion of chromosome 22q11.2 is now recognized as the cause for the condition of the majority of patients previously described as having the DiGeorge, velocardiofacial syndromes, and conotruncal anomalies face syndromes. Common features include cardiac malformations (70%), cleft palate or velopharyngeal insufficiency (48%), neonatal hypocalcemia (63%), thymic hypoplasia (65%), dysmorphic face (95%), and mental retardation (50%).

Epidemiology At least 1 in 2500 (M1:F1). Women are more likely to be identified as affected parents in familial cases, although the reason for this is not clear. The severity in males and females appears to be similar.

Embryology The conotruncal outflow tract of the heart, the thymus, and the parathyroid glands are all derived from neural crest cells that have migrated from the developing neural tube in the first month of development. This suggests involvement of this early cell population in the genesis of this syndrome. Deletion 22q11.2 was found in 50% of children with interrupted aortic arch, 35% of children with truncus arteriosus, and 16% of children with tetralogy of Fallot. No cases of transposition of the great vessels in one study have had deletion 22q11.2. It is commonly found in children with isolated cleft palate or velopharyngeal insufficiency with development delays.

Inheritance Patterns Chromosome microdeletion showing autosomal dominant inheritance, with the majority of cases being new mutations. Because of only mild to moderate developmental disabilities, however, affected parents are found in 10 to 15% of cases and are at 50% risk of having affected offspring.

Teratogens None.

Prognosis Significant neonatal morbidity and mortality related to the cardiac defects and sequelae of the immunodeficiency. Extensive cardiac and cleft palate surgery may be needed depending on associated malformations. Thereafter, the mild to moderate mental retardation is the most disabling feature. Although 50% of patients have IQs above 70, they all have significant cognitive impairment compared with other members of their families. Ten to 15% of adults are diagnosed with psychiatric illness, with one third of those individuals having had at least one episode of psychosis.

Sonography

FINDINGS

1. **Fetus:**
   a. Conotruncal abnormalities such as tetralogy of Fallot, truncus arteriosus, and interrupted aortic arch.
   b. Facial abnormalities include micrognathia and facial clefts.
   c. Renal obstruction with hydronephrosis or multicystic dysplastic kidney disease is sometimes present. In some instances, the hydronephrosis is due to a ureterocele.
   d. Thymic disorders. The thymus may be absent. Cystic replacement of the thymus has been seen.
   e. There may be a diaphragmatic hernia.
2. **Amniotic Fluid:** Polyhydramnios is often present.
3. **Placenta:** Normal.
4. **Measurements Data:**
   a. Microcephaly may be present.
   b. There are often shortened long bones, particularly the femur and humerus.
5. **When Detectable:** The cardiac abnormalities can be detected at about 16 weeks' gestation.

Differential Diagnosis

1. The combination of cardiac and limb abnormalities may suggest thrombocytopenia-absent radius syndrome or Holt-Oram syndrome.
2. Short limbs with a cardiac defect raise the question of Down syndrome.

Where Else to Look The presence of a conotruncal cardiac abnormality is an indication for a thorough survey of the entire fetus. Additional abnormalities would make chromosomal analysis for deletion 22 important.

Pregnancy Management

Investigations and Consultations Required The presence of any conotruncal abnormality and/or cleft palate detected in utero should prompt chromosome evaluation to include karyotype and fluorescent in situ hybridization studies for the 22q11.2 deletion. Fetal blood sampling to assess fetal T-cell function can be performed to assess immune function. Because of the significant risk of neonatal complications, consultation with a neonatologist is essential. Other consultations will depend on what other structural malformations are present.

Fetal Intervention This multisystem disorder is not amenable to in utero therapy.

Monitoring   Polyhydramnios is a frequent complication, and both clinical and sonographic assessment of amniotic fluid volume should be done regularly. Significant polyhydramnios may result in preterm labor.

Pregnancy Course   Generally unremarkable unless complicated by polyhydramnios.

Pregnancy Termination Issues   If a cytogenetic diagnosis has been established, there are no special autopsy requirements.

Delivery   The site of delivery must be a tertiary center where the multiple neonatal complications can be managed.

Neonatology

Resuscitation   In general, management of the onset of respiration and need for assistance is influenced by the nature of the associated cardiac defect. If a ductus dependent lesion has been identified or is suspected, oxygen supplementation may be limited to 40 to 60% while oxygen saturation is monitored to avoid hyperoxemia. Immediate infusion of prostaglandin E_1 should be instituted. Other abnormalities affecting onset of respiration include orofacial clefts, Pierre Robin variants, and diaphragmatic hernia, although these are infrequent in occurrence, except with the velocardiofacial syndrome within this complex of anomalies.

Transport   Immediate transport to a tertiary center with pediatric cardiac diagnostic and surgical capabilities is essential. During transport, the infusion of prostaglandin E_1 should be maintained. Because apnea is a frequent side effect of prostaglandin infusion, intubation and assisted ventilation during transport may be necessary. Supplemental oxygen should be limited to that necessary to maintain an acceptable oxygen saturation.

Testing and Confirmation   The complete delineation of the cardiac defect is accomplished by echocardiography in the majority of cases. Cardiac catheterization may be indicated if early surgical intervention is required. Additional laboratory testing should include serum calcium concentrations on a frequent basis, quantification of the T lymphocytes, and high-resolution chromosomal studies, if not obtained prenatally.

Nursery Management   The specific defects present will dictate the direction of care. The key issues are airway adequacy, hemodynamic stability and oxygen delivery, and identification of concomitant problems such as immunodeficiency and hypocalcemia. Seizures from the hypocalcemia may manifest in the absence of careful monitoring and maintenance of adequate serum calcium concentrations. All blood for transfusion should be irradiated prior to transfusion until there is evidence of T-cell sufficiency to avoid the risks of graft-versus-host reactions.

REFERENCES

Conley ME, Beckwith JB, Mancer JFK, Tenckhoff L: The spectrum of the DiGeorge syndrome. J Pediatr 1979;94:883.

Davidson A, Khandelwal M, Punnett HH: Prenatal diagnosis of the 22q11 deletion syndrome. Prenat Diagn 1997;17:380–383.

DeVriendt K, van Schouboeck D, Eyskens B, et al: Polyhydramnios as a prenatal symptom of the DiGeorge/Velo-cardio-facial syndrome. Prenat Diagn 1998;18:68–72.

Goldmuntz E, Clark BJ, Mitchell LE, et al: Frequency of 22q11 deletions in patients with conotruncal defects. J Am Coll Cardiol 1998;32:492–498.

Goodship J, Cross I, LiLing J, Wren C: A population study of chromosome 22q11 deletions in infancy. Arch Dis Child 1998;79:348.

Goodship J, Robson SC, Sturgiss S, et al: Renal abnormalities on obstetric ultrasound as a presentation of DiGeorge syndrome. Prenat Diagn 1997;17:867–870.

Leana-Cox J, Pangkanon S, Eanet KR, et al: Familial DiGeorge/velocardiofacial syndrome with deletions of chromosome area 22q11.2: Report of five families with a review of the literature. Am J Med Genet 1996;65:309–316.

Mehraein Y, Wippermann C-F, Michel-Behnke I, et al: Microdeletion 22q11 in complex cardiovascular malformations. Hum Genet 1997;99:433.

Ryan AK, Goodship JA, Wilson DI, et al: Spectrum of clinical features associated with interstitial chromosome 22q11 deletions: A European collaborative study. J Med Genet 1997;34:798–804.

Thomas JA, Graham JM Jr: Chromosomes 22q11 deletion syndrome: An update and review for the primary pediatrician. Clin Pediatr (Phila) 1997;36:253–266.

Van Hemel JO, Schaap C, Van Opstal D, et al: Recurrence of DiGeorge syndrome: Prenatal detection by FISH of a molecular 22q11 deletion. J Med Genet 1995;32:657.

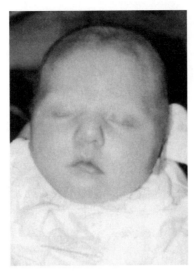

A 6-month-old infant with deletion 22q11.2 syndrome and interrupted aortic arch, type B. Note the downslanting palpebral fissures and prominent nose.

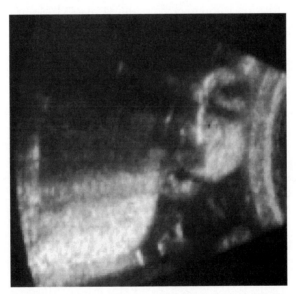

Facial sonogram of a 23-week fetus with deletion 22q11.2 syndrome, with interrupted aortic arch showing typical facies.

11.3 Fryns Syndrome

Epidemiology

Definition Autosomal recessive genetic condition characterized by diaphragmatic hernia or defects and other malformations with high lethality.

Epidemiology Rare, with an estimated incidence of 0.7 in 10,000 births.

Embryology In addition to diaphragmatic hernia or defects, which occur in 90% of cases, other common abnormalities include central nervous system malformations (Dandy-Walker malformation, agenesis of corpus callosum; 50%), cystic kidneys (55%), microretrognathia (92%), genitourinary abnormalities (86%), distal digital hypoplasia (100%), and cleft lip with or without cleft palate (70%). There are two reports of Fryns syndrome presenting antenatally with cystic hygroma.

Inheritance Patterns Autosomal recessive with a 25% recurrence risk in future pregnancies. The gene responsible for the disorder has not yet been identified.

Teratogens None.

Prognosis Poor, with most cases ending in stillbirth or early neonatal death due to pulmonary hypoplasia. Rare survivors without diaphragmatic involvement have all had mental retardation.

Sonography

FINDINGS

1. **Fetal:**
   a. Nuchal thickening has been found at 11 to 14 weeks' gestation. Cystic hygromas have also been described.
   b. A diaphragmatic hernia is a feature seen in most but not all cases.
   c. Facial changes include micrognathia, broad nasal bridge, cleft lip and palate, abnormal ear shape, and occasionally microphthalmia.
   d. Cranial changes include Dandy-Walker malformation, agenesis of the corpus callosum, and ventriculomegaly.
   e. Genitourinary abnormalities include renal cysts, uterine abnormalities, cryptorchidism, and hypospadias.
   f. Limb abnormalities, including club feet and absent digits, are sometimes found.
2. **Amniotic Fluid:** Polyhydramnios is usual.

3. **Placenta:** Normal.
4. **Measurement Data:** There may be a small abdominal circumference, since some stomach contents are in the chest in the diaphragmatic hernia.
5. **When Detectable:** Detection at 12 weeks' gestation on the basis of the nuchal thickening has been reported. Diagnosis at 20 weeks from the diaphragmatic hernia and other abnormalities is possible.

Differential Diagnosis Includes syndromes with diaphragmatic hernia such as trisomy 18, chromosome 4p- (Wolf-Hirschhorn) syndrome, tetrasomy 12p (Pallister-Killian) syndrome, Simpson-Golabi-Behmel syndrome, Cornelia de Lange syndrome, and lethal multiple pterygium syndrome. Also includes other multiple malformation syndromes with brain and genital abnormalities, such as the Walker-Warburg syndrome and Smith-Lemli-Opitz syndrome.

Where Else to Look Cardiac abnormalities have occasionally been reported.

Pregnancy Management

Investigations and Consultations Required This syndrome is most likely to be detected because of the sonographic finding of diaphragmatic hernia and will generally be a diagnosis of exclusion. Therefore, chromosomal studies and fetal echocardiography are essential to exclude other conditions. It is especially important that the chromosomal studies be done on amniotic fluid, not fetal blood, and that fluorescent in situ hybridization be done on uncultured cells to exclude the Pallister-Killian syndrome (iso-12p).

Fetal Intervention Because of the lethality of the condition, in utero repair should not be considered in cases of diaphragmatic hernia if there are limb or renal abnormalities suggestive of Fryns syndrome.

Monitoring No additional monitoring other than routine obstetric care is indicated.

Pregnancy Course Usually uncomplicated, unless polyhydramnios develops secondary to the diaphragmatic hernia.

Pregnancy Termination Issues The subtle physical features seen in Fryns syndrome make labor induction the best alternative, if a precise diagnosis is to be made.

Delivery A precise prospective diagnosis is unlikely before birth. Therefore, standard obstetric care is indicated, including appropriate fetal surveillance.

Neonatology

Resuscitation A full discussion with the parents about the limited prognosis for fetuses with this syndrome is essential prior to delivery. The decision to attempt resuscitation should be based on the spectrum of organ malformations present, since the majority of infants reported in the literature have not survived the neonatal period. The absence of a diaphragmatic hernia or diaphragmatic abnormality seems to improve survival potential; however, significant neuroanatomic abnormalities have been reported in the survivors, with a high incidence of mental retardation. A decision for limited or no support following delivery is an option, particularly with evidence of severe diaphragmatic abnormality and other serious organ system malformations.

Transport If there is uncertainty about the survivability of the infant, transport by an experienced neonatal transport team to a tertiary center with multiple pediatric medical and surgical subspecialists and neonatal intensive care capabilities is indicated for diagnostic evaluation to facilitate the decisions concerning surgical intervention and long-term support.

Testing and Confirmation Careful physical examination will identify the characteristic facial features and limb abnormalities, and diagnostic imaging—echocardiography and cranial ultrasonography—will delineate the most significant other organ system malformations. Magnetic resonance imaging is the preferred technique for evaluation of intracranial malformations but must be deferred until the clinical course is stable.

Nursery Management Full ventilatory support from birth is required if diaphragmatic hernia is present. Often the accompanying pulmonary hypoplasia is the predominant factor dictating clinical management (see Chapter 5.2). If a cardiac malformation is also present, the management is further modified as needed for the specific abnormality.

REFERENCES

Cunniff C, Jones KL, Saal HM, Stern HJ: Fryns syndrome: An autosomal recessive disorder associated with craniofacial anomalies, diaphragmatic hernia, and distal digital hypoplasia. Pediatrics 1990;85:499–504.

Enns GM, Cox VA, Goldstein RB, et al: Congenital diaphragmatic defects and associated syndromes, malformations, and chromosome anomalies: A retrospective study of 60 patients and literature review. Am J Med Genet 1998;79:215–225.

Fryns JP: Fryns syndrome: A variable MCA syndrome with diaphragmatic defects, coarse face, and distal limb hypoplasia. J Med Genet 1987;24:271.

Fryns JP, Moerman F, Goddeeris P, et al: A new lethal syndrome with cloudy corneae, diaphragmatic defects and distal limb deformities. Hum Genet 1979;50:65.

Hosli IM, Tercanli S, Rehder H, Holzgreve W: Cystic hygroma as an early first-trimester ultrasound marker for recurrent Fryns' syndrome. Ultrasound Obstet Gynecol 1997;10:422–424.

Moerman P, Fryns JP, Vandenberghe K, et al: The syndrome of diaphragmatic hernia, abnormal face and distal limb anomalies (Fryns syndrome): Report of two sibs with further delineation of the multiple congenital anomaly (MCA) syndrome. Am J Med Genet 1988;31:805.

Samueloff A, Navot D, Birkenfeld A, Schenker JG: Fryns syndrome: A predictable, lethal pattern of multiple congenital anomalies. Am J Obstet Gynecol 1987;156:86–88.

Sheffield JS, Twickler DM, Timmons C, et al: Fryns syndrome: Prenatal diagnosis and pathologic correlation. J Ultrasound Med 1998;17:585–589.

Van Hove JLK, Spiridigliozzi GA, Heinz R, et al: Fryns syndrome survivors and neurologic outcome. Am J Med Genet 1995;59:334.

11.4 Meckel-Gruber Syndrome (Dysencephalia Splanchnocystica)

Epidemiology/Genetics

Definition Autosomal recessive genetic syndrome characterized by an occipital encephalocele (63%), polydactyly (55%), and cystic dysplasia of the kidneys (100%).

Epidemiology Rare (<1/100,000) with an increased incidence in the Finnish population (1/9000) (M1:F1).

Embryology Other features include microcephaly, Dandy-Walker cyst, hydrocephalus, microphthalmia, cleft lip with or without cleft palate, and genital abnormalities.

Inheritance Patterns Autosomal recessive with a 25% recurrence risk in future pregnancies. The gene has been mapped to chromosome 17q22-23 but has not yet been identified.

Teratogens None.

Prognosis Only rare survival of more than a few days or weeks.

Sonography

FINDINGS

1. **Fetus:**
   a. An occipital encephalocele is present in most cases (80%). The encephalocele varies greatly in size and can be very small.
   b. Postaxial polydactyly is present in 75% of cases but is often difficult to see because of the oligohydramnios.
   c. Cystic dysplasia of the kidneys is the most constant finding. The cysts can be discrete and readily visible or too small to see, resulting in enlarged echogenic kidneys. The bladder may be absent.
   d. Microcephaly is a consistent finding even if the encephalocele only contains fluid and despite the usual presence of ventriculomegaly.
   e. Other cranial findings that may be seen include cerebellar hypoplasia with Dandy-Walker abnormalities, Arnold-Chiari malformation, and agenesis of the corpus callosum.
   f. Facial features that may be present include microphthalmia, micrognathia, and cleft lip and/or palate (30%).
   g. Heart defects are occasionally seen.
   h. Cryptorchidism and hypoplastic genitalia may be present.
   i. Bilateral club feet are commonplace.
   j. An enlarged liver due to hepatic fibrosis may be seen.

2. **Amniotic Fluid:** Oligohydramnios is usual but not invariable secondary to the renal dysplasia. It can occur as early as 14 weeks' gestation.
3. **Placenta:** Normal.
4. **Measurement Data:** A small head size is usual, but there is an enlarged abdomen due to the renal enlargement.
5. **When Detectable:** At about 12 weeks' gestation.

Pitfalls

1. The encephalocele may be attached to the brain by a small stalk. It can be very small and may only be intermittently visible.
2. Oligohydramnios makes the polydactyly very difficult to see.
3. The renal appearance is highly variable. In some instances dysplastic large cysts are obvious, but in others the kidneys are overall enlarged and echogenic.

Differential Diagnosis

1. Trisomy 13, trisomy 18, and other syndromes with encephalocele and cystic renal dysplasia.
2. Infantile polycystic kidney disease, but encephalocele and polydactyly are absent.
3. Isolated encephalocele—These can be frontal or parietal rather than occipital and normally have a larger base than Meckel-Gruber encephaloceles. They may be due to amniotic band syndrome.
4. Cystic hygroma—These usually have internal septa and form an obtuse angle with the skull as opposed to the acute angle formed by an encephalocele.
5. Walker-Warburg syndrome—This syndrome features occipital encephalocele, lissencephaly, cerebellar abnormalities such as hypoplasia or Dandy-Walker, and eye abnormalities including microphthalmia and cataract.
6. Trisomy 13—Holoprosencephaly rather than encephalocele is the usual cranial finding in trisomy 13. The kidneys are smaller and contain fewer cysts than in Meckel-Gruber syndrome.

Where Else to Look This syndrome involves almost every organ in the body, so a comprehensive survey should be undertaken.

Pregnancy Management

Investigations and Consultations Required Chromosomal studies should be done to exclude trisomy 13. If continuation of the pregnancy is being considered, a consultation with a neonatologist is appropriate to develop a plan for management for the infant following delivery.

Fetal Intervention   Not applicable to this lethal condition.

Monitoring   Maternal status should be monitored in standard fashion. Fetal evaluation is not appropriate because emergency intervention is not indicated.

Pregnancy Course   Renal malformations may result in oligohydramnios, and if monitoring is used in labor, severe fetal heart rate deceleration may be seen. Therefore, fetal monitoring in labor is not recommended.

Pregnancy Termination Issues   Unless the features are classic for Meckel-Gruber syndrome, delivery of an intact fetus may be necessary to establish a precise diagnosis.

Delivery   Electronic fetal monitoring and cesarean section should be avoided unless requested by the family after a thorough discussion of the prognosis for infants with the Meckel-Gruber syndrome.

Neonatology

Resuscitation   The reported prognosis is uniformly lethal, with the majority of perinatal deaths occurring before delivery. Neonatal resuscitation with a known prenatal diagnosis is not indicated. When the birth of an involved infant is unexpected and resuscitation is initiated, the result is minimal prolongation of survival. The accompanying pulmonary hypoplasia associated with absent fetal renal function and/or central nervous system abnormalities limit the response to resuscitation.

Transport   Indicated only if diagnostic confirmation and counseling are not available locally.

Testing and Confirmation   The presence of an extracranial occipital mass, cystic dysplasia of the kidneys, and pan-polydactyly are the classic findings of Meckel-Gruber syndrome. Other intracranial malformations may occur, and in a limited number of cases polydactyly is absent. The concomitant occurrence of multiple organ systems abnormalities is frequent. Diagnostic imaging (sonography, magnetic resonance imaging) will elucidate the characteristics of the major organ abnormalities.

Nursery Management   Care is usually limited to provision of warmth, hygiene, and comfort once the diagnosis is confirmed. Support for parental grieving and genetic counseling for future pregnancies is essential.

REFERENCES

Agdab-Barmada M, Claassen D: A distinctive triad of malformations of the central nervous system in the Meckel-Gruber syndrome. J Neuropathol Exp Neurol 1990;49:610.

Braithwaite JM, Economides DL: First-trimester diagnosis of Meckel-Gruber syndrome by transabdominal sonography in a low-risk case. Prenat Diagn 1995;15:1168–1170.

Budorick NE, Pretorius DH, McGahan JP, et al: Cephalocele detection in utero: Sonographic and clinical features. Ultrasound Obstet Gynecol 1995;5:77.

Farag TI, Usha R, Uma R, et al: Phenotypic variability in Meckel-Gruber syndrome. Clin Genet 1990;38:176.

Maynor CH, Hertzberg BS, Ellington KS: Antenatal sonographic features of Walker-Warburg syndrome: Value of endovaginal sonography. J Ultrasound Med 1992;11:301–303.

Nyberg DA, Hallesy D, Mahony BS, et al: Meckel-Gruber syndrome: Importance of prenatal diagnosis. J Ultrasound Med 1990;9:691–696.

Paavola P, Salonen R, Baumer A, et al: Clinical and genetic heterogeneity in Meckel syndrome. Hum Genet 1997;101:88.

Salonen R: The Meckel syndrome: Clinicopathological finding in 67 patients. Am J Med Genet 1984;18:671–689.

Salonen R, Norio R: The Meckel syndrome in Finland: Epidemiologic and genetic aspects. Am J Med Genet 1984;18:691–698.

Saw PD, Rouse GA, DeLange M: Meckel syndrome: Sonographic findings. J Diagn Med Sonogr 1991;7:8–11.

Sepulveda W, Sebire NJ, Souka A, et al: Diagnosis of the Meckel-Gruber syndrome at eleven to fourteen weeks' gestation. Am J Obstet Gynecol 1997;176:316–319.

Wapner RJ, Kurtz AB, Ross RD, Jackson LG: Ultrasonographic parameters in the prenatal diagnosis of Meckel syndrome. Obstet Gynecol 1981;57:388–392.

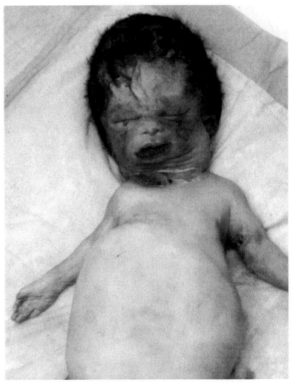

A 38-week stillborn with Meckel-Gruber syndrome. Note abdominal distension from polycystic kidneys. Small posterior encephalocele is not seen.

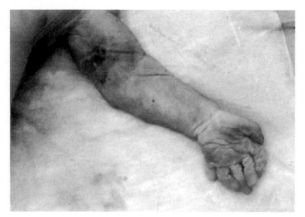

Left hand of a 38-week stillborn with Meckel-Gruber syndrome with postaxial polydactyly.

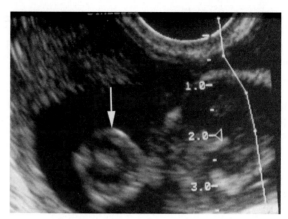

Occipital encephalocele (*arrow*) in a 13-week fetus with Meckel-Gruber syndrome (endovaginal view).

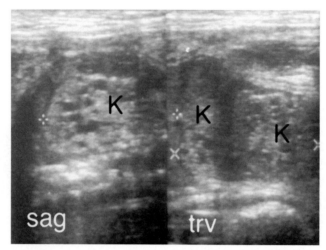

Sagittal (sag) and transverse (trv) views of the enlarged kidneys containing cysts (K) in a fetus with Meckel-Gruber syndrome.

11.5

Pena-Shokeir Phenotype (Fetal Akinesia/Hypokinesia Sequence)

Epidemiology/Genetics

Definition Heterogeneous group of disorders characterized by polyhydramnios, prenatal onset of growth restriction with head sparing, multiple joint contractures, characteristic facies, and pulmonary hypoplasia.

Epidemiology Rare (M1:F1).

Embryology Pena-Shokeir is best thought of as a number of separate neuromuscular disorders resulting in a similar phenotype. The phenotype consists of polyhydramnios, prenatal onset of growth restriction with head sparing, multiple joint contractures, webbed neck, closed hands, flexed wrists, absence of flexion creases, rocker-bottom feet, rigid expressionless face, hypertelorism, prominent eyes, short umbilical cord, and pulmonary hypoplasia. The common pathophysiology of the phenotypic features is thought to be decreased or absent fetal movement in utero. Pathologic findings have been heterogeneous and include congenital myopathies, anterior horn cell abnormalities, and abnormalities of the brain.

Inheritance Patterns Autosomal recessive inheritance has been seen in approximately one half of reported cases. Empiric recurrence risk for an isolated case with nonspecific pathology would be 10 to 15%.

Teratogens Maternal myasthenia gravis and any agent causing central nervous system damage, including infectious agents, fetal hypotension, or stroke.

Prognosis Cases with a classic phenotype are lethal and may be stillborn (30%) or die in the first few months of life of respiratory complications. Because of the heterogeneous nature of this phenotype, the prognosis is dependent on the etiology of the causative disorder.

Sonography

FINDINGS

1. **Fetus:**
   a. Limb abnormalities include the following:
      1. Flexion contractures of the arms, which are rigidly flexed at the elbows, and with the lower extremities flexed at the hips and hyperextended at the knees and feet.
      2. The fetal extremities are virtually immobile. Selective immobility of the upper limbs with normal movement of lower limbs has been reported.
      3. Clenched hands with ulnar deviation (camptodactyly).
      4. Clubbed feet.
      5. Diminished muscle bulk.
      6. The spine may be kyphotic, scoliotic, or lordotic.
   b. Facial abnormalities may include the following:
      1. Hypertelorism
      2. Micrognathia
      3. Depressed nasal bridge
      4. Malformed, low-set ears
      5. Persistently open small mouth (carp mouth)
   c. Other abnormalities may include the following:
      1. Cryptorchidism
      2. Cleft palate
      3. Cardiac anomalies
      4. Agenesis of the corpus callosum
      5. Hypoplastic cerebellum
      6. Small narrow chest
      7. Nuchal thickening at 11 to 14 weeks' gestation
      8. An absent stomach, presumably due to lack of swallowing
2. **Amniotic Fluid:** Severe, late-onset polyhydramnios is usually present.
3. **Placenta:** The placenta is small and thin with a relatively short umbilical cord.
4. **Measurement Data:** Intrauterine growth restriction is present.
5. **When Detectable:** The syndrome has been detected at 18 weeks' gestation.

Differential Diagnosis

1. Other multiple malformation syndromes with growth retardation such as trisomy 18.
2. Arthrogryposis, but the additional abnormalities in the face, brain, and heart are not present with the typical arthrogryposis case (see Chapter 8.4).
3. Smith-Lemli-Opitz—The limbs are mobile and are not subject to contractures (see Chapter 11.6).
4. Multiple pterygium syndrome—Similar and not easy to distinguish without a family history (see Chapter 8.12).
5. Freeman-Sheldon syndrome—Also hard to distinguish without a family history.

Pregnancy Management

Investigations and Consultations Required Chromosomal studies should be performed to exclude trisomy 18. Amniotic fluid cultures for cytomegalovirus and maternal serum for TORCH (toxoplasmosis, other infections, rubella, cytomegalovirus infection, and herpes simplex) titers should be considered. Fetal echocardiography should be performed to detect the associated cardiac malformations.

Fetal Intervention Not appropriate for this usually lethal condition.

Monitoring Prenatal growth deficiency and polyhydramnios are commonly seen as components of the fetal akinesia sequence. Ultrasonography may be useful to document these findings, but fetal surveillance is inappropriate for this condition.

Pregnancy Course Polyhydramnios and preterm labor are common findings in this disorder. Therapeutic amniocentesis and tocolytic agents are contraindicated to prolong the pregnancy.

Pregnancy Termination Issues The multiple etiologies for the fetal akinesia almost always require a complete pathologic examination of an intact fetus to establish a precise diagnosis.

Delivery Fetuses with a small chest and polyhydramnios are likely to die of pulmonary hypoplasia. After an in-depth discussion of the implications of the diagnosis, most couples will concur with the recommendation that fetal monitoring and intervention for "fetal distress" not be performed in labor.

Neonatology

Resuscitation Pulmonary hypoplasia and/or the underlying central nervous system defect are most likely the dominant abnormalities affecting survival potential for this group of infants. Because survival potential, as reported in the literature, is virtually nil, a prenatal discussion of the option for nonintervention should the infant be liveborn is appropriate. If intervention is elected, care should be exercised with positive pressure ventilation because barotrauma with air leak is a frequent complication in pulmonary hypoplasia.

Transport Transfer to a tertiary center with pediatric subspecialty capabilities is appropriate to confirm the diagnosis and provide counseling and support for the parents regarding prolonged life support, once the diagnosis is confirmed.

Testing and Confirmation There is no definitive diagnostic test antemortem, although magnetic resonance imaging and/or computed tomography may be helpful in delineating the underlying neurologic defect. Peripheral nerve and muscle biopsies may also be helpful.

Nursery Management At present, providing life support while proceeding with the diagnostic evaluation and facilitating the adjustment of the parents to the diagnosis

and likely prognosis are the primary components of care. There are no reported cases of long-term survival that could inform a long-term management approach.

REFERENCES

Ajayi RA, Keen CE, Knott PD: Ultrasound diagnosis of Pena-Shokeir phenotype at 14 weeks of pregnancy. Prenat Diagn 1995;15:762–764.

Chen H, Blumberg B, Immken L, et al: The Pena-Shokeir syndrome: Report of five cases and further delineation of the syndrome. Am J Genet 1983;16:213.

Erdl R, Schmidtke K, Jakobeit M, et al: Pena-Shokeir phenotype with major CNS-malformations: Clinicopathological report of two siblings. Clin Genet 1989;36:127.

Genkins SM, Hertzberg BS, Bowie JD, Blow O: Pena-Shokeir type I syndrome: In utero sonographic appearance. J Clin Ultrasound 1989; 17:56–61.

Hageman G, Willemse J: The heterogeneity of the Pena-Shokeir Syndrome. Neuropediatrics 1987;18:45.

Hall JG: Analysis of Pena-Shokeir phenotype. Am J Med Genet 1986; 25:99–117.

Lindhout D, Hageman G, Beemer FA, et al: The Pena-Shokeir syndrome: Report of nine Dutch cases. Am J Med Genet 1985;21:655.

Muller LM, de Jong G: Prenatal ultrasonographic features of Pena-Shokeir I syndrome and the trisomy 18 syndrome. Am J Med Genet 1986;25:119–129.

Ohlsson A, Fong KW, Rose TH, Moore DC: Prenatal sonographic diagnosis of Pena-Shokeir syndrome type I, or fetal akinesia deformation sequence. Am J Med Genet 1988;29:59–65.

Paladini D, Tartaglione A, Agangi A: Pena Shokeir phenotype with variable onset in three pregnancies. Ultrasound Obstet Gynecol 2001;17: 163–165.

Pena SDJ, Shokeir MHK: Syndrome of camptodactyly, multiple ankyloses, facial anomalies, and pulmonary hypoplasia: A lethal condition. J Pediatr 1974;85:373.

Shenker L, Reed K, Anderson C, et al: Syndrome of camptodactyly, ankyloses, facial anomalies, and pulmonary hypoplasia (Pena-Shokeir syndrome): Obstetric and ultrasound aspects. Am J Obstet Gynecol 1985;152:303–307.

Tongsung T, Chanprapaph P, Khunamornpong S: Prenatal ultrasound of regional akinesia with Pena-Shokeir phenotype. Prenat Diagn 2000; 20:422–425.

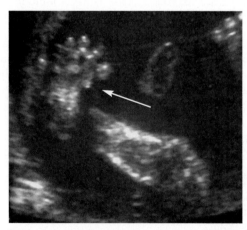

Clubhand with ulnar deviation (*arrow*) in a fetus with Pena-Shokeir syndrome.

11.6 Smith-Lemli-Opitz Syndrome

Epidemiology/Genetics

Definition A multiple congenital anomaly syndrome caused by a defect in cholesterol synthesis.

Epidemiology Occurs in 1 in 20,000 to 40,000 births (M1:F1). It is more common among northern Europeans, with a lower frequency in Africans and Asians.

Embryology This disorder is an inborn error in cholesterol metabolism due to mutations in the 7-dehydrocholesterol reductase gene on chromosome 11q12-q13. It is characterized by prenatal onset of growth restriction with microcephaly (90%) and moderate to severe mental retardation. Characteristic abnormalities include cleft palate (40–50%), cardiac defects (40%), hypospadias and/or cryptorchidism (50%), postaxial polydactyly (25–50%), and two-three-toe syndactyly. Atrioventricular canal defects and anomalous pulmonary venous return are more common than expected based on unselected series of patients. Diagnosis is based on a consistent clinical phenotype with demonstration of elevated serum 7-dehydrocholesterol.

Inheritance Patterns Autosomal recessive with 25% recurrence risk in families with a previously affected child.

Teratogens None.

Screening Carrier testing is becoming available on a research basis in families with identified gene mutations. Prenatal ultrasonography looking for anomalies and 7-dehydrocholesterol testing is recommended for families with a previously affected child and a 25% recurrence risk. Elevated 7-dehydrocholesterol levels in amniotic fluid or in chorionic villi tissue samples are diagnostic. A low uE3 as part of a maternal serum screen, especially combined with low human chorionic gonadotropin (beta HCG?) and alpha-fetoprotein levels, should prompt further investigation when seen with abnormal sonographic findings.

Prognosis May be lethal if associated with severe anomalies. Otherwise moderate to severe mental retardation can be expected. Modest postnatal growth and behavioral improvement is seen following oral cholesterol supplementation.

Sonography

FINDINGS

1. **Fetus:**
   a. Microcephaly with the cranial size below the 10th percentile is typical.
   b. Abnormal genitalia with hypospadias, cryptorchidism, micropenis, ambiguous genitalia, or female-appearing genitalia with a male karyotype.
   c. Limb abnormalities include syndactyly of the second and third toes, postaxial polydactyly, clenched hands, and valgus deformity of the feet.
   d. Renal abnormalities are often seen and include hydronephrosis, cystic kidneys, or hypoplastic kidneys.
   e. Nuchal thickening occurs in the first trimester at 11 to 13 weeks' gestation.
   f. Occasional findings include hydrops, cleft palate, heart defects, cerebellar hypoplasia, cataracts, and micrognathia.
2. **Amniotic Fluid:** Oligohydramnios may be present.
3. **Placenta:** Normal.
4. **Measurement Data:** There is often severe intrauterine growth retardation.
5. **When Detectable:** The diagnosis has been established as early as 11 weeks by the finding of nuchal lucency in an at-risk fetus. Abnormalities of the limbs, such as polydactyly, have been detected at 12 weeks.

Differential Diagnosis Includes trisomy 18, trisomy 13, Noonan syndrome, and other multiple malformation phenotypes with congenital heart disease.

Where Else to Look This condition affects the entire fetus, so a thorough fetal survey is recommended.

Pregnancy Management

Investigations and Consultations Required Because a precise diagnosis is not possible by ultrasonography, a complete evaluation of the fetus, including chromosomal studies and fetal echocardiography, is essential. A presumptive diagnosis can be made if maternal serum screening reveals a low serum unconjugated estriol value. Precise diagnostic testing is available using either chorionic villi or amniotic fluid cells and measuring 7-dehydrocholesterol.

Fetal Intervention At present, no fetal intervention is known to be effective. Current trials of dietary therapy in childhood may provide insights into possible fetal therapies.

Monitoring Prenatal growth deficiency and an increased incidence of stillbirth are found in this condition. Thorough discussion with the family and consultation with a pediatric geneticist should be undertaken before embarking on an intensive course of fetal surveillance.

Pregnancy Course Obstetric complications, such as intrauterine growth deficiency, stillbirth, and breech presentation are not uncommon in fetuses affected with Smith-Lemli-Opitz syndrome.

Pregnancy Termination Issues A precise biochemical diagnosis should be obtained before choosing the method of pregnancy termination.

Delivery The significant incidence of neonatal complications makes delivery in a tertiary center the most appropriate option.

Neonatology

Resuscitation Given the severe prognosis for early infancy death, moderate to severe mental retardation in survivors, and, as yet, no effective treatment of the metabolic defect, consideration of nonintervention in the event of respiratory depression at birth is appropriate when the prenatal diagnostic findings indicate the severe form (type II) of the disorder. There are no specific technical requirements for initiating respiration in an involved infant.

Transport Transfer of the newborn to a tertiary center with pediatric subspecialty diagnostic capabilities for confirmation of the diagnosis is appropriate.

Testing and Confirmation A defect in cholesterol biosynthesis has been identified. The characteristic plasma findings are abnormally low plasma cholesterol and elevated precursor, 7-dehydrocholesterol, concentrations. Ambiguous or female-appearing genitalia with a 46,XY karyotype occurs frequently.

Nursery Management No definitive therapy for the metabolic defect has been reported. In general, management consists of supportive care with attention to appropriate management of the associated renal and cardiac anomalies. Supporting the parents in long-term care planning for severely impaired infants is essential.

REFERENCES

Abuelo DN, Tint GS, Kelley R, et al: Prenatal detection of the cholesterol biosynthetic defect in the Smith-Lemli-Opitz syndrome by the analysis of amniotic fluid sterols. Am J Med Genet 1995;56:281.

Bick DP, McCorkle D, Stanley WS, et al: Prenatal diagnosis of Smith-Lemli-Opitz syndrome in a pregnancy with low maternal serum oestriol and a sex-reversed fetus. Prenat Diagn 1999;19:68–71.

Cunniff C, Kratz LE, Moser A: Clinical and biochemical spectrum of patients with the RSH/Smith-Lemli-Opitz syndrome and abnormal cholesterol metabolism. Am J Med Genet 1997;68:263–269.

Dallaire L, Mitchell G, Giguere R, et al: Prenatal diagnosis of Smith-Lemli-Opitz syndrome is possible by measurement of 7-dehydrocholesterol in amniotic fluid. Prenatal Diagn 1995;15:855–858.

Elias ER, Irons MB, Hurley AD, et al: Clinical effects of cholesterol supplementation in six patients with the Smith-Lemli-Opitz syndrome (SLOS). Am J Med Genet 1997;68:305–310.

Irons MD, Tint GS: Prenatal diagnosis of Smith-Lemli-Opitz syndrome. Prenat Diag 1998;18:369–372.

Johnson JA, Aughton DJ, Comstock CH, et al: Prenatal diagnosis of Smith-Lemli-Opitz syndrome, type II. Am J Med Genet 1994;49:240.

Kratz LE, Kelley RI: Prenatal diagnosis of the RSH/Smith-Lemli-Opitz syndrome. Am J Med Genet 1999;82:376–381.

Lin AE, Ardinger HH, Ardinger RH Jr, et al: Cardiovascular malformations in Smith-Lemli-Opitz syndrome. Am J Med Genet 1997;68:270–278.

Maymon R, Ogle RF, Chitty L: Smith-Lemli-Opitz syndrome presenting with persistent nuchal edema and non-immune hydrops. Prenat Diagn 1999;19:105–107.

McGaughran JM, Clayton PT, Mills KA, et al: Prenatal diagnosis of Smith-Lemli-Opitz syndrome. Am J Med Genet 1995;56:269.

Mills K, Mandel H, Montemagno R, et al: First trimester prenatal diagnosis of Smith-Lemli-Opitz syndrome (7-dehydrocholesterol reductase deficiency). Pediatr Res 1996;39:816–819.

Opitz J: RSH/SLO (Smith-Lemli-Opitz) syndrome: Historical, genetic, and developmental considerations. Am J Med Genet 1994;50:344.

Pierquin G, Peeters P, Roels F, et al: Severe Smith-Lemli-Opitz syndrome with prolonged survival and lipid abnormalities. Am J Med Genet 1995;56:276–280.

Rossiter JP, Hofman KJ, Kelley RJ: Smith-Lemli-Opitz syndrome: Prenatal diagnosis by quantification of cholesterol precursors in amniotic fluid. Am J Med Genet 1995;56:272.

Seller MJ, Russell J, Tint GS: Unusual case of Smith-Lemli-Opitz syndrome type II. Am J Med Genet 1995;56:265.

Smith DW, Lemli L, Opitz JM: A newly recognized syndrome of multiple congenital anomalies. J Pediatr 1964;64:210.

Tint GS: The cholesterol biosynthesis defect in the Smith-Lemli-Opitz syndrome. Am J Med Genet 1994;50:336.

Tint GS, Abuelo D, Tille M, et al: Fetal Smith-Lemli-Opitz syndrome can be detected accurately and reliably by measuring amniotic fluid dehydrocholesterols. Prenat Diagn 1998;18:651–658.

Tint GS, Irons M, Elias ER, et al: Defective cholesterol biosynthesis associated with the Smith-Lemli-Opitz syndrome. N Engl J Med 1994;330:107.

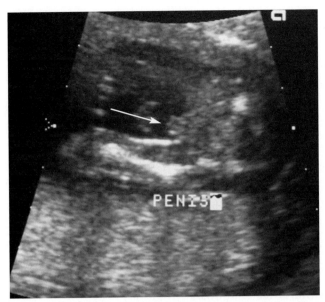

Sonogram of a fetus with Smith-Lemli-Opitz syndrome with ambiguous genitalia. This view shows a rudimentary scrotum and penis (*arrow*). (Courtesy of Sandi Isbister, MD, Ultrasound Institute of Baltimore.)

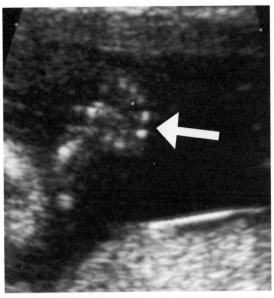

Same fetus showing appearances consistent with labia (*arrow*). (Courtesy of Sandi Isbister, MD, Ultrasound Institute of Baltimore.)

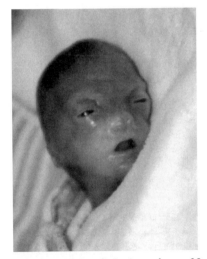

A 20-week fetus with Smith-Lemli-Opitz syndrome. Note the eyelid ptosis, broad nasal bridge, and short upturned nose.

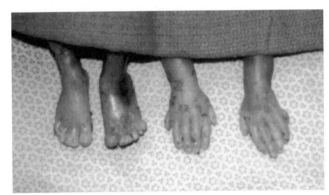

Hands and feet of a 20-week fetus with Smith-Lemli-Opitz syndrome. Note the 2-3 toe syndactyly and postaxial polydactyly of hands.

11.7 Tuberous Sclerosis

Epidemiology/Genetics

Definition Neurocutaneous syndrome characterized by cutaneous and central nervous system hamartomas, seizures, mental retardation, and cardiac rhabdomyomas.

Epidemiology About 1 in 10,000 births (M1:F1).

Embryology Postnatally, tuberous sclerosis is characterized by facial angiofibromas (83%); seizures (93%); mental retardation (62%); renal angiomyolipomas and cysts (60%); dental pitting (7%); cardiac rhabdomyomas; intracranial calcification (50%); brain, retina, optic nerve, and periungual hamartomas; and hypopigmented macules (60%). Antenatally, cardiac rhabdomyomas are the most common feature, and it is estimated that more than 50% of children with tuberous sclerosis have antenatal cardiac rhabdomyoma. The majority (50–85%) of children with cardiac rhabdomyomas have tuberous sclerosis.

Inheritance Patterns Autosomal dominant with great variability. Approximately 60 to 85% of cases represent new mutations. Individuals with tuberous sclerosis have a 50% chance of passing the condition to each child. Gonadal mosaicism has been reported in some families. Two genetic loci on chromosomes 9q34 and 16p13 have been identified that account for the vast majority of cases. Genetic testing in suspected cases may be available on a research or clinical basis.

Teratogens None.

Prognosis Seizures and mental retardation are the most important contributors to the morbidity associated with tuberous sclerosis. Childhood brain tumors and kidney failure are uncommon complications. Cardiac rhabdomyomas almost always regress on their own.

Sonography

FINDINGS

1. **Fetus:**
   a. Intracranial changes reported include asymmetrical lateral ventricles with abnormally shaped choroid plexus. Agenesis of the corpus callosum is common. A tuber has been detected in utero. An echogenic mass impinging on a dilated lateral ventricle was seen.
   b. With magnetic resonance imaging, poor gyral formation has been reported. Hyperintense nodules on T1-weighted sequences correlate with periventricular and subcortical tubers.
   c. Cardiac changes—Cardiac rhabdomyomas are common. An echogenic mass in the heart is seen. Hydrops fetalis with pleural and pericardial effusions and ascites may develop if the rhabdomyoma is located at a critical site
2. **Amniotic Fluid:** Normal.
3. **Placenta:** Normal unless there is hydrops.
4. **Measurement Data:** Normal.
5. **When Detectable:** Cardiac rhabdomyoma have been detected at 20 weeks' gestation.

Differential Diagnosis

1. Rhabdomyoma not related to tuberous sclerosis.
2. Cystic adenomatoid malformation if the rhabdomyoma is pedunculated and extends outside the cardiac border. Rhabdomyoma will pulsate with the heart.
3. Other rare cardiac tumors such as teratoma, osteoma, and hemangioma.

Where Else to Look Look in the brain for other features of tuberous sclerosis: the presence of tubers, asymmetric ventricles, abnormally shaped choroid plexus, and agenesis of the corpus callosum.

Additional Investigations Careful physical examination of parents and siblings looking for skin manifestations of tuberous sclerosis is warranted to refine recurrence risk and help confirm the diagnosis. Further evaluation of the family with renal ultrasonography or computed tomography can also be considered.

Pregnancy Management

Investigation and Consultation Required Additional investigations depend on what structural malformations are present. As noted previously, careful evaluation of the parents for signs of tuberous sclerosis is necessary if a presumptive diagnosis of fetal tuberous sclerosis is made. Additional consultation, such as cardiology, will depend on the malformations seen.

Fetal Intervention None is indicated unless cardiac complications develop (hydrops or arrhythmia). Management would follow usual guidelines for these complications.

Monitoring Serial sonographic examinations should be performed to detect signs of arrhythmia or hydrops secondary to cardiac rhabdomyomas. If these complications arise, consideration can be given to early delivery, but only after full discussion with the family regarding the significant complications associated with tuberous sclerosis.

Pregnancy Course No specific obstetric complications are to be expected, unless fetal hydrops develops.

Pregnancy Termination Issues Unless the diagnosis has been made in one of the parents, an intact fetus is necessary for a complete autopsy.

Delivery Site of delivery will depend on the type of malformations seen and fetal status. In general, delivery is best accomplished in a tertiary center.

Neonatology

Resuscitation Management of the onset of respiration is determined by the spectrum of fetal abnormalities identified. Hydrops fetalis either from cardiac arrhythmia or from intracavital obstruction of blood flow may be present. If so, interventions must be directed at reducing impingement of lung expansion by serosal fluid collections and pleural and/or peritoneal effusions (see Chapter 13.2). The specific arrhythmic type will determine the appropriate antiarrhythmic therapy. The presence of intracranial tubers rarely affects onset of respiration.

Transport Transfer to a tertiary center with the appropriate pediatric and surgical subspecialists and diagnostic capabilities is determined by the clinical presentation of the disorder. Immediate transfer is recommended with any evidence of hemodynamic instability or neurologic symptomatology. The neonate who has an uneventful adaptation and remains asymptomatic may be referred for outpatient evaluation within the first few weeks following birth.

Testing and Confirmation Appropriate evaluation of cardiac tumors includes electrocardiography, echocardiography, and, in selected cases, cardiac catheterization and/or cardiothoracic magnetic resonance imaging. Appropriately weighted magnetic resonance imaging is the modality of choice for demonstration of intracranial lesions, although both ultrasonography and computed tomography have been used.

Nursery Management Interventions should be directed at amelioration and correction of any hemodynamic abnormalities and cardiac arrhythmias (see Chapter 13.2). Most reports of fetal/neonatal rhabdomyomas indicate resolution of the tumors during the first several months, leading to the recommendation that surgical ex-

cision of the tumor in early infancy be limited to cases with persistent symptoms and the lack of evidence of tumor regression. The onset of seizures in early infancy from tuberous sclerosis has been reported, and, if present, requires anticonvulsant therapy.

REFERENCES

Axt-Fliedner R, Qush H, Hendrik H: Prenatal diagnosis of cerebral lesions and multiple intracardiac rhabdomyomas in a fetus with tuberous sclerosis. J Ultrasound Med 2001;20:63–67.

Brackley KJ, Farndon PA, Weaver JB, et al: Prenatal diagnosis of tuberous sclerosis with intracerebral signs at 14 weeks' gestation. Prenat Diagn 1999;19:575–579.

Christophe C, Bartholome J, Blum D, et al: Neonatal tuberous sclerosis: US, CT, and MR diagnosis of brain and cardiac lesions. Pediatr Radiol 1989;19:446.

Franz DN: Diagnosis and management of tuberous sclerosis complex. Semin Pediatr Neurol 1998;5:253–268.

Guerta LG, Burgueros M, Elorza MC, et al: Cardiac rhabdomyoma presenting as fetal hydrops. Pediatr Cardiol 1986;7:171.

Gushiken BJ, Callen PW, Silverman N: Prenatal diagnosis of tuberous sclerosis in monozygotic twins with cardiac masses. J Ultrasound Med 1999;18:165–168.

Hahn JS, Bejar R, Gladson CL: Neonatal subependymal giant cell astrocytoma associated with tuberous sclerosis: MRI, CT, and ultrasound correlation. Neurology 1991;41:124.

Harding CO, Pagon RA: Incidence of tuberous sclerosis in patients with cardiac rhabdomyoma. Am J Med Genet 1990;37:443–446.

Hwa J, Ward C, Nunn G, et al: Primary intraventricular cardiac tumors in children: Contemporary diagnostic and management options. Pediatr Cardiol 1994;15:233.

Jones AC, Shyamsundar MM, Thomas MW, et al: Comprehensive mutation analysis of TSC1 and TSC2 and phenotypic correlations in 150 families with tuberous sclerosis. Am J Hum Genet 1999;64:1305–1315.

Komori S, Bessho T, Fukuda H, Kanazawa K: A report on the perinatal diagnosis of 4 cases of cardiac tumors. Arch Gynecol Obstet 1995;256:213.

Krapp M, Baschat AA, Gembruch U, et al: Tuberous sclerosis with intracardiac rhabdomyoma in a fetus with trisomy 21: Case report and review of literature. Prenat Diagn 1999;19:610–613.

Roach ES, DiMario FJ, Kandt RS, Northrup H: Tuberous sclerosis consensus conference: Recommendations for diagnostic evaluation. National Tuberous Sclerosis Association. Child Neurol 1999;14:401–407.

Scurry J, Watkins A, Acton C, Drew J: Tachyarrhythmia, cardiac rhabdomyomata, and fetal hydrops in a premature infant with tuberous sclerosis. J Paediatr Child Health 1992;28:260.

Sgro M, Barrozzino T, Toi A, et al: Prenatal detection of cerebral lesions in a fetus with tuberous sclerosis. Ultrasound Obstet Gynecol 1999;14:356–359.

Sonigo P, Elmaleh A, Fermont L, et al: Prenatal MRI diagnosis of fetal cerebral tuberous sclerosis. Pediatr Radiol 1996;26:1.

Sugita K, Itoh K, Takeuchi Y, et al: Tuberous sclerosis: Report of two cases studied by computer-assisted tomography within one week after birth. Brain Dev 1985;7:438.

Wallace G, Smith HC, Watson GH, et al: Tuberous sclerosis presenting with fetal and neonatal cardiac tumors. Arch Dis Child 1990;65:377.

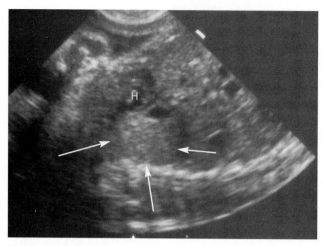

Massive exophytic rhabdomyoma (*arrows*) that lies alongside the heart (H) in a 24-week pregnancy. Initially thought to be a chest mass, it was recognized as having a cardiac origin because it pulsated with the heart. Tuberous sclerosis was diagnosed after birth.

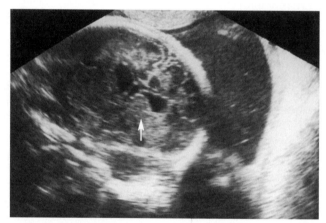

Coronal image of fetus with tuberous sclerosis showing a cranial tuber (*arrow*) located at the foramen of Monro. Note the bilateral ventriculomegaly. (From Sgro M, Barozzino T, Toi A, et al: Prenatal detection of cerebral lesions in a fetus with tuberous sclerosis. Ultrasound Obstet Gynecol 1999;14:356–359.)

11.8 VACTERL Association

Epidemiology/Genetics

Definition Acronym for a nonrandom association of birth defects, including vertebral anomalies (60%), anal atresia (60%), cardiac defects (60%), tracheoesophageal fistula (85%), renal anomalies (60%), and radial limb abnormalities (65%). Diagnosis is based on the presence of at least three of these defects.

Epidemiology Rare (M1:F1).

Embryology Unknown. May result from a single early defect in fetal blastogenesis or fetal mesoderm formation.

Inheritance Patterns Sporadic. There is a VACTERL-like syndrome with hydrocephalus that has autosomal recessive or X-linked inheritance.

Teratogens None known. Diabetic embryopathy may result in a similar pattern of malformations.

Prognosis There is a 75% survival rate. Central nervous system abnormalities are rare and most children have normal intelligence.

Sonography

FINDINGS

1. **Fetus:**
   a. Polydactyly.
   b. Vertebral anomalies:
      1. Caudal regression—Shortened spine with absent vertebral bodies, often with scoliosis (see Chapter 2.5).
      2. Hemivertebrae or absent vertebrae—These are not easy to detect with ultrasonography. There will be an inability to see posterior elements with slight angulation of the spine at the abnormal area. Two or more posterior elements may be fused.
   c. Anal atresia—Anal atresia is rarely diagnosable in utero. Occasionally, dilated large bowel will be visible. The anus can be seen as a small echogenic spot posterior to the genitalia. Absence of this spot may indicate atresia (see Chapter 6.1).
   d. Esophageal atresia—The stomach will be either small or absent. Polyhydramnios will be present (see Chapter 5.3).
   e. Renal abnormalities—There may be hydronephrosis or multicystic kidney (see Chapters 4.4 and 4.8).
   f. Radial ray problems—The radius may be absent or small, with accompanying loss of portions of the hand (see Chapter 8.15).
   g. Congenital heart defects may be found.
2. **Amniotic Fluid:** With gut atresia, polyhydramnios will be present.
3. **Placenta:** Normal placenta.
4. **Measurement Data:** Normal.
5. **When Detectable:** None of the findings are easy to detect, but they should be visible at 16 to 18 weeks.

Differential Diagnosis

1. Many of these findings are also seen with chromosomal anomalies.
2. Multiple malformation syndromes, including the Holt-Oram syndrome (autosomal dominant) and thrombocytopenia-absent radius syndrome, may have similar manifestations.
3. The overall good long-term prognosis for infants with Jarcho-Levin syndrome consists of multiple vertebral segmentation defects coupled with fusion deformities of the ribs. Associated anomalies include renal abnormalities, spina bifida, clubfeet, renal atresia, and cleft palate.

Where Else to Look A thorough survey of the entire fetus is desirable, since the syndrome involves multi-organ systems.

Pregnancy Management

Investigations and Consultations Required As with all multiple malformation cases, chromosomal evaluation is essential, even though VACTERL itself is not associated with a chromosomal abnormality. Fetal echocardiography should be performed to delineate the severity of the cardiac defect. A pediatric surgeon should be consulted to discuss surgical management with the family.

Monitoring In the absence of polyhydramnios, no specific changes in obstetric care are required. Serial ultrasonograms to detect increasing amniotic fluid volumes are appropriate.

Pregnancy Course Polyhydramnios may be a complicating factor and may result in preterm labor.

Pregnancy Termination Issues To establish a precise diagnosis, an intact fetus must be delivered and appropriate morphologic, radiologic, and pathologic examinations performed.

Delivery The site of delivery should be a tertiary center with appropriate medical and surgical specialists available to deal with the multiple malformations that are a part of this "syndrome." The mode of delivery should be based on obstetric indications.

Neonatology

Resuscitation The special management issues at birth are based on the specific organ defects known to be present. Among the ones included in the VACTERL association, tracheoesophageal fistula and cardiac defects have an impact on the onset of respiration and early adaptation. Resuscitation and stabilization of cardiorespiratory function measures to be instituted are discussed in the chapters concerned with those specific defects.

Transport Referral to a tertiary perinatal center with multiple pediatric and surgical subspecialists is always indicated. Care during transport should include the specific measures for each of the defects known or suspected to be present.

Testing and Confirmation A diagnosis can be made at birth. Radiographic studies are recommended to look for associated spinal abnormalities.

Nursery Management Priority in management is determined by the specific malformations known to be pres-

ent. Thus, immediate diagnostic evaluation to identify the defects the infant manifests should be instituted. The next step is to coordinate the various surgical interventions. The long-term prognosis is governed by the potential correctability of the cardiac defect; therefore, prompt, accurate diagnosis by echocardiography is essential initially.

Both tracheoesophageal fistula and anal atresia require urgent surgical intervention to alleviate their life-threatening impact once the cardiac defect is determined to be correctable. In general, the vertebral, extremity, and renal defects are not associated with significant dysfunction in the neonatal period and therefore have lesser influence on the plan of care.

REFERENCES

Czeizel A, Ludanyi I: An aetiological study of the VACTERL-association. Eur J Pediatr 1985;144:331–337.

Hull AD, James G, Pretorius DH: Detection of Jarcho-Levin syndrome at 12 weeks gestation by nuchal translucency screening and three dimensional ultrasound. Prenat Diagn 2001;21:390–394.

McGahan JP, Leeba JM, Lindfors KK: Prenatal sonographic diagnosis of VATER association. J Clin Ultrasound 1988;16:588–591.

Oneije CI, Sherer DM, Hankwerker Shah L: Prenatal diagnosis of sirenomelia with bilateral hydrocephalus: Report of a previously undocumented form of VACTERL-H association. Am J Perinatol 1998;15:193–197.

Tongsong T, Wanapirak C, Piyamongkol W, Sudasana J: Prenatal sonographic diagnosis of VATER association. J Clin Ultrasound 1999;27:378–384.

Weaver DD, Mapstone CL, Yu PL: The VATER association. Analysis of 46 patients. Am J Dis Child 1986;140:225–229.

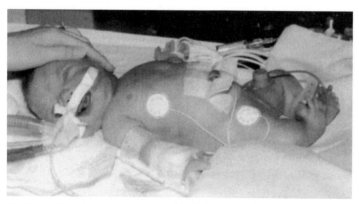

Newborn with truncus arteriosus, vertebral abnormalities, femoral hypoplasia, and bifid great toes resulting from maternal diabetic embryopathy.

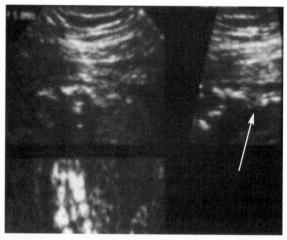

Transverse, sagittal, and C-scan three-dimensional views of anomalous vertebra in a 20-week pregnancy in a diabetic woman. Arrow points to missing hemivertebra. The adjacent vertebra is fused.

Twins

12

12.1 Intrauterine Growth Restriction or Retardation (IUGR) in Twins

Epidemiology/Genetics

Definition Generally defined as weight less than the 10th percentile for gestational age. Should be based on a growth chart for twins, not singleton pregnancies.

Epidemiology

Overall Twins occur once in 100 births, more common in people of African origin than in people of European origin, among whom in turn it is more common than in people of Asian origin. Increasing incidence with the increased use of fertility medications.

Monozygotic One in 250, with one third being diamniotic/dichorionic and two thirds being diamniotic/monochorionic; 1% monoamniotic/monochorionic; conjoined twins are rare.

Dizygotic One in 160 in European and European American populations; 1 in 100 in African Americans; 1 in 25 in parts of Nigeria. All are diamniotic and dichorionic. Increased risk in women 35 to 39 years old (10-fold over teenaged females) as well as multiparous females.

Intrauterine growth restriction (IUGR) is reported to occur in 12 to 47% of twin pregnancies, in contrast to 5 to 7% in singleton pregnancies. The higher rate is thought to be due to competition for available nutrients. More commonly, however, only one of the twins is growth retarded, which may be due to abnormalities such as the twin-to-twin transfusion syndrome (TTTS) or some genetic disorders in the growth-retarded twin and not an intrinsic placental problem.

Embryology

Monozygotic Due to division of the developing cell mass in two during the first 17 days of development. Diamniotic/dichorionic, 0–3 days; diamniotic/monochorionic, 4–8 days; monoamniotic/monochorionic, 9–14 days; conjoined 15–17 days; Monozygotic twinning is a malformative process with a two to three times increased risk of major malformations.

Dizygotic Due to the release and subsequent fertil-

ization of two separate eggs during a single menstrual cycle. Only at increased risk for fetal deformations. Discordance in fetal growth can result from a nutritional, genetic, chromosomal, infectious, or other cause.

Inheritance Pattern Dizygotic twinning, but not monozygotic, has some genetic component, occurring more often in certain families and more commonly in women of African-American ancestry. Familial clustering has been associated with dizygotic twins (expressed in females only), but not with monozygotic twins. Recurrence risk for dizygotic twins is approximately 2% in the European population. Risk of a twin pregnancy in a female twin is 1 in 58.

Prognosis The overall rate of both fetal mortality and neonatal morbidity is significantly increased for the growth-restricted fetus. In the TTTS, severe polyhydramnios may result in preterm delivery with increased rates of mortality and morbidity.

Sonography

FINDINGS

1. **Fetus:** One or both twins will be too small for gestational age. Intrauterine growth restriction (IUGR) is as common in dizygotic twins as in monozygotic twins.
2. **Amniotic Fluid:** Fluid around the smaller fetus or fetuses will be decreased. An attempt to determine the amniotic fluid index around each twin is of value.
3. **Placenta:** The placenta related to the smaller twin will be decreased in size. Establish whether the twins are dichorionic diamniotic or monochorionic diamniotic. With diamniotic diachorionic twins there will be four components to the membrane between the two sacs and the twin peak sign will be present. A triangular projection of placental tissue extends between the intratwin chorionic membranes. If the twins are of different gender, a dichorionic diamniotic twin pregnancy is present.
4. **Measurement Data:** The abdominal circumference

measurement will be decreased, and other measurement data (head and limb measurements) may or may not be decreased.

5. **When Detectable:** Growth restriction in twins may be detected as early as 14 weeks' gestation but usually presents in the third trimester.

Pitfalls If one twin lies anterior to the other, abdominal circumference measurements may be unobtainable.

Differential Diagnosis The vast majority of the reports indicate IUGR affecting only one twin, and in monozygotic twinning many of these cases represent variants of the TTTS. However, discrepancy in placental support is the probable cause of most discordant IUGR in multiple gestation.

Where Else to Look

1. Look for evidence of hydrops as in the TTTS.
2. If there is apparently a diamniotic monochorionic pregnancy, make sure that there is not a "stuck" twin with the amniotic membrane apparently "shrink-wrapped" around the smaller fetus.
3. A biophysical profile and cord Doppler studies should be performed.

Pregnancy Management

Investigations and Consultations Required IUGR in one of the twins should prompt evaluations of chromosome status of that fetus and a determination of maternal serology for TORCH (toxoplasmosis, other infection, rubella, cytomegalovirus infection, herpes simplex), which may present in a discordant manner. IUGR involving both twins requires a thorough evaluation of the patient for lifestyle factors or underlying medical conditions that cause growth restriction.

Fetal Intervention Not indicated except in cases of TTTS.

Monitoring The twin pregnancy with IUGR or growth discordance is a high-risk situation that should be managed by a perinatologist. Non-stress testing appears to be a good method of fetal assessment and can be used in a fashion similar to that for singleton pregnancies for management of IUGR. Discordant findings on non-stress testing requires additional testing, and the biophysical profile appears to be the best alternative.

Pregnancy Termination Issues Not applicable to this situation.

Delivery The pregnancy with discordant twins is an extremely high-risk situation requiring delivery and management in a tertiary center.

Neonatology

Resuscitation IUGR twins and the smaller of discordant twins are at very high risk for developing fetal distress during labor and for requiring resuscitation. Two resuscitation teams should be present for every twin delivery. No special techniques are required unless twin-twin transfusion has occurred.

Transport Referral to a tertiary perinatal center is determined by the degree of prematurity and the level of care required.

Nursery Management The discordant twin with IUGR is at risk for complications of hypoglycemia, respiratory distress, polycythemia, hyperbilirubinemia, and postasphyxial syndromes of organ injury and malfunction. Management is determined by the degree of prematurity, the birth weight, and the presence of complications.

REFERENCES

Blickstein I, Lancet M: The growth discordant twin. Obstet Gynecol Surv 1988;43:509–515.

Bronsteen R, Goyert G, Bottoms S: Classification of twins and neonatal morbidity. Obstet Gynecol 1989;74:98–101.

Hill LM, Krohn M, Lazebnik N, et al: The amniotic fluid index in normal twin pregnancies. Am J Obstet Gynecol 2000;182:950–954.

Naeye RL, Benirschke K, Hagstrom JW, Marcus CC: Intrauterine growth of twins as estimated from liveborn birth-weight data. Pediatrics 1966;37:409–416.

Sherer DM: Is less intensive fetal surveillance of dichorionic twin gestations justified? Ultrasound Obstet Gynecol 2000;15:167–173.

Trop I: The twin peak sign. Radiology 2001;220:68–69.

12.2

Acardiac Twin
(Acardiac Monster; Holoacardius)
Twin Reversed
Arterial Perfusion Sequence

Epidemiology/Genetics

Definition Acardia is a complex malformation associated with monozygotic, monochorionic twins or triplets, in which one twin has a severe abnormality involving malformations of the head and upper body with an absent or rudimentary, nonfunctioning heart.

Epidemiology One in 35,000 births, or 1 in 100 monozygotic twin pairs.

Embryology Most likely caused by placental, anastomotic, vascular connections between twins leading to reversal of blood flow to one twin. The "perfused" twin receives unoxygenated blood, which results in aplasia or hypoplasia of the heart, head, and upper limbs. The "pump" twin is usually morphologically normal but may show signs of congestive heart failure, including hydrops.

Inheritance Patterns Sporadic.

Teratogens None known.

Prognosis All of the perfused twins die. The pump twins have a 50% mortality rate, with death most often caused by heart failure or death of the co-twin.

Sonography

FINDINGS

1. **Fetus:** In addition to a normal fetus, a second fetus is seen that has an absent or nonfunctioning heart—the acardiac fetus.
   a. Acardiac twin—This twin obtains its blood supply from the normal pump twin. The acardiac twin either has no head, or there is anencephaly with only the base of the brain present. There will be gross skin thickening of the upper trunk and neck areas. Large cystic hygroma-like spaces in the skin are seen. An omphalocele may be present. Sometimes the upper limbs are absent. Club feet and absent toes are often seen. Although there are no cardiac pulsations, lower limb movements are visible.
   b. The pump twin—The normal twin may show signs of hydrops with hepatosplenomegaly, pleural and pericardial effusions, and skin thickening. The heart may be enlarged, with a prominent right atrium.
   c. In a rare variant an incomplete parasitic twin is attached to the host twin (twinning epigastric heteropagus). In a typical case, lower limbs and lower abdomen are present attached to the host by a long twisted pedicle—the cord. An omphalocele is often present in the host twin in such cases.

2. **Amniotic Fluid:** Polyhydramnios is present. No membrane or a thin membrane may be seen between the two fetuses. If a membrane is present, polyhydramnios may develop around the pump twin, with oligohydramnios around the acardiac twin. The blood flow in the umbilical arteries in the acardiac twin can be shown by color flow Doppler sonography to be toward the fetal abdomen of the acardiac twin—the reverse of normal. A single umbilical artery is seen in 50% of cases. The umbilical vein may be markedly dilated.
3. **Placenta:** Single placenta. Placental thickening may develop if hydrops occurs.
4. **Measurement Data:** Usually normal in the pump twin, but the abdominal circumference may increase in the pump twin if there is impending hydrops due to hepatosplenomegaly.
5. **When Detectable:** At about 11 to 12 weeks' gestation by vaginal sonography.

Differential Diagnosis The acardiac twin may be mistaken for a dead anencephalic twin fetus. The skin thickening, absence of the heart, cystic hygroma, and presence of leg movement give the diagnosis away. Misdiagnosis may be associated with significant fetal and maternal risks.

Where Else to Look Look in the normal fetus for signs of hydrops: cardiomegaly with right atrial dilation and tricuspid regurgitation, hepatosplenomegaly, pleural effusion, ascites, and abnormal Doppler findings.

Pregnancy Management

Investigations and Consultations Required

1. A follow-up sonogram showing interval growth should establish the diagnosis.
2. Chromosomal studies on the pump twin should be done, because one study found a 9% risk of chromosomal abnormality.
3. The high risk of prematurity requires that a consultation be obtained with a neonatologist to discuss management options with the family.

Fetal Intervention A number of therapeutic approaches have been attempted, including maternal digitalization, serial amniocentesis, maternal indomethacin therapy, endoscopic ligation of the umbilical cord, thrombosis of the umbilical artery using the percutaneous placement of a thrombogenic coil or laser therapy, and hysterotomy with selective delivery of the affected twin. When the weight of the acardiac twin exceeds 50% of the weight of the normal twin, there is more than a 60% percent chance of death of the pump twin.

Currently there are two major approaches to therapy that

should be considered and discussed with the patient. Ultrasonographically guided ablation of the arterial supply within the fetus, either with alcohol or thermocoagulation, is technically easier but does not ligate the vessels. Fetoscopic approaches have also been successful, using bipolar cautery or ligation of the cord, depending on the gestational age.

Monitoring The extremely high risk of pregnancy complications requires that care be coordinated by a perinatologist and that serial ultrasonographic examinations be performed every 1 to 2 weeks to assess fetal status.

Pregnancy Course There is a high risk of polyhydramnios and cardiac failure in the pump twin, with a mortality rate of 50 to 75%.

Pregnancy Termination Issues Should this option be chosen, a complete evaluation of an intact fetus and placenta should be made to confirm the diagnosis.

Delivery Delivery should occur in a tertiary center because of the high risk of prematurity and of delivering a compromised infant.

Neonatology

Resuscitation Anticipate difficulty with spontaneous onset of respiration as well as problems associated with preterm delivery in the pump twin. The team must be prepared to deal with congestive heart failure early in the course.

Transport Transfer to a tertiary center for neonatal intensive care is necessary in the majority of cases. Respiratory assistance, as well as support of myocardial function with continuous infusion of inotropic medication, may be required during transport.

Nursery Management Respiratory support, relief of myocardial stress, reduction of congestive heart failure, and correction of perinatal asphyxia are usually needed,

and thus it is necessary to institute measures to accomplish these goals immediately following birth. Because most twin reversed arterial perfusion sequence pregnancies are delivered prematurely, respiratory distress syndrome may also further complicate the clinical course. Early administration of surfactant replacement therapy may hasten the resolution of the latter.

REFERENCES

Al-Malt A, Ashmead G, Judge N, et al: Color-flow and Doppler velocimetry in prenatal diagnosis of acardiac triplet. J Ultrasound Med 1991;10:341–345.

Benson CB, Bieber FR, Genest DR, Doubilet PM: Doppler demonstration of reversed umbilical blood flow in an acardiac twin. J Clin Ultrasound 1989;17:291–295.

Fries MH, Goldberg JD, Golbus MS: Treatment of acardiac-acephalus twin gestations by hysterotomy and selective delivery. Obstet Gynecol 1992;79:601–604.

Langlotz H, Sauerbrei E, Murray S: Transvaginal Doppler sonographic diagnosis of an acardiac twin at 12 weeks gestation. J Ultrasound Med 1991;10:175–179.

McCurdy CM Jr, Childers JM, Seeds JW: Ligation of the umbilical cord of an acardiac-acephalus twin with an endoscopic intrauterine technique. Obstet Gynecol 1993;82:708–711.

Milner R, Crombleholme TM: Trouble with twins: Fetoscopic therapy. Semin Perinatol 1999;23:474–483.

Osborn P, Gross T, Shah JJ, Lindsay M: Prenatal diagnosis of fetal heart failure in twin reversed arterial perfusion syndrome. Prenat Diagn 2000;20:615–617.

Petit T, Taynal P, Ravasse P: Prenatal sonographic diagnosis of a twinning epigastric heteropagus. Ultrasound Obstet Gynecol 2001;17:534–535.

Pretorius DH, Leopold GR, Moore TR, et al: Acardiac twin: Report of Doppler sonography. J Ultrasound Med 1988;7:413–416.

Rodeck C, Deans A, Jauniaux E: Thermocoagulates for the early treatment of pregnancy with an acardiac twin. N Engl J Med 1998;339:1293–1295.

Schwarzler P, Ville Y, Moscosco G, et al: Diagnosis of twin reversed arterial perfusion sequence in the first trimester by transvaginal color Doppler ultrasound. Ultrasound Obstet Gynecol 1999;13:143–146.

Sepulveda W, Bower S, Hassan J, Fish NM: Ablation of acardiac twin by alcohol ingestion into the intra-abdominal umbilical artery. Obstet Gynecol 1995;86:680–681.

Van Allen MI, Smith DW, Shepard TH: Twin reversed arterial perfusion (TRAP) sequence: A study of 14 twin pregnancies with acardius. Sem Perinatol 1983;7:285–293.

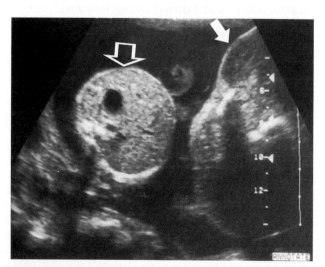

Normal "pump" twin (*open arrow*) alongside the acardiac acephalic twin (*closed arrow*). Note the discrepancy in size between the twins. There is no evidence as yet of hydrops in the "pump" twin.

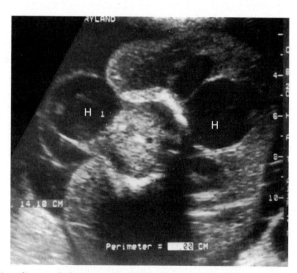

Acardiac acephalic twin. There is massive skin thickening around the fetal trunk, and several large cystic spaces (H) can be seen in the thickened skin resembling cystic hygroma. No fetal head was present, although moving lower limbs were seen.

12.3 Conjoined Twins

Epidemiology/Genetics

Definition *Conjoined twins* refers to incomplete anatomic separation at some location between monozygotic twins. Fusion at the thorax/abdomen (thoracopagus) accounts for 70% of cases.

Epidemiology The incidence is estimated to be 1 in 33,000 to 1 in 165,000 births, accounting for approximately 1% of monozygotic twins. Of note is the striking female prevalence (75% or greater).

Embryology Conjoined twins are thought to be an incomplete separation of a single embryo. The precise etiology for this event has not been established.

Inheritance Patterns Sporadic, with no increased recurrence risk in subsequent pregnancies.

Prognosis Potential for separation with optimal survival of both infants is directly related to the location of the union, the status of shared vital organs, and the presence of associated organ malformations.

Sonography

FINDINGS

1. **Fetus:** Twin fetuses lie adjacent to each other and do not move apart with fetal movement. The twins can be joined at the head (craniopagus), rump (ischiopagus), thorax/abdomen (thoracopagus), or some combination (e.g., cephalothoracopagus). There can be two heads (dicephalus), but all other structures are single. Three-dimensional ultrasonography and magnetic resonance imaging (MRI) are of help in showing the details of the malformation.
2. **Amniotic Fluid:** Polyhydramnios is frequent. There is a monoamniotic cavity.
3. **Placenta:** Normal. This malformation occurs only with monochorionic, monoamniotic placentation. The umbilical artery may contain more than three vessels.
4. **Measurement Data:** Normal where the fetus is not joined.
5. **When Detectable:** The syndrome has been detected as early as 8 weeks' gestation.

Pitfalls

1. Precise definition of joined areas may be difficult due to fetal lie.
2. Small zones of fusion may permit the twins to rotate 180 degrees; a vertex breech presentation does not exclude the diagnosis.
3. With extreme degrees of fusion, the twins may be mistaken for a singleton.

Differential Diagnosis Two normal fetuses that are relatively immobile and lie adjacent to each other.

Where Else to Look Look in detail at the fusion site; for example, establish with color Doppler sonography whether there is common liver arterial circulation or common cardiac system. Cardiac and gastrointestinal anomalies are common.

Pregnancy Management

Investigations and Consultations Required Fetal echocardiography should be performed to assess cardiac structure. Consultations with a pediatric surgeon and a neonatologist are essential to assess prognosis for separation and to plan perinatal management.

Fetal Intervention None is indicated.

Monitoring If the diagnosis is made early, the option of pregnancy termination should be offered to the parents. Serial sonographic examinations, every 3 to 4 weeks, should be done to monitor growth, to detect fetal hydrops, and to detect fetal demise.

Pregnancy Course Polyhydramnios is a complicating feature in up to 75% of cases. Nearly one third of conjoined twins will be stillborn.

Pregnancy Termination Issues No special considerations are necessary. Delivery by a destructive procedure is appropriate to avoid hysterotomy.

Delivery A planned caesarean delivery with appropriate personnel in attendance should be performed in a tertiary center.

Neonatology

Resuscitation The onset of respiration may be complicated by the site of attachment, particularly for thoracic and/or abdominally conjoined pairs. A very skilled intubator will be required if mechanical respiratory support is needed. Bag and mask ventilation should be provided to the lesser depressed infant, if mechanically feasible, while an endotracheal tube is placed in the more depressed one initially. Performing chest compressions may not be possible for twins conjoined at the chest.

Transport   Transfer to a tertiary center, with comprehensive pediatric diagnostic and surgical capabilities, after stabilization, is important to facilitate evaluation for potential for separation. Provision of a reliable airway, warmth, and intravenous fluids is essential to a safe transport. Frequently, prematurity mandates special care.

Nursery Management   The major objective is to establish the proper priority for diagnostic and treatment interventions, as follows:

1. Establish appropriate cardiorespiratory adaptation.
2. Maintain basic support: warmth, nutrition, protection from infection.
3. Maintain family confidentiality.
4. Plan diagnostic studies for optimum delineation of organ structure, by order of organ importance for survival first and separation potential second. The timing of surgical separation must be individualized for each conjoined twin pair. The majority experience seems to favor delay beyond the immediate neonatal period in the absence of either a life-threatening anomaly or complication forcing surgical separation on an emergency basis.

Surgery

Preoperative Assessment   The specific diagnosis of the type of conjoined twins should follow the postnatal resuscitation. An accurate diagnosis of the type of twinning is essential for any perioperative assessment.

There are four types of conjoined twins and subclasses based on a spectrum of malformations. Thoracopagus twins are joined at the sternum, diaphragm, and liver. As such, they face each other. Approximately half the cases have fused gastrointestinal tracts, and in an additional 25% the biliary tract is fused. Thoracopagus twins and variants of this form represent approximately 75% of all conjoined twins. As with most problems of embryogenesis, there is a spectrum of fusion defects that characterize thoracopagus twins. The omphalopagus variant involves union from the xiphoid to the umbilicus. This is the most common type of conjoined twins. Sternopagus twins are joined only at the sternum and represent the second variation of thoracopagus twins. Ischiopagus twins are connected from the umbilicus to a fused pelvis and account for 5% of all forms of conjoined twins. These twins have three or four legs. In addition, ischiopagus twins share a lower gastrointestinal tract. Pygopagus twins are joined both at the lower back and at the sacrum and therefore the twins are back to back. The incidence of pygopagus twins is approximately 18%. Again, there is one rectum and one anus, but usually separate spinal cords. Craniopagus twins are fused at the skull and represent the most rare twin malformation, with an incidence of 2%. There are separate brains but frequently a common venous drainage.

In general, survival rates are better if the twins are allowed to grow and develop. However, emergency separation procedures are indicated if one twin is stillborn or in full cardiac arrest. Associated malformations such as ruptured omphalocele, obstructive uropathy, cloacal exstro-

phy, imperforate anus, or severe intracardiac defects may also necessitate emergency separation.

A systematic approach to the work-up is predicated on the diagnosis of the twins. In general, priority is given to the cardiac status in the event that emergency separation is required for deteriorating heart function. Electrocardiography, echocardiography, and cardiac catheterization are all useful to evaluate the cardiac system. The gastrointestinal tract is best evaluated with a contrast study, and the biliary tree should be studied separately with isotopic tracers (DISIDA scans). Excellent hepatopancreaticobiliary detail can be obtained from ultrasonography. Selective angiography is helpful to obtain information about the vascular contribution of liver lobes. Computed tomographic (CT) scans are helpful for pelvic and perineal musculature and the bony pelvis architecture. Plain radiographs are helpful for architecture of the extremities. The nervous system is best evaluated using electroencephalography, CT scans, and MRI. Contrast studies of both the vagina and the urethra are best performed in conjunction with cystoscopy to determine the extent of shared organs of the reproductive and genitourinary tracts. Ultrasonography, CT, MRI, and intravenous pyelography are all also helpful for the shared components of the genitourinary tract alone.

Ultimately, two separate operative teams consisting of surgeons, anesthesiologists, and nurses should all be aware of the planned procedure preoperatively. A diagram of the anatomy is essential, as is an algorithm of the planned separation. If necessary, multiple rehearsals should be performed of the entire separation and definitive repair. The monitoring apparatus should also be discussed preoperatively.

Operative Indications   All conjoined twins will require separation for long-term survival. In general, survival rates after surgery are close to 50% in the first 3 weeks of life, whereas operation during weeks 4 to 14 approaches a survival rate of 90%. Therefore, most surgical teams prefer to perform separation in the second or third month of life. If necessary, gastrointestinal decompression (colostomy or ileostomy) or genitourinary diversion (pyeloplasty or vesicostomy) may be performed long before definitive repair.

Types of Procedures   The choice of operative procedures depends on the complexity of the malformation. In general, shared organs must be divided such that functional integrity is maintained for each twin. If residual organ function is not possible, then innovative bypass techniques should be considered. Such is the case with the extrahepatic biliary tree. If vascular and anatomic integrity to these structures cannot be maintained, then one twin may require a portoenterostomy for biliary drainage into the gastrointestinal tract. In addition, muscle and bone defects must be covered. Skin can be a major problem, and therefore serious consideration should be given to prior insertion of tissue expanders.

Thoracopagus twins require attention to the heart, pericardium, chest cavity, abdominal wall, and potentially fused abdominal organs. Thoracopagus twins have a spectrum of cardiac defects ranging from two hearts and a shared pericardium to one muscle system for the conjoined twins. Frequently, cardiopulmonary bypass must be employed for this step in the procedure. The liver in these twins usually requires separation, and in one quarter of cases a decision must be made about the biliary tree. The gastrointestinal tract is frequently fused at the second portion of the duodenum, again making it a difficult decision to bypass one twin and render the entire extrahepatic biliary system to the other.

Ischiopagus twin separation involves division of a fused pelvis, abdominal wall, and lower gastrointestinal tract. In addition, complex separation of the genitourinary tract is required. Here again, following separation a decision is made about who gets what. One twin will have a normal anus and rectum and the other will require reconstruction using the proximal colon. Each twin will require some type of pelvic bone reconstruction, such as an iliac osteotomy, which can be performed at the time of separation or as a secondary procedure. Vertebral body and hip support may also be required and may involve prosthetic parts. For orthopedic and gastrointestinal reasons, the anatomy of the pelvis must be restored. The ischiopagus tetrapus variant is easier to reconstruct, in contrast to the tripus type of twin. Skin coverage is also a problem with the ischiopagus twins. As expected, inadequate skin coverage may lead to infection, evisceration, and often sacrifice of the tripus third limb. Preoperative tissue expansion usually takes 8 to 12 weeks, for a total of 12 to 20 cm of tissue expansion.

Pygopagus twins require division at the level of the sacrum, spinal canal, rectum, and, on occasion, bladder, vagina, and urethra. Perineal musculature can be a problem for the shared rectum, especially if there is a sacral plexus defect, thereby denervating a portion of the levator diaphragm musculature. Skin coverage is usually not a problem for the pygopagus twin separation and closure.

Craniopagus twin separation requires division of the calvaria. Usually there are two whole brains but a shared venous sinus, despite the use of hypothermic circulatory arrest. Division of this shared venous sinus makes the operative procedure a very high risk for exsanguination. Again, the preoperative use of tissue expanders facilitates closure of the scalp for both children.

The twins are subject to life-threatening as well as chronic debilitating complications. Intraoperative bleeding represents the most insidious life-threatening problem. This complication occurs when large shared hepatic and perineal vessels are emptied in favor of the larger twin, thus producing hypovolemic shock in the smaller of the twins. Preoperative recognition of these large low-resistance shunts facilitates prompt separation of these vessels prior to other procedures. This is a potential problem for the thoracopagus variants as well as the ischiopagus twins. Inadequate skin coverage for either of the conjoined twins at separation may lead to evisceration and cardiopulmonary collapse in the postoperative period. Infection may occur at any time, especially if prosthetic material becomes infected. Spinal communication at any level may predispose to meningitis. This potential neurologic complication can accompany separation of ischiopagus and pygopagus twins.

Surgical Results/Prognosis   There is a paucity of morbidity and mortality data for separation of conjoined twins. In general, results are dependent on the complexity of the malformation, the extent of shared organs, and the general condition of the infants at the time of separation. Results are best in situations in which there is no life-threatening operative division of shared organs, such as the heart and brain. Therefore, good results are expected for thoracopagus twins (omphalopagus and xiphopagus) who do not share hearts and pygopagus separation. Ischiopagus twin separation involves separation and reconstruction of the gastrointestinal, genitourinary, and reproductive tracts as well as the skeleton. As expected, significant morbidity and long-term disability in all these systems is certainly possible. Craniopagus separation outcome is improved if there is no required venous division and reconstruction.

Ethical and moral decisions abound for all members of the multidisciplinary team, including the parents, at all stages of the evaluation process and actual operative procedure. At each step in the algorithm of the separation of conjoined twins, there is the potential for life-and-death decisions.

REFERENCES

Barth RA, Filly RA, Goldberg JD, et al: Conjoined twins: Prenatal diagnosis and assessment of associated malformations. Radiology 1990; 177:201–207.

Filler RM: Conjoined twins and their separation. Semin Perinatal 1986; 10:82–91.

Hoyle RM: Surgical separation of conjoined twins. Surg Gynecol Obstet 1990;170:549–562.

Kingston CA, McHugh K, Kumaradevan J: Imaging in the preoperative assessment of conjoined twins. Radiographics 2001;21:1187–1208.

Lipsky K: Conjoined twins: Psychosocial aspects. AORN J 1982;35: 58–61.

Mann MD, Coutts JP, Kaschula RO, et al: The use of radionuclides in the investigation of conjoined twins. J Nucl Med 1983;24:479–484.

Maymon R, Halperin R, Weinraub Z, et al: Three-dimensional transvaginal sonography of conjoined twins at 10 weeks: A case report. Ultrasound Obstet Gynecol 1998;11:292–294.

Miller D, Columbani P, Buck JR, et al: New techniques in the diagnosis and operative management of Siamese twins. J Pediatr Surg 1983; 18:373–376.

O'Neill JA, Holcomb GW, Schnaufer L, et al: Surgical experience with thirteen conjoined twins. Ann Surg 1988;208:299–312.

Ricketts R, Gray SW, Skandalakis JE: Conjoined twins. In Skandalakis JE, Gray SW (eds): Embryology for Surgeons, 2nd ed. Baltimore, Williams & Wilkins, 1994, pp 1066–1078.

Schnaufer L: Conjoined twins. In Raffensperger JG (ed): Swenson's Pediatric Surgery, 5th ed. Norwalk, CT, Appleton & Lange, 1990, pp 969–978.

Tongsong T, Chanprapaph P, Pongsatha S: First-trimester diagnosis of conjoined twins: A report of three cases. Ultrasound Obstet Gynecol 1999;14:434–437.

Votteler TP: Conjoined twins. In Welch KJ, Randolph JG, Ravitch MM, et al (eds): Pediatric Surgery, 4th ed. Chicago, Mosby-Year Book, 1986, pp 771–779.

Wong KC, Ohimura A, Roberts TH, et al: Anesthesia management for separation of craniopagus twins. Anesth Analg 1980;59:883–886.

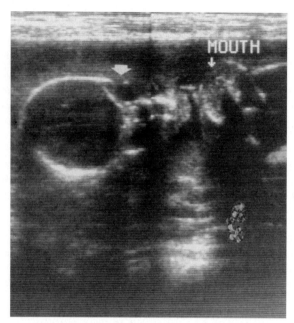

Conjoined twins joined at the thorax (thoracopagus). There were two fetal heads present that faced each other. *Broad arrow*, orbit of A; *small arrow*, mouth of B.

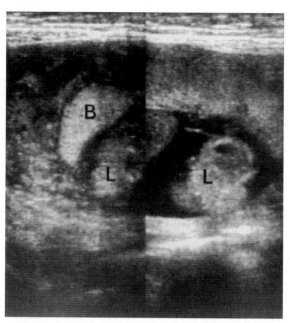

Conjoined twins. Single fetal abdomen with ascites and two livers within it. Although spines were visible in the thorax, caudal regression was present and there was no spine present in the abdomen. *B*, placenta; *L*, liver.

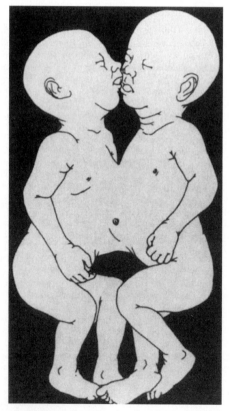

Thoracoomphalopagus twins. (Reprinted with permission from Vottler TP: Surgical separation of conjoined twins. AORN J 1982; pp. 36–38. Copyright © AORN, Inc.)

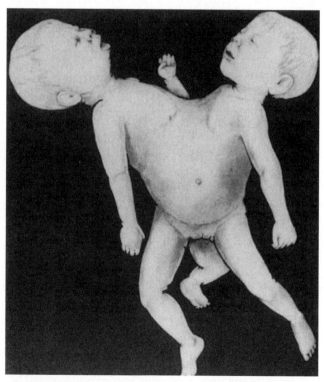

Ischiopagus tripus twins. (Reprinted with permission from Vottler TP: Surgical separation of conjoined twins. AORN J 1982; pp. 36–38. Copyright © AORN, Inc.)

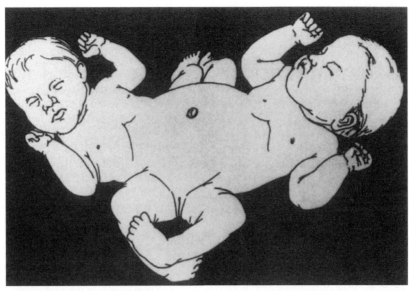

Ischiopagus tetrapus twins. (Reprinted with permission from Vottler TP: Surgical separation of conjoined twins. AORN J 1982; pp. 36–38. Copyright © AORN, Inc.)

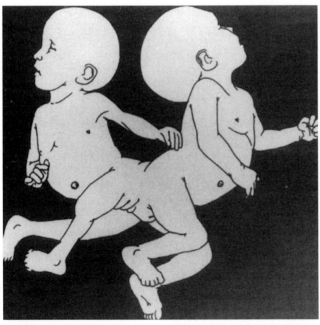

Pygopagus twins. (Reprinted with permission from Vottler TP: Surgical separation of conjoined twins. AORN J 1982; pp. 36–38. Copyright © AORN, Inc.)

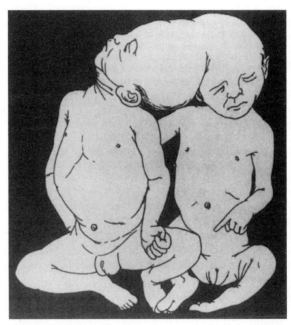

Craniopagus twins. (Reprinted with permission from Vottler TP: Surgical separation of conjoined twins. AORN J 1982; pp. 36–38. Copyright © AORN, Inc.)

12.4 Monoamniotic, Monochorionic Twins

Epidemiology/Genetics

Definition The presence of two fetuses in one pregnancy. Monozygotic twins are genetically identical twins originating from a single fertilized egg via an early embryonic split. Dizygotic twins are the result of the release and fertilization of two separate eggs during one menstrual cycle and are genetically full siblings, sharing 50% of their genetic material.

Epidemiology One in 250, with one third being diamniotic/dichorionic and two thirds being diamniotic/monochorionic; 1% are monoamniotic/monochorionic.

Embryology

Monozygotic Due to division of the developing cell mass in two during the first 17 days of development. Monozygotic twinning is a malformative process with a two to three times increased risk of major malformations.

Inheritance Patterns Familial clustering has been associated with dizygotic twins (expressed in females only), but not with monozygotic twins. Recurrence risk for dizygotic twins is approximately 2% in the European population. Risk of a twin pregnancy in a female twin is 1 in 58.

Teratogens None known.

Prognosis

Overall Increased risk for loss of one or both fetuses, prematurity, and low birth weight. Risk of intrauterine fetal demise highest (50–70%) for monoamniotic/monochorionic twins due to intertwining of the umbilical cords. Prognosis for conjoined twins is variable and is discussed in Chapter 12.3.

Monozygotic Increased (two to three times) risk of structural malformations, including neural tube defects and congenital heart defects; increase highest for monoamniotic/monochorionic twins. Also increased risk of vascular connections and twin-to-twin transfusions, as discussed in Chapter 12.6.

Dizygotic Increased risk for deformational abnormalities such as club feet due to in utero crowding.

Sonography

FINDINGS

1. **Fetus:**
   a. If the twin-to-twin transfusion is present, one twin may develop signs of hydrops with pleural effusion, ascites, pericardial effusion, and skin thickening.

   b. Bradycardia may occur related to cord entanglement.
2. **Amniotic Fluid:**
   a. Only a single amniotic cavity is present. There may be polyhydramnios.
   b. The cords may be entangled, showing numerous twists. Doppler sonography may show high-resistance flow with low or no diastolic flow if the cord twist is jeopardizing the fetus.
3. **Placenta:** A single placenta is present.
4. **Measurement Data:** Growth discrepancy between the twins may be present if the twin-to-twin transfusion syndrome is present. The donor twin will be small and the recipient twin large. IUGR not associated with twin-to-twin transfusion syndrome may also occur.
5. **When Detectable:** Cord entanglement has been detected in the first trimester at 10 weeks. Cord entanglement is thought to take place early, when fetal movement is the greatest.

Pitfalls The membrane between monochorionic diamniotic twins is easy to overlook, particularly in the first trimester and in the stuck twin syndrome. Make sure both twins can be moved by gravity and one is not fixed in position by placing the mother on the side and examining the amniotic cavity. The membrane between monochorionic diamniotic twins may not be evident until 12 to 14 weeks' gestation. In obese patients or in cases of doubt, CT amniography can be helpful. The demonstration of different distinct arterial waveforms with Doppler in two entwined cords can also prove that there is a monoamniotic cavity.

Differential Diagnosis Monochorionic, diamniotic twins. See Pitfalls.

Additional Investigations Detailed ultrasonography looking for possible malformations or deformations as well as determination of amnion and chorion status. DNA zygosity testing is available, although not necessarily considered routine in a prenatal setting.

Pregnancy Management

Investigations and Consultations Required Consultation with a perinatologist and neonatologist is essential for developing a plan of management.

Fetal Intervention If one fetus has an anomaly, fetoscopic cord ligation has been proposed. The cord must be divided after ligation to prevent entanglement of the surviving twin.

Monitoring No firm conclusion can be made regarding optimal surveillance. Some authors have recommended serial ultrasonograms every 2 weeks after 24 weeks' gestation to evaluate fetal biometry, size discordance, amniotic fluid volume, biophysical profile, and umbilical cord mapping with color flow Doppler sonography. Non-stress testing has been advocated as often as daily beginning at 25 to 26 weeks' gestation to look for variable decelerations or bradycardia. Unfortunately, none of these approaches would prevent death from sudden, severe cord compression. If an institution uses weekly steroids in high-risk circumstances, then this approach should begin as soon as intensive monitoring begins (24–25 weeks).

Pregnancy Course   As noted in the Monitoring section, there is a high risk of sudden fetal death secondary to cord entanglement. Usually both fetuses will die. Even if a twin survives the death of the co-twin, the survivor remains at risk for severe neurologic injury, thought to be secondary to acute hypotension following the death of the co-twin.

Pregnancy Termination Issues   The high risk of fetal morbidity and mortality mandates that this option be discussed with the family.

Delivery   Some studies have suggested that deaths do not occur after 32 weeks, but most authors do report deaths as late as 35 weeks. Delivery at 32 weeks at a site with excellent neonatal intensive care services would appear to offer the optimal outcome, although there is little scientific evidence to support this approach.

Neonatology

Resuscitation   With chronic in utero twin-to-twin transfusion, both infants frequently are depressed at birth and require immediate attention to facilitate the onset of respiration and resolution of birth asphyxia. Two skilled resuscitation teams are required, and each must be prepared to deal with the resultant blood and red cell volume problem unique to the respective infant: severe anemia in the donor and severe polycythemia/hypervolemia in recipient. Either

one or both twins could present with hydrops. Monoamniotic, monochorionic twins are frequently extremely preterm at time of birth, either from spontaneous preterm labor or from planned induction of labor, and therefore often need extensive support from delivery forward for a successful transition to extrauterine life.

Transport   Transfer of both infants to a tertiary perinatal center is indicated when there is preterm delivery, respiratory distress, or distress secondary to anemia or polycythemia. In utero transfer is the best transfer technique.

Nursery Management   Issues of respiratory support, transfusion, cardiac failure, perinatal asphyxia, hypoglycemia, and prematurity are frequently encountered. Partial exchange transfusions, to correct both anemia and polycythemia, are usually safer than simple transfusion and phlebotomy, as there is less stress on circulating blood volume and myocardial function with that approach.

REFERENCES

Aisenbrey GA, Catanzarite VA, Hurley TJ, et al: Monoamniotic and pseudomonoamniotic twins: Sonographic diagnosis, detection of cord entanglements, and obstetric management. Obstet Gynecol 1995,86:218–222.

Beasley E, Megerian G, Gerson A, Roberts NS: Monoamniotic twins: Case series and proposal for antenatal management. Obstet Gynecol 1999,93:130–134.

Carr SR, Aronson MP, Coustan DR: Survival rates of monoamniotic twins do not decrease after 30 weeks gestation. Am J Obstet Gynecol 1990,163:719–722.

Daniel Y, Ochshorn Y, Fait G, et al: Analysis of 104 twin pregnancies conceived with assisted reproductive technologies and 193 spontaneously conceived twin pregnancies. Fertil Steril 2000;74:683–689.

Gaziano E, De Lia J, Kuhlmann R: Diamniotic monochorionic twin gestations: An overview. J Matern Fetal Med 2000;9:89–96.

Jenkins T, Wapner R: The challenge of prenatal diagnosis in twin pregnancies. Curr Opin Obstet Gynecol 2000;12:87–92.

Little J, Bryan E: Congenital anomalies in twins. Semin Perinatol 1986;10:50–64.

Milner R, Crombleholme TM: Trouble with twins: Fetoscopic therapy. Semin Perinat 1999;23:474–483.

Rodis JF, McIlveen PF, Egan JFX, et al: Monoamniotic twins: Improved perinatal survival with accurate prenatal diagnosis and antenatal surveillance. Am J Obstet Gynecol 1997;177:1046–1049.

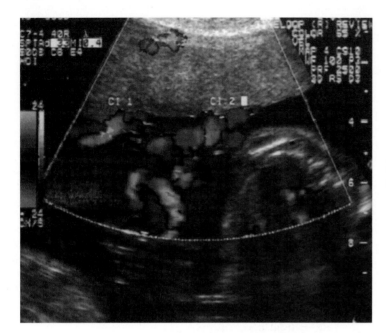

Monoamniotic monochorionic twins. Single placenta with adjacent cord insertions (C1 & C2). Only minimal cord entanglement has occurred so far. (See color figure following p. x).

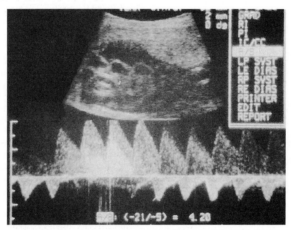

Entangled cord with at least 5 twists (*arrowheads*). The umbilical artery Doppler is still normal and the twins survived.

12.5 Stuck Twin

Epidemiology/Genetics

Definition *Stuck twin* is described as a diamniotic pregnancy in which one fetus resides against the uterine wall in a severely oligohydramniotic sac, and the co-twin is in a severely polyhydramniotic sac.

Epidemiology This problem complicates up to 8% of twin pregnancies and as many as 35% of monochorionic diamniotic gestations.

Embryology Most cases probably represent the severe end of the twin-to-twin transfusion syndrome. The condition has been described in dichorionic and even dizygotic pregnancies, however. The etiology for these cases remains unknown.

Inheritance Patterns Stuck twin is a sporadic event, limited to the current pregnancy.

Prognosis Fetal/neonatal mortality and morbidity rates are high. Fetal death and preterm delivery are the most common complications.

Sonography

FINDINGS

1. **Fetus:**
   a. On the initial study there is apparently no membrane between the twins, although detailed inspection may show a small portion of a membrane close to the smaller twin. The membrane is actually "shrink-wrapped" around the smaller twin, since there is almost no fluid in the smaller sac. The twins are of different sizes. The smaller twin lies adjacent to the uterine border and will not move away from the myometrium if the mother's position is changed, even if the twin is then in a nondependent position; this twin is "stuck."
   b. In most instances, the syndrome is related to twin-to-twin transfusion syndrome; the large twin may show evidence of hydrops with skin thickening, ascites, pleural effusion, and so on.
   c. Absent or reversed diastolic flow in the donor umbilical artery and a pulsatile umbilical vein in the recipient are associated with a poor prognosis if, as is usual, stuck twin syndrome is related to twin-to-twin transfusion syndrome (TTTS).
2. **Amniotic Fluid:** There will be polyhydramnios around the larger twin, and, although not immediately apparent, there is oligohydramnios with little or no fluid in the smaller sac. Membranes within the small cavity around the stuck twin may be seen and represent infolded adherent amniotic membrane, which may form a sling or adhesions.
3. **Placenta:** In most instances, a single placenta is present. The syndrome is thought to relate to a shared circulation through the single placenta, with excessive blood going to the larger twin and too little blood perfusing the smaller twin, leading to an imbalance in amniotic fluid quantity in the two sacs. The segment of the placenta supplying the stuck twin may be much more echogenic than the area of the placenta supplying the twin with normal growth. The cord insertion of the stuck twin may be velamentous at the edge of the placenta, perhaps accounting for the poor blood supply to the smaller twin.
4. **Measurement Data:** There is a marked discrepancy in size, with the smaller twin almost always the equivalent of at least 2 weeks smaller than the larger twin.
5. **When Detectable:** The syndrome has been reported as early as 15 weeks' gestation but usually develops at about 22 weeks.

Pitfalls Growth discrepancy in diamniotic twins is common, but the amniotic fluid volumes should be only mildly discrepant, with IUGR in one dizygotic twin. No polyhydramnios should surround the larger twin.

Differential Diagnosis

1. Diamniotic twins, with IUGR in one twin.
2. Monoamniotic twins, with IUGR in one.
3. Twin-to-twin transfusion without stuck twin syndrome.

Where Else to Look

1. Look hard for findings of hydrops in both twins. The donor twin may eventually become the recipient. Early findings of hydrops include hepatosplenomegaly and a small pericardial effusion.
2. Look in the stuck twin for renal anomalies causing oligohydramnios, since not all cases of stuck twin relate to twin-to-twin transfusion syndrome.
3. In particular, the stuck twin may show signs of embolization or infarction, before repeated amniocenteses have been performed. Intracranial echogenic areas or hydrocephalus may develop more often in the stuck twin but they can occur in the recipient twin.

Pregnancy Management

Investigations and Consultations Required Congenital malformations, including chromosomal abnormalities resulting in severe IUGR in one fetus also must be ruled out. Fetal echocardiography should be done to assess both cardiac structure and function. Maternal serum and amniotic fluid studies should be done to rule out fetal infections.

Fetal Intervention   Selective fetal reduction of the stuck twin is contraindicated unless it can clearly be delineated that the fetuses are dizygotic. In monozygotic twins, vascular anastomosis between the placenta may result in significant neurologic damage to or death of the surviving twin. Only those procedures involving ligation or cautery of the affected twin's umbilical cord should be used if a decision is made to selectively reduce the stuck twin. In cases of stuck twin on the basis of TTTS, therapy with serial amniocentesis reductions or laser oblation of anastomotic vessels may result in normalization of the amniotic fluid volume.

Repeated amniocenteses to drain off the excess amniotic fluid in the sac with polyhydramnios are required. Fluid in this sac should be kept at a low volume. This may require daily or every other day removal of liters of fluid when the diagnosis is first made. Fluid will sometimes spontaneously return to the anhydramniac sac.

Monitoring   Weekly assessments of fetal and fluid status are essential to institute appropriate therapy. In the absence of therapy, mortality is extremely high for the stuck twin, and there is a significant risk of death or severe morbidity in the surviving twin.

Pregnancy Course   Without the use of repeated amniocenteses, fetal mortality with the stuck twin syndrome is approximately 80%. Preterm labor occurs in a majority of cases in which there is polyhydramnios in one sac. Mortality for one or both fetuses is quite high despite therapy, with only 50 to 60% of fetuses surviving to delivery.

Pregnancy Termination Issues   If termination is an option, morphologic evaluation of the fetuses and placentas should be made to confirm the diagnosis.

Delivery   The extremely high risk of neonatal complications mandates that delivery occur in a tertiary center.

Neonatology

Resuscitation   Preterm delivery either electively secondary to deteriorating fetal condition or secondary to preterm labor is frequently associated with early-onset respiratory distress. In the stuck twin, the concomitant occurrence of in utero compromise increases the likelihood of severe depression following delivery, necessitating aggressive resuscitation and early initiation of mechanical ventilatory support. In the polyhydramniac twin, congestive heart failure/hypervolemia may be present, contributing to the need for resuscitation. In both instances, early surfactant replacement therapy in conjunction with respiratory support may be indicated.

Transport   Transfer to a tertiary perinatal center will be dependent on the degree of prematurity and the concomitant problems of respiratory distress syndrome, and prematurity-related conditions.

Nursery Management   As noted, the management issues are determined by the degree of prematurity and its concomitant problems. Anemia in the stuck twin and polycythemia in the other can be seen and, when present, requires appropriate early correction to facilitate appropriate cardiorespiratory transition. The latter may also require inotropic therapy if congestive heart failure is a significant clinical feature.

REFERENCES

Al-Kouatly HB, Skupski DW: Intrauterine sling: A complication of the stuck twin syndrome. Ultrasound Obstet Gynecol 1999;14:419–421.

Bruner JP, Rosemond RL: Twin-to-twin transfusion syndrome: A subset of the twin oligohydramnios-polyhydramnios sequence. Am J Obstet Gynecol 1993;169:925–930.

Elliott JP: Amniocentesis for twin-twin transfusion syndrome. Contemp Obstet Gynecol 1992;Aug:30–47.

Lees CC, Schwarzler P, Ville Y, Campbell S: Stuck twin syndrome without signs of twin-to-twin transfusion. Ultrasound Obstet Gynecol 1998;12:211–214.

Mahony BS, Petty CN, Nyberg DA, et al: The stuck twin phenomenon: Ultrasonographic findings, pregnancy outcome, and management with serial amniocenteses. Am J Obstet Gynecol 1990;163:1513–1522.

Myles JO, Denbow DL, Duncan R, et al: Antenatal factors at diagnosis that predict outcome in twin-twin transfusion syndrome. Am J Obstet Gynecol 2000;183:1023–1028.

Patten RM, Mack LA, Harvey D, et al: Disparity of amniotic fluid volume and fetal size: Problem of the stuck twin—US studies. Radiology 1989;172:153–157.

Reisner DP, Mahony BS, Petty CN, et al: Stuck twin syndrome: Outcome in thirty-seven consecutive cases. Am J Obstet Gynecol 1993;169:991–995.

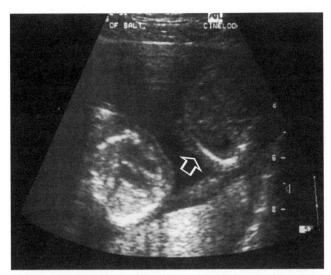

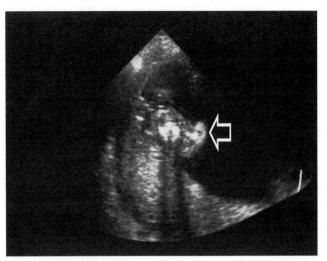

"Stuck" twins. There was polyhydramnios with an apparently monoamniotic pregnancy. The smaller twin was immobile, and with detailed views a membrane adherent to the smaller twin was seen (*arrow*).

Right-side-up view. The "stuck" twin (*arrow*) remains adherent to the uterine wall and does not drop into a dependent position.

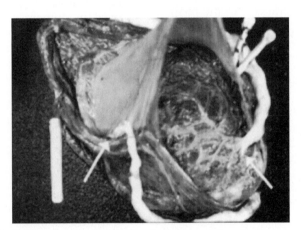

Single placenta in a case of stuck twin syndrome. Note the velamentous insertion of the cord on the left (*arrows*).

12.6 Twin-to-Twin Transfusion (TTTS)

Epidemiology/Genetics

Definition Twin-to-twin transfusion syndrome describes a continuum of complications that are seen in monozygotic, monochorionic twins, resulting from transplacental vascular communications.

Epidemiology The incidence of twin-to-twin transfusion ranges from 5 to 15% of all twin pregnancies. However, the acute, severe form is seen in only approximately 1% of monochorionic gestations.

Embryology This pregnancy complication results from transplacental arteriovenous communications. Blood is shunted from one twin, the donor, who develops anemia, growth retardation, and oligohydramnios, to the recipient, who becomes plethoric, macrosomic, and occasionally hydropic with severe polyhydramnios.

Inheritance This is a sporadic event unique to the monozygotic, monochorionic gestation.

Prognosis Mortality rates of 50 to 100% have been reported. Complications include intrauterine death of one or both fetuses and a high risk of preterm labor. For a surviving twin, there is significant risk of central nervous system and other malformations, now thought to be on the basis of acute hemodynamic and ischemic changes at the time of the death of the co-twin.

Sonography

FINDINGS

1. **Fetus:**
   a. Monozygotic twins of discrepant size. One twin (the recipient) is larger and one (the donor) smaller than expected by gestational age.
   b. The larger twin may become hydropic; there may be pleural effusion, ascites, pericardial effusion, and skin thickening. Hepatosplenomegaly may be present. The stomach and bladder will be larger in the recipient twin.
   c. Donor twins may show biventricular hypertrophy with a hyperechogenic left ventricular wall. Some recipient twins may also show biventricular hypertrophy and cardiac enlargement.
      Right ventricular hypertrophy, pulmonary stenosis, and tricuspid regurgitation may occur in the recipient twin.
   d. Absent or reversed diastolic flow in the donor umbilical artery and a pulsatile umbilical vein in the recipient are associated with a poor prognosis.

2. **Amniotic Fluid:**
   a. Membrane—The syndrome occurs only if the twins are monochorionic, but there may be two amniotic sacs. The membrane will have only two components.
   b. Fluid—The amniotic sacs may be unequal, with the smaller twin having less fluid around it and the larger twin with polyhydramnios (see Chapter 12.5).
3. **Placenta:** With a monochorionic diamniotic pregnancy, there is only one placenta and the membrane between the two amniotic cavities is thin, since it only has two components. The gender of the two fetuses is the same. The cord of the larger twin will be larger than the cord to the smaller twin. A difference in the echogenicity of the areas of the placenta supplying each twin may be seen. The smaller twin may be supplied by a more echogenic placental area. Arterial communications between the two fetuses' placental circulations are present and can be visualized with color-flow Doppler on the surface of the placenta. Mapping the arterial communications helps in planning laser ablation therapy. The communications may be best observed using three-dimensional Doppler.
4. **Measurement Data:** One twin shows evidence of IUGR. As follow-up studies are performed, the smaller twin may become the recipient and the growth pattern may reverse. The larger twin may have a spuriously large abdominal circumference if there is ascites.
5. **When Detectable:** The syndrome has been detected at 8 weeks but is usually seen between 16 and 25 weeks. If it presents in the third trimester, the syndrome develops less rapidly, but significant weight (15%) and hematocrit (7.5 g/dL) differences may exist.

Pitfalls

1. Apparent TTTS in monozygotic, monoamniotic twins may be diamniotic, monozygotic twins with a stuck twin.
2. Oligohydramnios around one twin may not relate to TTTS.
3. Hydrops in twins may occur not related to the TTTS.

Differential Diagnosis IUGR is common in all forms of twins without the TTTS.

Where Else to Look

1. Look carefully for diamniotic dizygotic twins. Findings that indicate diamniotic dizygotic twins are (a) the "twin peak" sign in the placenta—a portion of placenta pokes into the space between the fused amniotic membranes; (b) more than two components to the intersac membrane; (c) different fetal gender. These findings eliminate the possibility of TTTS, since they establish

a diagnosis of diamniotic dizygotic twins. Two placentas make monozygotic twins unlikely but not impossible, since a succenturiate lobe could be present.

2. Make sure the smaller twin is not stuck by placing the mother in positions that force the smaller twin to fall into a dependent position and look for evidence of a membrane.

3. Look for other causes of hydrops, such as cardiac problems or infection.

Pregnancy Management

Investigations and Consultations Required Because of the difficulty that arises in distinguishing TTTS from other causes of stuck twin, some authors have recommended a full evaluation of both fetuses for chromosome abnormalities and TORCH studies on maternal blood to exclude fetal infection. Fetal echocardiography should be done to assess both cardiac structure and function. Because of the high risk of prematurity, a neonatologist should be consulted.

Fetal Intervention Because of the extremely high mortality rate, a number of treatment approaches have been attempted, with serial amnioreduction and endoscopic laser surgery the two options providing improved outcomes. The study by Hecher et al found that overall survival was not different between the two approaches, but laser therapy resulted in a higher proportion of cases with more than one surviving twin. The major benefit to laser therapy is the decreased risk of neurologic complications in the event of the death of one twin. Because of the limited availability of centers providing laser therapy, initial therapy with amnioreduction may be the best approach, with referral for laser therapy reserved for cases not responding to serial amniocentesis. Selective reduction of one twin should only be done by a method that ligates or coagulates the umbilical cord.

Monitoring Weekly sonographic studies with Doppler assessment are necessary to detect cases that may benefit from therapeutic intervention. Serial assessment of cardiac function may be helpful in deciding an appropriate course of therapy. Early detection of preterm labor and appropriate therapy are essential components of pregnancy management.

Pregnancy Termination Issues If diagnosis is made early, this option should be discussed with the family, given the significant risk of fetal mortality and morbidity in surviving fetuses.

Delivery Delivery must occur in a tertiary center with full neonatal capabilities.

Neonatology

Resuscitation With chronic in utero twin-to-twin transfusion, both infants frequently are depressed at birth and require immediate attention to facilitate the onset of respiration and resolution of birth asphyxia. Two skilled resuscitation teams are required, and each must be prepared to deal with the resultant blood and red blood cell volume problem unique to the respective infant: severe anemia in the donor and severe polycythemia/hypervolemia in recipient. Either one or both twins could present with hydrops.

Transport Transfer of both infants to a tertiary perinatal center is indicated when there is preterm delivery, respiratory distress, or distress secondary to anemia or polycythemia. In utero transfer is the best transfer technique.

Nursery Management Issues of respiratory support, transfusion, cardiac failure, perinatal asphyxia, hypoglycemia, and prematurity are frequently encountered. Partial exchange transfusions, to correct both anemia and polycythemia, are usually safer than simple transfusion and phlebotomy, as there is less stress on circulating blood volume and myocardial function with that approach.

REFERENCES

Achiron R, Rabinovitz R, Aboulafia Y, et al: Intrauterine assessment of high-output cardiac failure with spontaneous remission of hydrops fetalis in twin-twin transfusion syndrome: Use of two-dimensional echocardiography, Doppler ultrasound, and color flow mapping. J Clin Ultrasound 1992;20:271–277.

Brown DL, Benson CB, Driscoll SG, Doubilet PM: Twin-twin transfusion syndrome: Sonographic findings. Radiology 1989;170:61–63.

Dickinson JE, Evans SF: Obstetric and perinatal outcomes from the Australian and New Zealand twin-twin transfusion syndrome registry. Am J Obstet Gynecol 2000;182:706–712.

Elliott JP, Urig MA, Clewell WH: Aggressive therapeutic amniocentesis for treatment of twin-twin transfusion syndrome. Obstet Gynecol 1991;77:537–540.

Fesslova V, Villa L, Nava S, et al: Fetal and neonatal echocardiographic findings in twin-twin transfusion syndrome. Am J Obstet Gynecol 1998;179:1056–1062.

Hecher K, Plath H, Bregenzer T, et al: Endoscopic laser surgery versus serial amniocentesis in the treatment of severe twin-twin transfusion syndrome. Am J Obstet Gynecol 1999;180:717–724.

Klebe JG, Inogomar CJ: The fetoplacental circulation during parturition illustrated by the interfetal transfusion sydrome. Pediatrics 1972;49:112–116.

Mari G, Detti L, Oz U, Abuhamad AZ: Long-term outcome in twin-twin transfusion syndrome treated with serial aggressive amnioreduction. Am J Obstet Gynecol 2000;183:211–217.

McCulloch K: Neonatal problems in twins. Clin Perinatol 1988;15:141–158.

Milner R, Crombleholme TM: Trouble with twins: Fetoscopic therapy. Semin Perinatal 1999;23:474–483.

Nizard J, Bonnet D, Fermont L, et al: Acquired right heart outflow tract anomaly without systemic hypertension in recipient twin in twin twin transfusion syndrome. Ultrasound Obstet Gynecol 2001;18:669–672.

Pharoah POD, Adi Y: Consequences of in-utero death in a twin pregnancy. Lancet 2000;355:1597–1602.

Rodis JF, Vintzileos AM, Campbell WA, Nochimson DJ: Intrauterine fetal growth in discordant twin gestations. J Ultrasound Med 1990;9:443–448.

Tan KL, Tan R, Tan SH, Tan AM: The twin transfusion sydrome: Clinical observations on 35 affected pairs. Clin Pediatr 1979;18:111–114.

Urig MA, Clewell WH, Elliott JP: Twin-twin transfusion syndrome. Am J Obstet Gynecol 1990;163:1522–1526.

Welsh AW, Taylor D, Cosgrove D, et al: Freehand three-dimensional Doppler demonstration of monochorionic vascular anastomoses in vivo: Preliminary report. Ultrasound Obstet Gynecol 2001;18:317–324.

Yamada A, Kasugai M, Ohno Y, et al: Antenatal diagnosis of twin-twin transfusion syndrome by doppler ultrasound. Obstet Gynecol 1991;78:1058–1061.

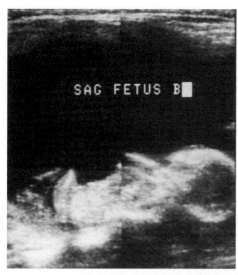

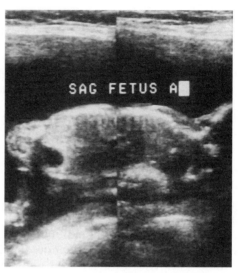

Twin-twin transfusion syndrome. Fetus B is small with little soft tissue. There was moderate polyhydramnios. This was a monoamniotic pregnancy, but the syndrome may develop in monochorionic diamniotic pregnancies.

Fetus A is larger than expected and there is mild skin thickening. Hydrops may occur in more severe examples.

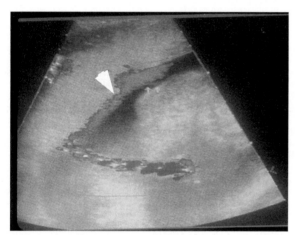

Color flow view showing large communicating vessel between the placental circulations of identical twins, running along the surface of the placenta (*arrowhead*). (See color figure following p. x.)

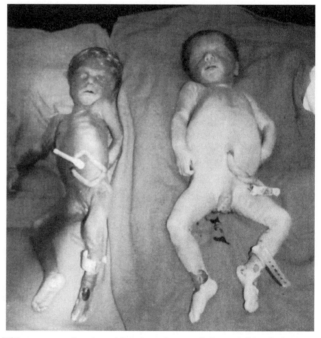

Thirty-two-week twins with twin-twin transfusion resulting in in-utero demise. Note discordant size.

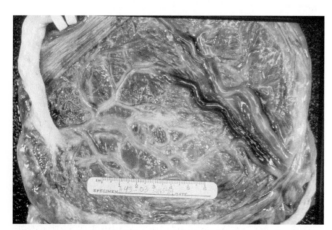

Placenta from a case of twin-twin tranfusion with a stuck twin showing large communicating vessels between the twins.

Miscellaneous Abnormalities 13

13.1 Chorioangioma

Epidemiology/Genetics

Definition Chorioangiomas are benign vascular tumors of the placenta. They are most commonly encapsulated, round, and intraplacental.

Epidemiology Chorioangiomas are found in approximately 1% of placentas examined at term.

Embryology Chorioangiomas are the most common primary tumor of the placenta.

Inheritance These tumors are sporadic, with no increased risk in future pregnancies.

Prognosis Most chorioangiomas are incidental findings. Very rarely, secondary fetal hydrops may develop.

Sonography

FINDINGS

1. **Fetus:** Usually the fetus is normal. On rare occasions, severe fetal anemia may develop because the placental mass shunts blood and acts as an arteriovenous malformation. Hydrops may develop. The earliest signs are hepatosplenomegaly and small pericardial effusions. Pleural effusion, ascites, and skin thickening follow.
2. **Amniotic Fluid:** The amniotic fluid volume is almost always increased if a large mass is present.
3. **Placenta:** A mass is present in the placenta that has many arteries within it. The mass usually protrudes into the amniotic cavity and is often located near the cord insertion. Tumor vascularity varies. Color flow Doppler sonography may demonstrate arterial flow compatible with an arteriovenous malformation. The more arterial flow there is in a mass, the more likely it is that there will be complications such as polyhydramnios and hydrops.
4. **Measurement Data:** If there is fetal anemia, intrauterine growth retardation is usual. Chorioangiomas are usually not associated with any complications if they are less than 6 cm in diameter.

5. **When Detectable:** Earliest detection reported is at 15 weeks' gestation, but chorioangiomas often develop later in pregnancy.

Pitfalls

1. Venous lakes—Venous flow within a venous lake may not be visible with Doppler and color flow sonography. Look intently with real-time imaging and subtle red blood cell movement will be seen. Venous lakes often lie at the edge of the placenta and protrude into the amniotic fluid.
2. The chorioangioma may lie alongside the fetus and be mistaken for a fetal mass such as a sacrococcygeal teratoma.

Differential Diagnosis

1. Preplacental hematoma—A mass with a similar appearance to a chorioangioma arising from the placental surface. No flow will be seen on real time or with Doppler imaging.
2. Placental lake on placental surface—The apparent mass will show venous flow with real time and no flow with Doppler imaging.
3. Placental cyst—Cysts arising from the placental surface often have a solid component at the base. A round, thin membrane outlining the echo-free component of the cyst will be seen. These cysts may represent resolving hematoma.

Where Else to Look Look at the fetus for intrauterine growth restriction and for evidence of fetal heart failure.

Pregnancy Management

Investigations and Consultations Required No further investigation is required. Additional consultation will be necessary only if fetal complications develop.

Fetal Intervention None is indicated.

Monitoring Serial sonographic examinations are essential to detect early signs of fetal hydrops and to monitor fluid volumes. Fetal growth also must be assessed regularly. The development of hydrops should prompt early delivery. In the absence of complications, aggressive intervention is contraindicated, as many of these lesions will spontaneously regress.

Pregnancy Course Chorioangiomas are, in rare instances, associated with an increased risk of intrauterine growth retardation, fetal hydrops, and polyhydramnios.

Pregnancy Termination Issues If pregnancy termination is chosen, an intact fetus and placenta must be delivered to confirm the sonographic diagnosis.

Delivery In the absence of fetal complications, delivery at a tertiary center is not necessary. Pregnancies with polyhydramnios and/or fetal hydrops are likely to be delivered preterm, and delivery should occur at a tertiary center.

Neonatology

Resuscitation There are no specific measures required unless fetal anemia and/or hydrops fetalis is present (see Chapter 13.2).

Transport Unless there has been concurrent fetal illness, transfer of the newborn is not indicated.

Nursery Management There are no special care requirements for the newborn except for the infant who has developed hydrops fetalis (see Chapter 13.2).

REFERENCES

Chazotte C, Girz B, Koenigsberg M, Cohen WR: Spontaneous infarction of placental chorioangioma and associated regression of hydrops fetalis. Am J Obstet Gynecol 1990;163:1180–1181.

Dao AH, Rogers CW, Wong SW: Chorioangioma of the placenta: Report of 2 cases with ultrasound study in 1. Obstet Gynecol 1981;57: 46S–48S.

Jauniaux E, Ogle R: Color Doppler imaging in the diagnosis and management of chorioangiomas. Ultrasound Obstet Gynecol 2000;15: 463–467.

Tonkin IL, Setzer ES, Ermocilla R: Placental chorioangioma: A rare cause of congestive heart failure and hydrops fetalis in the newborn. Am J Roentgenol 1980;134:181–183.

Van Wering JH, Van Der Slikke JW: Prenatal diagnosis of chorioangioma associated with polyhydramnios using ultrasound. Eur J Obstet Gynecol Reprod Biol 1985;19:255–259.

Wolfe BK, Wallace JHK: Pitfall to avoid: Chorioangioma of the placenta simulating fetal tumor. J Clin Ultrasound 1987;15:405–408.

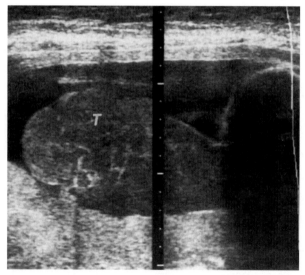

Huge mass arising from the placenta (T). Arteries could be seen within the mass using color flow ultrasonography. Despite the large size, no fetal hydrops developed.

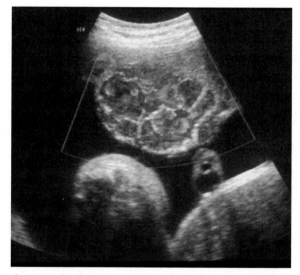

Another example of a chorioangioma. This mass, which arose from the placenta, had numerous arteries within it visible with real-time ultrasonography and confirmed on color flow.

13.2 Nonimmune Hydrops Fetalis

Epidemiology/Genetics

Definition *Hydrops fetalis* refers to fluid accumulation in serous cavities and/or edema of soft tissues in the fetus. It is characterized as nonimmune if there is no indication of a fetomaternal blood group incompatibility. Most series include isolated fetal ascites in the definition of hydrops.

Epidemiology The incidence is approximately 1 in 2500 to 1 in 3500 neonates.

Embryology The causes are diverse and include numerous maternal, fetal, and placental disorders. Table 1, modified from Holzgreve et al., outlines some of the diverse conditions that have been associated with hydrops fetalis.

Inheritance The heterogeneous nature of the etiologic conditions ranges from those that are sporadic to mendelian disorders with a 25% risk of recurrence. In cases for which no cause can be determined, an empiric risk of recurrence of 5% is appropriate for counseling purposes.

Sonography

FINDINGS

1. **Fetus:** More than two of the following findings need to be present: fetal ascites, pleural effusion, pericardial effusion, or skin thickening. Usually, the earliest finding is pericardial effusion.
2. **Amniotic Fluid:** Polyhydramnios is commonly seen, depending on the cause of the hydrops.
3. **Placenta:** Placentomegaly is often present, depending on the cause of hydrops, such as Rh disease, chorioangioma, and so on.
4. **Measurement Data:** Variable, depending on the cause of the hydrops.
5. **When Detectable:** Depends on the cause—it can occur at 13 weeks' gestation with cystic hygroma.

Pitfalls

1. Isolated fetal ascites, pericardial effusion, skin thickening, or pleural effusion have a different prognosis and causation but may precede hydrops.
2. Pseudopericardial effusion—The fat pad around the heart may be mistaken for an early pericardial effusion.
3. Pseudoascites—Apparent small amounts of intra-abdominal fluid may represent periabdominal fat or muscle rather than fluid.

Differential Diagnosis None, if more than two of the four basic components are present. Rh disease, which

Table 13-2-1 Conditions Associated With NIHF

Conditions	Individual Conditions
Cardiovascular	Tachyarrhythmia
	Congenital heart block
	Anatomic defects
	Cardiomyopathy
	Myocarditis (Coxsackie virus or CMV)
Chromosomal	Down syndrome (trisomy 21)
	Other trisomies
	Turner's syndrome
	Triploidy
Malformation syndromes	Thanatophoric dwarfism
	Arthrogryposis multiplex congenita
	Osteogenesis imperfecta
	Achondrogenesis
	Neu-Laxova syndrome
	Recessive cystic hygroma
Twin pregnancy	Twin-twin transfusion syndrome
Hematologic	Alpha-thalassemia
	Arteriovenous shunts (e.g., large vascular tumors)
	G6PD deficiency
	Pleural effusion
Respiratory	Diaphragmatic hernia
	Cystic adenoma of the lung
	Mediastinal teratoma
Gastrointestinal	Jejunal atresia
	Midgut volvulus
	Meconium peritonitis
Liver	Polycystic disease of the liver
	Biliary atresia
	Hepatic vascular malformations
Maternal	Severe diabetes mellitus
	Severe anemia
	Hypoproteinemia
Placenta-umbilical cord	Chorioangioma
	Fetomaternal transfusion
	Placental and umbilical vein thrombosis
	Angiomyxoma of the umbilical cord
Medications	Antepartum indomethacin (taken to stop premature labor, causing fetal ductus closure and secondary NIHF)
Infections	CMV
	Toxoplasmosis
	Syphilis
	Congenital hepatitis
	Herpes simplex, type 1
	Rubella
Miscellaneous	Congenital lymphedema
	Congenital hydrothorax or chylothorax
	Sacrococcygeal teratoma

Modified from Holzgreve W, Holzgreve B, Curry CI: Nonimmune hydrops fetalis: diagnosis and management. Semin Perinatol 1985;9:57. CMV, cytomegalovirus; G6PD, glucose-6-phosphate dehydrogenase; NIHF, nonimmune hydrops fetalis.

presents with hydrops, is considered elsewhere (see Chapter 13.3).

It is essential to exclude blood group incompatibility and other conditions for which fetal transfusions would be therapeutic. Likewise, other treatable conditions, such as cardiac arrhythmia, must be differentiated before obstetric management plans are formulated.

Where Else to Look Every structure in the body may be abnormal in association with hydrops. Possible causes include the following:

1. Cystic hygroma—The skin thickening will have septation and cystic spaces within.
2. Cardiac—Many examples of hydrops are caused by a cardiac abnormality. Pay particular attention to the heart rhythm and rate, since abnormalities of these structures are usually correctable.
3. Masses in any site, particularly sacrococcygeal teratoma and cystic adenomatoid malformations.
4. Infection, such as stigmata of cytomegalovirus.
5. Chorioangioma in the placenta.
6. Chromosomal abnormalities, particularly Down syndrome.
7. Twin-to-twin transfusion syndrome in twins.

Pregnancy Management

Investigations and Consultations Required Karyotyping and fetal echocardiography. A protocol for the diagnostic evaluation of the pregnancy complicated by hydrops is outlined in Table 2. Other consultations will depend on the etiology that is determined.

Fetal Intervention Intervention should be reserved for those cases in which a precise diagnosis has been established. Intrauterine transfusion has been successful for anemia secondary to parvovirus infection. Fetuses with a primary lung lesion treated by shunt placement have been reported to have resolution of hydrops. Control of fetal cardiac arrhythmias has been the most successful intervention for associated fetal hydrops.

Fetal hydrops may be diagnosed in the first trimester. In these cases, chromosomal studies should be done by chorionic villus sampling. If aneuploidy is not found, and the maternal serologic evaluation is negative, a detailed ultrasonographic evaluation and fetal echocardiography should be done at 18 weeks' gestation.

Monitoring Every attempt must be made to establish a diagnosis. The aggressiveness of the management approach will be highly dependent on the overall prognosis for the fetus. In general, a nonaggressive approach is warranted for idiopathic hydrops because the mortality rate is high and is not improved by early delivery. These high-risk pregnancies should be managed by a perinatologist who is familiar with the diverse causes for hydrops. If the cause is unknown, reexamine at frequent intervals, such as every 2 weeks. A cause may become apparent.

Pregnancy Course There is a significant risk of polyhydramnios and preeclampsia associated with fetal hy-

Table 13-2-2   Diagnostic Steps in the Prenatal Evaluation of NIHF

Levels of Invasiveness	Diagnostic Test
Noninvasive	Complete blood count and indices
	Hemoglobin electrophoresis
	Kleihauer-Betke stain
	Syphilis (VDRL) and TORCH titers
	Fetal echocardiography
Amniocentesis	Fetal karotype
	Amniotic fluid viral cultures
	Alpha-fetoprotein
	Specific metabolic tests
Fetal blood sampling	Rapid karyotype
	Hemoglobin chain analysis, if indicated
	Fetal plasma analysis for specific IgM
	Fetal plasma albumin

IgM, immunoglobulin-M; TORCH, toxoplasmosis, other, rubella, cytomegalovirus, and herpes simplex virus; VDRL, Veneral Disease Research Laboratory (test for syphylis).

drops. Fetal mortality rates have been reported to range from 75 to 90%.

Pregnancy Termination Issues Unless a precise diagnosis has been made antenatally, an intact fetus must be delivered for a complete pathologic evaluation.

Delivery Delivery must occur at a tertiary center because of the complicated neonatal resuscitation likely to be required. The mode of delivery should be based on obstetric indications, but the high risk of "fetal distress" will mean a high rate of cesarean section for fetuses with hydrops.

Neonatology

Resuscitation Fetuses with hydrops tolerate labor poorly. They develop asphyxia secondary to the accompanying placental pathologic lesions, as well as from the disorder causing the hydrops. Except in very uncommon cases, extensive resuscitation with immediate respiratory support is required. Both thoracentesis and paracentesis may be needed following delivery to permit adequate ventilatory excursions. Manipulation of circulating blood volume, without the capability to monitor both arterial and venous pressure, is fraught with the risk of fetal deterioration.

Transport Referral to a tertiary perinatal center is mandatory both because of the very high mortality risk and because of the extensive technical support required for diagnostic evaluation and management.

Nursery Management The management approach is determined by two factors: the effects on cardiorespiratory function of the hydropic state and the underlying cause. Mobilization of the hydropic fluid without concomitant further hemodynamic compromise is the initial goal. Fluid restriction, diuresis, dialysis, and exchange transfusion have all been used successfully.

If not established prenatally, determining the cause is imperative both to facilitate therapeutic intervention and to provide accurate counseling regarding prognosis and recurrence risk.

REFERENCES

Holzgreve W, Curry CJ, Golbus MS, et al: Investigation of nonimmune hydrops fetalis. Am J Obstet Gynecol 1984;150:805–812.

Holzgreve W, Holzgreve B, Curry CJ: Nonimmune hydrops fetalis: Diagnosis and management. Semin Perinatol 1985;9:52–67.

Hutchinson AA, Drew JH, Yu VY, et al: Nonimmunologic hydrops fetalis: A review of 61 cases. Obstet Gynecol 1982;59:347–352.

Iskarps K, Jauniaix E, Rodeck C: Outcome of nonimmune hydrops fe-talis diagnosed during the first half of pregnancy. Obstet Gynecol 1997;90:321–325.

Jauniaux E: Diagnosis and management of early nonimmune hydrops fetalis. Prenat Diagn 1997;17:1261–1268.

Jauniaux E, Van Maldergem L, De Munter C, et al: Nonimmune hydrops fetalis associated with genetic abnormalities. Obstet Gynecol 1990;75:568–572.

Machin GA: Hydrops revisited: Literature review of 1,414 cases published in the 1980s. Am J Med Genet 1989;34:366–390.

McGillivray BC, Hall JG: Nonimmune hydrops fetalis. Pediatr Rev 1987;9:197–202.

Saltzman DH, Frigoletto FD Jr, Harlow BL, et al: Sonographic evaluation of hydrops fetalis. Obstet Gynecol 1989;74:106–111.

Santolaya J, Alley D, Jaffe R, Warsof SL: Antenatal classification of hydrops fetalis. Obstet Gynecol 1992;79:256–259.

Van Maldergem L, Jauniaux E, Fourneau C, Gillerot Y: Genetic causes of hydrops fetalis. Pediatrics 1992;89:81–86.

Watson J, Campbell S: Antenatal evaluation and management of non-immune hydrops fetalis. Obstet Gynecol 1986;67:589–593.

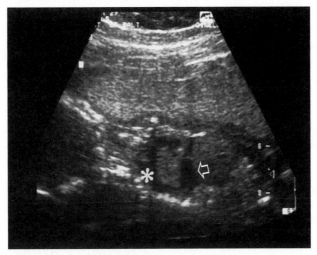

Sagittal view of the fetal trunk. Pleural effusion (*) surrounds the fetal lung. Fetal ascites is present (*arrow*).

13.3 Rhesus Incompatibility (Red Blood Cell Alloimmunization)

Epidemiology/Genetics

Definition *Rh disease* refers to the hemolytic process in the fetus that results from Rh blood group incompatibility between the mother and the fetus.

Epidemiology Before the advent of passive immunization with Rh immune globulin, erythroblastosis fetalis occurred in approximately 1% of pregnancies. However, the use of Rh immune globulin has markedly decreased the incidence of this disorder.

Embryology The pathophysiology of this condition is a direct result of severe anemia secondary to red blood cell hemolysis caused by maternal anti-Rh antibodies. These antibodies may be directed at any of the components of the Rh system; C, D, and E are the more common immunizing antigens.

Inheritance The genetic component is the inheritance of one of the Rh antigen complex by the fetus of a mother who lacks that antigen. If the father is homozygous for the antigen, all offspring will inherit it. If he is heterozygous, there is a 50% risk for each fetus to inherit the sensitizing antigen. The manifestations in succeeding "positive fetuses" in a sensitized mother tend to have more severe disease. This occurs most frequently with D (Rh positive) sensitization.

Prognosis In experienced centers, intravascular transfusion will result in better than 95% survival rate in nonhydropic fetuses. Survival falls to 80 to 85% in fetuses with hydrops.

Sonography

FINDINGS

1. **Fetus:**
   a. Hydrops is seen with severe Rh incompatibility. The more severe the hydrops, the worse the prognosis. There is skin thickening, a pleural effusion, a pericardial effusion, and ascites. The liver and spleen are enlarged. Tracking liver length is a technique for assessing the severity of anemia.
   b. Tricuspid regurgitation may be present. There is hypertrophy of ventricular walls and the intraventricular septum.
   c. There is increased blood velocity in the left ventricle and aorta.
   d. Middle cerebral artery Doppler velocimetry has been used to predict the risk of fetal anemia. The peak systolic velocity is increased in anemic fetuses.

The timing of transfusions can be monitored by tracking middle cerebral artery peak systolic velocity.
2. **Amniotic Fluid:** The amniotic fluid volume may be increased.
3. **Placenta:** The placenta is enlarged, with an evenly echogenic texture.
4. **Measurement Data:** Growth is less than expected, although the trunk circumference may be spuriously large because of hepatosplenomegaly and fetal ascites.
5. **When Detectable:** The earliest the syndrome has been detected is 16 weeks' gestation. With repeated affected infants, the syndrome develops earlier.

Pitfalls A normal slim echopenic area around the heart may be confused with a pericardial effusion. Pericardial effusions are often not symmetrical.

Differential Diagnosis There are numerous other causes of hydrops (nonimmune hydrops). For a discussion of the other potential causes, see Chapter 13.2.

Where Else to Look Look for other causes of hydrops: (1) cardiac causes; (2) infectious causes; and (3) chromosomal causes (see Chapter 13.2).

Pregnancy Management

Investigations and Consultations Required Maternal antibody screens and assessment of fetal hematologic status by cordocentesis are the essential components of the work-up.

Fetal Intervention Intravascular transfusions should be performed in a center with significant experience in the management of Rh disease. Transfusion therapy should be instituted when the fetal hematocrit is less than 30%. The procedure involves a simple transfusion of packed red blood cells (70% or greater hematocrit) into the umbilical vein. Paralysis of the fetus with pancuronium (0.3 mg/kg estimated fetal weight intravenously) to prevent fetal movement is preferable.

The final fetal hematocrit should be between 45 and 50%. Repeat transfusions are based on the loss of 1% hematocrit per day, but more frequent transfusions may be necessary initially until the fetal red cell mass is essentially all Rh-negative transfused red blood cells.

Monitoring Once transfusion therapy has been initiated, weekly sonographic evaluations should be performed, looking for subtle signs of fetal hydrops. Management must be under the direction of a perinatologist.

Pregnancy Course In severe cases of hydrops, poly-hydramnios may be a late manifestation. Without transfusion, fetal death will occur in cases of severe hydrops.

Delivery Delivery must occur in a tertiary center. The mode of delivery will depend on the predicted hemoglobin levels. Moderately to severely anemic fetuses may not tolerate labor well and may benefit from elective caesarian section.

Neonatology

Resuscitation In general, the majority of fetuses who have been affected by Rh isoimmunization do not experience distress in labor and thus do not require assistance with the onset of respiration. Only those with anemia of a profound degree and those with hydrops fetalis are the exception. (See Chapter 13.2 for the specific details of management.)

Transport Indications for referral to a tertiary perinatal center immediately following birth include hydrops fetalis, severe anemia (hemoglobin less than 10 g/dL), anticipated need for exchange transfusion in the first 24 hours of life (rise in bilirubin of greater than 1.5 mg/dL per hour). (See Chapter 13.2 for the specific details of management.)

Testing and Confirmation Other causes of hydrops not associated with anemia, and therefore not treatable by transfusion, must be excluded. The severity of the isoimmunization should be assessed early by obtaining hemoglobin, reticulocyte count, albumin, and fractionated bilirubin concentrations on admission.

Nursery Management Prompt and efficient cardiorespiratory adaptation is the initial focus of management. Restoring adequate oxygen-carrying capacity promptly without hemodynamic stress is important if there is significant anemia. A prehydropic state should be suspected with hypoalbuminemia. Bilirubin accumulation is controllable with phototherapy in mild cases and exchange transfusion in moderate to severe ones. (See Chapter 13.2 for specific details of management of hydrops.)

REFERENCES

Bahado-Singh RO, Oz AU, Hsu DC, et al: Middle cerebral artery Doppler velocimetric deceleration angle as a predictor of fetal anemia in Rh-alloimmunized fetuses without hydrops. Am J Obstet Gynecol 2000;183:746–749.

Benacerraf BR, Frigoletto FD Jr: Sonographic sign for the detection of early fetal ascites in the management of severe isoimmune disease without intrauterine transfusion. Am J Obstet Gynecol 1985;152:1039–1041.

Bloom RS: Delivery room resuscitation of the newborn. In Fanaroff AA, Martin RJ: Neonatal-Perinatal Medicine: Diseases of the Fetus and Infant. St. Louis: Mosby-Year Book, 2001; pp. 416–439.

Diffi L, Oz V, Guney I: Doppler ultrasound velocimetry for timing the second intrauterine transfusion in fetuses with anemia from red cell alloimmunisation. Am J Obstet Gynecol 2001;185:1048–1051.

Kamp IL, Klumper JCM, Bakkum RSLA: The severity of immune fetal hdrops is predictive of fetal outcome after treatment. Am J Obstet Gynecol 2001;185:668–673.

Oberhoffer R, Grab D, Keckstein J, et al: Cardiac change in fetuses secondary to immune hemolytic anemia and their relation to hemoglobin and catecholamine concentrations in fetal blood. Ultrasound Obstet Gynecol 1999;13:396–400.

Queenan JT: Management of Rh-immunized pregnancies. Prenat Diagn 1999;19:852–855.

Roberts A, Mitchell JM, Lake Y: Ultrasonographic surveillance in red blood cell alloimmunization. Am J Obstet Gynecol 2001;184:1251–1255.

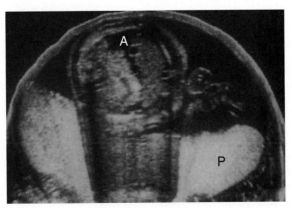

Transverse view of a fetus with severe hydrops due to Rh incompatibility. Note much enlarged placenta (P), fetal ascites (A), and severe skin thickening.

Abnormal Sonographic Findings

14

14.1 Amniotic Membranes

Epidemiology/Genetics

Definition A thin echogenic line surrounded on either side by echo-free amniotic fluid.

Epidemiology Common.

Embryology See description of membrane types.

Sonography

FINDINGS

1. **Fetus:** Normal, except when the membranes are caused by amniotic band syndrome.
2. **Amniotic Fluid:** Several types of membranes can be seen in the amniotic fluid:
   a. Amniotic bands—Thin, curving membranes attached to the fetus. Very difficult to see.
   b. The border of a marginal bleed—This is a relatively thick, slightly curved membrane that ends at the uterine border. It usually starts at the edge of the placenta. When the ultrasound gain control is increased, low-level echoes are visible within the area enclosed by the membrane. Old blood may become more or less sonolucent, but since there is proteinaceous material present, the echogenicity is slightly greater than in normal amniotic fluid and can be made visible by increasing the gain.
   c. Twin gestational sac membrane—The sac border remains when a blighted ovum occurs with a twin pregnancy. The remaining gestational sac border is smooth and curved and encloses a small space. The "twin peak" sign with placenta growing into the placental origin of the intrasac membranes may be seen.
   d. Amniotic sheet—If there is a pre-existing synechia prior to pregnancy, the gestational sac implants on the membrane. This membrane has a double layer, since the amnion and chorion surround the synechiae. A small circle is seen at the amniotic border of the membrane, presumably enclosing the synechiae. Amniotic sheets have, so far, had no pathologic significance.
   e. Placental cyst—Placental cysts arise from the amniotic border of the placenta and extend into the amniotic fluid. A solid component may be seen at the placental aspect of the cyst. These cysts are thought to be the sequela to a placental bleed.
   f. Unfused amniotic sac—The amnion and chorion are normally unfused until about 12 to 13 weeks' gestation. Occasionally, they remain unfused until as late as 17 weeks. In some patients following amniocentesis, blood is introduced into the space between the amnion and chorion, at the time of amniocentesis. This mishap is associated with prematurity.
   g. Subchorionic lucent space—An echopenic area, just below the placental surface, represents either Wharton's jelly deposition or a venous lake. Low-level echoes will be seen within the suspect area, which will show movement on real-time imaging, if they are due to a venous lake.
3. **Placenta:** May extend into the base of the membrane with a diamniotic dichorionic pregnancy.
4. **Measurement Data:** Normal.
5. **When Detectable:** With an endovaginal probe, at about 13 weeks' gestation.

Where Else to Look Look for stigmata of the amniotic band syndrome and the limb-body wall complex.

Pregnancy Management

Investigations and Consultations Required In the absence of other structural malformations, no additional evaluation is necessary. Additional consultations should be dictated by the specific malformations seen.

Monitoring No change in standard obstetric management is warranted.

Pregnancy Termination Issues Not indicated unless a severe structural malformation is seen in the fetus.

Delivery Site is dependent on the presence, or absence, of a fetal structural malformation.

REFERENCES

Benacerraf BR, Frigoletto FD Jr: Sonographic observation of amniotic rupture without amniotic band syndrome. J Ultrasound Med 1992;11: 109–111.

Burrows PE, Lyons EA, Phillips HJ, Oates I: Intrauterine membranes: Sonographic findings and clinical significance. J Clin Ultrasound 1982;10:1–8.

Burton DJ, Filly RA: Sonographic diagnosis of the amniotic band syndrome. Am J Roentgenol 1991;156:555–558.

Finberg HJ: Uterine synechiae in pregnancy: Expanded criteria for recognition and clinical significance in 28 cases. J Ultrasound Med 1991;10:547–555.

Herbert WN, Seeds JW, Cefalo RC, Bowes WA: Prenatal detection of intraamniotic bands: Implications and management. Obstet Gynecol 1985;65:36S–38S.

Jeanty P, Lacirica R, Luna SK: Extra-amniotic pregnancy: A trip to the extraembryonic coelom. J Ultrasound Med 1990;9:733–736.

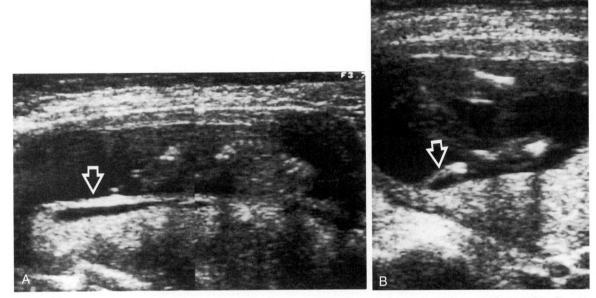

Amniotic sheet. The amniotic sheet has a double component derived from the amnion and chorion, wrapping around a synechia. On sagittal views (*left*), it can be quite lengthy, but the transverse view (*right*) is short because it ends with a small circle at the site of the synechia (*arrows*).

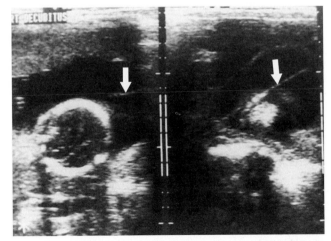

Amniotic band. The thin amniotic band can be seen approaching the fetus and attached to one arm (*arrows*). This type of band follows a disruption of the amnion in the early first trimester.

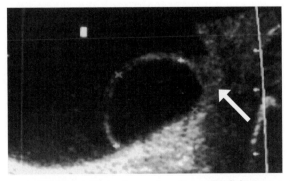

Empty sac following a blighted ovum in a diamniotic dichorionic twin. Note the twin peak sign with the placenta invaginating into the area between the chorionic membranes (*arrow*). This apparent single-thickness membrane has 4 components—2 amniotic and 2 chorionic membranes.

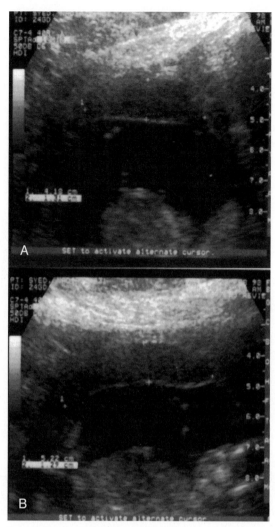

Membrane related to subchorionic bleed (*arrow*). These bleeds develop alongside the placenta. The blood changes appearance with time and may be echo-free unless the gain is raised. Note the subtle echoes enclosed by the membrane related to the bleed.

14.2 Cord Cyst

Epidemiology/Genetics

Definition   Cyst arising from the cord.

Epidemiology   Rare. No epidemiologic survey has been performed.

Embryology   Cysts in the cord may represent (1) remnant of the primitive allantois present when the cord is formed; (2) cystic expansion of the omphalomesenteric duct, also an embryologic remnant; or (3) cystic degeneration of Wharton's jelly, the material that surrounds the cord.

Inheritance Patterns   Not recurrent.

Prognosis   If isolated, of no consequences, but associated with fetal and cord abnormalities.

Sonography

FINDINGS

1. **Fetus:** None.
2. **Amniotic Fluid:** Normal.
3. **Placenta:** Normal. One or more echo-free cysts are present arising from the cord, generally located close to the fetal trunk. Size varies from a few millimeters to 5 cm.
4. **Measurement Dat**a: Normal.
5. **When Detectable:** In the second trimester.

Pitfalls   Wharton's jelly can be very prominent and form a thick echopenic area around the cord in some normal individuals.

Differential Diagnosis

1. Cord tumors—Will have internal echoes and show flow on color flow sonogram. Cystic areas may be present within the mass.
2. Umbilical artery aneurysm—Nonpulsatile and turbulent flow will be present on color flow Doppler image. There may be a calcified wall to the "cyst."
3. Cord pseudocyst—Cavity formed by degeneration of Wharton's jelly; there is no epithelial lining. Not distinguishable from allantoic cyst by sonographic appearance if there is only one. Pseudocysts are often multiple and carry a poor prognosis. They are associated with intrauterine growth restriction (IUGR) and chromosomal anomalies, particularly trisomy 18. Pseudocysts often develop in the second trimester but may not be present until after 24 weeks' gestation.

Cysts occurring transiently in the first trimester are not associated with an adverse pregnancy outcome.

4. Omphalomesenteric cyst—An enteric-lined cyst that connects to the region of the Meckel diverticulum.
5. Vesicoallantoic cyst—An umbilical cord cyst that communicates with the fetal bladder. A dumbbell-shaped cystic mass at the basal part of the umbilical cord extending into the fetus is seen.
5. Hemangioma of the umbilical cord—Densely echogenic cord mass with overall cord edema.
6. Angiomyxoma—Mass involving the cord with cystic center but thick irregular echogenic rind. Overall thickening of the cord occurs.
7. Hematoma of the cord—Usually there is a history of an amniocentesis or percutaneous umbilical cord blood sampling. Irregularly shaped mass arising from the cord with internal echoes. Vibrates with cord pulsation.

Where Else to Look

1. There is an association with omphalocele and chromosomal anomalies.
2. Urachal cysts are often seen with allantoic cysts. A cyst will be present in the fetal trunk located between the bladder and the umbilicus. The allantoic cyst may appear to communicate with the urachal cyst.

Pregnancy Management

Investigations and Consultations Required   If an omphalocele as well as the allantoic cyst is seen, the fetal karyotype should be obtained.

Monitoring   Follow-up sonograms are worthwhile. Cord compression by an enlarging allantoic cyst, as evidenced by abnormal Doppler patterns with low diastolic values, has been reported.

Pregnancy Course   Unremarkable.

Delivery   Ensure that the cord is sent for pathologic analysis.

REFERENCES

Battaglia C, Artini PG, D'Ambrogio G, Genazzani AR: Cord vessel compression by an expanding allantoic cyst: Case report. Ultrasound Obstet Gynecol 1992;2:58–60.

Casola G, Scheible W, Leopold GR: Large umbilical cord: A normal finding in some fetuses. Radiology 1985;156:181–182.

Fortune DW, Ostor AG: Umbilical artery aneurysm. Am J Obstet Gynecol 1978;131:339–340.

Frazier HA, Guerrieri JP, Thomas RL, Christenson PJ: The detection of a patent urachus and allantoic cyst of the umbilical cord on prenatal ultrasonography. J Ultrasound Med 1992;11:117–120.

Ghidini A, Romero R, Eisen RN, et al: Umbilical cord hemangioma: Prenatal identification and review of the literature. J Ultrasound Med 1990;9:297–300.

Harp J, Rouse GA, De Lange M: Sonographic prenatal diagnosis of allantoic cyst. J Dent Maxillofac Surg 1992;8:28–32.

Iaccarino M, Baldi F, Persico O, Palagiano A: Ultrasonographic and pathologic study of mucoid degeneration of umbilical cord. J Clin Ultrasound 1986;14:127–129.

Jauniaux E, Campbell S, Vyas S: The use of color Doppler imaging for prenatal diagnosis of umbilical cord anomalies: Report of three cases. Am J Obstet Gynecol 1989;161:1195–1197.

Jauniaux E, Moscoso G, Chitty L, et al: An angiomyxoma involving the whole length of the umbilical cord: Prenatal diagnosis by ultrasonography. J Ultrasound Med 1990;9:419–422.

Jeanty P: Fetal and funicular vascular anomalies: Identification with prenatal US. Radiology 1989;173:367–370.

Jones TB, Sorokin Y, Bhatia R, et al: Single umbilical artery: Accurate diagnosis? Am J Obstet Gynecol 1993;169:538–540.

Kalter CS, Williams MC, Vaughn V, Spellacy WN: Sonographic diagnosis of a large umbilical cord pseudocyst. J Ultrasound Med 1994;13:487–489.

Middleton MA, Middleton WD, Wiele K: Case Report 2: Allantoic cyst of the umbilical cord. Am J Roentgenol 1989;152:1324–1325.

Morin LR: Sonography of umbilical cord hematoma. Am J Roentgenol 1991;156:1115.

Nyberg DA, Mahony BS, Luthy D, Kapur R: Single umbilical artery: Prenatal detection of concurrent anomalies. J Ultrasound Med 1991;10:247–253.

Nyberg DA, Shepard T, Mack LA, et al: Significance of a single umbilical artery in fetuses with central nervous system malformations. J Ultrasound Med 1988;7:265–273.

Pollack MS, Bound LM: Hemangioma of the umbilical cord: Sonographic appearance. J Ultrasound Med 1989;8:163–166.

Rempen A: Sonographic first-trimester diagnosis of umbilical cord cyst. J Clin Ultrasound 1989;17:53–55.

Resta RG, Luthy DA, Mahony BS: Umbilical cord hemangioma associated with extremely high alpha-fetoprotein levels. Obstet Gynecol 1988;72:488–491.

Rosenberg JC, Chervenak FA, Walker BA, et al: Antenatal sonographic appearance of omphalomesenteric duct cyst. J Ultrasound Med 1986;5:719–720.

Ruvinsky ED, Wiley TL, Morrison JC, Blake PG: In utero diagnosis of umbilical cord hematoma by ultrasonography. Am J Obstet Gynecol 1981;140:833–834.

Sachs L, Fourcroy JL, Wenzel DJ, et al: Prenatal detection of umbilical cord allantoic cyst. Radiology 1982;145:445–446.

Satge DCL, Larcmund M, Chenad MR: An umbilical cord teratoma in a 17-week-old fetus. Prenat Diagn 2001;21:284–288.

Sepulveda W, Gutierrez J, Sanchez J, et al: Pseudocyst of the umbilical cord: Prenatal sonographic appearance and clinical significance. Obstet Gynecol 1999;93:377–381.

Sepulveda W, Leible S, Ulloa A, et al: Clinical significance of first trimester umbilical cord cysts. J Ultrasound Med 1999;18:95–99.

Shukanami K, Tsuji T, Kostsuji F: Prenatal sonographic features of vesicoalloantoic cyst. Ultrasound Obstet Gynecol 2000;15:545–546.

Siddiqi TA, Bendon R, Schultz DM, Miodovnik M: Umbilical artery aneurysm: Prenatal diagnosis and management. Obstet Gynecol 1992;80:530–533.

Sutro WH, Tuck SM, Loesevitz A, et al: Prenatal observation of umbilical cord hematoma. Am J Roentgenol 1984;142:801–802.

Vesce F, Guerrini P, Perri G, et al: Ultrasonographic diagnosis of ectasia of the umbilical vein. J Clin Ultrasound 1987;15:346–349.

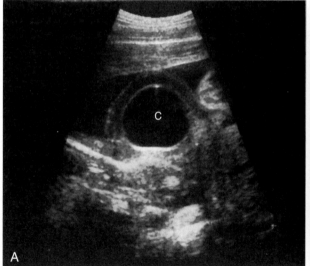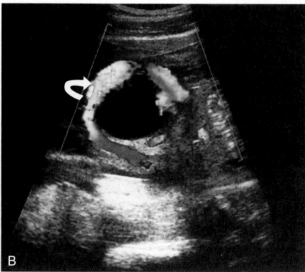

Left, Allantoic cyst associated with the cord. A cyst is completely echo-free and single. It is located quite close to the fetal abdominal wall (C). *Right,* View of the cord cyst with color flow used to demonstrate the cord (*arrow*).

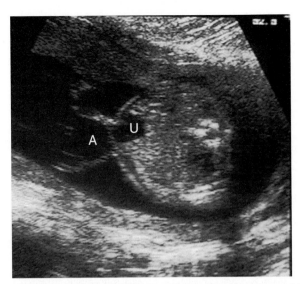

Vesicoallantoic cyst. An allantoic cyst (A) lies adjacent to the cord insertion and to a urachal cyst (U) within the fetal abdomen.

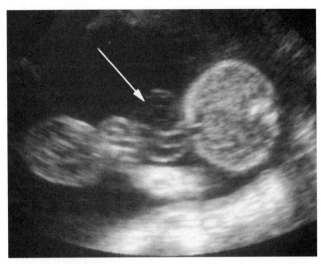

Very thick cord with much Wharton's jelly with cord cyst (*arrow*), in a case of trisomy 18.

14.3 Intrauterine Growth Restriction (IUGR)

Epidemiology/Genetics

Definition There is considerable variability in the definition of what constitutes a growth-retarded infant. Definitions include a birth weight below 2500 g at term, a birth weight below the 3rd percentile for gestational age, a birth weight below the 10th percentile for gestational age, or a birth weight more than two standard deviations below the mean for gestational age. The most commonly used definition is a birth weight below the 10th percentile for gestational age.

Epidemiology IUGR affects 3 to 10% of all pregnancies, depending on the definition used.

Embryology Subnormal fetal growth may result from chronic uteroplacental insufficiency, exposure to drugs or environmental agents, congenital infections, or intrinsic genetic limitations of growth potential. Fetuses with growth restriction due to nutritional compromise tend to have sparing of head growth (asymmetrical growth retardation). Early or symmetric IUGR should suggest chromosomal abnormalities such as trisomy 18 or triploidy, maternal uniparental disomy for chromosomes 7 or 14, or a lethal skeletal dysplasia. Microcephaly may indicate either in utero infection or central nervous system malformations.

Inheritance Recurrent IUGR most commonly represents an underlying maternal medical condition. There is no genetic basis for true IUGR. Healthy but small for gestational age infants may be the result of as yet unknown genetic factors.

Prognosis Perinatal mortality is four to eight times higher for the growth-retarded fetus, and significant morbidity is noted in up to 50% of the survivors. Prolonged severely reduced blood flow with IUGR shown by absent or reversed flow in the umbilical artery is associated with long-term impairment of intellectual development and small stature.

Sonography

FINDINGS

1. **Fetus:** Diminished soft tissue mass. Decreased liver size. There may be echogenic bowel.
2. **Amniotic Fluid:** Usually diminished. If the fluid is increased, consider the possibility of a chromosomal anomaly.
3. **Placenta:**
   a. Usually thin and small.
   b. If enlarged and thickened or "molar" in appearance, consider triploidy.
   c. Grade 3 placenta occurring prior to 34 to 36 weeks' gestation often heralds or accompanies IUGR of vascular origin, as with maternal hypertension or placental infarcts.
4. **Measurement Data:** Estimated fetal weight is based on ultrasonic measurement of (a) abdominal circumference; (b) biparietal diameter and head circumference; and (c) femur length. Various formulas use the abdominal circumference in combination with other parameters to determine weight. Three different growth patterns are seen:
   a. Symmetrical—All measurement data are small compared with known dates either established by early sonogram, known conception date, or early clinical examination.
   b. Asymmetrical—Head measurements are consistent with dates or not far behind, whereas abdomen measurements are at least 2 weeks less and below the 10th percentile (this type is associated with more anomalies and a greater risk of neonatal complications).
   c. Femur sparing—Head and abdomen measurements are small, whereas the femur and cerebellar measurements are consistent with dates. If dates are unclear and all other measurements are 3 to 4 weeks less than the femur, IUGR is likely.
5. **When Detectable:** Very early, such as 15 weeks' gestation, in association with karyotypic abnormalities; or at 28 to 32 weeks with preeclampsia and hypertension.

Pitfalls

1. Distinction from wrong dates is difficult when a patient presents late with uncertain menstrual dates. Oligohydramnios and an abnormal umbilical artery Doppler finding and biophysical profile favor true IUGR.
2. Distinction from the familially small baby is difficult. A family history of small children and normal fluid, biophysical profile, and umbilical artery Doppler findings suggest a normal fetus.
3. Quality views of the abdominal circumference are crucial, since weight estimates are so dependent on this measurement. Weight estimation errors are less with small fetuses but are, in the best of hands, ±1 to 200 g/1000 g.
4. The long thin fetus is easily overlooked with ultrasonographic measurements.

Differential Diagnosis

1. Wrong dates and normal fetus.
2. Normal small fetus.

Where Else to Look

1. Do tests of fetal well-being: (a) Biophysical profile including the non-stress test; (b) umbilical artery and

middle cerebral artery Doppler imaging; and (c) amniotic fluid index.

2. With early IUGR look for:

A. Stigmata of chromosomal anomalies: (1) trisomy 18—choroid plexus cyst, clenched hands and club feet, neural crest anomaly, and congenital heart defects; (2) stigmata of triploidy—large placenta with molar aspects, asymmetrical IUGR, micrognathia, cleft palate, hand and feet deformities, hydrocephalus and neural crest anomalies; (3) trisomy 13—holoprosencephaly, facial deformities, omphalocele, renal cystic dysplasia, hand and feet abnormalities, and congenial heart defects.

B. Nonchromosomal syndromes: (1) cytomegalovirus infection—hepatosplenomegaly, microcephaly with lateral ventricular dilation with echogenic borders, and hydrops; (2) Neu-Laxova syndrome—microcephaly, micrognathia, protruding eyeballs, joint contractures, edematous skin, heart defects, cleft lip, and polyhydramnios; (3) Cornelia de Lange syndrome—micrognathia, clinodactyly, micromelia, hypospadias, and undescended testes; (4) fetal alcohol syndrome—cardiac abnormalities, microcephaly, micrognathia, and cleft lip and palate (see Chapter 10.1).

Pregnancy Management

Investigations and Consultations Required Chromosomal evaluation of the fetus and maternal TORCH (toxoplasmosis, other infection, rubella, cytomegalovirus infection, herpes simplex) titers should be performed in cases of otherwise unaccounted for IUGR.

Fetal Intervention Experimental work evaluating methods of increasing fetal "nutrition" by instillation of amino acids into the amniotic fluid or by direct intravascular injections have been attempted. However, at present these methods are not appropriate for clinical management.

Monitoring The management of the fetus with IUGR should be in the hands of a perinatologist. The timing of fetal assessment methods such as non-stress testing and biophysical profile must be individualized, depending on the clinical circumstances. Early delivery is often the treatment of choice when fetal lung maturity has been attained.

Pregnancy Course IUGR places the fetus at significant risk for stillbirth or hypoxic damage to the central nervous system. Oligohydramnios is a later manifestation of severe IUGR.

Pregnancy Termination Issues Not applicable to this clinical circumstance.

Delivery The site for delivery must be one with the capabilities to manage premature and/or compromised infants.

Neonatology

Resuscitation Growth-retarded fetuses, in general, are less tolerant of the stress of labor and are more prone to experience asphyxia than normally grown fetuses. They are, therefore, more likely to require immediate resuscitation, particularly if delivery is either preterm or postterm. The more severe the growth retardation, the greater the risk for severe asphyxia. Any special techniques required relate to the cause of the growth retardation.

Transport Indications for referral to a tertiary perinatal center are very low birth weight (less than 1.5 kg), very early gestation (less than 32 weeks), concomitant illness or life-threatening complications, or associated organ malformations. Care during transport will be determined by the indication for referral.

Testing and Confirmation Establishing an etiologic diagnosis, if such was not completed prior to delivery, is important and difficult, as there are myriad causes, many of which cannot be excluded definitively. In some large series of IUGR, a definite cause cannot be determined in more than half of the cases. A careful physical examination and review of the maternal social, medical, and obstetric history are the first and most important diagnostic steps. Further evaluations—serologic testing, radiographic imaging, chemical analysis, karyotyping—will be determined by the information from the history and physical assessment.

Nursery Management Care following birth is directed toward stabilization of cardiorespiratory function and recovery from perinatal asphyxia. As a group, IUGR infants are more prone to postasphyxial cardiovascular and central nervous system syndromes, hypoglycemia, polycythemia, and coagulopathies. Other neonatal problems are dependent on the cause of the growth retardation, and thus care requirements will vary with the specific diagnoses.

REFERENCES

Barros FC, Huttly SR, Victora CG, et al: Comparison of the causes and consequences of prematurity and intrauterine growth retardation: A longitudinal study in southern Brazil. Pediatrics 1992;90:238–244.

Benson CB, Boswell SB, Brown DL, et al: Improved prediction of intrauterine growth retardation with use of multiple parameters. Radiology 1988;168:7–12.

Brown HL, Miller JM Jr, Gabert HA, Kissling G: Ultrasonic recognition of the small-for-gestational-age fetus. Obstet Gynecol 1987;69:631–635.

Dashe J, McIntire DD, Lucas MJ, Leveno KJ: Effects of symmetric and asymmetric fetal growth on pregnancy outcomes. Obstet Gynecol 2000;96:321–328.

Davies BR, Casanueva E, Arroyo P: Placentas of small-for-dates infants: A small controlled series from Mexico City, Mexico. Am J Obstet Gynecol 1984;149:731–736.

Gembruch U, Gortner L: Perinatal aspects of preterm intrauterine growth restriction. Ultrasound Obstet Gynecol 1998;11:233–239.

Gulmezoglu AM, Ekici E: Sonographic diagnosis of Neu-Laxova syndrome. J Clin Ultrasound 1994;22:48–51.

Khoury MJ, Erickson JD, Cordero JF, McCarthy BJ: Congenital malformations and intrauterine growth retardation: A population study. Pediatrics 1988;82:83–90.

Kramer MS, Olivier M, McLean FH, et al: Impact of intrauterine growth retardation and body proportionality on fetal and neonatal outcome. Pediatrics 1990;86:707–713.

Langlois S, Yong SL, Wilson RD, et al: Prenatal and postnatal growth failure associated with maternal heterodisomy for chromosome 7. J Med Genet 1995;32:871–875.

Medchill MT, Peterson CM, Kreinick C, Garbaciak J: Prediction of estimated fetal weight in extremely low birth weight neonates (500–1000 g). Obstet Gynecol 1991;78:286–290.

Miyoshi O, Hayashi S, Fujimoto M, et al: Maternal uniparental disomy for chromosome 14 in a boy with intrauterine growth retardation. J Hum Genet 1998;43:138–142.

Ott WJ: Defining altered fetal growth by second-trimester sonography. Obstet Gynecol 1990;75:1053–1059.

Tretter AE, Sanders RC, Meyers CM, et al: Antenatal diagnosis of lethal skeletal dysplasias. Am J Med Genet 1998;75:518–522.

Villar J, de Onis M, Kestler E, et al: The differential neonatal morbid-ity of the intrauterine growth retardation syndrome. Am J Obstet Gynecol 1990;163:151–157.

Warshaw JB: Intrauterine growth retardation. Pediatr Rev 1986;8:107–114.

Weinerroither A, Steiner H, Tomaselli J: Intrauterine blood flow and long-term intellectual, neurologic and social development. Obstet Gynecol 2001;97:449–453.

Yogman MW, Kraemer HC, Kindlon D, et al: Identification of intrauterine growth retardation among low birth weight preterm infants. J Pediatr 1989;115:799–807.

14.4 Macrosomia

Epidemiology/Genetics

Definition *Macrosomia* is defined as a birth weight of 4500 g or greater (4000 g or greater in diabetic mothers) at term or as a weight that is over the 90th percentile for gestational age.

Epidemiology Macrosomic infants account for 1 to 2% of all deliveries. Significant risk factors are advanced maternal age, multiparity, obesity, maternal diabetes, and gestational age greater than 42 weeks.

Embryology The mechanisms that result in excessive fetal growth are unknown. Patients with glucose intolerance (gestational diabetes or overt diabetes) are at significant risk for this complication.

Inheritance Although no precise genetic mechanism has been elucidated, a previous delivery of a macrosomic infant is associated with a markedly increased risk in subsequent pregnancies.

Prognosis Providing delivery problems, such as birth trauma, do not occur and there is no syndrome diagnosis such as the Beckwith-Wiedemann syndrome, the long-term prognosis is good.

Sonography

FINDINGS

1. **Fetus:** Skin thickening, without a central echopenic component as is seen in hydrops, is usually present. The fetus has large cheeks, with an enlarged cheek-to-cheek diameter.
2. **Amniotic Fluid:** Mild polyhydramnios is usually present and may be the presenting finding.
3. **Placenta:** The placenta is usually unaffected. The placenta may be enlarged if the macrosomia is secondary to maternal diabetes.
4. **Measurement Data:**
   a. All measurement data, especially the abdominal circumference, are larger than usual (above the 90th percentile).
   b. The cheek-to-cheek ratio is helpful; babies with fat cheeks are usually macrosomic. A study at 35 weeks' gestation may be valuable in deciding on early induction at 38 weeks.
   c. Fetal soft tissue in the arm or thigh and the ratio of the thigh soft tissue thickness to femur length can be measured but have not proved very reliable as predictors of macrosomia.
5. **When Detectable:** Increased fetal size first becomes apparent at about 28 weeks. Polyhydramnios may precede enlarged fetal size in fetuses subsequently shown to be macrosomic.

Pitfalls Measurement data for large babies is often inaccurate in weight estimation by as much as 700 g.

Differential Diagnosis

1. Hydropic skin thickening—There will be an echopenic subdermal area with hydrops. Pleural effusion and ascites will be seen.
2. Although several of the genetic syndromes with excessive fetal growth (Beckwith-Wiedemann syndrome, Weaver syndrome, Sotos syndrome) may be confused with "benign" macrosomia, the obstetric management would not be modified in most circumstances. A prospective diagnosis is possible for Beckwith-Wiedemann syndrome if an omphalocele is present but unlikely for the other overgrowth syndromes.

Where Else to Look

1. Macrosomic fetuses of diabetic mothers therefore have a greater risk of multiple malformations, i.e., heterotaxia syndrome, VACTERL association, complex congenital heart defects, caudal regression/dysplasia. Therefore, a detailed look at the heart, spine, gut, and kidneys is required (see Chapter 11.8).
2. Look for large tongue and enlarged liver and kidneys, the features of Beckwith-Wiedemann syndrome (see Chapter 11.1).

Pregnancy Management

Investigations and Consultations Required Fetal echocardiography should be performed to exclude cardiac malformations. Consultation with a neonatologist to plan perinatal management is appropriate. Assessment of maternal glucose tolerance should be done to exclude diabetes.

Fetal Intervention None is indicated.

Monitoring If the patient is found to have gestational diabetes, maternal dietary control may slow the rate of fetal growth. By definition, however, this diagnosis will not be made until late in pregnancy, at which time management options are limited.

Pregnancy Course There is a significant risk of birth trauma and shoulder dystocia, long-term neurologic complications, and perinatal death.

Pregnancy Termination Issues Not applicable.

Delivery Some authors have recommended pursuing cae-sarian section if estimated fetal weight is 4700 g or more. If vaginal delivery is attempted, a physician experienced in the management of shoulder dystocia should be present and ap-propriate anesthesia and pediatric support should be avail-able. Delivery should occur in a tertiary center.

Neonatology

Resuscitation The risk for fetal distress is higher than for infants of normal birth weight and is related both to pregnancy complications resulting in fetal overgrowth and to the size of the infant. A resuscitation team should be present for the delivery of any infant anticipated to weigh 4.5 kg or more. No special techniques are required. Ten-sion on the neck and upper extremities should be avoided until brachial plexus injury has been excluded by careful physical examination.

Transport Referral to a tertiary perinatal center is in-dicated only if neonatal complications develop or con-genital malformations are suspected.

Nursery Management Admission to a special care nursery for observation during the early transition period is advisable and mandatory if maternal diabetes or post-term delivery (after 42 completed weeks) are etiologic fac-tors. Soft tissue injury, bruising, brachial plexus injury, respiratory distress, hypoglycemia, polycythemia, and hy-perbilirubinemia are the more common neonatal prob-lems irrespective of the maternal factors present. In addi-tion, postasphyxial organ injury syndromes are more likely with postmaturity. Cyanosis unrelieved by oxygen in a macrosomic infant should be considered a neonatal emer-gency requiring immediate evaluation for cardiac defects. In the absence of pregnancy or intrapartum complications, the nursery course is usually benign.

REFERENCES

Abramowicz JS, Robischon K, Cox C: Incorporating sonographic cheek-to-cheek diameter, biparietal diameter and abdominal circumference improves weight estimation in the macrosomic fetus. Ultrasound Ob-stet Gynecol 1997;9:409–413.

Abramowicz JS, Sherer DM, Woods JR Jr: Ultrasonographic measure-ment of cheek-to-cheek diameter in fetal growth disturbances. Am J Obstet Gynecol 1993;169:405–408.

Ballard JL, Rosenn B, Khoury JC, Miodovnik M: Diabetic fetal macro-somia: Significance of disproportionate growth. J Pediatr 1993;122:115–119.

Benson CB, Doubilet PM, Saltzman DH: Sonographic determination of fetal weights in diabetic pregnancies. Am J Obstet Gynecol 1987;156:441–444.

Chauhan SP, West DJ, Scardo JA, et al: Antepartum detection of macro-somic fetus: Clinical versus sonographic, including soft-tissue mea-surements. Obstet Gynecol 2000;95:639–642.

Chervenak JL, Divon MY, Hirsch J, et al: Macrosomia in the postdate pregnancy: Is routine ultrasonographic screening indicated? Am J Ob-stet Gynecol 1989;161:753–756.

Jovanovic-Peterson L, Peterson CM, Reed GF, et al: Maternal post-prandial glucose levels and infant birth weight: National Institute of Child Health and Human Development—Diabetes in Early Preg-nancy study. Am J Obstet Gynecol 1991;164:103–111.

Leikin EL, Jenkins JH, Pomerantz GA, Klein L: Abnormal glucose screening tests in pregnancy: A risk factor for fetal macrosomia. Ob-stet Gynecol 1987;69:570–573.

Lubchenco LO: The infant who is large for gestational age. In The High Risk Infant. Philadelphia, WB Saunders, 1976.

Ranzini AC, Day-Salvatore D, Turner T, et al: Intrauterine growth and ultrasound findings in fetuses with Beckwith-Wiedemann syndrome. Obstet Gynecol 1997;89:538–542.

Sacks DA: Fetal macrosomia and gestational diabetes: What's the prob-lem? Obstet Gynecol 1993;81:775–781.

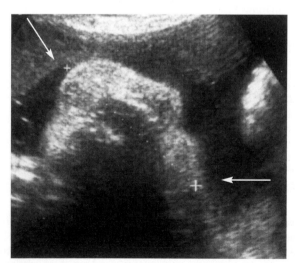

Macrosomia. View of the face. The fetal skin is thick and the cheeks are prominent (*arrows*).

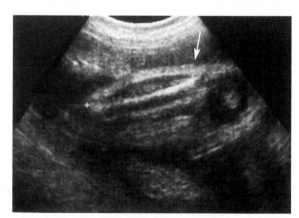

View of the thigh. Note the thick skin (*arrow*).

14.5 Oligohydramnios

Epidemiology/Genetics

Definition Diminished amniotic fluid volume for a given gestational age.

Epidemiology Common.

Teratogens Indomethacin, used to inhibit labor, can induce oligohydramnios.

Screening Increased maternal serum alpha-fetoprotein may be due to oligohydramnios.

Prognosis Poor with first- and second-trimester oligohydramnios. Oligohydramnios in a normally grown fetus, occurring for the first time in the third trimester, usually carries a good prognosis.

Sonography

FINDINGS

1. **Fetus:** Severe oligohydramnios may be accompanied by the features of Potter's syndrome. Check for club feet, deviated hands, and limb contractures.
2. **Amniotic Fluid:** The severity of the oligohydramnios depends on the underlying process. Normal standards for amniotic fluid exist, based on the amniotic fluid index. The amniotic fluid index is measured in the following fashion: the pregnant uterus is divided into four quadrants, a vertical measurement is made of the deepest uninterrupted fluid pocket in each quadrant, and the four measurements are added together. A measurement of less than 5 cm is considered to indicate oligohydramnios. An alternative approach is to measure a single vertical pocket. Less than 2 cm is considered by most to be the threshold for oligohydramnios.
3. **Placenta:** Appearance varies, depending on the underlying cause.
4. **Measurement Data:**
   a. If the oligohydramnios is associated with IUGR, all measurements, particularly the abdominal circumference, will be decreased.
   b. Often the fetal head is dolichocephalic—The head shape is long and thin.
5. **When Detectable:** Maternal control of amniotic fluid volume exists until somewhere between 14 and 18 weeks' gestation, so oligohydramnios of fetal origin may not be evident until 18 weeks. Oligohydramnios related to premature rupture of membranes, chorionic villus sampling, and severe IUGR can present early in the second trimester.

Pitfalls

1. Amniotic fluid volume normally decreases markedly in the late third trimester.
2. The amniotic fluid index is a subjective method of measuring the amount of fluid. Two examiners can come up with different results, depending on the fetal alignment, within a short time interval.
3. Areas filled with cord may be mistaken for amniotic fluid. Use color flow Doppler sonography on questionable areas to see if they are actually umbilical cord.
4. Maternal hydration affects amniotic fluid volume. Make sure the patient is well hydrated before diagnosing oligohydramnios.
5. The presence of particulate matter within the amniotic fluid is of uncertain significance but makes it difficult to obtain an amniotic fluid index.

Where Else to Look

1. Renal causes—Look for absence of the kidneys, obstructed or dysplastic kidneys, and abnormally large kidneys, as with infantile polycystic kidney or adult polycystic kidney disease.
2. All measurement data may be decreased if there is IUGR.
3. Check the cervix for cervical incompetence. The bladder should be empty. A translabial or endovaginal approach should be used, so the whole length of the cervix can be seen. If there is premature rupture of membranes, the cervix will be short (less than 3.5 cm) and the internal os will have some fluid within it showing funneling.
4. The presence of fetal breathing is reported to decrease the likelihood of pulmonary hypoplasia. If the oligohydramnios is first discovered in the late second or third trimester, perform the biophysical profile and umbilical cord Doppler measurements.
5. Because of the decreased amniotic fluid, club feet and deviated hands develop. Limb changes are hard to see because they develop only when there is almost no fluid.

Pregnancy Management

Investigations and Consultation Required Amnioinfusion—If the cause of the decreased fluid is not apparent with sonography and there is little or no fluid present, instillation of a mixture of Ringer's solution, dextrose, and indigo carmine may be helpful. About 150 to 250 mL is instilled. The increased "amniotic fluid" will allow better visualization of the fetus; if there is an amniotic fluid leak, the indigo carmine will stain a tampon left in the vagina; and the fetus will drink the fluid and the stomach and bladder will fill, if the kidneys are functioning. A false-positive diagnosis of ruptured membranes may occur if fluid is instilled in the extra-amniotic space.

Monitoring

1. Renal—If fluid disappears altogether, lung development is impaired or absent. If there is severe bilateral obstructive renal disease, sonograms every 2 to 3 weeks are required to check fluid volume.
2. Premature rupture of membranes—The prognosis is very poor, and the likelihood of hypoplastic lungs and limb contractures is high. In some cases of premature rupture of membranes, however, resealing of membranes has been reported. Sonograms every 2 weeks will show whether there is increased fluid accumulation.
3. IUGR—Severe IUGR and oligohydramnios at an early stage, such as 23 weeks' gestation, portend a poor prognosis, and usually fetal death ensues. Sonograms every 2 weeks, accompanied by twice-weekly biophysical profiles, are recommended. Timing for delivery will depend on the findings of the parameters of fetal well-being such as biophysical profile, non-stress testing, and Doppler imaging (see Chapter 14.3).

Delivery   Delivery should occur in a tertiary center.

REFERENCES

Barss VA, Benacerraf BR, Frigoletto FD Jr: Second trimester oligohydramnios, a predictor of poor fetal outcome. Obstet Gynecol 1984;64:608–610.

Blott M, Greenough A, Nicolaides KH, Campbell S: The ultrasonographic assessment of the fetal thorax and fetal breathing movements in the prediction of pulmonary hypoplasia. Early Human Devel 1990;21:143–151.

Bronshtein M, Blumenfeld Z: First- and early second-trimester oligohydramnios: A predictor of poor fetal outcome except in iatrogenic oligohydramnios post chorionic villus biopsy. Ultrasound Obstet Gynecol 1991;1:245–249.

Fisk NM, Ronderos-Dumit D, Soliani A, et al: Diagnostic and therapeutic transabdominal amnioinfusion in oligohydramnios. Obstet Gynecol 1991;78:270–278.

Hill LM, Breckle R, Gehrking WC: The variable effects of oligohydramnios on the biparietal diameter and the cephalic index. J Ultrasound Med 1984;3:93–95.

Horsager R, Nathan L, Leveno KJ: Correlation of measured amniotic fluid volume and sonographic preductions of oligohydramnios. Obstet Gynecol 1994;83:955–958.

Mandell J, Peters CA, Estroff JA, Benacerraf BR: Late onset severe oligohydramnios associated with genitourinary abnormalities. J Urol 1992;148:515–518.

Mercer LJ, Brown LG: Fetal outcome with oligohydramnios in the second trimester. Obstet Gynecol 1986;67:840–842.

Moore TR, Longo J, Leopold GR, et al: The reliability and predictive value of an amniotic fluid scoring system in severe second-trimester oligohydramnios. Obstet Gynecol 1989;73:739–742.

Sherer D, Langer O: Oligohydramnios: Use and misuse in clinical management. Ultrasound Obstet Gynecol 2001;18:411–419.

14.6 Polyhydramnios

Epidemiology/Genetics

Definition   Excess amniotic fluid for the stage of pregnancy.

Epidemiology   Polyhydramnios is present in about 1% of pregnancies. It is particularly common in women with diabetes mellitus and in obese women. In about 20% of cases, it is associated with a serious fetal anomaly.

Embryology   In many instances, it is due to defective or obstructed fetal ingestion of amniotic fluid.

Prognosis   Dependent on underlying cause.

Sonography

FINDINGS

1. **Fetus:** With polyhydramnios related to maternal obesity or diabetes mellitus, the fetus is enlarged (macrosomic). Polyhydramnios may precede the macrosomia.
2. **Amniotic Fluid:** The amniotic fluid volume is increased and there will be an amniotic fluid index of over 24. An alternative technique is to measure the largest fluid pocket. A fluid pocket measuring greater than 8 cm in transverse and longitudinal section is considered abnormal. In the late third trimester, an amniotic fluid index of 15 or more is suggestive of polyhydramnios, since the fluid volume normally decreases.
3. **Placenta:** Often appears thin, since it is spread over a wider area.
4. **Measurement Data:** Depends on the underlying cause, but often increased.
5. **When Detectable:** Polyhydramnios may be seen at about 16 weeks' gestation but is rare before 25 weeks' gestation.

Pitfalls:

1. The amniotic fluid normally decreases in the third trimester, so polyhydramnios may be present with indices of under 20 in the late third trimester.
2. A single, large, transversely aligned pocket may give a spuriously low amniotic fluid index, since only one or two vertical fluid measurements will be counted in the amniotic fluid index.

Where Else to Look

1. Look in the gastrointestinal tract for obstruction—There will be dilated loops of bowel at most levels of obstruction. The most severe polyhydramnios occurs with proximal obstruction above the ligament of Treitz, as with tracheoesophageal atresia when the stomach may not be seen.
2. Look in the chest or abdomen for a mass that compresses the esophagus, stomach, or small bowel, such as cystic adenomatoid malformation, diaphragmatic hernia, or severe ureteropelvic junction obstruction.
3. Look for intracranial or facial malformations that result in defective swallowing, such as anencephaly or cleft lip and palate.
4. Look for short-limbed dwarfism—The limbs will be very short and the chest will be small, so there will be secondary esophageal compression.
5. Muscular problems associated with defective swallowing such as myotonic dystrophy should be sought. Look for limb contractures in multiple pterygium syndrome and congenital arthrogryposis.
6. All measurement data may be increased, as in macrosomia. This is the most common association of polyhydramnios.

Pregnancy Management

Investigations and Consultation Required   The presence of structural malformations or fetal growth restriction and polyhydramnios is an indication for chromosomal studies. The incidence of karyotypic abnormalities is quite low in cases of isolated polyhydramnios. Fetal echocardiography should be done to exclude cardiac malformations. If the mother has not been screened for diabetes, this should be done. Consideration should be given to assessing the mother for the presence of the myotonic dystrophy gene, as one study showed almost 10% of the cases of idiopathic polyhydramnios to be due to congenital myotonic dystrophy. Fetal karyotyping is indicated in cases of polyhydramnios combined with fetal growth restriction.

Fetal Intervention   Severe polyhydramnios that results in maternal respiratory compromise may require serial amnioreductions of large volumes of fluid. In cases of preterm labor, amnioreduction may be beneficial in delaying delivery until steroids can be administered to stimulate fetal pulmonary maturity. Indomethacin has been shown to decrease fetal urine output and secondarily to decrease amniotic fluid volume. It may be useful in some cases to delay delivery, but only with careful monitoring of the fetal ductus arteriosus, because premature closure is a side effect of treatment. Additional reported side effects are necrotizing enterocolitis and neonatal oliguria.

Monitoring   Depending on the severity of the polyhydramnios, serial ultrasonograms every 1 to 3 weeks may be useful for monitoring amniotic fluid volume and instituting early treatment for preterm labor.

Delivery The site of delivery should be a tertiary center in all cases with severe polyhydramnios. In the absence of structural malformation, mild polyhydramnios should not alter obstetric management.

REFERENCES

Biggio JR, Wenstrom KD, Duband MB, Cliver SP: Hydramnios prediction of adverse prenatal outcome. Obstet Gynecol 1999;94:773–777.

Carlson DE, Platt LD, Medearis AL, Horenstein J: Quantifiable polyhydramnios: Diagnosis and management. Obstet Gynecol 1990;75:989–992.

Devriendt K, van Schoubroeck D, Eyskens B, et al: Polyhydramnios as a prenatal symptom of DiGeorge/velo-cardio-facial syndrome. Prenat Diagn 1998;18:68–72.

Esplin MS, Hallan S, Farrington PF, et al: Myotonic dystrophy is a significant cause of idiopathic polyhydramnios. Am J Obstet Gynecol 1998;179:974–977.

Hill LM, Breckle R, Thomas ML, Fries JK: Polyhydramnios: Ultrasonically detected prevalence and neonatal outcome. Obstet Gynecol 1987;69:21–25.

Sickler GK, Nyberg DA, Sohaey R, Luthy DA: Polyhydramnios and fetal intrauterine growth restriction: Ominous combination. J Ultrasound Med 1997;16:609–614.

Sivit CJ, Hill MC, Larsen JW, Lande IM: Second-trimester polyhydramnios: Evaluation with US. Radiology 1987;165:467–469.

Stoll CG, Alembik Y, Dott B: Study of 156 cases of polyhydramnios and congenital malformations in a series of 118,265 consecutive births. J Obstet Gynecol 1991;165:586–590.

Appendices

Differential Diagnoses of Abnormal in Utero Sonographic Findings

Abdomen

ABDOMINAL CYST OR FLUID COLLECTION

Dilated bladder
Dilated bowel
Hydroureter
Ovarian cyst (in females)
Renal cystic lesions, particularly ureteropelvic junction with anterior pelvis or pelvic dysplastic kidney (see separate differential diagnosis)
Adrenal cyst or hemorrhage
Choledochal cyst
Duodenal atresia, anal atresia, gut atresia
Enteric duplication cyst
Hepatic arteriovenous malformation
Hepatic cyst
Hydrometrocolpos
Liver cyst
Lymphangioma
Meckel's diverticulum
Meconium pseudocyst
Mesenteric cyst
Rectal dilation
Sacrococcygeal (cystic) teratoma
Splenic cyst
Umbilical vein varix
Urachal cyst

ABDOMINAL WALL PROCESS

Omphalocele
Gastroschisis
Physiologic gut herniation (8 to 12 weeks' gestation)
Limb-body wall complex
Umbilical hernia
Bladder exstrophy
Cloacal exstrophy (OEIS complex)
Pentalogy of Cantrell
Vesicoallantoic cyst
Urachal cyst

STOMACH NONVISUALIZATION

Diaphragmatic hernia (left-sided)
Normal variant
Tracheoesophageal atresia or fistula/esophageal atresia
Central nervous system problems that prevent swallowing
Facial cleft
Hiatus hernia
Micrognathia

ASCITES (ISOLATED)

Renal obstruction
Chylous fluid—Turner syndrome
Meconium peritonitis

DILATED STOMACH AND DUODENUM

Duodenal atresia
Normal variant
Annular pancreas
Antral web
Diabetic embryopathy
Gut malrotation

ECHOGENIC AREA IN ABDOMEN

Echogenic Mass
Adrenal hemorrhage
Dysplastic second collecting system
Extralobar sequestration
Hepatic tumor
Neuroblastoma
Ovarian cyst with hemorrhage
Sacrococcygeal teratoma
Fetus-in-fetu
Echogenic Bowel
Cystic fibrosis
Intragut or intra-abdominal bleed
Meconium in the third trimester
Normal variant at term
Trisomy 21
Intrauterine growth retardation
Fetal infections (cytomegalovirus)
Meconium peritonitis
Other chromosomal abnormality
Calcification
Normal variant
Fetal infections (cytomegalovirus infection, toxoplasmosis)
Gallstones

Idiopathic arterial calcification
Teratoma (intrapelvic or in adrenal region)
Intraluminal calcification—imperforate anus/anal atresia

LARGE BOWEL DILATION

Anorectal malformation or atresia
Meconium plug syndrome
Hirschprung's disease

OMPHALOCELE

Chromosome anomaly—trisomy 13, 12p, 18, 21, triploidy
Isolated
Umbilical hernia
Amniotic band syndrome
Beckwith-Wiedemann syndrome
Carpenter's syndrome
CHARGE association
Meckel-Gruber syndrome
Pentalogy of Cantrell
Valproate
Short-rib–polydactyly syndromes, various types

SMALL BOWEL DILATION

Jejunoileal atresia
Volvulus
Meconium ileus
Meconium peritonitis
Enteric duplications
Gastroschisis
Massive bilateral ureteropelvic junction obstruction
Cystic fibrosis

Genitourinary

ABSENT BLADDER

Following voiding
Renal agenesis (bilateral)
Technical—obese patient and prone fetus
Bilateral renal dysplasia
Bladder exstrophy
Caudal regression
Cloacal exstrophy
Infantile polycystic kidney disease
Severe intrauterine growth retardation
Sirenomelia
Meckel-Gruber syndrome

CYSTS IN KIDNEYS

Multicystic dysplastic kidney
Severe hydronephrosis in single or double systems
Meckel-Gruber syndrome
Chromosomal—trisomy 13
Adult polycystic kidney
Chromosomal—trisomy 18
Ellis-van Creveld syndrome
Fryns syndrome
Infantile polycystic kidney disease
Jeune's asphyxiating thoracic dystrophy
Joubert syndrome
Marden-Walker syndrome
McKusik-Kaufman syndrome
Orofacial-digital syndrome, various types (microcysts)
Roberts' syndrome
Short-rib-polydactyly syndromes, various types
Smith-Lemli-Opitz syndrome

Tuberous sclerosis
Zellweger syndrome

ENLARGED KIDNEYS OR KIDNEY

Autosomal recessive (infantile polycystic) kidney disease
Autosomal dominant (adult) polycystic kidney disease
Compensatory hypertrophy
Crossed renal ectopia
Double collecting system
Hydronephrosis
Multicystic dysplastic kidney disease
Beckwith-Wiedemann syndrome
Meckel-Gruber syndrome
Trisomy 13
Mesoblastic nephroma

GENITAL ABNORMALITIES

Smith-Lemli-Opitz syndrome
Camptomelic dysplasia
Cloacal extrophy
Chromosomal abnormalities, various
CHARGE association
Cornelia de Lange syndrome
Ectrodactyly-ectodermal-dysplasia-clefting (EEC) syndrome
Fanconi's syndrome
Fraser syndrome
Noonan syndrome
Pallister-Killian syndrome
Pena-Shokeir syndrome
Short-rib-polydactyly syndrome
Fryns syndrome
MURCS (müllerian duct aplasia, renal aplasia, cervicothoracic
    somite dysplasia)

HYDRONEPHROSIS ASSOCIATIONS

Ectopic ureter
Multicystic dysplastic kidney (hydronephrotic form)
Posterior urethral valves
Reflux
Ureterocele and ectopic ureter
Ureteropelvic junction obstruction
Ureterovesical junction obstruction
Bladder exstrophy
Chromosomal—trisomy 13 and 21
Cloacal exstrophy
Ectrodactyly-ectodermal-dysplasia-clefting (EEC) syndrome
Hemifacial microsomia (Goldenhar's syndrome)
McKusik-Kaufman syndrome
Megacystis megaureter
Megacystis microcolon
Sacrococcygeal teratoma

POSSIBLE SUPRARENAL MASS

Adrenal hematoma
Multicystic duplicated collecting system
Extrapulmonary sequestration (left side)
Neuroblastoma
Hepatic mass
Liver cyst

RENAL AGENESIS

Isolated
VACTERL association
Caudal regression/sirenomelia
Chromosomal—trisomy 21 (Down syndrome)
Diabetic embryopathy

Fraser syndrome (cryptophthalmos)
Hemifacial microsomia (Goldenhar's syndrome)
Limb-body wall complex
MURCS (müllerian duct aplasia, renal aplasia, cervicothoracic somite dysplasia)
Short rib polydactyly
Townes-Brock syndrome

Cardiac

ENLARGED HEART

Cardiomyopathy
Hydrops
Anemia
Small chest (normal size heart appears large—dwarfing syndromes)
Bilateral atrioventricular valve regurgitation
Pronounced bradycardia
Severe mitral valve regurgitation
Pericardial effusion

LEFT HEART ENLARGEMENT

Aortic stenosis
Cardiomyopathy

RIGHT HEART ENLARGEMENT

Coarctation of the aorta (particularly relative to left heart)
Hypoplastic left heart syndrome (particularly if tricuspid regurgitation)
Dysplastic pulmonary valve syndromes (with severe pulmonary regurgitation)
Premature closure of the ductus (e.g., nonsteroidal anti-inflammatory drugs such as indomethacin and aspirin)
Tetralogy of Fallot

RIGHT ATRIAL ENLARGEMENT

Ebstein anomaly
Tricuspid regurgitation
Tricuspid stenosis
Total anomalous pulmonary venous return (left atrial hypoplasia, so right atrium appears large)

BRIGHT ECHOES IN THE HEART

Chordae tendineae (normal variant)
Papillary muscle (normal variant)
Rhabdomyoma (tuberous sclerosis)
Dystrophic calcification syndrome
Angioma
Endocardial fibroelastosis (linear echogenic border to left ventricle)
Critical aortic stenosis and aortic atresia
Myocarditis

CARDIAC ABNORMALITY ASSOCIATIONS

Chromosome abnormalities
Noonan syndrome
VACTERL association
Diabetic embryopathy
Deletion 22q syndrome (DiGeorge/velocardiofacial syndrome)
Adams-Oliver syndrome
Campomelic dysplasia
Cornelia de Lange syndrome
Cri-du-chat syndromes

Ellis-van Creveld syndrome (chondroectodermal dysplasia)
Fanconi's syndrome
Fetal alcohol syndrome
Fetal infections
Hemifacial microsoma (Goldenhar's syndrome)
Holt-Oram syndrome
Heterotaxy syndrome—situs inversus (Ivemark syndrome)
Hydrolethalis
McKusik-Kaufman syndrome
Maternal phenylketonuria
Meckel-Gruber syndrome
Neu-Laxova syndrome
Retinoic acid embryopathy
Rubenstein-Taybi syndrome
Roberts' syndrome
Short-rib-polydactyly syndromes
Smith-Lemli-Opitz syndrome
Thrombocytopenia-absent radius syndrome (TAR)
Tuberous sclerosis (rhabdomyoma)
Williams syndrome
Zellweger syndrome

CARDIAC MASS

Rhabdomyoma (tuberous sclerosis)
Hypertrophic cardiomyopathy
Pericardiac masses (e.g., thymus, teratoma)
Basal cell nevus syndrome

PERICARDIAL EFFUSION

Infections

- Cytomegalovirus
- Parvovirus
- Myocarditis

Valvular aortic stenosis (especially if mitral regurgitation is present)
Cardiomyopathy
Pronounced bradycardia
Tachycardia
Early sign of anemia—Rh, parvovirus, and α-thalassemia
Early sign of hydrops
Pericardial cyst
Normal echopenic rim (pseudopericardial effusion)
Cardiac tumor
Chromosomal—45XO (Turner syndrome)
Confusion with pleural effusion

REVERSED ATRIAL SHUNT (LEFT ATRIUM TO RIGHT ATRIUM)

Critical mitral stenosis, mitral atresia
Severe left ventricular dysfunction
Severe left ventricular hypoplasia
Critical aortic stenosis/atresia
Hypoplastic left heart syndrome

REVERSED DUCTAL FLOW (AORTA-PULMONARY ARTERY)

Tricuspid atresia
Tetralogy of Fallot with severe pulmonary stenosis or atresia
Critical pulmonary stenosis or atresia

RETROGRADE FLOW IN THE AORTIC ARCH

Critical mitral stenosis, mitral atresia
Severe left ventricular dysfunction

Severe left ventricular hypoplasia
Critical aortic stenosis/atresia
Hypoplastic left heart syndrome
Interrupted aortic arch

ABSENT DUCTUS

Tetralogy of Fallot/pulmonary atresia
Tetralogy of Fallot with dysplastic pulmonary valve
syndrome

BRADYCARDIA

Sinus node dysfunction
Atrioventricular node block (secondary or tertiary)
(complete heart block)
Blocked premature atrial contractions

TACHYCARDIA

Sinus tachycardia
Supraventricular tachycardia
Atrial flutter
Atrial fibrillation with rapid ventricular response
Ventricular tachycardia
Sepsis
Anemia
Thyrotoxicosis

Chest

FLUID COLLECTION IN CHEST

Pleural effusion
Bronchogenic cyst
Cystadenomatoid malformation of lung
Diaphragmatic hernia (stomach)
Bronchial atresia
Cystic hygroma
Duplication cyst
Enlarged cardiac chamber
Hiatus hernia (stomach)
Pericardial cyst
Mediastinal teratoma
Neuroenteric cyst

SOLID MASS IN CHEST

Cystadenomatoid malformation of lung
Pulmonary sequestration
Cardiac tumor-rhabdomyoma
Chest-wall hematoma
Mediastinal teratoma
Neuroblastoma metastases
Normal thymus

DIAPHRAGMATIC HERNIA ASSOCIATIONS

Fryns syndrome
Trisomy 18 and other chromosomal abnormalities
Jarcho-Levin syndrome
Deletion 4p (Wolf-Hirshorn syndrome)
Pallister-Kinlein (tetrasomy 12p)

PLEURAL EFFUSION

Chylothorax
Early sign of hydrops (secondary to hydrops)
Hemothorax
Secondary to pulmonary sequestration, cystadenomatoid
malformation, tracheal atresia
Lung agenesis

SMALL CHEST

Osteogenesis imperfecta type II
Thanatophoric dysplasia
Achondrogenesis, all types
Achondroplasia
Atelosteogenesis, all types
Camptomelic dysplasia
Chondrodyoplasia punctata
Ellis-van Creveld syndrome (chondroectodermal dysplasia)
Fibrochondrogenesis
Hypophosphatasia
Jeune's asphyxiating thoracic dystrophy
Multiple pterygium syndrome
Short-rib-polydactyly syndromes, all types
Spondyloepiphyseal dysplasia congenita

Central Nervous System

AGENESIS OF THE CORPUS CALLOSUM ASSOCIATIONS

Dandy-Walker cyst
Isolated
Aicardi syndrome
Acrocallosal syndrome
Apert syndrome
Chromosomal—trisomy 13
Chromosomal—trisomy 18
Chromosomal—trisomy 21 (Down syndrome)
Encephalocele
Fetal alcohol syndrome
Fetal infections
Fryns syndrome
Hydrolethalus
Meckel-Gruber syndrome
Neu-Laxova syndrome
Smith-Lemli-Opitz syndrome
Walker-Warburg syndrome
Zellweger syndrome

BRAIN TOO EASILY SEEN (UNDEROSSIFICATION OF BONE)

Osteogenesis imperfecta, type II
Achondrogenesis, some types
Acrania
Atelosteogenesis
Hypophosphatasia
Short-rib-polydactyly syndrome

CEREBELLAR HYPOPLASIA

Dandy-Walker cyst
Spinal dysraphism
Chromosomal—trisomy 13
Chromosomal—trisomy 18
Chromosomal—trisomy 21 (Down syndrome)
Cri-du-chat syndrome
Fetal infections
Joubert syndrome
Meckel-Gruber syndrome
Neu-Laxova syndrome
Smith-Lemli-Opitz syndrome
Walker-Warburg syndrome

DANDY-WALKER CYST

Cornelia de Lange syndrome
Chromosomal—triploidy
Chromosomal—trisomy 13
Chromosomal—trisomy 18

Chromosomal—trisomy 21
Joubert syndrome
Aicardi syndrome
Fetal alcohol syndrome
CHARGE syndrome
Maternal diabetic embryopathy
Fryns syndrome
Meckel-Gruber syndrome
Neu-Laxova syndrome
Neural tube defect
Fetal infections
Smith-Lemli-Opitz syndrome
Walker-Warburg syndrome

ECHOGENIC BRAIN FOCUS OR FOCI

Cerebellar vermis (normal)
Choroid plexus (normal)
Fetal infections (cytomegalovirus infection [wall of lateral
   ventricles] and toxoplasmosis)
Gyri in third trimester
Intrabrain hemorrhage when fresh
Intracranial tumor (teratoma and lipoma of the corpus
   callosum)
Tuberous sclerosis

ENCEPHALOCELE

**Amniotic band syndrome—asymmetrical top of the head
   lesions**
Isolated
Adams-Oliver syndrome
Chromosomal—trisomy 13
Chromosomal—trisomy 18
Dandy-Walker cyst
Dysegmental dysplasia
Meckel-Gruber syndrome
Roberts' syndrome (pseudothalidomide)
Walker-Warburg syndrome

FLUID COLLECTION IN THE HEAD

Bilateral
Choroid plexus cyst
Ventriculomegaly
Single
Cavum septum pellucidum and/or vergae (normal)
Quadrageminal cistern (normal)
Choroid plexus cyst
Third ventricular enlargement
Arachnoid cyst
Bleed
Porencephalic cyst
Schizencephaly
Tumor (cystic teratoma)
Dandy-Walker cyst
Mega cisterna magna
Aneurysm of vein of Galen
Holoprosencephaly
Intrahemispheric cyst with agenesis of the corpus callosum
Cystic encephalomalacia and periventricular encephalomalacia
Posterior fossa extra-axial cyst
Subdural hygroma
Unilateral hydrocephalus

HOLOPROSENCEPHALY

Chromosomal—trisomy 13
Isolated
Aicardi syndrome
Campomelic dysplasia

CHARGE association
Chromosomal—triploidy
Chromosomal—trisomy 18
Chromosomal—18p−
Diabetic embryopathy
DiGeorge syndrome
Maternal diabetic embryopathy
Frontonasal dysplasia
Fryns syndrome
Short-rib-polydactyly syndrome
Smith-Lemli-Opitz syndrome

HYDRANENCEPHALY CAUSES

Isolated
Fetal infections
Stuck twin (death of co-twin)
Cocaine embryopathy
Familial hydranencephaly (autosomal recessive)

KLEEBLATTSCHÄDEL DEFORMITY OF SKULL (CLOVERLEAF SKULL)

Apert syndrome
Pfeiffer syndrome
Thanatophoric dysplasia
Amniotic band syndrome
Campomelic dysplasia
Crouzon syndrome

MACROCEPHALY

Familial macrocephaly
Ventriculomegaly
Achondrogenesis, all types
Achondroplasia
Basal cell nevus syndrome
Beckwith-Wiedemann syndrome
Chromosomal—triploidy (relative enlargement)
Greig's cephalopolysyndactyly syndrome
Intracranial tumor
Sotos syndrome
Thanatophoric dysplasia

MICROCEPHALY

Drugs (alcohol, hydantoin, aminopterin)
**Fetal infections (cytomegalovirus infection, toxoplasmosis,
   rubella)**
Isolated (including autosomal and X-linked recessive forms)
Spinal dysraphism
Cerebral atrophy
Chromosome abnormalities (especially trisomy 18)
Adams-Oliver syndrome
Cornelia de Lange syndrome
Craniosynostosis
Cri-du-chat syndrome
Encephalocele
Freeman-Sheldon syndrome
Holoprosencephaly
Lenz syndrome
Lissencephaly (including Miller-Diecker syndrome)
Maternal phenylketonuria
Meckel-Gruber syndrome
Neu-Laxova syndrome
Roberts' syndrome
Rubenstein-Taybi syndrome
Seckel syndrome
Smith-Lemli-Opitz syndrome
Teratogens
Walker-Warburg syndrome

POSTERIOR FOSSA CYST

Arachnoid cyst (extra-axial cyst)
Dandy-Walker cyst
Dilated cisterna magna
Porencephalic cyst
Quadrageminal cyst
Vein of Galen aneurysm

VENTRICULOMEGALY

Aqueduct stenosis
Arnold-Chiari malformation (neural tube defect)
Dandy-Walker malformation
Encephalocele
Hydrocephalus ex vacuo (atrophy)
Normal variant (mild)
Achondroplasia (third trimester)
Agenesis of the corpus callosum (colpocephaly)
Amniotic band syndrome
Arachnoid cyst
Baller-Gerold syndrome
Campomelic dysplasia
CHARGE
Chromosomal abnormalities
Craniosynostosis
Fetal alcohol syndrome
Fetal infections (cytomegalovirus infection and toxoplasmosis)
Fryns syndrome
Holoprosencephaly
Hydrolethalis
Intracranial bleed
Meckel-Gruber syndrome
Lissencephaly including Miller-Diecker syndrome
Neoplasms
Neu-Laxova syndrome
Roberts' syndrome (pseudothalidomide)
Short-rib-polydactyly syndromes
Smith-Lemli-Opitz syndrome
Thanatophoric dysplasia
Vein of Galen aneurysm
Walker-Warburg syndrome
Zellweger syndrome

Spine
SHORT SPINE

Iniencephaly
Caudal regression/sirenomelia
Jarcho-Levin syndrome
Klippel-Feil syndrome

SPINAL DYSRAPHISM ASSOCIATIONS

Chromosome abnormalities (triploidy and trisomy 18)
Maternal diabetic embryopathy
Aminopterin
Amniotic band syndrome
Anencephaly
Cataract
Caudal regression
Cloacal exstrophy (OEIS syndrome)
Diastematomyelia
Encephalocele
Valproic acid embryopathy
Retinoic acid embryopathy
Iniencephaly
Limb-body wall complex
Rachischisis

Roberts' syndrome (pseudothalidomide)
Sacrococcygeal teratoma

VERTEBRAL ABNORMALITIES

Maternal diabetic embryopathy
Neural tube defect
VACTERL association
Cloacal extrophy (OEIS syndrome)
Diastomatomyelia
Hemifacial microsomia (Goldenhar's syndrome)
Jarcho-Levin syndrome
Klippel-Feil syndrome
Kniest syndrome
Larsen syndrome
MURCS
Noonan syndrome
Skeletal dysplasia, many types

Eyes
EXOPHTHALMOS/PROPTOSIS/PROMINENT EYES

Craniosynostosis
Apert syndrome (acrocephalosyndactyly, type I)
Carpenter's syndrome
Crouzon syndrome
Jackson-Weiss syndrome
Melnick-Needles syndrome
Neu-Laxova syndrome
Pfeiffer syndrome

CATARACT

Fetal infections
Neu-Laxova syndrome
Walker-Warburg syndrome
Zellweger syndrome

HYPERTELORISM

Aarskog syndrome
Acrocallosal syndrome
Atelosteogenesis
Craniosynostosis syndromes
Chromosomal—4p− (Wolf-Hirschhorn syndrome)
Frontal encephalocele
Frontonasal dysplasia
Larsen syndrome
Marden-Walker syndrome
Melnick-Needles syndrome
Noonan syndrome
Neu-Laxova syndrome
Pena-Shokeir syndrome
Otopalatodigital syndrome
Opitz hypertelorism hypospadias syndrome
Robinow syndrome (fetal face syndrome)

HYPOTELORISM

Holoprosencephaly
Chromosomal abnormalities, particularly trisomy 13
Trigonocephaly
Baller-Gerald syndrome

MICROPHTHALMIA OR ANOPHTHALMIA

Chromosomal abnormalities, especially trisomy 13
Isolated
CHARGE
Fetal infections (rubella, varicella, toxoplasmosis)

Fraser syndrome—cryptophthalmos
Goldenhar's syndrome (hemifacial microsomia)
Hydrolethalis
Lenz syndrome
Neu-Laxova syndrome
Oculodentodigital syndrome
Walker-Warburg syndrome

Face

ASYMMETRY

Goldenhar's syndrome (hemifacial microsomia)
Amniotic band syndrome with facial cleft
Craniosynostosis and associated syndromes
CHARGE syndrome
Greig's cephalopolysyndactyly syndrome
Jackson-Weiss syndrome
Saethre-Chotzen syndrome
Townes-Brock syndrome

CLEFT LIP AND PALATE*

Isolated
Amniotic band syndrome (L)
Chromosome abnormalities, especially trisomy 13 (M,L,P)
Holoprosencephaly (M,L)
Stickler syndrome (P)
Atelosteogenesis (P)
Campomelic dysplasia (P)
CHARGE association (P)
Cri-du-chat syndrome
Diastrophic dysplasia (P)
Ectrodactyly-ectodermal-dysplasia-clefting syndrome (L,P)
Fetal anticonvulsant syndrome (L)
Hydrolethalus
Maternal phenylketonuria (P)
Meckel-Gruber syndrome (M,L,P)
Mohr's syndrome (M)
Multiple pterygium syndrome, lethal (P)
Orofacial-digital syndrome, various types (M,L,P)
Otopalatodigital syndrome
Retinoic acid embryopathy (L,P)
Roberts' syndrome (L,P)
Robinow syndrome (L,P)
Short-rib-polydactyly syndromes, various types (L,P)
Spondyloepiphyseal dysplasia congenita (P)
Stickler syndrome
Treacher-Collins syndrome (P)
Velocardiofacial syndrome/DiGeorge sequence (P)
Smith-Lemli-Opitz syndrome
Gorlin syndrome
Pierre Robin sequence

MACROGLOSSIA

Beckwith-Wiedemann syndrome
Chromosomal—trisomy 21 (Down syndrome)
Oral teratoma

MALFORMED EARS

Chromosome abnormalities, especially trisomy 18
Acrofacial dysostoses (microtia)
Branchio-otorenal syndrome

*M = midline cleft lip and/or palate, L = lateral cleft and/or palate, P = cleft palate only

CHARGE association
Hemifacial microsomia (Goldenhar's syndrome) (tags, microtia)
Retinoic acid embryopathy
Townes-Brock syndrome (tags)
Treacher-Collins syndrome (tags) (microtia)

MICROGNATHIA

Chromosomal abnormalities, especially trisomy 18
Pierre Robin sequence
Short-rib-polydactyly syndrome
Stickler syndrome
Acrofacial dysostoses, various types
Atelosteogenesis
Campomelic dysplasia
CHARGE association
Cri-du-chat syndrome
Fetal teratogens (alcohol, valproic acid, retinoic acid)
Freeman-Sheldon syndrome (whistling facies)
Hemifacial microsomia (Goldenhar's syndrome)
Hypoglossia, hypodactyly
Joubert syndrome
Larsen syndrome
Melnick-Needles syndrome
Multiple pterygium syndrome
Marden-Walker syndrome
Neu-Laxova syndrome
Nager syndrome
Orofacial-digital syndrome, various types
Otocephaly
Retinoic acid embryopathy
Seckel syndrome
Skeletal dysplasias, various types
Smith-Lemli-Opitz syndrome
Sotos syndrome
Treacher-Collins syndrome

MIDFACE HYPOPLASIA/DEPRESSED NASAL BRIDGE/MAXILLARY HYPOPLASIA

Achondroplasia (third trimester)
Atelosteogenesis
Campomelic dysplasia
Chondrodysplasia punctata (third trimester)
Cleidocranial dysostosis
Thanatophoric dysplasia
Apert syndrome
Carpenter syndrome
Fetal alcohol syndrome
Fetal warfarin syndrome
Larsen syndrome
Osteogenesis imperfecta, type II
Pfeiffer syndrome
Holoprosencephaly sequence
Pena-Shokeir syndrome
Smith-Lemli-Opitz syndrome
Stickler syndrome

Limbs

ABNORMAL THUMB

Diabetic embryopathy
Holt-Oram syndrome
VACTERL association
Acrofacial dysostoses, various types
Apert syndrome (acrocephalosyndactyly, type I)
Baller-Gerold syndrome

Carpenter syndrome (acrocephalopolysyndactyly, type II)
Chromosomal—trisomy 18
Cornelia de Lange syndrome
Diastrophic dysplasia
Ectrodactyly-tibial aplasia syndrome
Fanconi's syndrome
Greig's cephalopolysyndactyly syndrome
Hemifacial microsomia (Goldenhar's syndrome)
Orofacial-digital syndrome, various types
Pfeiffer syndrome (acrocephalosyndactyly, type V)
Poland anomaly
Rubinstein-Taybi syndrome
Townes-Brock syndrome

ABSENT DIGITS

Amniotic band syndrome
Poland anomaly
Terminal transverse limb defect
Acrofacial dysostoses, various types
Atelosteogenesis
Adams-Oliver syndrome
Baller-Gerold syndrome
Various chromosomal abnormalities
Cornelia de Lange syndrome
Ectrodactyly-ectodermal-dysplasia-clefting syndrome
Ectrodactyly-tibial aplasia syndrome
Fanconi's syndrome
Fryns syndrome
Holt-Oram syndrome
Nager's acrofacial dystosis
Oromandibular limb hypogenesis
Pfeiffer syndrome (acrocephalosyndactyly, type V)
Poland anomaly
Roberts' syndrome (pseudothalidomide)
Townes-Brock syndrome
VACTERL association

ASYMETRIC LIMBS

Amniotic band syndrome
Osteogenesis imperfecta
Femoral hypoplasia
Terminal transverse limb deficiency
Femur-fibula-ulna syndrome
Proteus syndrome
Klippel-Trenaunay-Weber syndrome
Rubenstein-Taybi syndrome

ABSENT LIMBS

Amniotic band syndrome
Diabetic embryopathy
Limb-body wall complex
Terminal transverse limb deficiency
Acrofacial dysostoses, various types
Atelosteogenesis
Cornelia de Lange syndrome
Ectrodactyly-ectodermal-dysplasia-clefting syndrome
Grebe syndrome
Holt-Oram syndrome
Oromandibular limb hypogenesis
Poland anomaly
Retinoic acid embryopathy
Roberts' syndrome (pseudothalidomide)
Sirenomelia
Thalidomide embryopathy
Thrombocytopenia-absent radius syndrome

BONE HYPOMINERALIZATION

Achondrogenesis
Hypophosphatasia
Osteogenesis imperfecta

BOWING

Campomelic dysplasia—particularly tibia and femur
Osteogenesis imperfecta, type II—particularly tibia and femur
Thanatophoric dysplasia
Achondrogenesis
Boomerang dysplasia
Diabetic embryopathy
Dyssegmental dysplasia
Fibrochondrogenesis
Focal femoral deficiency—only involves tibia and femur
Hypophosphatasia
Melnick-Needles syndrome
Normal (if femur scanned from medial aspect)
Oligohydramnios sequence
Roberts' syndrome

CLENCHED HANDS

Arthrogryposis, various types
Chromosomal abnormalities, especially trisomy 18
Amniotic band syndrome
Apert syndrome
Congenital muscular dystrophy, various types
Freeman-Sheldon syndrome
Harlequin icthyosis
Multiple pterygium syndrome
Neu-Laxova syndrome
Pena-Shokeir syndrome
Smith-Lemli-Opitz syndrome
X-linked hydrocephalus (thumb)

CLINODACTYLY

Chromosomal abnormalities, especially trisomy 18 and trisomy 21
Normal variant
Acrocephalosyndactyly syndromes
Amniotic band syndrome
Campomelic dysplasia
Cornelia de Lange syndrome
Ectrodactyly-ectodermal-dysplasia-clefting syndrome
Harskog syndrome
Holt-Oram syndrome
Miller-Dieker syndrome
Orofacial-digital syndrome, various types
Poland anomaly
Roberts' syndrome
Russell-Silver syndrome
Seckel syndrome
Saetre-Chotzen syndrome
Townes-Brock syndrome

CLUB FOOT

Arthrogryposis, various types
Chromosomal abnormalities, especially trisomy 18
Isolated
Neural tube defect
Adam-Oliver syndrome
Amniotic band syndrome
Amyloplasia congenita
Atelosteogenesis
Campomelic dysplasia

Caudal regression, especially diabetic embryopathy
Chondrodysplasia punctata (rhizomelic type), lethal
Diabetic embryopathy
Ellis-van Creveld syndrome
Diastrophic dysplasia
Freeman-Sheldon syndrome (whistling face)
Fryns syndrome
Hydrolethalus
Larsen syndrome
Meckel-Gruber syndrome
Multiple pterygium syndrome
Pena-Shokeir syndrome
Seckel syndrome
Short-rib-polydactyly syndromes, various types
Smith-Lemli-Opitz syndrome
Thrombocytopenia-absent radius syndrome (TAR)
Zellweger syndrome

FRACTURES

Osteogenesis imperfecta, all types
Achondrogenesis
Hypophosphatasia

JOINT CONTRACTURES—CONTRACTURES OF THE EXTREMITIES

Arthrogryposis, various types
Caudal dysplasia sequence (diabetic embryopathy)
Chromosomal abnormalities, especially trisomy 18
Neural tube defect (lower limbs)
Amniotic band syndrome
Amyloplasia congenita
Apert syndrome (acrocephalosyndactyly, type I)
Beals' syndrome (contractual arachnodactyly)
Cornelia de Lange syndrome
Diastrophic dysplasia
Focal femoral deficiency
Freeman-Sheldon syndrome
Larsen syndrome
Multiple pterygium syndrome, various types
Neu-Laxova syndrome
Oligohydramnios sequence
Pena-Shokeir syndrome
Roberts' syndrome
Seckel syndrome
Zellweger syndrome

LIMB SHORTENING

Achondrogenesis
Osteogenesis imperfecta, types II, III
Thanatophoric dysplasia
Achondroplasia
Campomelic dysplasia
Diastrophic dysplasia
Ellis-van Creveld syndrome
Hypophosphatasia
Kniest syndrome
Roberts' syndrome
Short-rib-polydactyly syndrome
Spondyloepiphyseal dysplasia congenita
Other rare dysplasias
Rhizomelic Shortening
Asphyxiating thoracic dysplasia (Jeune's syndrome)
Achondroplasia
Early intrauterine growth retardation
Thanatophoric dysplasia
Atelosteogenesis

Chondrodysplasia punctata, rhizomelic type
Diabetic embryopathy
Familial
Fetal warfarin syndrome
Fibrochondrogenesis
Focal femoral deficiency (diabetic embryopathy)
Neu-Laxova syndrome
Short-rib-polydactyly syndromes
Selected Limbs
Amniotic band syndrome
Caudal regression (diabetic embryopathy)
Focal femoral deficiency (diabetic embryopathy)
Osteogenesis imperfecta
Campomelic dysplasia
Cornelia de Lange syndrome
Fanconi's syndrome
Femur-fibula-ulna syndrome
Holt-Oram syndrome
Roberts' syndrome
Thrombocytopenia-absent radius syndrome
VATER syndrome

MUSCLE WASTING

Arthrogryposis, various types
Congenital muscular dystrophy, various types
Amyoplasia congenita
Freeman-Sheldon syndrome
Neural tube defect, various types (lower limbs only)
Multiple pterygium syndrome (lethal)
Pena-Shokeir syndrome

POLYDACTYLY

Preaxial
Carpenter's syndrome
Diabetic embryopathy
Greig's cephalopolysyndactyly syndrome (feet)
Townes-Brock syndrome
Fanconi's anemia
Postaxial
Chromosome abnormalities, especially trisomy 13
Familial, especially African American
Acrocallosal syndrome
Atelosteogenesis
Carpenter's syndrome
Ellis-van Creveld syndrome (chondroectodermal dysplasia)
Grebe syndrome
Greig's cephalopolysyndactyly syndrome (hands)
Hydrolethalis
Joubert syndrome
McKusik-Kaufman syndrome
Meckel-Gruber syndrome
Mohr's syndrome
Orofacial-digital syndrome
Pallister-Hall syndrome
Short-rib-polydactyly syndromes
Smith-Lemli-Opitz syndrome

RADIAL HYPOPLASIA/SHORT RADIAL RAY

Chromosomal abnormalities, especially trisomy 18
Cornelia de Lange syndrome
Holt-Oram syndrome
VACTERL association
AASE syndrome
Acrofacial dysostoses, various types
Amniotic band
Baller-Gerold syndrome

Fanconi's syndrome
Hemifacial microsomia (Goldenhar's syndrome)
Roberts' syndrome (pseudothalidomide)
Thrombocytopenia-absent radius syndrome (TAR)
Townes-Brock syndrome

ROCKER-BOTTOM FEET

Arthrogryposis, various types
Chromosomal abnormalities, especially trisomy 18
Syndromes with severe neurologic impairment, including
Fryns syndrome, multiple pterygium syndromes, Neu-
Laxova syndrome

SOFT TISSUE MASS

Fibrosarcoma
Hemangioma
Infantile myofibromatosis
Klippel-Trenaunay-Weber syndrome
Mafucci syndrome
Proteus syndrome
Teratoma, including sacrococcygeal teratoma
Turner syndrome

STIPPLED EPIPHYSES

Chondrodysplasia punctata
Chromosome anomalies, especially trisomy 18
Vitamin K deficiency
Warfarin syndrome
Zellweger syndrome

SYNDACTYLY

Neu-Laxova syndrome
Ectrodactyly-ectodermal-dysplasia-clefting syndrome
Apert syndrome
Cephalopolysyndactyly syndromes
Fraser syndrome
Mohr syndrome
Smith-Lemli-Opitz syndrome (second and third toes)
Chromosomal syndromes, especially triploidy

Neck

CYSTIC HYGROMA

Chromosomal abnormalities, especially Turner syndrome,
trisomy 21
Regression to normal (common)
Acardiac, acephalic twin
Achondrogenesis
Multiple pterygium syndrome
Neu-Luxova syndrome
Noonan syndrome
Pena-Shokeir syndrome
Roberts' syndrome

HYPEREXTENDED NECK

Anterior lymphangioma
Cervical neural tube defect (iniencephaly)
Cervical teratoma
Goiter
Neuromuscular disorder
Normal variant
Neu-Laxova syndrome

NUCHAL THICKENING OR INCREASED NUCHAL TRANSLUCENCY (MEMBRANE)

Chromosomal abnormalities, especially Turner syndrome
and trisomy 21

Cardiac anomalies
Normal variant
Achondrogenesis
Apert syndrome
Cri-du-chat syndrome
Jacobson syndrome
Joubert syndrome
Multiple pterygium syndrome
Roberts' syndrome
Spinal muscular atrophy
Noonan syndrome
Smith-Lemli-Opitz syndrome
Zellweger syndrome

NECK MASS

Amniotic band syndrome
Anterior lymphangioma
Branchial cleft cyst
Cervical neural tube defect (iniencephaly)
Cystic hygroma (bilateral)
Cystic hygroma (unilateral)
Encephalocele
Goiter
Hemangioma
Nuchal thickening
Teratoma of neck
Thyroglossal duct cyst

Other

AMNIOTIC MEMBRANE

Amniotic band syndrome
Amniotic sheet
Subamniotic or subchorionic bleed
Twin membrane
Unfused amniotic membrane
Amniotic membrane displacement following amniocentesis
Limb-body wall complex (amniotic disruption sequence)
Placental cyst

CHROMOSOMAL ANOMALY SONOGRAPHIC FINDINGS

Central nervous system anomalies
  Holoprosencephaly
  Dandy-Walker malformation, cerebellar hypoplasia
  Hydrocephalus
  Spina bifida
  Agenesis of the corpus callosum
Choroid plexus cysts—large or associated with other
  abnormalities
Hypotelorism, cleft lip and palate, single nostril, absent nose
Cystic hygroma
Nuchal thickening/translucency
Cardiac malformations
Duodenal atresia
Gut atresia
Omphalocele
Genitourinary anomalies
  Obstructive uropathy (obstruction at or distal to the
  urethrovesical junction)
  Renal cystic dysplasia with other abnormalities
Hydrops
Hydrothorax
Club foot, rocker-bottom foot
Club hand or clenched hand
Severe early intrauterine growth retardation
Polyhydramnios or oligohydramnios

Single umbilical artery
Multiple cord cysts

CORD MASS

Allantoic cyst
Wharton's jelly
Aneurysm
Angiomyxoma
Cord cyst
Cord knot
Hemangioma
Hematoma
Mucoid degeneration of the cord
Omphalomesenteric cyst
Teratoma
Thrombosis of umbilical vessels
Umbilical vein varix
Urachal cyst

HYDROPS

Anemia, including Rh disease and α-thalassemia
Cardiac malformation (congenital heart disease)
Chromosomal abnormalities, especially Turner syndrome
    and trisomy 21
Chest masses, including cystadenomatoid malformation
Cystic hygroma
Fetal infections (cytomegalovirus infection, parvovirus
    infection, syphilis, toxoplasmosis)
Twin-to-twin transfusion syndrome
Achondrogenesis
Cardiac tumor-rhabdomyoma-tuberous sclerosis
Chondrodysplasia punctata
Chorioangioma
Congenital nephrotic syndrome, Finnish type
Cornelia de Lange syndrome
Cystadenomatoid malformation of lung
Diabetic embryopathy
Meconium peritonitis
Diaphragmatic hernia
Dysrhythmia
Extralobar pulmonary sequestration
Fetomaternal transfusion
Fibrochondrogenesis
Glycogen storage disease
Hypophosphatasia
Hepatic tumor
Hypophosphatasia
Lymphangioma
Multiple pterygium syndrome, lethal
Neu-Laxova syndrome
Noonan syndrome
Osteogenesis imperfecta, various types
Pena-Shokeir syndrome
Teratomas, including sacrococcygeal teratoma
Short-rib-polydactyly syndromes, various types
Tracheal atresia

INTRAUTERINE GROWTH RETARDATION

Chromosomal abnormalities, especially triploidy and
    trisomy 18
Poor quality measurements
Small normal fetus
Skeletal dysplasias, various types
CHARGE association
Cornelia de Lange syndrome
Fetal infections (cytomegalovirus, varicella, rubella)
Fetal alcohol syndrome

Fetal aminopterin/methotrexate syndrome
Fetal warfarin syndrome
Fibrochondrogenesis
Fryns syndrome
Harlequin syndrome (asymmetric)
Hypophosphatasia
Neu-Laxova syndrome
Osteogenesis imperfecta, various types
Pena-Shokeir syndrome
Roberts' syndrome (pseudothalidomide)
Russel-Silver syndrome
Seckel syndrome
Short-rib-polydactyly syndromes, various types
Smith-Lemli-Opitz syndrome
Spondyloepiphyseal dysplasia congenita

MACROSOMIA

Diabetic embryopathy
Familial
Poor-quality measurements
Wrong dates
Beckwith-Wiedemann syndrome
Simpson-Golabi-Behmel syndrome
Sotos syndrome
Weaver syndrome

OLIGOHYDRAMNIOS

Bilateral dysplastic kidney
Bilateral renal agenesis (see Renal agenesis)
Bilateral ureteral obstruction
Infantile polycystic kidney disease
Intrauterine growth restriction (retardation)
Normal in late third trimester
Posterior urethral valves
Postmaturity
Premature rupture of membranes
Stuck twin
Congenital infections
Sirenomelia and caudal regression
Chromosomal—various, especially triploidy

PLACENTAL MASS

Chorioangioma
Venous lake
Wharton's jelly deposition
Fetal lobulation
Partial molar changes
Mole and normal fetus
Placental cyst
Placental infarct

PLACENTAL THICKENING

Normal variant
Chorioangioma
Chromosome various, especially triploidy
Diabetic embryopathy
Fetal infections (cytomegalovirus, rubella, syphilis,
    toxoplasmosis)
Hydrops, especially Rh incompatibility
Beckwith-Wiedemann syndrome

POLYHYDRAMNIOS

Associated with fetal hydrops
Fetal infections—parvovirus
Diabetic embryopathy
Duodenal atresia
Gut atresias
Macrosomia

Tracheoesophageal fistula (esophageal atresia)
Twins
Chromosomal—various, especially Turner syndrome and
    trisomy 13
Anemias (thalassemia)
Cardiac malformation—heart failure, various types
Severe/lethal skeletal dysplasias, various types
Obstructing rhabdomyoma (tuberous sclerosis)
Chorioangioma
Congenital nephrotic syndrome, Finnish type
Cystadenomatoid malformation of lung
Diaphragmatic hernia
Epignathus
Fetal goiter

Fryns syndrome
Hydrolethalus
Idiopathic
Intra-abdominal mass (e.g., mesoblastic nephroma)
Large ovarian cysts
Megacystis microcolon
Micrognathia—severe, e.g., otocephaly
Multiple pterygium syndrome
Neck teratoma
Osteogenesis imperfecta, various types
Otocephaly
Sacrococcygeal teratoma
Short-rib-polydactyly
Twin-to-twin transfusion syndrome

Appendices

Sonographic Features of Less Common Fetal Abnormalities

Aarskog Syndrome

Hypertelorism
Short nose
Clinodactyly

AASE Syndrome

Radial hypoplasia

Acrocallosal Syndrome

Agenesis of corpus callosum
Hypertelorism
Polydactyly—postaxial

Acrofacial Dysostosis

Malformed ears
Micrognathia
Abnormal thumb
Absent digits
Radial hypoplasia

Acromesomelic Dysplasia

Mesomelic shortness
Adams-Oliver syndrome
Absent digits
Encephalocele
Microcephaly
Cardiac defects
Clubfoot

Aicardi Syndrome

Agenesis of corpus callosum
Arachnoid cyst
Dandy-Walker syndrome
Holoprosencephaly

Alpha-Thalassemia

Hydrops

Amyloplasia Congenita

Abdominal-wall process
Club foot
Joint contractures

Atelosteogenesis

Small chest
Hypertelorism
Cleft lip and palate
Micrognathia
Absent limbs
Club foot
Polydactyly—postaxial
Rhizomelic shortening
Intrauterine growth retardation

Baller-Gerold Syndrome

Malformed kidney
Mild ventriculomegaly
Hypotelorism
Absent digits
Abnormal thumb
Radial hypoplasia

Basal Cell Nevus Syndrome

Macrocephaly
Cardiac mass

Beals' Syndrome

Joint contractures

Boomerang Dysplasia

Bowing

Branchiootorenal Syndrome

Malformed ears

CHARGE Association

Omphalocele
Cardiac abnormality
Holoprosencephaly
Cleft palate
Micrognathia
Intrauterine growth retardation
Genital hypoplasia

Chondrodysplasia Punctata

Small chest
Club foot
Rhizomelic shortening
Hydrops
Stippled epiphyses

Chromosome—18p−

Holoprosencephaly
Hypotelorism
Club foot

Chromosome—18q−

Microphthalmia/anophthalmia

Chromosome—47,XXY

Cystic hygroma

Chromosome—4p− (Wolf-Hirschorn)

Hypertelorism
Cardiac abnormality
Malformed ears (tags)

Chromosome—Duplication 20p

Hypertelorism

Cleidocranial Dysplasia

Partial or total asplasia of the clavicles
Brachycephaly

Congenital Muscular Dystrophy

Clenched hands
Muscle wasting

Congenital Nephrotic Syndrome

Polyhydramnios
Hydrops

Cornelia de Lange Syndrome

Cardiac abnormality
Dandy-Walker cyst
Microcephaly
Short nose
Abnormal thumb
Absent digits
Absent limbs
Clinodactyly
Radial hypoplasia
Short limbs
Hydrops
Intrauterine growth retardation

Cri-du-Chat Syndrome

Microcephaly
Micrognathia
Cardiac malformation
Facial abnormalities such as cleft lip and palate
Hypoplastic cerebellum
Increased nuchal translucency

Diabetic Embryopathy

Duodenal atresia
Malformed kidney
Renal agenesis
Cardiac abnormality
Holoprosencephaly
Spinal dysraphism
Abnormal thumb
Absent limbs
Thick placenta
Bowing
Club foot
Joint contractures
Polydactyly—preaxial
Rhizomelic shortening
Vertebral defects
Hydrops
Macrosomia
Polyhydramnios

Dyssegmental Dysplasia

Bowing

Ectrodactyly-Ectodermal-Dysplasia-Clefting Syndrome

Hydronephrosis
Cleft lip and palate
Absent digits
Absent limbs
Clinodactyly

Ectrodactyly-Tibial Aplasia Syndrome

Abnormal thumbs
Absent digits

Ellis-Van Creveld Syndrome

Renal cystic structure
Cardiac abnormality

Small chest
Club foot
Polydactyly—postaxial
Short limbs
Intrauterine growth retardation

Fanconi's Syndrome

Cardiac abnormality
Abnormal thumb
Absent digits
Radial hypoplasia

Fetal Aminopterin/Methotrexate Syndrome

Mesomelic shortness
Intrauterine growth retardation

Fetal Infections

Echogenic area in abdomen (cytomegalovirus)
Cardiac mass
Agenesis of the corpus callosum
Cerebellar hypoplasia
Dandy-Walker cyst
Echogenic brain foci
Microcephaly
Mild ventriculomegaly
Cataract
Microphthalmia or anophthalmia
Hydrops
Intrauterine growth retardation
Thick placenta

Fetal Warfarin Syndrome

Short nose
Rhizomelic shortening
Intrauterine growth retardation
Stippled epiphyses

Fibrochondrogenesis

Small chest
Rhizomelic shortening
Hydrops
Intrauterine growth retardation

Fraser Syndrome

Microphthalmia or anophthalmia
Syndactyly
Genital abnormalities
Laryngeal atresia
Malformations of the nose and ear
Renal agenesis
Cardiac defects
Skeletal defects

Freeman-Sheldon Syndrome

Micrognathia
Clenched hands
Club foot
Joint contractures
Muscle wasting

Frontonasal Dysplasia

Holoprosencephaly
Hypertelorism

Grebe Syndrome

Absent limbs
Polydactyly—preaxial

Greig's Cephalopolysyndactyly Syndrome

Macrocephaly
Hypertelorism
Facial asymmetry
Abnormal thumb
Polydactyly—preaxial/postaxial

Harlequin Icthyosis

Open mouth with large tongue
Amniotic fluid debris with intra-amniotic membrane
Clenched or fixed hands

Holt-Oram Syndrome

Cardiac abnormality
Abnormal thumb
Absent digits
Absent limbs
Clinodactyly
Radial hypoplasia

Hydrolethalus

Agenesis of the corpus callosum
Microphthalmia or anophthalmia
Polydactyly—postaxial
Ventriculomegaly
Polyhydramnios
Micrognathia
Cleft palate
Heart defect
Club foot

Hypophosphatasia

Small chest
Easily seen brain
Bowing
Moderate to severe bone shortening
Hydrops
Intrauterine growth retardation
Diffuse hypomineralization

Ivemark Syndrome

Situs inversus
Complex heart defect
Polysplenia

Jackson-Weiss Syndrome

Exophthalmos/proptosis/prominent eyes
Facial asymmetry

Jacobsen Syndrome

Increased nuchal translucency
Trigonocephaly
Hypertelorism
Micrognathia
Cardiac defects

Jarcho-Levin Syndrome (Spondylocostal Dysostosis)

Increased nuchal translucency
Malaligned and malformed vertebra
Fan-shaped ribs

Joubert Syndrome

Increased nuchal thickening
Multicystic kidneys
Micrognathia
Polydactyly
Cerebellar hypoplasia and Dandy-Walker cyst

Klippel-Feil Syndrome

Vertebral defects

Kniest Syndrome

Short limbs
Kyphoscoliosis
Platyspondyly
Epiphyseal splaying

Larsen Syndrome

Club foot
Abnormal vertebral segmentation with kyphoscoliosis
Hypertelorism
Depressed nasal bridge
Micrognathia
Prominent forehead
Joint dislocation

Lenz Syndrome

Microcephaly
Renal dysgenesis
Microphthalmia

Marden-Walker Syndrome

Micrognathia
Hypertelorism
Joint contractures
Renal cysts

Marfan Syndrome

Aortic widening
Unduly long bones

Maternal Phenylketonuria

Cardiac abnormality
Microcephaly
Cleft palate

McKusik-Kaufman Syndrome

Hydronephrosis
Cardiac abnormality
Polydactyly—postaxial
Vaginal atresia or duplication
Hydrometrocolpos
Other genitourinary anomalies
Anorectal atresia

Megacystis Megaureter

Hydronephrosis
Large bladder
Dilated ureters
Mostly male

Megacystis Microcolon

Large bladder
Polyhydramnios
Dilated small bowel
Mostly female

Melnick-Needles Syndrome

Hypertelorism
Micrognathia
Bowing
Exophthalmos

Miller-Dieker Syndrome

Short nose
Clinodactyly
Lissencephaly

MURCS (müllerian duct aplasia, renal aplasia, cervicothoracic somite dysplasia)

Upper spine vertebral deformities
Renal agenesis or ectopia
Hypoplasia of uterus

Nager Acrofacial Dysostosis

Micrognathia
Deformed ears
Absent digits

Neu-Laxova Syndrome

Malformed ears
Cystic hygroma
Congenial heart disease
Agenesis of the corpus callosum
Cerebellar hypoplasia

Lissencephaly
Microcephaly with sloping forehead
Cataract
Exophthalmos/proptosis/prominent eyes with
    hypertelorism
Microphthalmia or anophthalmia
Clenched hands
Joint contractures
Rocker-bottom feet
Micrognathia with flat nose

Noonan Syndrome

Cardiac abnormality—pulmonary stenosis
Hypertelorism
Cystic hygroma
Cryptorchidism
Hemivertebrae

Oculodentodigital Syndrome

Microphthalmia or anophthalmia

Opitz Hypertelorism Hypospadias Syndrome

Hypertelorism

Orofacial-Digital Syndrome

Renal cystic structure
Cleft lip and palate
Micrognathia
Abnormal thumb
Clinodactyly
Polydactyly—postaxial
Males only

Oromandibular Limb Hypogenesis

Absent digits
Absent limbs

Otocephaly

Hypoplasia or absence of the mandible and tongue
Very severe micrognathia
Polyhydramnios
Absence of stomach

Otopalatodigital Syndrome

Hypertelorism
Cleft lip and palate

Pallister-Hall Syndrome

Intracranial tumor—hypothalamic mass
Polydactyly—postaxial

Poland Anomaly

Absent digits

Absent limbs
Clinodactyly

Proteus Syndrome

Macrodactyly
Soft tissue masses
Variable-sized limbs

Retinoic Acid Embryopathy

Absent limbs
Cardiac abnormality
Cerebellar hypoplasia
Spinal dysraphism
Lateral cleft lip
Cleft palate
Malformed ears
Micrognathia

Roberts' Syndrome

Cardiac abnormality
Encephalocele
Mild ventriculomegaly
Spinal dysraphism
Cataract
Lateral cleft lip and cleft palate
Absent digits
Absent limbs
Clinodactyly
Short limbs
Intrauterine growth retardation
Phocomelia
Genitourinary anomaly

Robinow Syndrome

Hypertelorism
Lateral cleft lip and cleft palate
Short nose

Rubinstein-Taybi Syndrome

Abnormal thumb
Microcephaly
Beaked nose
Cardiac defects

Russell-Silver Syndrome

Asymmetrical intrauterine growth retardation with
    normal-sized head
Asymmetric short long bones
Syndactyly and clinodactyly

Saethre-Chotzen Syndrome

Exophthalmos/proptosis/prominent eyes
Facial asymmetry
Clinodactyly

Seckel Syndrome

Microcephaly
Micrognathia

Clinodactyly
Club foot
Joint contractures
Intrauterine growth retardation

Short-Rib-Polydactyly Syndromes

Omphalocele
Renal dysplasia
Cardiac abnormality
Holoprosencephaly
Mild ventriculomegaly
Lateral cleft lip and cleft palate
Micrognathia
Club foot
Polydactyly—postaxial
Rhizomelic shortening
Short limbs
Hydrops
Intrauterine growth retardation
Polyhydramnios

Simpson-Golabi-Behnel Syndrome

Macrosomia

Sotos Syndrome

Dolichocephaly
Macrocephaly
Macrosomia
Hypertelorism

Spondyloepiphyseal Dysplasia Congenita

Small chest
Cleft palate
Short limbs
Intrauterine growth retardation
Short, mildly bowed femurs

Stickler Syndrome

Cleft palate
Micrognathia
Short nose
Cataracts
Scoliosis

Thalidomide Embryopathy

Absent limbs
Phocomelia

Thrombocytopenia—Absent Radius (TAR) Syndrome

Cardiac abnormality
Absent limbs
Club foot
Radial hypoplasia

Townes-Brock Syndrome

Duodenal atresia
Renal agenesis
Facial asymmetry
Malformed ears
Abnormal thumb
Absent digits
Clinodactyly
Polydactyly—preaxial/radial hypoplasia

Warburg Syndrome (Walker-Warburg)

Agenesis of the corpus callosum
Dandy-Walker cyst
Encephalocele
Lissencephaly
Mild ventriculomegaly
Cataract
Microphthalmia or anophthalmia

Weaver Syndrome

Macrosomia
Cardiac defects

Williams Syndrome

Cardiac defects—supravalvular aortic stenosis

Zellweger Syndrome

Renal cystic structure
Cataract
Club foot
Joint contractures
Increased nuchal translucency
Colpocephaly
Agenesis of the corpus callosum
Cardiac defects
Decreased or absent movement
Stippled epiphyses

Index

Note: Page numbers followed by the letter f refer to figures; those followed by the letter t refer to tables.